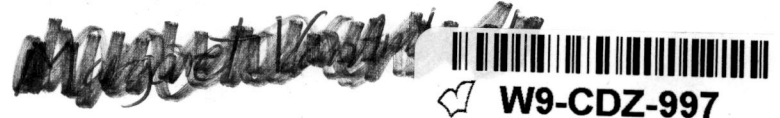

THE DAVIS BOOK OF MEDICAL ABBREVIATIONS: A DECIPHERING GUIDE

Sarah Lu Mitchell-Hatton, CMT

F. A. DAVIS Company • Philadelphia

Printed in the United States of America

Last digit indicates print number: 10 9 8

NOTE: As new scientific information becomes available through basic and clinical research, recommended treatments and drug therapies undergo changes. The author(s) and publisher have done everything possible to make this book accurate, up-to-date, and in accord with accepted standards at the time of publication. The authors, editors and publisher are not responsible for errors or omissions or for consequences from application of the book, and make no warranty, expressed or implied, in regard to the contents of the book. Any practice described in this book should be applied by the reader in accordance with professional standards of care used in regard to the unique circumstances that may apply in each situation. The reader is advised always to check product information (package inserts) for changes and new information regarding dose and contraindications before administering any drug. Caution is especially urged when using new or infrequently ordered drugs.

DEDICATION

This book is dedicated to Jim, my husband, for his patience, to Sidney Franz, a friend and teacher beyond compare, and to the memory of my Aunt Laura Trine, a very special lady.

PREFACE

Abbreviations are both a boon and a bane in this increasingly complicated and technical world. Each of us uses abbreviations daily to simplify our lives. From grocery lists to correspondence and from friendly discussions to professional speeches, avoiding abbreviations is all but impossible.

This book is tailored to the needs of medical transcriptionists who are required daily to decipher a wide range of abbreviations and acronyms as well as to the needs of other medical personnel who also deal with abbreviations. As this group requires reference works which are simple to use and logical in format, this book is compiled alphabetically by abbreviation and alphabetically by definition under each abbreviation.

A Deciphering Guide is an appropriate subtitle for this work as it is intended as a key to decipher medical codes just as spies need secret code lists to scramble and decipher messages. The key for this book is found in the medical specialty listings which appear after the definitions. It should be stressed that these specialty listings are a guide only as medical specialties overlap and diseases often touch many specialties. While diabetes is an endocrinological disease, its effects range from ophthalmology to neurology and from nephrology to orthopedics so DM (diabetes mellitus) will be listed as endocrinology but it may be used by many different specialties.

Every specialty has its own definitions and usages for abbreviations, just as each of us uses abbreviations differently in notes to ourselves and in grocery lists. To denote one specialty as having the preferred abbreviation and definition degrades all other specialties. This book does not list one abbreviation as being preferred over another or one definition as being preferred over another because of the different specialties' usages.

Included are many odd, obsolete, profane, slang, and utterly stupid abbreviations because they *are* in use. Sports abbreviations are included due to their usage in sports medicine. Many nonmedical abbreviations such as FBI and NAACP are listed because of their use in psychiatry. Slang abbreviations are included as they are often found in dictation, particularly when a physician is quoting a patient.

Pronunciations of acronyms and words created from abbreviations are included in the alphabetical listing of abbreviations. This feature will enable the user to more easily identify an unknown word (i.e., "pock" for "POC" [products of conception]).

Pronunciations of and listings of prefixes and suffixes are included in this book as physicians will abbreviate a word by its prefix or suffix, especially after using the complete word several times. They are also used in such cases as "hypo and hyperthyroidism."

The use of punctuation in abbreviations and in general language is changing in both medical and English grammar. Very few periods are being used now. Even MD (medical doctor) is missing its periods. I have included both forms in this book as persons reading a patient's older charts will need to know both usages.

There is a great misuse of abbreviations today; however, they are a fact of life with which we must deal by learning as much as we can about them. The medical community will not change its usage of abbreviations but will continue to create abbreviations to simplify its work and thus increase the work of the medical transcriptionists, medical records personnel, and others who need to read the medical record as well as increasing the dangers of misinterpretation. Continuing education about abbreviations is vital to those who read medical records and those who transcribe them. This book has attempted to condense numerous sources of abbreviations and definitions into one compact reference book with the hope of furthering knowledge of abbreviations throughout the medical community.

All abbreviations are **dangerous** unless each person **knows** exactly what is meant. I have noted a few dangerous abbreviations in the book but the medical specialty listings should help the researcher decipher which definition is intended in each case. If the correct abbreviation and/or definition is not known, it is prudent not to guess at such vital information but to question the appropriate party concerning the item.

The field of medical transcription is becoming more complex daily. With the advent of medical transcription companies who handle the work of many hospitals, the medical transcriptionist must be conversant with far more terminology than would be expected in a single hospital setting. Unfortunately, abbreviations are not standardized throughout the world and are continually changed by physicians for ease of usage whether it be in their dictation or their written notes.

The Joint Commission on Accreditation of Hospitals requires that medical reports do *not* contain abbreviations in their diagnoses. The medical transcriptionist is thus required to decipher any abbreviations which are dictated as a part of the diagnoses. The Joint Commission also requires each hospital to have available a list of abbreviations which has been approved by the medical staff but has not compiled an approved list to be adopted by all hospitals. The lists I have from several major hospitals and from which I have garnered information show a wide variety of differences in their approved abbreviations, including several abbreviations with more than one definition which shows the complexity of the abbreviation problem within each hospital.

ACKNOWLEDGMENTS

I wish to thank most of all Jean-François Vilain, my editor, who has been extremely patient with my work as well as encouraging me to keep going. I also want to thank the many transcriptionists around the nation who have expressed enthusiasm in this project and who have been asking when I will be finished with the book. While this book began over twenty-one years ago, they were the ones who brought it to fruition by believing in me. This book has progressed from a small notebook to a huge card file, to a large notebook, to many computer disks, to these pages, a progression which could not have been possible without my many friends.

I also wish to thank the people who reviewed this work:

Juanita Bryant, CMA-AC
Sidney Franz, CMT
Barbara Gylys, MEd, CMA-A
Theresa Indovina, RMA, CMA
Emily Kogan-Ulibarri, CMT
Betty Warrenfeltz, RN
Mary-Ellen Wedding, M.Ed., MT(ASCP), CMA

The immensity of the project was eased by their helpful comments. They spent a great many hours reviewing these pages and ensuring their correctness. I am very grateful to them for their assistance.

It would have been impossible to produce this book without the assistance of Jim, my husband, and Sidney Franz, my constant teacher, who believed in me and this project. They both deserve more thanks than I can possibly express.

HOW TO USE THIS BOOK

The alphabetical listing of abbreviations, acronyms, prefixes, suffixes, and pronunciations is designed as a simple usage tool based on the more familiar dictionaries. The abbreviations are listed in the following order:

AA	All capital letters.
AA.	All capital letters with punctuation.
AA2	All capital letters with Arabic numbers.
AA+	All capital letters with symbols.
Aa	Combinations of capital letters and lower case letters.
aa	All lower case letters.

Numerals
Arabic numerals in abbreviations are found only under the letters included in the abbreviations. **49er** is found under **er** rather than under **forty-niner.**

Roman numerals are listed alphabetically by the letters of which they are comprised. V (five [Roman numeral]) is found under the letter V in the abbreviation listings. This is done to alleviate the need to search for spellings rather than single letters or combinations of letters.

Definitions
Following each abbreviation are found its various definitions which also include listings of the medical specialties in which they are found and their pronunciations where applicable as follow:

> **OR**
> operating room (surgery) {pronounced "oh-are"}
> **O.R.**
> operating room (surgery) {pronounced "oh-are"}
> **"oh-are"**
> {pronunciation of OR and O.R. [operating room]} (surgery) {not an abbreviation}

Specialties
The listing of specialties is wide; however, some specialties have been combined due to their interworkings and common usage of abbreviations. Two such combinations are psychiatry and psychology which are generally listed underneath **psychiatry** and physical therapy, occupational therapy, speech and language therapy, and rehabilitation which are most often listed under **rehabilitation.**

Pronunciations

Rather than using the pronunciation symbols in current use which are rather confusing for those who have not studied them, I have listed the pronunciations as if they were words such as "max-E" and "oh-are."

It is my hope that the reader will find this work a helpful resource tool. As medicine changes so rapidly, I know that tomorrow I will find a new abbreviation to include in the next edition. I also know that you will find many new abbreviations that have not been included in this book but should be included in the next edition. I hope that you will share with me any abbreviations you feel need to be included. To send in information regarding this book and/or new abbreviations, please include your name and address, the abbreviation, the sentence in which it was used, its definition, and the medical specialty it is most frequently used in. Send the information to me at:

Sarah Lu Mitchell-Hatton, CMT
c/o Lynn Borders Caldwell,
Associate Editor
F. A. Davis Company
1915 Arch Street
Philadelphia, PA 19103

I thank you for your assistance.

TABLE OF CONTENTS

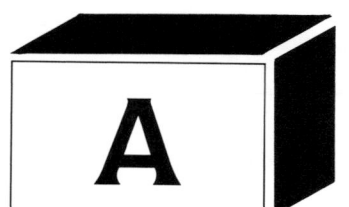

α
alpha [first letter of Greek alphabet]

A

absolute temperature
absorbance (radiology)
acceptor (chemistry)
accommodation (electricity, neurology, and ophthalmology)
acetum [vinegar] (pharmacology)
Actinomyces [a fungus] (laboratory)
adenine (chemistry and laboratory)
adenosine (genetics and laboratory)
adrenalin(e) [also called *epinephrine*] (cardiovascular, endocrinology, laboratory, pharmacology, and surgery)
adult
age
akinetic (cardiovascular, neurology, and radiology)
alive
allergist (allergy)
allergy
alveolar (laboratory and respiratory)
alveolar gas (laboratory and respiratory)
ambulatory (orthopedics and rehabilitation)
ampere (electricity and measurement)
amphetamine (chemical dependency and pharmacology)
angstrom [also ångström] (physics)
Angstrom unit (physics)
annum [year]
anode (radiology)
Anopheles [a mosquito genus] (entomology)
ante [before]
anterior
antrum [maxillary sinus] (otorhinolaryngology)
apical
aqua [water]
aqueous
area
argon (chemistry)
arteria [artery] (cardiovascular)

arteriolar (cardiovascular and ophthalmology)
assessment
atrium (cardiovascular)
atropine (cardiovascular, laboratory, ophthalmology, and pharmacology)
auricle (cardiovascular and otorhinolaryngology)
auris [ear] (otorhinolaryngology)
average
axial
mass number (chemistry)
start of anesthesia (anesthesiology)
total acidity (laboratory)

A
alveolar gas (laboratory and respiratory)
[*NOTE: The abbreviation is subscripted.*]

A.

absolute temperature
absorbance (radiology)
acceptor (chemistry)
accommodation (electricity, neurology, and ophthalmology)
acetum [vinegar] (pharmacology)
Actinomyces [a fungus] (laboratory)
activity [radiation] (radiology)
adenine (chemistry and laboratory)
adenosine (genetics and laboratory)
admit
admittance
adrenalin(e) [also called *epinephrine*] (cardiovascular, laboratory, pharmacology, and surgery)
adult
age
alanine (genetics and laboratory)
allergy
alveolar gas (laboratory and respiratory)
ampere (electricity and measurement)
amphetamine (chemical dependency and pharmacology)
anaphylaxis (allergy)

1

anesthesia (anesthesiology)
annum [year]
anode (radiology)
Anopheles [a mosquito genus] (entomology)
anterior
aqueous
area
argon (chemistry)
arteria [artery] (cardiovascular)
atomic weight (chemistry)
atropine (cardiovascular, laboratory, ophthalmology, and pharmacology)
axial
point A (radiology)
start of anesthesia (anesthesiology)
total acidity

Å

angstrom (physics)
Angstrom unit (physics)

Ã

cumulated activity

A1

aortic component of the first heart sound [also called *aortic first sound* and *first aortic sound*] (cardiovascular)

A₁

A₁ segment (neurology)
aortic component of the first heart sound [also called *aortic first sound* and *first aortic sound*] (cardiovascular)

A2

aortic component of the second heart sound [also called *aortic second sound* and *second aortic sound*] (cardiovascular)

A₂

aortic component of the second heart sound [also called *aortic second sound* and *second aortic sound*] (cardiovascular)

A-2371

{not an abbreviation} (chemotherapy, oncology, and pharmacology)

A-4

[pulley] (orthopedics)

A-8103

{not an abbreviation} [also called *piperazine*] (chemotherapy, oncology, and pharmacology)

μA

gamma A immunoglobulin (laboratory)
immunoglobulin A (laboratory)
microampere (electricity)

a

accommodation (electricity, neurology, and ophthalmology)
acid
after
agar (laboratory)
ampere (electricity and measurement)
anode (radiology)
ante [before]
anterior
apical
aqua [water]
area
arteria [artery] (cardiovascular)
arterial in the blood phase (laboratory and respiratory)
asymmetric
atto- {not an abbreviation} [prefix meaning 10^{-18}] (measurement)
axial
thermodynamic activity (chemistry)
total acidity

a

arterial blood (cardiovascular and laboratory) [*NOTE: The abbreviation is subscripted.*]
alveolar gas (laboratory and respiratory)

a.

absorptivity (chemistry, laboratory, psychiatry, and radiology)
acceleration
accommodation (electricity, neurology, and ophthalmology)
acid
acidity (laboratory)
ampere (electricity and measurement)

annum [year]
anode (radiology)
anterior
aqua [water]
area
arteria [artery] (cardiovascular)
arterial blood (cardiovascular and laboratory)
asymmetric
atto- {not an abbreviation} [prefix meaning 10^{-18}] (measurement)
axial

ā

ante [before]

AA

acetic acid (laboratory and pharmacology)
achievement age (pediatrics and psychiatry)
active-assistive [range of motion] (orthopedics and rehabilitation)
Addicts Anonymous (chemical dependency, psychiatry, and rehabilitation)
adenylic acid (genetics and laboratory)
aggregated albumin (gastroenterology, laboratory, and nephrology)
Alcoholics Anonymous (chemical dependency, psychiatry, and rehabilitation)
alveolar-arterial (laboratory and respiratory)
aminoacetone (endocrinology and laboratory)
amino acid (chemistry, genetics, and laboratory)
amyloid-associated protein (laboratory)
ana [of each] (pharmacology)
anesthesiologist's assistant (anesthesiology)
anticipatory avoidance (psychiatry)
antiprotein accumulator (physics)
aortic aneurysm (cardiovascular)
arachidonic acid (chemistry, laboratory, and pharmacology)
arm-ankle [pulse ratio] (cardiovascular)
arteries (cardiovascular)
ascending aorta (cardiovascular)
Association of Anaesthetists (anesthesiology)
atomic absorption (chemistry)

Australia antigen (gastroenterology, infectious diseases, and laboratory)
authorized absence
automobile accident

A.A.

achievement age (pediatrics and psychiatry)
Alcoholics Anonymous (chemical dependency, psychiatry, and rehabilitation)

A̅A̅

ana [of each] (pharmacology)

A & A

aid and attendance (rehabilitation)
awake and aware (neurology)

A-a

alveolar-arterial [gradient] (laboratory and respiratory)
aortic artery [gradient] (cardiovascular and radiology)

aa

ana [of each] (pharmacology)
arteries (cardiovascular)

a̅a̅

ana [of each] (pharmacology)

aa.

arteriae [arteries] (cardiovascular)

AAA

abdominal aortic aneurysm (cardiovascular)
abdominal aortic aneurysmectomy (cardiovascular)
acute anxiety attack (psychiatry)
amalgam (chemistry, dentistry, and psychiatry)
American Academy of Allergy (allergy)
American Academy of Anatomists (anatomy)
androgenic anabolic agent (endocrinology, laboratory, and pharmacology)

A.A.A.
American Academy of Allergy (allergy)
American Association of Anatomists
(anatomy)

aaa
amalgama [obsolete variant of *amal-gam*] (chemistry, dentistry, and psychiatry)

aaa.
amalgama [obsolete variant of *amal-gam*] (chemistry, dentistry, and psychiatry)

AAAA
American Academy of Anesthesiologist's Assistants (anesthesiology)

AAAE
amino acid–activating enzymes (genetics and laboratory)

AAAHE
American Association for the Advancement of Health Education (education)

AAALAC
American Association for Accreditation of Laboratory Animal Care (laboratory and veterinary medicine)

AAAM
American Association for Automotive Medicine

AA-AMP
amino acid adenylate [also called *adenomonophosphate*] (laboratory)

AAAS
American Association for the Advancement of Science

A.A.A.S.
American Association for the Advancement of Science

AAATP
Association for Anesthesiologist's Assistants Training Programs (anesthesiology and education)

AAB
American Association of Bioanalysts

A.A.B.
American Association of Bioanalysis

AABB
American Association of Blood Banks (hematology and laboratory)

A.A.B.B.
American Association of Blood Banks (hematology and laboratory)

AAC
antibiotic-associated pseudomembranous colitis (gastroenterology)
antimicrobial agent–associated colitis (gastroenterology)
antimicrobial agents and chemotherapy (chemotherapy, pharmacology, and oncology)

AACAHPO
American Association of Certified Allied Health Personnel in Ophthalmology (ophthalmology)

AACC
American Association for Clinical Chemistry (chemistry and laboratory)

A.A.C.C.
American Association for Clinical Chemistry (chemistry and laboratory)

AACCN
American Association of Critical Care Nurses (nursing)

AACE
antigen-antibody crossed electrophoresis (laboratory)

AACHP
American Association for Comprehensive Health Planning

A.A.C.I.A.
American Association for Clinical Im-

munology and Allergy (allergy and immunology)

AACJC
American Association of Community and Junior Colleges (education)

AACO
American Association of Certified Orthoptists (ophthalmology)

AACP
American Academy of Child Psychiatry (pediatrics and psychiatry)
American Association of Colleges of Pharmacy (pharmacology)

A.A.C.P.
American Academy of Cerebral Palsy (genetics and neurology)

AACPDM
American Academy for Cerebral Palsy and Developmental Medicine (genetics and neurology)

AAD
alloxazine adenine dinucleotide [FAD] (laboratory)

A–a Do$_2$
alveolar–arterial oxygen difference (laboratory and respiratory)

AADP
American Academy of Dental Prosthetics (dentistry)
amyloid-A degrading protease (laboratory)

A.A.D.P.
American Academy of Dental Prosthetics (dentistry)

AADR
American Academy of Dental Radiology (dentistry and radiology)

A.A.D.R.
American Academy of Dental Radiology (dentistry and radiology)

AADS
American Academy of Dental Schools (dentistry and education)
American Association of Dental Schools (dentistry and education)

A.A.D.S.
American Academy of Dental Schools (dentistry)
American Association of Dental Schools (dentistry)

AAE
active assistive exercise (rehabilitation)
acute allergic encephalitis (allergy, infectious diseases, and neurology)
American Association of Endodontists (dentistry)

A.A.E.
American Association of Endodontists (dentistry)

A.A.E.E.
American Association of Electromyography and Electrodiagnosis (neurology)

AAEH
Association to Advance Ethical Hypnosis (psychiatry)

AAF
acetic-alcohol-formalin (laboratory and pharmacology)
acetylaminofluorine (chemistry and laboratory)
Army Air Force (armed forces)
ascorbic acid factor (laboratory)

AAFP
American Academy of Family Physicians (family practice)

A.A.F.P.
American Academy of Family Physicians (family practice)

AAGP
American Academy of General Practice
American Association for Geriatric Psychiatry (psychiatry)

A.A.G.P.
American Academy of General Practice

AAGS
adult adrenogenital syndrome (endocrinology, gynecology, and urology)

AAHA
American Academy of Health Administration (administration)

AAHC
Association of Academic Health Centers (administration and education)

AAHD
American Association of Hospital Dentists (dentistry)

AAHE
Association for the Advancement of Health Education (education)

AAHPER
American Academy for Health, Physical Education and Recreation (education)
American Association for Health, Physical Education and Recreation (education)

AAI
arm-ankle indices (cardiovascular)
American Association of Immunologists (immunology)

A.A.I.
American Association of Immunologists (immunology)

AAIA
acquired artery immune augmentation (cardiovascular)

AAID
American Academy of Implant Dentistry (dentistry)

A.A.I.D.
American Academy of Implant Dentistry (dentistry)

AAIDS
adult acquired immunodeficiency syndrome (immunology and infectious diseases)

AAIN
American Association of Industrial Nurses (nursing)

A.A.I.N.
American Association of Industrial Nurses (nursing)

AAL
anterior axillary line (anatomy)

AALAS
American Association of Laboratory Animal Science (laboratory, research, and veterinary medicine)

A.A.M.
American Academy of Microbiology (laboratory and microbiology)

AAMA
American Academy of Medical Administrators (administration)
American Association of Medical Assistants

A.A.M.A.
American Association of Medical Assistants

AAMC
American Association of Medical Clinics
American Association of Medical Colleges (education)
Association of American Medical Colleges (education)

A.A.M.C.
American Association of Medical Clinics
American Association of Medical Colleges (education)

AAME
acetylarginine methyl ester (laboratory)

AAMFT
American Association for Marriage and Family Therapy (psychiatry)

AAMI
Association for the Advancement of Medical Instrumentation

A.A.M.I.
Association for the Advancement of Medical Instrumentation

AAMIH
American Association for Maternal and Infant Health (neonatology, obstetrics, and pediatrics)

AAMMC
American Association of Medical Milk Commissioners (laboratory)

AAMP
American Academy of Medical Preventics

AAMR
American Academy of Mental Retardation (genetics and neurology)

AAMRA
American Association of Medical Record Administrators [formerly the *American Association of Medical Record Librarians*] (medical records)

AAMRL
American Association of Medical Record Librarians [obsolete; now called *American Association of Medical Record Administrators*] (medical records)

A.A.M.R.L.
American Association of Medical Record Librarians [obsolete; now called *American Association of Medical Record Administrators*] (medical records)

AAMT
American Association for Medical Transcription (medical records' transcription)
American Association for Music Therapy (psychiatry and rehabilitation)

A.A.M.T.
American Association for Medical Transcription (medical records' transcription)

AAN
alpha amino nitrogen [also called *alpha amino acid nitrogen*] (laboratory)
American Academy of Neurology (neurology)
American Academy of Nursing (nursing)
American Academy of Nutrition (dietary)
analgesic abuse nephropathy (nephrology)
analgesic-associated nephropathy (nephrology)
attending's admission notes

A.A.N.
American Association of Neuropathologists (neurology and pathology)

AANA
American Association of Nurse Anesthetists (anesthesiology and nursing)

AANM
American Association of Nurse-Midwives (nursing and obstetrics)

AANPI
American Association for Nurses Practicing Independently (nursing)

AANS
American Association of Neurological Surgeons (neurosurgery)

AAO
American Academy of Ophthalmology (ophthalmology)
American Academy of Optometry (ophthalmology)
American Academy of Osteopathy (osteopathy)
American Association of Ophthalmologists (ophthalmology)
American Association of Ophthalmology (ophthalmology)
American Association of Orthodontists (dentistry)

amino acid oxidase (laboratory)
awake, alert, and oriented (neurology)

A.A.O.
American Academy of Osteopathy (osteopathy)
American Academy of Otolaryngology (otorhinolaryngology)
American Association of Orthodontists (dentistry)

A-aO$_2$
alveolar–arterial oxygen gradient (laboratory and respiratory)

A-a O$_2$
alveolar–arterial oxygen gradient (laboratory and respiratory)

AAO X 3
awake and oriented to time, place, and person (neurology)

AAofA
Ambulance Association of America (emergency medicine)

AAOHN
American Association of Occupational Health Nurses (nursing)

AAOO
American Academy of Ophthalmology and Otolaryngology (ophthalmology and otorhinolaryngology)

A.A.O.O.
American Academy of Ophthalmology and Otolaryngology (ophthalmology and otorhinolaryngology)

AAOP
American Academy of Oral Pathology (pathology)
American Academy of Orthotists and Prosthetists (orthopedics)

A.A.O.P.
American Academy of Oral Pathology (pathology)

AAOS
American Academy of Orthopaedic Surgeons (orthopedics)

AAP
air at atmospheric pressure (respiratory)
American Academy of Pediatrics (pediatrics)
American Academy of Psychoanalysis (psychiatry)
assessment adjustment pass (psychiatry)

A.A.P.
American Academy of Pediatrics (pediatrics)
American Academy of Pedodontics (dentistry)
American Academy of Periodontology (dentistry)
American Academy of Psychoanalysts (psychiatry)
American Academy of Psychotherapists (psychiatry)
American Association of Pathologists (pathology)
Association for the Advancement of Psychoanalysis (psychiatry)
Association for the Advancement of Psychotherapy (psychiatry)
Association of American Physicians

AAPA
American Academy of Physician Assistants (nursing)
American Association of Physicians' Assistants (nursing)

A.A.P.A.
American Academy of Physician Assistants (nursing)
American Association of Pathologist Assistants (pathology)

AAPB
American Association of Pathologists and Bacteriologists (bacteriology, laboratory, and pathology)

A.A.P.B.
American Association of Pathologists and Bacteriologists (bacteriology, laboratory, and pathology)

AAPC
antibiotic-acquired pseudomembranous colitis (gastroenterology)

(A–a)P$_{CO_2}$
alveolar–arterial carbon dioxide difference (laboratory and respiratory)

AAPHD
American Association of Public Health Dentists (dentistry)

AAPHP
American Association of Public Health Physicians

A.A.P.H.P.
American Association of Public Health Physicians

AAPL
American Academy of Psychiatry and Law (psychiatry)

AAPMC
antibiotic-associated pseudomembranous colitis (gastroenterology)

AAPMR
American Academy of Physical Medicine and Rehabilitation (physical medicine and rehabilitation)
American Association of Physical Medicine and Rehabilitation (physical medicine and rehabilitation)

A.A.P.M.R.
American Academy of Physical Medicine and Rehabilitation (physical medicine and rehabilitation)

AAPS
American Association of Plastic Surgeons (plastic surgery)
Arizona Articulation Proficiency Scale (speech and language therapy)
Association of American Physicians and Surgeons

A.A.P.S.
American Academy of Plastic Surgeons (plastic surgery)
American Association of Physicians and Surgeons

AAPSC
American Association of Psychiatric Services for Children (pediatrics and psychiatry)

AAR
antigen-antiglobulin reaction (laboratory)

AARC
American Association for Respiratory Care (respiratory)

AAROM
active-assistive range of motion (rehabilitation)

AARP
American Association of Retired Persons

AART
American Association for Rehabilitation Therapy (rehabilitation)
American Association for Respiratory Therapy (respiratory)

A.A.R.T.
American Association for Respiratory Therapy (respiratory)

AAS
American Academy of Sanitarians
anthrax antiserum (pharmacology)
atlantoaxical subluxation (neurology and orthopedics)
aortic arch syndrome (cardiovascular)
atomic absorption spectrophotometry (laboratory)

AASCU
American Association of State Colleges and Universities (education)

AASD
American Academy of Stress Disorders (psychiatry)

AASH
adrenal androgen stimulating hormone (endocrinology and laboratory)

AASP
American Association of Senior Physicians

AAT
alanine aminotransferase (endocrinology, laboratory, nephrology, and rheumatology)
alpha-1-antitrypsin (endocrinology, gastroenterology, gynecology, laboratory, obstetrics, oncology, and respiratory)
auditory apperception test (otorhinolaryngology)

AATA
American Art Therapy Association (psychiatry and rehabilitation)

AATS
American Association for Thoracic Surgery (cardiovascular, gastroenterology, respiratory, and surgery)

AAU
Association of American Universities (education)

AAV
adeno-associated virus (laboratory)

AAVMC
Association of American Veterinary Medicine Colleges (education and veterinary medicine)

AAVP
American Association of Veterinary Parasitologists (veterinary medicine)

AAVV
accumulated alveolar ventilatory volume (laboratory and respiratory)

AB
abnormal
aborta [abortions] (obstetrics)
abortus [abortion] (obstetrics)
Aid to the Blind (ophthalmology)
alcian blue [a dye; also called *8GX*] (laboratory)
American Board
antibody (laboratory)
antigen-binding (laboratory)
apex beat (cardiovascular)

apnea-bradycardia [spells] (cardiovascular, neonatology, pediatrics, and respiratory)
Artium Baccalaureus [Bachelor of Arts] (education)
asbestos body (laboratory and respiratory)
asthmatic bronchitis (respiratory)
axiobuccal (dentistry)

A.B.
Assembly Bill (government)
Artium Baccalaureus [Bachelor of Arts] (education)

A & B
apnea and bradycardia (neonatology and respiratory)

A/B
acid-base [ratio] (laboratory)

A>B
air greater than bone [conduction] (otorhinolaryngology)

AB-100
{not an abbreviation} (chemotherapy, oncology, and pharmacology) {obsolete}

AB-132
{not an abbreviation} (chemotherapy, oncology, and pharmacology)

Ab
aborta [abortions] (obstetrics)
abortus [abortion] (obstetrics)
antibody (laboratory)

ab
aborta [abortions; followed by numerals indicating the number of abortions] (obstetrics)
abortus [abortion; followed by the numeral *1*, indicating one abortion] (obstetrics)
about
antibody (laboratory)
axiobuccal (dentistry)
form

ABA
abscissic acid (chemistry)
allergic bronchopulmonary aspergillosis
(respiratory)
antibacterial activity (pharmacology)

A2B+ A2B
Rhesus positive [blood group] (hematology and laboratory)

A.B.B.
American Board of Bioanalysis (laboratory)

abbrev
abbreviated
abbreviation

ABC
absolute band count (laboratory)
absolute basophil count (laboratory)
aconite, belladonna, chloroform (pharmacology)
Adriamycin, 1,3-bis(2-chloroethyl)-1-ni-
trosourea [*BCNU*; also called *carmustine*], and cyclophosphamide (chemotherapy, oncology, and pharmacology)
airway, breathing, and circulation (cardiovascular, emergency medicine, and
respiratory)
American Blood Commission
alternate birthing center (OB/GYN)
antigen-binding capacity (laboratory)
apnea, bradycardia, cyanosis (cardiovascular, emergency medicine, and respiratory)
artificial beta cells (laboratory)
aspiration biopsy cytology (hematology,
laboratory, and oncology)
atomic, biological, chemical [war fare]
(armed forces)
axiobuccocervical (dentistry)

A.B.C.
American Blood Commission (hematology)

A-B-C
airway, breathing, and circulation (cardiovascular, emergency medicine, and
respiratory)

ABCC
Atomic Bomb Casualty Commission
(government and radiation medicine)

ABCDE
botulism toxoid pentavalent (laboratory)

ABCIL
antibody-mediated cell-dependent immune lympholysis (laboratory)

ABCM
Adriamycin, bleomycin, cyclophosphamide, and mitomycin C (chemotherapy, oncology, and pharmacology)

A.B.C. method
alum, blood, clay method [for treatment
of raw sewage] (chemistry)

ABCP
American Board of Cardiovascular Perfusion (cardiovascular and radiology)

ABCX
Adriamycin, bleomycin, cisplatin, and
radiation therapy (chemotherapy, oncology, pharmacology, and radiation
therapy)

ABD
abdomen
abdominal
abdominal [fluid] (laboratory)
abdominal [pad] (orthopedics)
abduction (neurology and orthopedics)
aged, blind, disabled

Abd
abdomen
abdominal

abd
abdomen
abdominal
abduct (neurology and orthopedics)
abduction (neurology and orthopedics)
abductor (neurology and orthopedics)

abdc
abduct (neurology and orthopedics)
abduction (neurology and orthopedics)

ABDCT
atrial bolus dynamic computer tomography (cardiovascular and radiology)

ABD HYST
abdominal hysterectomy (gynecology)

Abd hyst
abdominal hysterectomy (gynecology)

ABDOM
abdomen
abdominal

Abdom
abdomen
abdominal

abdom
abdomen
abdominal

abd poll
abductor pollicis [muscle] (neurology and orthopedics)

"A-B-duck-tor"
{pronunciation of *A-B-ductor* [abductor muscle]} (neurology and orthopedics) {not an abbreviation}

A-B-duct
abduct (neurology and orthopedics) {pronounced "A-B-duct"}
abduction (neurology and orthopedics) {pronounced "A-B-duct"}

"A-B-duct"
{pronunciation of *A-B-duct* [abduct, abduction]} (neurology and orthopedics) {not an abbreviation}

A-B-ductor
abductor [muscle] (neurology and orthopedics) {pronounced "A-B-duck-tor"}

ABDV
Adriamycin, bleomycin, vinblastine, and dacarbazine [*DTIC*] (chemotherapy, oncology, and pharmacology)

ABE
acute bacterial endocarditis (cardiovascular)
botulism equine trivalent antitoxin (laboratory)

abe
abequose residue (laboratory)

ABEP
auditory brain-stem-evoked potential (neurology)

A.B.E.P.P.
American Board of Examiners in Professional Psychology (psychiatry)

ABFP
American Board of Forensic Psychiatry (psychiatry)

ABG
arterial blood gas(es) (laboratory and respiratory)
axiobuccogingival (dentistry)

abg
addictive behavior group (psychiatry)

a-b gap
air-bone gap (otorhinolaryngology)

ABG's
arterial blood gases (laboratory and respiratory)

ABHP
American Board of Health Physics (physics)

ABI
ankle-brachial index (cardiovascular)
atherothrombotic brain infarction (cardiovascular and neurology)

ABIG
absence of immunoglobulin G (laboratory)

ABL
a-beta-lipoproteinemia (gastroenterol-

ogy, laboratory, neurology, and ophthalmology)
allograft-bound lymphocytes (laboratory)
Army Biological Laboratory (armed
forces and laboratory)
Automated Biological Laboratory (laboratory)
axiobuccolingual (dentistry)

ABLB
alternate binaural loudness balance
(otorhinolaryngology)
Alternate Binaural Loudness Balance
[Test] (otorhinolaryngology)

ABMS
Advisory Board for Medical Specialties

A.B.M.S.
Advisory Board for Medical Specialties

ABMT
autologous bone marrow transplantation
(hematology and oncology)

ABN
abnormal
abnormality(ies)

Abn
abnormal
abnormality(ies)

abn
abnormal
abnormality(ies)

A2BN A2B
Rhesus negative, Rhesus-variant [D^u]
negative [blood group] (hematology
and laboratory)

ABNC
abnormal curve (laboratory)

ABN F%
abnormal forms percent [sperm count]
(laboratory and urology)

ABNG
AB negative [blood type] (hematology
and laboratory)

abnl
abnormal

A.B.N.M.
American Board of Nuclear Medicine
(radiology)

abnor
abnormal
abnormality(ies)

ABNORM
abnormal
abnormality(ies)

ABO
absent bed occupant
absent bed occupancy
abortion (obstetrics)
antibodies (laboratory)
{not an abbreviation} [refers to the blood
groups, A, AB, B, and O] (hematology
and laboratory)

Abor
abortion (obstetrics)

Abort.
abortion (obstetrics)

ABOS
American Board of Orthopaedic Surgery
(orthopedics)

ABP
Adriamycin, bleomycin, and prednisone
(chemotherapy, oncology, and pharmacology)
androgen-binding protein (endocrinology and laboratory)
arterial blood pressure (cardiovascular)

ABPA
allergic bronchopulmonary aspergillosis
(respiratory)

ABPN
American Board of Psychiatry and Neurology (neurology and psychiatry)

ABR
abortus Bang ring [probe or test] [also called *Abortus Bang Ringprobe test*] (laboratory and veterinary medicine)
abrasion
absolute bed rest
auditory brain response (neurology)
auditory brain stem response (neurology)

ABr
agglutination test for brucellosis (laboratory)

abr
abrasion(s)

abras
abrasion(s)

ABRET
American Board of Registration of Electroencephalographic Technicians (neurology)

ABR test
abortus Bang ring test [also called *Abortus Bang Ringprobe test*] (laboratory and veterinary medicine)

ABr test
abortus Bang ring test [also called *Abortus Bang Ringprobe test*] (laboratory and veterinary medicine)

ABS
absorbed
absorption
acrylonitrile-butadiene-styrene (chemistry)
acute brain syndrome (neurology)
admitting blood sugar (endocrinology and laboratory)
alkylbenzene sulfonate (chemistry)
at bedside (pharmacology)

1:5 ABS
1:5 Absorption-Reiter-Strain [cerebrospinal fluid test] (laboratory and neurology)

Abs
absorption

abs
absent
absolute

abs.
absent
absolute
away from

ABS FEB
absente febre [while fever is absent] (pharmacology)

abs. feb.
absente febre [while fever is absent] (pharmacology)

A.B.S. pill
aloin, extract of belladonna, and strychnine pill [a laxative] (gastroenterology and pharmacology)

ABST
absent (laboratory)

abst.
abstract

abstr.
abstract

ABT
aminopyrine breath test (gastroenterology, laboratory, and pharmacology)

abt
about

ABV
actinomycin D, bleomycin, and vincristine (chemotherapy, oncology, and pharmacology)

ABVD
Adriamycin [doxorubicin], bleomycin, Velban [vinblastine], and dacarbazine [DTIC] (chemotherapy, oncology, and pharmacology)

ABW
actual body weight

ABx
antibiotics (pharmacology)

ABY
acid bismuth yeast [agar] (laboratory)

AC
abdominal circumference (neonatology
　and pediatrics)
acetate (laboratory and pharmacology)
acetylcholine (laboratory, neurology,
　and pharmacology)
acromioclavicular [joint] (orthopedics)
acupuncture clinic (neurology)
acute
adrenal cortex (endocrinology)
adrenal corticoid (endocrinology and
　laboratory)
Adriamycin and cyclophosphamide
　(chemotherapy, oncology, and phar-
　macology)
air conditioning
air conduction (otorhinolaryngology)
all culture [broth] (laboratory)
alternating current (electricity)
anchored catheter (urology)
anodal closure (cardiovascular)
ante cibum [before meals] (pharmacol-
　ogy)
antecubital (cardiovascular and orthope-
　dics)
anterior chamber (ophthalmology)
anterior cruciate [ligament] (orthope-
　dics)
anticoagulant (cardiovascular, hematol-
　ogy, and pharmacology)
anticomplementary
anti-inflammatory corticoid (pharmacol-
　ogy)
aortic closure (cardiovascular)
assist control
atriocarotid (cardiovascular)
auriculocarotid (cardiovascular)
axiocervical (dentistry)

A.C.
acromioclavicular (orthopedics)
air conduction (otorhinolaryngology)
alternating current (electricity)
anodal closure (cardiovascular)
aortic closure (cardiovascular)
axiocervical (dentistry)

A/C
ambulatory care
anterior chamber [of eye] (ophthalmol-
　ogy)

5-AC
azacitidine (pharmacology)

Ac
accelerator
acetyl (chemistry)
acryl group (chemistry)
actinium (chemistry)
anterior chamber [of eye] (ophthalmol-
　ogy)

ac
acute
ante cibum [before meals] (pharmacol-
　ogy)

a.c.
alternating current (electricity)
ante cibum [before meals] (pharmacol-
　ogy)

a̅c̅
ante cibum [before meals] (pharmacol-
　ogy)

ACA
acyclovir (pharmacology)
adenocarcinoma (oncology)
adult child of alcoholic (psychiatry)
American Chiropractic Association (chi-
　ropractic medicine)
American College of Allergists (allergy)
American College of Anesthesiologists
　(anesthesiology)
American College of Angiology (cardio-
　vascular)
American College of Apothecaries
　(pharmacology)
American Council on Alcoholism (chem-
　ical dependency)
anterior cerebral artery (cardiovascular
　and neurology)
anticentromere antibody (genetics and
　laboratory)
automatic clinical analyzer (laboratory)

A.C.A.
adenocarcinoma (oncology)
American Chiropractic Association (chiropractic medicine)
American College of Allergists (allergy)
American College of Anesthesiologists (anesthesiology)
American College of Angiology (cardiovascular)
American College of Apothecaries (pharmacology)
American Council on Alcoholism (chemical dependency)

ΣACA
epsilon-aminocaproic acid (chemistry)

ACACB
American Council of Applied Clinical Nutrition (dietary)

AcAcOH
acetoacetic acid (laboratory)

ACAD
academy

acad
academy

acad.
academy

ACAN
acanthrocytes (laboratory)

ACANTH
acanthrocytes (laboratory)

ACAT
automated computerized axial tomography (radiology)

ACB
alveolar-capillary block (cardiovascular and respiratory)
antibody-coated bacteria (laboratory)
aortocoronary bypass (cardiovascular)

AC & BC
air conduction and bone conduction (otorhinolaryngology)

ACBE
air-contrast barium enema (gastroenterology and radiology)

ACBG
aortocoronary bypass graft (cardiovascular)

ACC
accommodation (electricity, neurology, and ophthalmology)
acinic cell carcinoma (oncology)
acute care center
adenoid cystic carcinoma (oncology)
administrative control center
adrenocortical carcinoma (oncology)
ambulatory care center
American College of Cardiology (cardiovascular)
American Critical Care
anodal closure contraction (cardiovascular)

A.C.C.
American College of Cardiology (cardiovascular)

Acc
adenoid cystic carcinoma (oncology)

Acc.
accommodation (electricity, neurology, and ophthalmology)

acc
acceleration
accident
accommodation (electricity, neurology, and ophthalmology)
according

acc.
acceleration
accident
accommodation (electricity, neurology, and ophthalmology)
according

ACCESS
American College of Cardiology Ex-

tended Study Services (cardiovascular)

AcCh
acetylcholine (laboratory)

AcChR
acetylcholine receptor (laboratory)

AcCHS
acetylcholinesterase (laboratory)

ACCl
accident

accid
accident

ACCL
anodal closure clonus (cardiovascular)

ACCl
anodal closure clonus (cardiovascular)

AcCoA
acetylcoenzyme A (laboratory)

accom
accommodation (electricity, neurology,
and ophthalmology)

accom.
accommodation (electricity, neurology,
and ophthalmology)

ACCP
American College of Chest Physicians
(cardiovascular and respiratory)
American College of Clinical Pharmacology (pharmacology)

accur
accurately
accuratissime [most carefully]

accur.
accurately
accuratissime [most carefully]

ACD
absolute cardiac dullness (cardiovascular)
acid-citrate-dextrose [solution] (pharmacology)

allergic contact dermatitis (allergy and
dermatology)
American College of Dentists (dentistry)
anterior chamber diameter (ophthalmology)
anterior chest diameter (respiratory)
area of cardiac dullness (cardiovascular)
dactinomycin (chemotherapy, pharmacology and oncology)

A.C.D.
acid-citrate-dextrose (pharmacology)

AC-DC
alternating current/direct current (electricity)
bisexual [heterosexual and homosexual]
(psychiatry and infectious disease)

ACDF
adult child of a dysfunctional family
(psychiatry)
anterior cervical diskectomy and fusion
(neurosurgery and orthopedics)

ACD&F
anterior cervical diskectomy and fusion
(neurosurgery and orthopedics)

ACD solution
citric acid, trisodium citrate, and dextrose solution (pharmacology)

ACE
acetonitrile (chemistry)
actinium emanation (radiation therapy
and radiology)
adrenal cortical extract (endocrinology
and pharmacology)
adrenocortical extract (endocrinology
and pharmacology)
Adriamycin [doxorubicin], cyclophosphamide, and etoposide [VP-16] (chemotherapy, oncology, and pharmacology)
alcohol, chloroform, ether [mixture] (anesthesiology and pharmacology)
angiotensin-converting enzyme [inhibi-
tor] (laboratory)
{not an abbreviation} [brand name for
the Ace bandage]

ACe
Adriamycin [doxorubicin] and cyclophosphamide [Cytoxan] (chemotherapy, oncology, and pharmacology)

ACEH
acid cholesterol ester hydrolase (laboratory)

ACE-I
angiotensin-I converting enzyme [inhibitor] (laboratory and pharmacology)

ACE-II
Adriamycin [doxorubicin], cyclophosphamide, and etoposide [VP-16] in high dose infusion (chemotherapy, oncology, and pharmacology)

A.C.E. mixture
alcohol, chloroform, ether mixture (anesthesiology and pharmacology)

ACEP
American College of Emergency Physicians (emergency medicine)

acetyl-CoA
acetylcoenzyme A (laboratory)

ACF
accessory clinical findings
acid-fast culture (laboratory)
acute care facility

ACFO
American College of Foot Orthopedists (orthopedics)

A.C.F.O.
American College of Foot Orthopedists (orthopedics)

ACFS
American College of Foot Surgeons (orthopedics)

A.C.F.S.
American College of Foot Surgeons (orthopedics)

ACFUCY
actinomycin D, 5-fluorouracil, and cyclophosphamide (chemotherapy, oncology, and pharmacology)

ACG
American College of Gastroenterology (gastroenterology)
angiocardiography (cardiovascular and radiology)
apexcardiogram (cardiovascular)

A.C.G.
American College of Gastroenterology (gastroenterology)
angiocardiography (cardiovascular and radiology)

AcG
accelerator globulin [factor V] (hematology and laboratory)

Ac-G
accelerator globulin [factor V] (hematology and laboratory)

AC globulin
accelerator globulin [factor V] (hematology and laboratory)

ACGME
Accreditation Council on Graduate Medical Education (education)

A.C.G.P.
American College of General Practitioners

ACGPOMS
American College of General Practitioners in Osteopathic Medicine and Surgery (osteopathy)

ACH
acetylcholine (laboratory)
adrenal cortical hormone (laboratory)
adrenocortical hormone {obsolete} (laboratory)
after coming head (obstetrics)
arm, chest, height
arm girth, chest depth, hip width [index of nutritional condition of children] (dietary and pediatrics)

ACh
acetylcholine (laboratory and neurology)

ACHA
American College Health Association
American College of Hospital Administrators (administration)

A.C.H.A.
American College of Hospital Administrators (administration)

ACHE
acetylcholinesterase (laboratory)

AChE
acetylcholinesterase (laboratory)

AChR
acetylcholine receptor (laboratory)

AChRab
acetylcholine receptor antibody (neurology and laboratory)

AC&HS
before meals and at bedtime (pharmacology)

AChS
Association of the Society of Chiropodists (podiatry)

ACI
acoustic comfort index (otorhinolaryngology)
adenylate cyclase inhibitor (laboratory)
adrenal cortical insufficiency (endocrinology and laboratory)
after-care instructions
anticlonus index (neurology)

A.C.I.
after-care instructions

ACID
Adriamycin, cyclophosphamide, dacarbazine [DTIC], and actinomycin D (chemotherapy, oncology, and pharmacology)

"acid-foss"
{pronunciation of *acid phos* [acid phosphatase]} (laboratory) {not an abbreviation}

acid phos
acid phosphatase (laboratory) {pronounced "acid-foss"}

acid p'tase
acid phosphatase (laboratory)

ACIP
Advisory Committee on Immunization Practices

ACIR
Automotive Crash Injury Research

A.C.J.
acromioclavicular joint (orthopedics)

ACL
acromioclavicular line (orthopedics)
anterior cruciate ligament (orthopedics)

ACl
aspiryl chloride (laboratory)

A.C.L.A.
American Clinical Laboratory Association (laboratory)

ACLC
Assessment of Children Language Comprehension (speech and language therapy)

ACLD
Association for Children with Learning Disabilities (education)

ACLM
American College of Legal Medicine

A.C.L.P.S.
Academy of Clinical Laboratory Physicians and Scientists

ACLS
advanced cardiac life support (cardiovascular)

Advanced Cardiac Life Support Program
(cardiovascular)

ACLU
American Civil Liberties Union

ACM
Adriamycin, cyclophosphamide, and
methotrexate [same as *CAM*] (chemotherapy, oncology, and pharmacology)
albumin-calcium-magnesium (laboratory)

ACME
Advisory Council on Medical Education
(education)

ACMS
American Chinese Medical Society

ACN
acute conditioned neuroses (psychiatry)
American College of Neuropsychiatrists
(neurology and psychiatry)
American College of Nutrition (dietary)

A.C.N.
American College of Neuropsychiatrists
(neurology and psychiatry)

ACNM
American College of Nuclear Medicine
(nuclear medicine and radiology)
American College of Nurse-Midwives
(nursing and obstetrics)

A.C.N.M.
American College of Nuclear Medicine
(nuclear medicine and radiology)
American College of Nurse-Midwives
(nursing and obstetrics)

A.C.N.P.
American College of Nuclear Physicians
(nuclear medicine and radiology)

ACO
American College of Otolaryngologists
(otorhinolaryngology)
anodal closing odor (cardiovascular)

ACOA
adult child of alcoholic (psychiatry)

ACOAP
Adriamycin, cyclophosphamide, vincristine, cytosine arabinoside, and prednisone (chemotherapy, oncology, and
pharmacology)

ACOG
American College of Obstetricians and
Gynecologists (gynecology and obstet-
rics)

A.C.O.G.
American College of Obstetricians and
Gynecologists (gynecology and obstet-
rics)

ACOHA
American College of Osteopathic Hospital Administrators (administration and
osteopathy)

A.C.O.H.A.
American College of Osteopathic Hospital Administrators (administration and
osteopathy)

ACO-HNS
American Council of Otolaryngology—
Head and Neck Surgery (otorhinolar-
yngology)

ACOI
American College of Osteopathic Inter-
nists (internal medicine)

A.C.O.I.
American College of Osteopathic Inter-
nists (internal medicine)

ACOMS
American College of Oral and Maxillofacial Surgeons (dentistry and surgery)

ACOOG
American College of Osteopathic Obstetricians and Gynecologists (gynecology, obstetrics, and osteopathy)

A.C.O.O.G.
American College of Osteopathic Obste-

tricians and Gynecologists (gynecology, obstetrics, and osteopathy)

ACOP
Adriamycin, cyclophosphamide, vincristine, and prednisone (chemotherapy, oncology, and pharmacology)
American College of Osteopathic Pediatricians (osteopathy and pediatrics)

A.C.O.P.
American College of Osteopathic Pediatricians (osteopathy and pediatrics)

ACOPP
Adriamycin [doxorubicin], cyclophosphamide, vincristine, prednisone, and procarbazine (chemotherapy, oncology, and pharmacology)

ACOS
American College of Osteopathic Surgeons (osteopathy and surgery)

A.C.O.S.
American College of Osteopathic Surgeons (osteopathy and surgery)

acous
acoustical
acoustics

ACP
acid phosphatase (laboratory)
acyl-carrier protein (laboratory)
American College of Pathologists (pathology)
American College of Pharmacists (pharmacology)
American College of Physicians
American College of Prosthodontists (dentistry)
American College of Psychiatrists (psychiatry)
Animal Care Panel (veterinary medicine)
anodal closing picture (cardiovascular)
aspirin, caffeine, phenacetin (pharmacology)
Association for Child Psychiatrists (pediatrics and psychiatry)
Association of Clinical Pathologists (laboratory and pathology)

Association of Correctional Psychologists (psychiatry)

AC P
acid phosphatase (laboratory)

A.C.P.
American College of Physicians
American College of Pathologists (laboratory and pathology)
Association of Clinical Pathologists (laboratory and pathology)

AC-PH
acid phosphatase (laboratory)

ACPM
American College of Preventive Medicine

A.C.P.M.
American College of Preventive Medicine

ACPP
adrenocorticopolypeptide (laboratory)

ACPP PF
acid phosphatase prostatic fluid (laboratory)

ACR
acriflavine [a dye] (laboratory)
adenomatosis of the colon and rectum (gastroenterology, oncology, and pathology)
American College of Radiology (radiology)
anticonstipation regimen (gastroenterology)

A.C.R.
American College of Radiology (radiology)

Acr
acrylic (chemistry)

ACS
American Cancer Society (oncology)
American Chemical Society (chemistry)

American College of Surgeons (surgery)
anodal closing sound (cardiovascular)
antireticular cytotoxic serum (pharmacology)
aperture current setting
arterial cannulation support (cardiovascular)
Association of Clinical Scientists

A.C.S.
American Cancer Society (oncology)
American Chemical Society (chemistry)
American College of Surgeons (surgery)
antireticular cytotoxic serum (pharmacology)
Association of Clinical Scientists

ACSM
American College of Sports Medicine (sports medicine)

A.C.S.M.
American College of Sports Medicine (sports medicine)

ACSP
Advisory Council on Scientific Policy

A.C.S.P.
Advisory Council on Scientific Policy

ACSV
aortocoronary-saphenous vein [graft] (cardiovascular)

ACSW
Academy of Certified Social Workers (social work)

ACT
achievement through counseling and treatment (psychiatry)
actinomycin (pharmacology)
activated clotting time (hematology, cardiovascular, and laboratory)
activated coagulation time (hematology and laboratory)
advanced coronary treatment (cardiovascular)
allergen challenge test (allergy and laboratory)
American Council on Transplantation (transplantation medicine and surgery)

anticoagulant therapy (hematology and laboratory)
automated computerized tomography (radiology)

act
active

ACTA
American Cardiovascular Technologists Association (cardiovascular)
American Corrective Therapy Association
Automatic Computerized Transverse Axial [x-ray system] (radiology)

act-C
actinomycin C (pharmacology)

ACT-D
actinomycin D [dactinomycin] (chemotherapy, oncology, and pharmacology)

act-D
actinomycin D [dactinomycin] (chemotherapy, oncology, and pharmacology)

ACTe
anodal closure tetanus (cardiovascular)

Act Ex
active exercise (rehabilitation)

ACTH
adrenocorticotropic hormone (endocrinology and laboratory)
automated computerized transverse [axial scanner] (radiology)

ACTH-RF
corticotropic [adrenocorticotropic] releasing factor (endocrinology and laboratory)

ACTIFD
Actifed (allergy, otorhinolaryngology, pharmacology and respiratory)

ACTIN-D
actinomycin D [also called *dactinomy-*

cin] (chemotherapy, oncology, and pharmacology)

ACTIV
activity

ACTN
adrenocorticotropin (endocrinology and laboratory)

ACTP
adrenocorticotropic polypeptide (endocrinology and laboratory)

ACTSEB
anterior chamber tube shunt encircling band (ophthalmology)

ACUT
acute phase (laboratory)

ACUTENS
acupuncture and transcutaneous electrical nerve stimulation (orthopedics and neurology)

ACV
acyclovir (pharmacology)
atrial/carotid/ventricular (cardiovascular)

ACVD
acute cardiovascular disease (cardiovascular)

ACVRD
arteriosclerotic cardiovascular renal disease (cardiovascular and nephrology)

Acyl–Co A
organic compound–coenzyme A ester (laboratory)

AD
accident dispensary
addict (chemical dependency)
adenoid degeneration [virus] (laboratory)
adenovirus (laboratory)
admitting diagnosis
alcohol dehydrogenase (laboratory)
Aleutian disease [of minks] (veterinary medicine)
Alzheimer's disease (neurology)

analgesic dose (pharmacology)
anodal duration (cardiovascular)
antigenic determinant (laboratory)
arthritic dose (pharmacology and rheumatology)
Associate Degree [Nursing Programs] (education and nursing)
auris dextra [right ear] (otorhinolaryngology)
autonomic dysreflexia (neurology)
average deviation
axiodistal (dentistry)
axis deviation (cardiovascular, ophthalmology, and radiology)
cytosine arabinoside and daunomycin [same as *DA*] (chemotherapy, oncology, and pharmacology)
diphenylchlorarsine [toxic smoke used in warfare; also called *Clark I*] (armed services and chemistry)

A.D.
auris dextra [right ear] (otorhinolaryngology)

A & D
ascending and descending
admission and disposition

Ad
adrenal (endocrinology)

Ad.
adrenal (endocrinology)

ad
adde [*addetur*, let them be added] (pharmacology)
auris dextra [right ear] (otorhinolaryngology)
axiodistal (dentistry)
{not an abbreviation} [Latin preposition meaning *to* or *up to*]

ad.
adde [*addetur*, let them be added] (pharmacology)

a.d.
alternis diebus [alternating days, every other day] (pharmacology)

auris dextra [right ear] (otorhinolaryngology)

ADA
adenosine deaminase (immunology and laboratory)
adult children of alcoholics (chemical dependency and psychiatry)
American Dental Association (dentistry)
American Dermatological Association (dermatology)
American Diabetes Association (endocrinology)
American Dietetic Association (dietary)
anterior descending artery (cardiovascular)

A.D.A.
American Dental Association (dentistry)
American Dermatological Association (dermatology)
American Diabetes Association (endocrinology)
American Dietetic Association (dietary)

ADA#
American Diabetes Association diet number (dietary and endocrinology)

ADAA
American Dental Assistants Association (dentistry)

ADAMHA
Alcohol, Drug Abuse and Mental Health Administration (chemical dependency and psychiatry)

A.D.A.M.H.A.
Alcohol, Drug Abuse and Mental Health Administration (chemical dependency and psychiatry)

ADAP
American Dental Assistant's Program (dentistry and education)
Assistant Director of Psychiatry [British] (psychiatry)

ADAU
adolescent drug abuse unit (chemical dependency)

ADB
accidental death benefit (insurance)

ADC
Aid to Dependent Children (government)
acquired immunodeficiency syndrome [AIDS] dementia complex (immunology and neurology)
albumin, dextrose, catalase [media] (laboratory)
ambulance design criteria (emergency medicine)
analog-to-digital converter (computer science)
anodal duration contraction (cardiovascular)
average daily census (administration)
axiodistocervical (dentistry)

A.D.C.
Aid to Dependent Children (government)

AdC
adrenal cortex (endocrinology)

ADCC
antibody-dependent cell-mediated cytotoxicity (laboratory)
antibody-dependent cellular cytotoxicity (laboratory)

ADCONFU
Adriamycin, cyclophosphamide, 5-fluorouracil, and actinomycin D (chemotherapy, oncology, and pharmacology)
Adriamycin, cyclophosphamide, vincristine, and 5-fluorouracil (chemotherapy, oncology, and pharmacology)

ADD
adduction (neurology and orthopedics)
adenosine deaminase (immunology and laboratory)
alcohol and drug dependency clinic (chemical dependency)
androstanediene (endocrinology and laboratory)
androstanedione (endocrinology and laboratory)

attention deficit disorder (pediatrics and psychiatry)

average daily dose (pharmacology)

Add
adduction (neurology and orthopedics)

add
adde [add] (pharmacology)
addantur [let them be added] (pharmacology)
addition
adduction (neurology and orthopedics)
adductor (neurology and orthopedics)

add.
adde [add] (pharmacology)
addetur [let there be added] (pharmacology)
addition
adduction (neurology and orthopedics)

add c trit
adde cum tritu [add triturition] (pharmacology)

add. c. trit.
adde cum tritu [add triturition] (pharmacology)

ADD/H
attention deficit disorder with hyperactivity (pediatrics and psychiatry)

ad def an
ad defectionem animi [to the point of fainting]

ad def. an.
ad defectionem animi [to the point of fainting]

ad deliq
ad deliquium [to fainting]

ad deliq.
ad deliquium [to fainting]

addend
addendus [to be added] (pharmacology)

ADDD/H
attention deficit and distractability disorder with hyperactivity (pediatrics and psychiatry)

addict
addiction (chemical dependency)

addn
addition

add poll
adductor pollicis [muscle] (orthopedics)

ADDS
American Digestive Disease Society (gastroenterology)

ADDU
alcohol and drug dependency unit (chemical dependency)

"A-D-duck-tor"
{pronunciation of *A-D-ductor* [adductor (muscle)]} (neurology and orthopedics) {not an abbreviation}

A-D-duct
adduct (neurology and orthopedics) {pronounced "A-D-duct"}
adduction (neurology and orthopedics) {pronounced "A-D-duct"}

"A-D-duct"
{pronunciation of *A-D-duct* [adduct, adduction]} (neurology and orthopedics) {not an abbreviation}

A-D-ductor
adductor [muscle] (neurology and orthopedics) {pronounced "A-D-duck-tor"}

ADD w H
attention deficit disorder with hyperactivity (pediatrics and psychiatry)

ADE
acute disseminated encephalitis (neurology)
apparent digestible energy (gastroenterology)

Ade
adenine (chemistry and laboratory)

Ade Cbl
adenosylcobalamin (laboratory)

ad effect
ad effectum [until effectual] (pharmacology)

ad effect.
ad effectum [until effectual] (pharmacology)

ADEM
acute disseminated encephalomyelitis (neurology)
acute disseminating encephalomyelitis (neurology)

adeno-CA
adenocarcinoma (oncology)

ADEQ
adequate

adeq
adequate

ad feb
adstante febre [fever being present]

ad. feb.
adstante febre [fever being present]

ADG
atrial diastolic gallop (cardiovascular)
axiodistogingival (dentistry)

ADGMS
Assistant Director General of Medical Services

ad gr acid
ad gratum aciditatem [to an agreeable acidity] (pharmacology)

ad gr. acid.
ad gratum aciditatem [to an agreeable acidity] (pharmacology)

ad grat. acid.
ad gratum aciditatem [to an agreeable acidity] {obsolete} (pharmacology)

ad gr gust
ad gratum gustum [to an agreeable taste] (pharmacology)

ad gr. gust.
ad gratum gustum [to an agreeable taste] (pharmacology)

ADH
alcohol dehydrogenase (laboratory)
antidiuretic hormone [also called *vasopressin*] (endocrinology, laboratory, and pharmacology)

ADHA
American Dental Hygienists' Association (dentistry)

ADHC
Adult Day Health Care [Center]

ADHIB
adhibendus [to be administered] (pharmacology)

adhib
adhibendus [to be administered] (pharmacology)

adhib.
adhibendus [to be administered] (pharmacology)

ADI
Academy of Dentistry, International (dentistry)
acceptable daily intake
atlantodens interval (neurosurgery and orthopedics)
axiodistoincisal (dentistry)

ADIC
Adriamycin and dacarbazine [DTIC] (chemotherapy, oncology, and pharmacology)

ad int
ad interim [meanwhile]

ad. int.
ad interim [meanwhile]

adj
adjunct

adj.
adjoining

ADL
activities of daily living (rehabilitation)

Ad. Lib.
ad libitum [as desired, at pleasure, as much as needed, freely] (pharmacology)

ad lib
ad libitum [as desired, at pleasure, as much as needed, freely] (pharmacology)

ad lib.
ad libitum [as desired, at pleasure, as much as needed, freely] (pharmacology)

ADM
abductor digiti minimi [muscles of hands or feet] (orthopedics and podiatry)
administrative medicine
administrator
admission
admit
Adriamycin [also called *doxorubicin*] (chemotherapy, oncology, and pharmacology)

AdM
adrenal medulla (endocrinology)

Adm
admission
admitted

adm
admission
admit

admin
administer (pharmacology)
administration

admit
admission

ADMOV
admove [*admoveatur*, apply, let it be applied] (pharmacology)

admov
admove [*admoveatur*, apply, let it be applied] (pharmacology)

admov.
admove [*admoveatur*, apply, let it be applied] (pharmacology)

ADMS
Assistant Director of Medical Services (administration)

ADN
Associate Degree in Nursing (nursing)

adn
adenoid (otorhinolaryngology)
adenoidectomy (otorhinolaryngology)

ad naus
ad nauseam [to the extent of producing nausea] (pharmacology)

ad naus.
ad nauseam [to the extent of producing nausea] (pharmacology)

ad neut
ad neutralizandum [to neutralization] (pharmacology)

ad neut.
ad neutralizandum [to neutralization] (pharmacology)

ADO
axiodisto-occlusal (dentistry)

ADOAP
Adriamycin [*doxorubicin*], cytosine arabinoside [*cytarabine*], vincristine, and prednisone (chemotherapy, oncology, and pharmacology)

Ad-OAP
Adriamycin [*doxorubicin*], cytosine arabinoside [*cytarabine*], vincristine, and

prednisone (chemotherapy, oncology, and pharmacology)

ADODM
adult-onset diabetes mellitus (endocrinology)

Adol
adolescent (pediatrics)

adol
adolescent (pediatrics)

ADP
Academy of Dental Prosthetics (dentistry)
adenosine diphosphate (laboratory)
Animal Disease and Parasite Research Division [United States Department of Agriculture] (agriculture, research, and veterinary medicine)
area diastolic pressure (cardiovascular)
automatic data processing (computer sciences)

ad part dolent
ad partes dolentes [to the painful parts]

ad part. dolent.
ad partes dolentes [to the painful parts]

ADPase
adenosine diphosphatase (laboratory)

ADPL
average daily patient load (administration)

ad pond om
ad pondus omnium [to the weight of the whole] (pharmacology)

ad pond. om.
ad pondus omnium [to the weight of the whole] (pharmacology)

ADQ
abductor digiti quinti [muscles of the hands or feet] (orthopedics and podiatry)

ADR
Accepted Dental Remedies (dentistry)
acute dystonic reaction (neurology)
Adriamycin [also called *doxorubicin*] (chemotherapy, oncology, and pharmacology)
adverse drug reaction

Adr
adrenalin(e) (laboratory and pharmacology)

adr
adrenalin(e) (laboratory and pharmacology)

ADRDA
Alzheimer's Disease and Related Disorders Association (neurology)

Adrenex.
adrenalectomy (endocrinology and surgery)

ADRIA
Adriamycin [also called *doxorubicin*] (chemotherapy, oncology, and pharmacology)

Adria
Adriamycin [also called *doxorubicin*] (chemotherapy, oncology, and pharmacology)

Adria + BCNU
Adriamycin [*doxorubicin*] and BCNU [*carmustine*] (chemotherapy, oncology, and pharmacology)

ADS
American Denture Society (dentistry)
anatomical dead space (anatomy)
anonymous donor's sperm (obstetrics)
antibody deficiency syndrome (immunology)
anticipate discharge tomorrow
antidiuretic substance (laboratory and pharmacology)
Army Dental Services (armed forces and dentistry)

ad sat
ad saturandum [to saturation] (pharmacology)

ad sat.
ad saturandum [to saturation] (pharmacology)

adst feb
adstante febre [when fever is present] (pharmacology)

adst. feb.
adstante febre [while fever is present] (pharmacology)

ADT
accepted dental therapeutics (dentistry)
adenosine triphosphate (laboratory)
agar-gel diffusion test (laboratory)
alternate-day treatment
any desired thing (pharmacology)
placebo (pharmacology)
{not an abbreviation} [a placebo, *A* meaning *any*, *D* meaning *what you desire*, and *T* meaning *thing* or *any desired thing*] (pharmacology)

ADTA
American Dance Therapy Association (rehabilitation)
American Dental Trade Association (dentistry)

ADTe
tetanic contraction (neurology)

ADTP
alcohol dependency treatment program (chemical dependency and rehabilitation)

ad us
ad usum [according to custom]

ad us.
ad usum [according to custom]

ad us ext
ad usum externum [for external use] (pharmacology)

ad us. ext.
ad usum externum [for external use] (pharmacology)

ADV
adenovirus (laboratory)
adversum [against]

A/DV
arterio/deep venous (cardiovascular and laboratory)

A-DV
arterio-deep venous [difference] (cardiovascular and laboratory)

Adv
advise

adv
advice
advise

adv.
adversum [adverse to, against]

ad 2 vic
ad duas vices [at two times, for two doses] (pharmacology)

ad 2 vic.
ad duas vices [at two times, for two doses] (pharmacology)

A5D5W
alcohol 5%, dextrose 5% in water (pharmacology)

ADX
adrenalectomized (endocrinology)

AE
above-elbow (orthopedics)
acrodermatitis enteropathica (dermatology, gastroenterology, and pediatrics)
air entry (respiratory)
anoxic encephalopathy (neurology)
antitoxineinheit [antitoxic unit] (laboratory)
apoenzyme (laboratory)

aryepiglottic
energy of activation

A.E.
antitoxineinheit [antitoxic unit] (laboratory)

A+E
Accident and Emergency [Ward or Department] (emergency medicine)
analysis and evaluation

AEA
above-elbow amputation (orthopedics)
alcohol, ether, acetone [solution] (laboratory)
Atomic Energy Authority (government)

AEC
at earliest convenience
Atomic Energy Commission (government)

A.E.C.
Atomic Energy Commission (government)

AED
automated external defibrillator (cardiovascular)

AEE
Atomic Energy Establishment (government)

AEG
aeger [*aegra*, the patient]
air encephalogram (neurology and radiology)

aeg
aeger [*aegra*, the patient]

aeg.
aeger [*aegra*, the patient]

AEI
acrylic eye illustrator (ophthalmology)

AEM
analytical electron microscope (laboratory)
analytical electron microscopy (laboratory)

AEMC
Albert Einstein Medical Center

AEMD
Albert Einstein Medical College (education)

AEMIS
Aerospace and Environmental Medicine Information System (aerospace medicine and ecology)

AEP
artificial endocrine pancreas (endocrinology)
auditory evoked potential (neurology)
average evoked potential (neurology)

AEq
age equivalent (pediatrics and psychiatry)

aeq
aequales [equal]

aeq.
aequales [equal]

AER
acoustic evoked response (neurology)
aldosterone excretion rate (endocrinology and laboratory)
auditory evoked response (neurology)
average evoked response (neurology)

AERE
Atomic Energy Research Establishment (government)

Aer. M.
aerosol mask (respiratory)

Aero
Aerobacter (laboratory)

Aero.
Aerobacter (laboratory)

Aer. T.
aerosol tent (respiratory)

AES
American Electroencephalographic Society (neurology)
American Encephalographic Society (neurology)
American Endocrine Society (endocrinology)
American Epidemiological Society (epidemiology and research)
antiembolic stockings (cardiovascular)
antral ethmoidal sphenoidectomy (otorhinolaryngology)

A.E.S.
American Encephalographic Society (neurology)
American Epidemiological Society (epidemiology and research)

AESP
applied extrasensory projection (parapsychology)

AESQ
Aeromedical Evacuation Squadron [Air Force] (armed forces)

AEST
Aeromedical Evacuation Support Team (armed forces)

AET
absorption equivalent thickness
aetatis [aged]
aetas [age]
2-amino-ethyl-isothiouronium bromide

aet
aetas [age]
aetiology [etiology]

aet.
aetas [age]

aetat
aetatis [age]

aetat.
aetatis [aged, of age]

aetiol
aetiology [etiology]

AF
abnormal frequency
acid-fast (laboratory)
aflatoxin [a toxic factor] (chemistry and laboratory)
Air Force (armed forces)
albumose-free [tuberculin] (infectious diseases, laboratory, pharmacology, and respiratory)
aldehyde fuchsin (laboratory)
amnionic fluid (obstetrics)
amniotic fluid (obstetrics)
angiogenesis factor (laboratory)
anterior fontanelle (neonatology and pediatrics)
antibody-forming (laboratory)
aortic flow (cardiovascular)
Armed Forces (armed forces)
Arthritis Foundation (orthopedics and rheumatology)
atrial fibrillation (cardiovascular)
atrial flutter (cardiovascular)
audiofrequency (otorhinolaryngology)
auricular fibrillation (cardiovascular)

A.F.
albumose-free [tuberculin] (infectious diseases, laboratory, pharmacology, and respiratory)

A-F
ankle-foot [orthosis] (orthopedics)
antifibrinogen (hematology and laboratory)

af
audiofrequency (otorhinolaryngology)

af.
audiofrequency (otorhinolaryngology)

AFAR
American Foundation for Aging Research (geriatrics and research)

AFB
acid-fast bacillus(i) (laboratory and respiratory)
aflatoxin B [a toxic factor] (chemistry and laboratory)

American foulbrood [of bees] (entomology and veterinary medicine)
American Foundation for the Blind (ophthalmology)
aortofemoral bypass (cardiovascular)

AFBG
aortofemoral bypass graft (cardiovascular)

AFC
air-filled cushions
antibody-forming cell (laboratory)

AFCR
American Federation for Clinical Research (research)

afeb
afebrile

AFDC
Aid to Families with Dependent Children (government)

AF/F
atrial fibrillation and/or flutter (cardiovascular)

aff
afferent
affinis [having an affinity with but not identical with]

aff.
afferent
affinis [having an affinity with but not identical with]

AFG
aflatoxin G [a toxic factor] (chemistry and laboratory)
alpha fetal globulin (laboratory)
amniotic fluid glucose (laboratory and obstetrics)

AFH
Air Force Hospital (armed forces)

AFI
amaurotic familial idiocy (genetics and neurology)

AFIB
atrial fibrillation (cardiovascular)

AFib
atrial fibrillation (cardiovascular)

A. fib.
atrial fibrillation (cardiovascular)

A fibers
{not an abbreviation} [myelinated fibers of the somatic nervous system (neurology)

AFIP
Air Force Institute of Pathology (armed forces, laboratory, and pathology)
Armed Forces Institute of Pathology (armed forces, laboratory, and pathology)

A.F.I.P.
Air Force Institute of Pathology (armed forces, laboratory, and pathology)
Armed Forces Institute of Pathology (armed forces, laboratory, and pathology)

AFL
aflatoxicol (chemistry)
antifatty liver [referring to factor in pancreatic tissue] (gastroenterology, laboratory, and pathology)
atrial flutter (cardiovascular)

AFM
aflatoxin M [a toxic factor] (chemistry and laboratory)

AFML
Armed Forces Medical Library (armed forces and library science)

A.F.M.L.
Armed Forces Medical Library (armed forces and library science)

AFMML
Air Force Medical Materials Letter (armed forces)

AFNC
Air Force Nurse Corps (armed forces and nursing)

AFO
ankle-foot orthosis (orthopedics)

AFP
alpha-fetoprotein (laboratory and oncology)
alpha$_1$-fetoprotein (laboratory and oncology)
anterior faucial pillar (otorhinolaryngology)
atrial filling pressure (cardiovascular)

aFP
alpha-fetoprotein (laboratory and oncology)

AFPP
acute fibrinopurulent pneumonia (respiratory)

AFQ
aflatoxin Q [a toxic factor] (chemistry and laboratory)

AFQT
Armed Forces Qualification Test (armed forces)

AFR
aqueous flare response
ascorbic free radical (laboratory)

AFRD
acute febrile respiratory disease (respiratory)

AFRI
acute febrile respiratory illness (respiratory)

AFS
acid-fast smear (laboratory)
American Fertility Society (obstetrics)

AFSAM
Air Force School of Aviation Medicine (aerospace medicine and armed forces)

AFSP
acute fibrinoserous pneumonia (respiratory)

AFT
aflatoxin [a toxic factor] (chemistry and laboratory)

AFTA
American Family Therapy Association (psychiatry)

AFTC
apparent free testosterone concentration (endocrinology and laboratory)

AFTN
autonomously functioning thyroid nodule (endocrinology)

AFV
amnionic fluid volume (obstetrics)

AFVSS
afebrile, vital signs stable

AG
albumin-globulin [ratio] (gastroenterology and laboratory)
aminoglycoside (endocrinology, laboratory, and pharmacology)
analytical grade (chemistry)
anion gap (endocrinology, gastroenterology, laboratory, and nephrology)
antiglobulin (immunology and laboratory)
antigravity
atrial gallop (cardiovascular)
axiogingival (dentistry)

A/G
albumin-globulin [ratio] (gastroenterology and laboratory)

A:G
albumin-globulin [ratio] (gastroenterology and laboratory)

Ag
antigen (laboratory)
argentum [silver] (chemistry)

AGA
accelerated growth area
acute gonococcal arthritis (infectious diseases and orthopedics)
American Gastroenterological Association (gastroenterology)
American Genetic Association (genetics)
American Geriatrics Association (geriatrics)
American Goiter Association (endocrinology)
appropriate for gestational age (neonatology)
at gestational age (neonatology)
average for gestational age (neonatology)

A.G.A.
American Gastroenterological Association (gastroenterology)
American Genetics Association (genetics)
American Geriatrics Association (geriatrics)

Ag-Ab
antigen-antibody [complex] (laboratory)

AGBAD
Alexander Graham Bell Association for the Deaf (otorhinolaryngology and speech and language therapy)

AGC
absolute granulocyte count (hematology and laboratory)
automatic gain control (radiology)

AGCT
Army General Classification Test (armed forces and psychiatry)

AGD
agar-gel diffusion (bacteriology and laboratory)
agarose diffusion [method] (cardiovascular and laboratory)

AGE
acrylamide gel electrophoresis (genetics and laboratory)
acute gastroenteritis (gastroenterology)

agarose gel electrophoresis (cardiovascular and laboratory)
angle of greatest extension (orthopedics and rehabilitation)

AGF
angle of greatest flexion (orthopedics and rehabilitation)

ag feb
aggredient febre [when fever increases]

ag. feb.
aggredient febre [when fever increases]

AGG
agammaglobulinemia (immunology)
agammaglobulinemia leukemia (hematology, immunology, and oncology)

agg
agglutinated
agglutination
aggravated
aggregate

agg.
agglutinated
agglutination
aggravated
aggregate

aggl.
agglutinated
agglutination

agglut
agglutinated
agglutination

aggred. feb.
aggrediente febre [when the fever increases]

AGGS
antigas gangrene serum (bacteriology and laboratory)

AGH
antihemophilic globulin [factor VIII] (hematology and laboratory)

AGI
Alan Guttmacher Institute

AgI
silver iodide (pharmacology)

agit
agita [shake, stir] (pharmacology)

agit.
agita [shake, stir] (pharmacology)

agit ante sum
agita ante sumendum [shake before taking] (pharmacology)

agit. ante sum.
agita ante sumendum [shake before taking] (pharmacology)

agit. vas.
agitato vase [the vial being shaken] (pharmacology)

AGL
acute granulocytic leukemia (hematology and oncology)
aminoglutethimide (cardiovascular, chemotherapy, endocrinology, oncology, and pharmacology)

AGLMe
N-alpha-acetylglycyl-L-lysine methyl ester (laboratory)

AGMK
African green monkey kidney (laboratory)

AGN
acute glomerulonephritis (nephrology)
agnosia (neurology)

agn.
agnosia (neurology)

AgNO₃
silver nitrate (pharmacology)

AgNOR
silver-staining nucleolar organizer region (laboratory)

Ag₂O
silver oxide (chemistry)

AGOS
American Gynecological and Obstetrical Society (gynecology and obstetrics)

AGP
acid glycoprotein (laboratory)
agar-gel precipitation [test] (bacteriology and laboratory)

AGPA
American Group Practice Association
American Group Psychotherapy Association (psychiatry)

AGPT
agar-gel precipitation test (bacteriology and laboratory)

AGR
anticipatory goal response (psychiatry)

A/G ratio
albumin-globulin ratio (gastroenterology and laboratory)

A/G ratio test
albumin-globulin ratio test (gastroenterology and laboratory)

AGS
adrenogenital syndrome (endocrinology)

A.G.S.
American Gynecological Society (gynecology)

AGT
antiglobulin test (immunology and laboratory)

agt
agent

AGTH
adrenoglomerulotropin hormone (endocrinology and laboratory)

AGTr
adrenoglomerulotropin (endocrinology and laboratory)

AGTT
abnormal glucose tolerance test (endocrinology and laboratory)

AGV
aniline gentian violet (pharmacology)

A.G.V.
aniline gentian violet (pharmacology)

AH
abdominal hysterectomy (gynecology)
accidental hypothermia (emergency medicine and sports medicine)
acetohexamide (endocrinology and pharmacology)
after-hyperpolarization (laboratory)
amenorrhea and hirsutism (endocrinology and gynecology)
aminohippurate (laboratory and nephrology)
antihyaluronidase (bacteriology and laboratory)
Army Hospital (armed forces)
arterial hypertension (cardiovascular)
artificial heart (cardiovascular)
ascites hepatoma (gastroenterology)
autonomic hyperreflexia (neurology)

A+H
Accident and Health [insurance]

Ah
hypermetropic astigmatism (ophthalmology)

ah
hyperopic astigmatism (ophthalmology)

AHA
acetohydroxamic acid (nephrology and pharmacology)
acquired hemolytic anemia (hematology)
American Heart Association (cardiovascular)
American Hospital Association (administration)
anterior hypothalamic area [of brain] (neurology)

aspartyl-hydroxamic acid (chemistry)
Associate, Institute of Hospital Administrators (administration)
autoimmune hemolytic anemia (hematology)
Australian hepatitis antigen (laboratory)

A.H.A.
American Heart Association (cardiovascular)
American Hospital Association (administration)

aha
acquired hemolytic anemia (hematology)

AHB
alpha-hydroxybutyric dehydrogenase (laboratory)

AHC
acute hemorrhagic conjunctivitis (ophthalmology)
acute hemorrhagic cystitis (urology)

AHD
arteriosclerotic heart disease (cardiovascular)
atherosclerotic heart disease (cardiovascular)
autoimmune hemolytic disease (hematology and laboratory)

AHDP
azacycloheptane-diphosphonate (pharmacology and radiology)

AHE
acute hemorrhagic encephalomyelitis (neurology)

AHES
artificial heart energy system (cardiovascular)

AHF
acute heart failure (cardiovascular)
American Health Foundation
American Hepatic Foundation (gastroenterology)

American Hospital Formulary (pharmacology)
antihemolytic factor (hematology and
laboratory)
antihemophilic factor [blood coagulation
Factor VIII] (hematology and laboratory)
Associated Health Foundation

AHFS
American Hospital Formulary Service
(pharmacology)

AHG
aggregated human globulin (laboratory)
antihemophilic globulin [blood coagulation Factor VIII] (hematology and laboratory)
antihuman globulin (hematology and
laboratory)

AHGS
acute herpetic gingival stomatitis (dentistry and otorhinolaryngology)

AHH
alpha-hydrazine analogue of histidine
(laboratory)
arylhydrocarbon hydroxylase (chemistry
and laboratory)
Association for Holistic Health

AHI
active hostility index (psychiatry)
Animal Health Institute (veterinary
medicine)
antihyaluronidase (bacteriology and laboratory)

AHIP
Assisted Health Insurance Plan (insurance)

AHLE
acute hemorrhagic leukoencephalitis
(neurology)

AHLS
antihuman lymphocyte serum (hematology)

AHM
ambulatory Holter monitoring (cardiovascular)

AHMA
American Holistic Medicine Association

AHMC
Association of Hospital Management
Committees (administration)

"ahm-nee-o"
{pronunciation of *amnio*
[amniocentesis]} (obstetrics) {not an
abbreviation}

AHN
Army Head Nurse (armed forces and
nursing)
assistant head nurse (nursing)

AHP
acute hemorrhagic pancreatitis (gastroenterology)
air at high pressure
American Health Professionals
Assistant House Physician

A.H.P.
Assistant House Physician

AHPA
American Health Planning Association

AHPI
American Health Professions Institute

AHR
Association for Health Records (medical
records)

AHRA
American Hospital Radiology Administrators (administration and radiology)

AHRF
American Hearing Research Foundation
(otorhinolaryngology and speech and
language therapy)

AHS
Academy of Health Sciences [Army]
(armed forces)
American Hearing Society (otorhi-

insemination husband donor and *homologous artificial insemination*] (obstetrics)

A.I.H.
American Institute of Homeopathy (homeopathic medicine)
artificial homologous insemination [also called *homologous artificial insemination*] (obstetrics)

AIHA
American Industrial Hygiene Association (industrial medicine)
autoimmune hemolytic anemia (hematology)

A.I.H.A.
American Industrial Hygiene Association (industrial medicine)

AIHC
American Industrial Health Conference (industrial medicine)

AII
angiotensin II (cardiovascular and laboratory)

AIII
angiotensin III (cardiovascular and laboratory)

AIIMS
All-India Institute of Medical Sciences [India]

AIL
angioimmunoblastic lymphadenopathy (dermatology, gastroenterology, hematology, infectious diseases, nephrology, and oncology)

AILD
angioimmunoblastic lymphadenopathy with dysproteinemia (dermatology, gastroenterology, hematology, infectious diseases, nephrology, and oncology)

AILT
amiloride inhibitable lithium transport (laboratory and psychiatry)

AIM
Amputees in Motion (orthopedics and rehabilitation)
Artificial Intelligence in Medicine (computer science)
L-asparaginase, ifosfamide, and methotrexate (chemotherapy, oncology, and pharmacology)

AIMS
abnormal involuntary movement scale (neurology)

AIN
acute interstitial nephritides (laboratory)
acute interstitial nephritis (nephrology)
American Institute of Nutrition (dietary)

AINS
anti-inflammatory nonsteroidal [agent or drug] (pharmacology)

AInsuf
aortic insufficiency (cardiovascular)

AIO
amyloid of immunoglobulin origin (immunology and laboratory)

AION
anterior ischemic optic neuropathy (neurology and ophthalmology)

AIP
acute intermittent porphyria (hematology)
aldosterone-induced protein (endocrinology and laboratory)
Anatuberculin, Petragnani's integral (laboratory, pharmacology, and respiratory)
automated immunoprecipitation [system] (immunology and laboratory)
automated immunoprecipitation (immunology and laboratory)
average intravascular pressure (cardiovascular)

AIPS
American Institute of Pathologic Science (pathology)

AIR
accelerated idioventricular rhythm (cardiovascular)
aminoimidazole ribonucleotide (laboratory)
artificial intelligence research (computer science)

AIS
androgen insensitivity syndrome (endocrinology)
anti-insulin serum (endocrinology and pharmacology)

AIS/MR
Alternative Intermediate Services for the Mentally Retarded (genetics and neurology)

AITT
arginine insulin tolerance test (endocrinology and laboratory)

AIU
absolute iodine uptake (endocrinology and radiology)

AIUM
American Institute of Ultrasound in Medicine (radiology)

AIVR
accelerated idioventricular rhythm (cardiovascular)

AJ
ankle jerk (neurology and orthopedics)

A.J.
ankle jerk (neurology and orthopedics)

A.J.C.C.S.
American Joint Committee on Cancer Staging (oncology)

AJCCS&ER
American Joint Committee for Cancer Staging and End Results (oncology)

AJDC
American Journal of Diseases of Children (pediatrics)

AJP
American Journal of Psychiatry (psychiatry)

AK
above-knee (orthopedics)
actinic keratosis (ophthalmology)
Alaska [Postal Service state abbreviation]

A/K
above-knee (orthopedics)

AKA
above-knee amputation (orthopedics)
alcoholic ketoacidosis (endocrinology and gastroenterology)
all known allergies
also known as

AK amp
above-knee amputation (orthopedics) {pronounced "A-kay-amp"}

"A-kay-amp"
{pronunciation of *AK amp* [above-knee amputation]} (orthopedics) {not an abbreviation}

AL
acute leukemia (hematology and oncology)
adaptation level
Alabama [Postal Service state abbreviation]
albumin (laboratory and pharmacology)
alcoholism (chemical dependency and psychiatry)
alignment mark [on cardiography] (cardiovascular)
axiolingual (dentistry)

A.L.
auris laeva [left ear] (otorhinolaryngology)

Al
aluminum (chemistry)

al
auris laeva [left ear] (otorhinolaryngology)

ALA
American Laryngological Association (otorhinolaryngology)
American Lung Association (respiratory)
aminolevulinic acid [for lead intoxication] (laboratory and toxicology)
axiolabial (dentistry)
delta-amino levulinic acid (laboratory)

A.L.A.
American Laryngological Association (otorhinolaryngology)

ALa
axiolabial (dentistry)

Ala
alanine (laboratory)

ALAD
abnormal left axis deviation (cardiovascular)
aminolevulinic acid dehydrase (laboratory)

ALAG
axiolabiogingival (dentistry)

ALaG
axiolabiogingival (dentistry)

"al-ah-non"
{pronunciation of *Al-Anon* [a part of Alcoholics Anonymous]} (psychiatry) {not an abbreviation}

"al-ah-teen"
{pronunciation of *Alateen* [a part of Alcoholics Anonymous]} (psychiatry) {not an abbreviation}

"al-ah-tot"
{pronunciation of *Alatot* [a part of Alcoholics Anonymous]} (psychiatry) {not an abbreviation}

ALAL
axiolabiolingual (dentistry)

ALaL
axiolabiolingual (dentistry)

Al-Anon
{not an abbreviation} [a part of Alcoholics Anonymous] (psychiatry) {pronounced "al-ah-non"}

ALAS
aminolevulinic acid synthetase (laboratory)
delta-aminolevulinic acid synthetase (laboratory)

ALAT
alanine aminotransferase [new name for *serum glutamic pyruvic transaminase* (SGPT)] (cardiovascular, gastroenterology, hematology, laboratory, and nephrology)
alanine transaminase (laboratory)

Alateen
{not an abbreviation} [a part of Alcoholics Anonymous] (psychiatry) {pronounced "al-ah-teen"}

Alatot
{not an abbreviation} [a part of Alcoholics Anonymous] (psychiatry) {pronounced "al-ah-tot"}

ALB
albumin (laboratory)

Alb
albus [white]

alb
albumin (laboratory and pharmacology)

alb.
albumin (laboratory and pharmacology)
albus [white]

ALB/GLOB
albumin/globulin [ratio] (gastroenterology and laboratory)

albus
{not an abbreviation} [Latin word meaning *white*]

ALC
acute lethal catatonia (neurology and psychiatry)
alcohol (chemical dependency, chemistry, laboratory, pharmacology, and psychiatry)
Alternative Lifestyle Checklist
approximate lethal concentration (pharmacology and radiology)
avian leukosis complex (veterinary medicine)
axiolinguocervical (dentistry)

alc
alcohol (chemical dependency, chemistry, laboratory, pharmacology, and psychiatry)
alcoholism (chemical dependency, chemistry, laboratory, pharmacology, and psychiatry)

ALCAR
phospho-ribosyl-5-amino-imidazole-carboxamide (laboratory) {pronounced "al-car"}

"al-car"
{pronunciation of *ALCAR* [phosphoribosyl-5-amino-imidaz-ole-carboxamide]} (laboratory) {not an abbreviation}

ALC R
alcohol rub (physical therapy)

AlCr
aluminum crown (dentistry)

AlcR
alcohol rub (physical therapy)

ALD
adrenoleukodystrophy (endocrinology, genetics, neurology, and pediatrics)
alcoholic liver disease (chemical dependency and gastroenterology)
aldolase (laboratory and neurology)

Ald
aldolase (laboratory and neurology)

ALD c̄ decomp.
alcoholic liver disease with decompensation (chemical dependency and gastroenterology)

aldo
aldosterone (endocrinology and laboratory) {pronounced "al-doe"}

"al-doe"
{pronunciation of *aldo* [aldosterone]} (endocrinology and laboratory) {not an abbreviation}

ALDOL
aldolase (laboratory and neurology)

ALDOS
aldosterone (endocrinology and laboratory)

ALDOST
aldosterone (endocrinology and laboratory)

ALEP
atypical lymphoepithelioid cell proliferation (hematology and laboratory)

ALF
American Liver Foundation (gastroenterology)

ALFT
abnormal liver function tests (gastroenterology and laboratory)

ALG
antilymphocyte globulin (hematology and laboratory)
antilymphocytic globulin (hematology and laboratory)
axiolinguogingival (dentistry)

A.L.G.
antilymphocyte globulin (hematology and laboratory)

ALGOL
{not an abbreviation} [acronym from *al-*

gorithmic oriented language] (computer science) {pronounced "al-gol"}

"al-gol"
{pronunciation of *ALGOL* [acronym from *al*gorithmic *o*riented *l*anguage]} (computer science) {not an abbreviation}

ALH
anterior lobe hormone (endocrinology, laboratory, and neurology)
anterior lobe of hypophysis (neurology)

A lines
{not an abbreviation} [refers to *Kerley's A lines*] (radiology and respiratory)

alk
alkaline (laboratory)

alk.
alkaline (laboratory)

ALKAPT
homogentistic acid [in urine] (genetics and laboratory)

"alk-foss"
{pronunciation of *alk. phos.* [alkaline phosphatase]} (laboratory) {not an abbreviation}

ALKISO
alkaline phosphatase isoenzymes (laboratory)

ALK-P
alkaline phosphatase (laboratory)

"alk-pea-tase"
{pronunciation of *alk p'tase* [alkaline phosphatase]} (laboratory) {not an abbreviation}

alk. phos.
alkaline phosphatase (laboratory) {pronounced "alk-foss"}

alk p'tase
alkaline phosphatase (laboratory) {pronounced "alk-pea-tase"}

ALL
acute lymphatic leukemia (hematology and oncology)
acute lymphoblastic leukemia (hematology and oncology)
acute lymphocytic leukemia (hematology and oncology)
allergy(ies)

All
allergy(ies)

all.
allergy(ies)

"all-ah-go"
{pronunciation of *oligo-* [a prefix meaning *few*, *little*, or *scanty*]} {not an abbreviation}

ALLO
atypical *Legionella*-like organisms (bacteriology and laboratory)

ALM
acral lentiginous melanoma (oncology)
alveolar lining material (respiratory)

ALMA
Adoptee's Liberty Movement Association {pronounced "al-mah"}

"al-mah"
{pronunciation of *ALMA* [Adoptee's Liberty Movement Association]} {not an abbreviation}

ALME
acetyl-lysine methyl ester (laboratory)

ALMe
acetyl-L-lysine methyl ester (laboratory)

ALMI
anterolateral myocardial infarction [also called *anterior lateral myocardial infarction*] (cardiovascular)

ALN
anterior lymph node

ALO
axiolinguo-occlusal (dentistry)

Al₂O₃
aluminum oxide (chemistry and pharmacology)

Al(OH)₃
aluminum hydroxide (chemistry and pharmacology)

ALOMAD
Adriamycin, chlorambucil, vincristine, methotrexate, actinomycin D, and dacarbazine [DTIC] (chemotherapy, oncology, and pharmacology)

ALOS
average length of stay [in health care institutions]

ALP
alkaline phosphatase (laboratory)
anterior lobe of pituitary (endocrinology)
antilymphocyte plasma (hematology and laboratory)

alpha-KG
alpha-ketoglutarate (laboratory)

alpha-LP
alpha-lipoprotein (cardiovascular and laboratory)

alpha-M
alpha₂-macroglobulin (hematology and laboratory)

ALPS
Aphasia Language Performance Scale (speech and language therapy)

ALRI
anterolateral rotational instability [also called *anterolateral rotary instability*] (orthopedics)

ALROS
American Laryngological, Rhinological, and Otological Society (otorhinolaryngology)

A.L.R.O.S.
American Laryngological, Rhinological, and Otological Society (otorhinolaryngology)

ALS
acute lateral sclerosis (neurology)
advanced life support (emergency medicine)
Advanced Life Support System (emergency medicine)
amyotrophic lateral sclerosis (neurology)
angiotensin-like substance (cardiovascular and laboratory)
anterolateral sclerosis (neurology)
anticipated life span (statistics)
antilymphatic serum (hematology and laboratory)
antilymphocyte serum (hematology and laboratory)
antilymphocytic serum (hematology and laboratory)

ALT
alanine aminotransferase [new name for *serum glutamic pyruvic transaminase* (SGPT)] (cardiovascular, gastroenterology, hematology, laboratory, and nephrology)
alanine transaminase (cardiovascular, gastroenterology, hematology, laboratory, and nephrology)
alternate
altitude
argon laser trabeculoplasty (ophthalmology)

alt
alternate
altitude

ALTB
acute laryngotracheobronchitis (otorhinolaryngology and respiratory)

alt dieb
alternis diebus [alternating days, every other day] (pharmacology)

alt. dieb.
alternis diebus [alternating days, every other day] (pharmacology)

alt diem
alternis diem [alternating days, every other day] (pharmacology)

ALTE
apparent life-threatening event (emergency and general medicine)

ALTEE
acetyl-L-tyrosine ethyl ester (laboratory)

alt hor
alternis horis [every other hour] (pharmacology)

alt. hor.
alternis horis [every other hour] (pharmacology)

alt noct
alternis nocta [every other night] (pharmacology)

alt. noct.
alternis nocta [every other night] (pharmacology)

ALU
arithmetic and logic unit (computer science)

ALV
avian leukosis virus (veterinary medicine)

alv
alveolar (respiratory)

alv.
alveolar (respiratory)

alv adst
alvo adstricta [when the bowels are constipated] (gastroenterology and pharmacology)

alv. adst.
alvo adstricta [when the bowels are constipated] (gastroenterology and pharmacology)

alv deject
alvi dejectiones [alvine dejections, discharge from the bowels] (gastroenterology and pharmacology)

alv. deject.
alvi dejectiones [alvine dejections, discharge from the bowels] (gastroenterology and pharmacology)

Alvx
alveolectomy (dentistry and maxillofacial surgery)

ALW
arch-loop-whorl

ALWMI
anterolateral wall myocardial infarction (cardiovascular)

A-LYM
atypical lymphocyte(s) (hematology and laboratory)

AM
actomyosin (laboratory)
aerospace medicine (aerospace medicine and armed forces)
alveolar macrophage (hematology and laboratory)
amalgam (dentistry)
ammeter (electricity)
amperemeter (electricity)
ampicillin [an antibiotic] (pharmacology)
amplitude modulation (cardiovascular, electricity, and neurology)
anovular menstruation (gynecology)
ante meridiem [before noon, in the morning]
anteromeatal (anatomy)
antibodies to cardiac myosin (cardiovascular and laboratory)
arithmetic mean (mathematics)
arousal mechanism (neurology)
arterial mean (cardiovascular)
Artium Magister [Master of Arts] (education)
atrial myxoma (cardiovascular and laboratory)

aviation medicine (aerospace medicine)
axiomesial (dentistry)
meter-angle (measurement)
myopic astigmatism (ophthalmology)

A.M.
ante meridiem [before noon, in the morning]
Artium Magister [Master of Arts] (education)

Am
amalgam (dentistry)
American [referring to nationality]
americium (chemistry)
amyl (chemistry)

am
ametropia (ophthalmology)
ante meridiem [before noon, in the morning]
meter-angle (measurement)
myopic astigmatism (ophthalmology)

a.m.
ante meridiem [before noon, in the morning]

AMA
against medical advice
American Medical Association
antimitochondrial antibody (laboratory)
Australian Medical Association

A.M.A.
against medical advice
American Medical Association
Australian Medical Association

AMA-DE
American Medical Association Drug Evaluation (pharmacology)

AMAL
Aeronautical-Medical Acceleration Laboratory (aerospace medicine and research)

AMAP
as much as possible

A-MAT
amorphous material (laboratory)

AMB
amphotericin B (pharmacology)

Amb
ambulate (rehabilitation)
ambulatory (rehabilitation)

amb
ambulance (emergency medicine)
ambulate (rehabilitation)
ambulatory (rehabilitation)

amb. care
ambulatory care (rehabilitation)

ambig
ambiguous

AMBL
acute myeloblastic leukemia (hematology and oncology)

AMBR
amber [color] (laboratory)

ambul
ambulation (rehabilitation)
ambulatory (rehabilitation)

AMC
Animal Medical Center (veterinary medicine)
antimalaria campaign (infectious diseases)
arm muscle circumference (neurology and orthopedics)
Army Medical Center (armed forces)
Army Medical Corps (armed forces)
arthrogryposis multiplex congenita (orthopedics)
axiomesiocervical (dentistry)

AMD
aeromedical data (armed forces)
Aerospace Medical Division [Air Force] (armed forces and aerospace medicine)
age-related macular degeneration (ophthalmology)
alpha-methyldopa (cardiovascular and pharmacology)

Army Medical Department (armed forces)
Association for Macular Diseases (ophthalmology)
axiomesiodistal (dentistry)

AMDS
Association of Military Dental Surgeons (armed forces and dentistry)

A.M.D.S.
Association of Military Dental Surgeons (armed forces and dentistry)

AME
agreed medical examiner

AMEA
American Medical Electroencephalographic Association (neurology)

A.M.E.A.
American Medical Electroencephalographic Association (neurology)

AMEBIA
amebiasis (laboratory)

AMEDS
Army Medical Service (armed forces) {pronounced "A-medz"}

"A-medz"
{pronunciation of *AMEDS* [Army Medical Service]} (armed forces) {not an abbreviation}

AMegL
acute megakaryoblastic leukemia (hematology)

AMEL
Aero-Medical Equipment Laboratory (manufacturer)

Amer
American [referring to nationality]

AMF
antimuscle factor (laboratory)

Amfre-G
Amfre-Grant, Incorporated [manufacturer] (pharmacology)

AMG
acoustic myography (otorhinolaryngology)
amyloglucoside [also called *glucoamylase*] (laboratory)
antimacrophage globulin (hematology and laboratory)
axiomesiogingival (dentistry)

AMH
automated medical history (medical records)

Amh
mixed astigmatism with myopia predominating (ophthalmology)

AMHA
Association of Mental Health Administrators (administration and psychiatry)

AMI
acute myocardial infarction (cardiovascular)
American Medical International Incorporated [hospital group]
amitriptyline hydrochloride [an antidepressant] (pharmacology and psychiatry)
anterior myocardial infarction (cardiovascular)
Association of Medical Illustrators (art and publishing)
axiomesioincisal (dentistry)

A.M.I.
Association of Medical Illustrators (art and publishing)

AMIIA
Army Medical Intelligence and Information Agency (armed forces)

AMINO
amino acid screen (laboratory)

AML
acute monocytic leukemia (hematology and oncology)

acute myeloblastic leukemia (hematology and oncology)
acute myelocytic leukemia (hematology and oncology)
acute myelogenous leukemia (hematology and oncology)
acute myeloid leukemia (hematology and oncology)
anterior mitral leaflet (cardiovascular)

AMLR
autologous mixed lymphocyte reaction (hematology and laboratory)

AMLS
antimouse lymphocyte serum (hematology and laboratory)

AMM
agnogenic myeloid metaplasia (hematology)
ammonia (chemistry, laboratory, and pharmacology)
antibodies to murine cardiac myosin (cardiovascular and laboratory)
Association Médicale Mondiale [World Medical Association]

AMML
acute monomyelocytic leukemia (hematology and oncology)
acute myelomonoblastic leukemia (hematology and oncology)

AMMOL
acute myelomonoblastic leukemia (hematology and oncology)

ammon
ammonia (chemistry, laboratory, and pharmacology)

AMN
alloxazine mononucleotide (laboratory)

amnio
amniocentesis (obstetrics) {pronounced "ahm-nee-oh"}

AMO
American Medical Optics [posterior chamber lens; manufacturer] (ophthalmology)
Assistant Medical Officer

Aviation Medical Officer (aerospace medicine)
axiomesio-occlusal (dentistry)

A.MOD.
behavior modification (psychiatry)

A-mode
amplitude modulation [a mode used in electroencephalography and ultrasound] (cardiovascular, neurology, obstetrics, and radiology)

AMOL
acute monoblastic leukemia (hematology and oncology)
acute monocytic leukemia (hematology and oncology)

AMO PC
American Medical Optics Posterior Chamber [lens] (ophthalmology)

AMOR
amorphous

amor
amorphous

AMORP
amorphous [sediment] (laboratory)

AMP
acid mucopolysaccharide (genetics and laboratory)
adenosine monophosphate [also called *adenylic acid*] (endocrinology and laboratory)
aminomonophosphate (laboratory)
amphetamine (chemical dependency, pharmacology, and psychiatry)
ampicillin [an antibiotic] (pharmacology) {pronounced "amp"}
ampule (pharmacology) {pronounced "amp"}
amputation (orthopedics)
average mean pressure (cardiovascular)

3′,5′-AMP
3′,5′-adenosine monophosphate (endocrinology and laboratory)

amp
ampere (electricity and measurement)
{pronounced "amp"}
amperage (electricity)
ampicillin [an antibiotic] (pharmacology) {pronounced "amp"}
amplification
ampule (pharmacology) {pronounced "amp"}
amputation (orthopedics)

amp.
ampere (electricity and measurement)
{pronounced "amp"}
amplification
ampule (pharmacology) {pronounced "amp"}
amputation (orthopedics)
amputee (orthopedics and rehabilitation)

"amp"
{pronunciation of *AMP* [ampicillin and ampule (pharmacology)] and *amp* [ampere (electricity and measurement), ampicillin (pharmacology), and ampule (pharmacology)]} {not an abbreviation}

AMPA
American Medical Publishers Association (publishing)

AMPH
amphetamine (chemical dependency, pharmacology, and psychiatry)

amph
amphoric [sound] (respiratory)

amp-hr
ampere-hour (electricity and measurement)

AMPIM
Animal Models of Protecting Ischaemic Myocardium (cardiovascular, research, and veterinary medicine)

ampl.
amplus [large]

AMPPPE
acute multifocal posterior placoid pigment epitheliopathy (dermatology)

A-M pr
Austin Moore prosthesis (orthopedics)

AM pros
Austin Moore prosthesis (orthopedics)

AMPS
abnormal mucopolysacchariduria (genetics and laboratory)
acid mucopolysaccharides (genetics and laboratory)

AMP-S
adenylosuccinic acid (laboratory, neurology, and orthopedics)

AMPT
Aminopterin (chemotherapy and oncology)

ampul.
ampulla [ampule] (pharmacology)

AMQ
American Medical Qualification [British]

AMR
activity metabolic rate
alternating motion rate (neurology)
alternating motion reflexes (neurology)
alternating motor rates (neurology)
Aviation Medical Reports (aerospace medicine)

AMRA
American Medical Record Association (medical records)

AMRI
anteromedial rotational instability (orthopedics)

AMRL
Aerospace Medical Research Laboratories (aerospace medicine and research)
Army Medical Research and Nutrition

Laboratory (armed forces, dietary, and research)

A.M.R.L.
Aerospace Medical Research Laboratories (aerospace medicine and research)

AMS
abortus, melitensis, suis
acute mountain sickness (cardiovascular, gastroenterology, neurology, and respiratory)
aggravated in military service (armed forces)
American Medical Systems [artificial urethral sphincter; manufacturer] (urology)
American Microscopical Society (laboratory)
amylase (laboratory)
antimacrophage serum (hematology and laboratory)
Army Medical Service [British] (armed forces)
Association of Military Surgeons (armed forces and surgery)
atypical measles syndrome (infectious diseases and pediatrics)
auditory memory span (neurology)
automated multiphasic screening (laboratory)
automicrobic system (laboratory)

A.M.S.
American Meteorological Society (meteorology)
American Microscopical Society (laboratory)
Army Medical Service (armed forces)
Association of Military Surgeons (armed forces and surgery)

ams.
amount of a substance

AMSA
acridinylamine methanesulphon-m-anisidide (chemotherapy, oncology, and pharmacology)
American Medical Society on Alcoholism (chemical dependency)
American Medical Students Association (education)

amsacrine (chemotherapy, oncology, and pharmacology)

AMSC
Army Medical Specialist Corps (armed forces)

AmSECT
American Society of Extra-Corporeal Technology (cardiovascular)

AMSIT
appearance, mood, sensorium, intelligence, and thought processes [a portion of the mental status examination] (neurology and psychiatry)

AMSRDC
Army Medical Service Research and Development Command (armed forces and research)

AMT
alpha-methyltyrosine (endocrinology and laboratory)
American Medical Technologists (laboratory)
amethopterin [also called *methotrexate*] (chemotherapy, oncology, and pharmacology)
amphetamine (chemical dependency, pharmacology, and psychiatry)

A.M.T.
American Medical Technologists (laboratory)

Amt
amount

amt
amount

am't
amount

amt.
amount

AMU
Army Medical Unit (armed forces)

amu
atomic mass unit (chemistry)

AMV
assisted mechanical ventilation (respiratory)

A.M.W.A.
American Medical Women's Association
American Medical Writer's Association
(publishing)

AMY
amylase (gastroenterology and laboratory)

AMYLAS
amylase (gastroenterology and laboratory)

AMY-SP
amylase urine spot [test] (gastroenterology and laboratory)

AN
anesthesia (anesthesiology)
aneurysm (cardiovascular)
anisometropia (ophthalmology)
anodal (chemistry, electricity, laboratory, and radiology)
anode (chemistry, electricity, laboratory, and radiology)
anorexia nervosa (gastroenterology and psychiatry)
antenatal (obstetrics)
aseptic necrosis (orthopedics)

A/N
Army-Navy [retractor] (surgery)
artery and nerve (cardiovascular and neurology)
artery and/or nerve (cardiovascular and neurology)
as needed (pharmacology)

6-AN
{not an abbreviation} [a topical cream] (dermatology and pharmacology)

An
actinon [also called *radon-219*] (chemistry and radiology)

A$_n$
normal atmosphere

An.
anisometropia (ophthalmology)
anodal (chemistry, electricity, laboratory, and radiology)
anode (chemistry, electricity, laboratory, and radiology)

an
anatomic (anatomy)

ANA
acetylneuraminic acid (laboratory)
American Narcolepsy Association (neurology)
American Neurological Association (neurology)
American Nurses' Association (nursing)
anesthesia (anesthesiology)
anesthetic (anesthesiology)
antinuclear antibody(ies) (gastroenterology, hematology, laboratory, oncology, respiratory, and rheumatology)
aspartyl naphthylamide (laboratory)

A.N.A.
American Neurological Association (neurology)
American Nurses' Association (nursing)

ana
so much of each [āā] (pharmacology)

ANAD
anorexia nervosa and associated disorders (gastroenterology and psychiatry)

ANAERO
anaerobe(s) (laboratory)

Anaes
anaesthesia [anesthesia] (anesthesiology)
anaesthetic [anesthetic] (anesthesiology)

Anaesth
anaesthesia [anesthesia] (anesthesiology)

anaesthetic [anesthetic] (anesthesiology)

ANA-FL
antinuclear antibody fluid (gastroenterology, hematology, laboratory, oncology, respiratory, and rheumatology)

anal
analgesic (pharmacology)
analyses
analysis

anal.
analgesic (pharmacology)
analysis
analyst

ANAP
agglutination negative, absorption positive (laboratory)

anast.
anastomosis (cardiovascular, gastroenterology, and surgery)

Anat
anatomical (anatomy)
anatomy

anat.
anatomical (anatomy)
anatomy

ANC
absolute neutrophil count (hematology and laboratory)
Army Nurse Corps (armed forces and nursing)

AnCC
anodal closure contraction (cardiovascular)

AND
anterior nasal discharge (otorhinolaryngology)

And
androgens (chemotherapy, endocrinology, laboratory, oncology, and pharmacology)

ANDA
Abbreviated New Drug Application (pharmacology)

ANDRO
androsterone (endocrinology, laboratory, and pharmacology)

ANDROS
androsterone (endocrinology, laboratory, and pharmacology)

AnDTe
anodal duration tetanus (cardiovascular)

ANEG
A negative [blood type] (hematology and laboratory)

Anes
anesthesia (anesthesiology)

anes
anesthesia (anesthesiology)

anes.
anesthesia (anesthesiology)
anesthesiology

Anesth
anesthesia (anesthesiology)
anesthetic (anesthesiology)

an ex
anode excitation (cardiovascular)

an. ex.
anode excitation (cardiovascular)

ANF
alpha-naphthoflavone (laboratory)
American Nurses' Foundation (nursing)
antinuclear factor [obsolete; now called *antinuclear antibody*] (gastroenterology, hematology, laboratory, oncology, respiratory, and rheumatology)
atrial natriuretic factor (cardiovascular, endocrinology, laboratory, and nephrology)

Ang
angiogram (cardiovascular and radiology)
angle

ang
angiogram (cardiovascular and radiology)
angle

"an-gee-oh"
{pronunciation of *angio* [angiocatheter, angiocatheterization, and angiography]} (cardiovascular and radiology) {not an abbreviation}

Ang GR
angiotensin generation rate (cardiovascular and laboratory)

angio
angiocatheter (cardiovascular and radiology) {pronounced "an-gee-oh"}
angiocatheterization (cardiovascular and radiology) {pronounced "an-gee-oh"}
angiography (cardiovascular and radiology) {pronounced "an-gee-oh"}

anh
anhydrous

anh.
anhydrous

ANIS
anisocytosis (hematology and laboratory)

ANISO
anisocytosis (hematology and laboratory)

Anisometr
anisometropia (ophthalmology)

ANIT
alpha-naphthylisothiocyanate (laboratory)

ank.
ankle (anatomy)

ANL
acute nonlymphoblastic leukemia (hematology and oncology)

ANLI
antibody-negative mice with latent infection (research and veterinary medicine)

ANLL
acute nonlymphoblastic leukemia (hematology and oncology)
acute nonlymphocytic leukemia (hematology and oncology)
acute nonlymphoid leukemia (hematology and oncology)

Ann
annals
annual

Annls
annals

AnOC
anodal opening contraction (cardiovascular)

ANOVA
analysis of variance

ANP
Adult Nurse Practitioner (nursing)
alpha-atrial natriuretic polypeptide [also called *atrial natriuretic factor* (ANF)] (cardiovascular, endocrinology, laboratory, and nephrology)
A-norprogesterone (endocrinology and laboratory)

ANP6-AN protocol
{not an abbreviation} [a topical cream] (dermatology and pharmacology)

ANRC
American National Red Cross (emergency medicine and hematology)

A.N.R.C.
American National Red Cross (emergency medicine and hematology)

ANRL
antihypertensive neutral renomedullary lipids (cardiovascular, laboratory, and nephrology)

ANS
American Nutrition Society (dietary)
answer
anterior nasal spine (otorhinolaryngology)
antineutrophilic serum (hematology and laboratory)
Army Nursing Service (armed forces and nursing)
arteriolonephrosclerosis (cardiovascular and nephrology)
Associate in Nursing Science (education and nursing)
autonomic nervous system (neurology)

ans
answer

ANSI
American National Standards Institute [previously called *ASA* (American Standards Association) and *USASI* (United States Standards Institute)] (measurement)

A.N.S.I.
American National Standards Institute [previously called *ASA* (American Standards Association) and *USASI* (United States Standards Institute)] (measurement)

ANT
acoustic noise test (otorhinolaryngology)
2-amino-5-nitro-thiazol [also called *aminonitrothiazole*] (chemistry, pharmacology, and veterinary medicine)
Animal Naming Test (speech and language therapy)
anterior

Ant
anterior
antimycin

ant
anterior

ant.
anterior

Ant A
antimycin A

antag
antagonistic (psychiatry)

ant ax line
anterior axillary line (anatomy)

ant. ax. line
anterior axillary line (anatomy)

ante
{not an abbreviation} [Latin word meaning *before*]

Anthrop
anthropology

ANTI
antibody (laboratory)

anticoag
anticoagulation (hematology)

anti-DNA
antibody to deoxyribonucleic acid [test] (laboratory and rheumatology)

anti-DNase B
antideoxyribonuclease B [antibody test for streptococcal infection] (laboratory)

anti-ENA
antibody to extractable nuclear antigen [test] (laboratory and rheumatology)

anti-GMB
antiglomerular basement membrane [antibodies] (cardiovascular)

anti-HA
anti-H antigen (bacteriology and laboratory)

anti-HAA
antibody hepatitis-associated antigen

(gastroenterology, infectious diseases, and laboratory)

anti-HB$_s$Ag
antibody to hepatitis B surface antigen (gastroenterology, infectious diseases, and laboratory)

anti-La
{not an abbreviation} [an antibody] (immunology and laboratory)

anti-log
antilogarithm (mathematics)

anti-RNP
antiribonucleoprotein (genetics and laboratory)

anti-Ro
{not an abbreviation} [an antibody] (immunology and laboratory)

anti-S
antisulfanilic acid (laboratory)

anti-Sm
anti-Smith [antibody] (hematology and laboratory)

anti-SM/RNP
antibody smooth muscle-ribonucleoprotein (genetics and laboratory)

ant jentac
ante jentaculum [before breakfast]

Ant pit
anterior pituitary [referring to anterior lobe of pituitary] (endocrinology and neurosurgery)

ANTR
apparent net transfer rate

Ant sup spine
anterior superior spine [of ilium] (orthopedics)

ANTU
alpha-naphthyl thiourea [a rodenticide] (chemistry, laboratory, and pharmacology)

ANUG
acute necrotizing ulcerative gingivitis (dentistry and otorhinolaryngology)

anx
anxiety (psychiatry)

anx. neur.
anxiety neurosis (psychiatry)

anx. reac.
anxiety reaction (psychiatry)

AO
acid output (gastroenterology)
acridine orange [test] (laboratory, oncology, and pathology)
American Optical [instruments and oximetry] (ophthalmology)
anodal opening (cardiovascular)
anterior oblique (radiology)
aorta (cardiovascular)
aortic (cardiovascular)
aortic opening (cardiovascular)
atomic orbital [contour] (chemistry and physics)
axio-occlusal (dentistry)
opening of the atrioventricular valves (cardiovascular)
{not an abbreviation} [a type of screw] (orthopedics)

A-O
acoustic-optic (ophthalmology and otorhinolaryngology)

A & O
alert and oriented (neurology and psychiatry)

A & O X 3
alert and oriented times three (neurology and psychiatry)
alert and oriented to person, place, and time (neurology and psychiatry)
awake and oriented times three (neurology and psychiatry)
awake and oriented to person, place, and time (neurology and psychiatry)

A & O X 4

alert and oriented times four (neurology and psychiatry)

alert and oriented to person, place, time, and date (neurology and psychiatry)

awake and oriented times four (neurology and psychiatry)

awake and oriented to person, place, time, and date (neurology and psychiatry)

Ao

aorta (cardiovascular)

AOA

abnormal oxygen affinity (hematology and laboratory)

American Optometric Association (ophthalmology)

American Orthopaedic Association (orthopedics)

American Orthopsychiatric Association (psychiatry)

American Osteopathic Association (osteopathic medicine)

A.O.A.

American Optometric Association (ophthalmology)

American Orthopaedic Association (orthopedics)

American Orthopsychiatric Association (psychiatry)

American Osteopathic Association (osteopathic medicine)

AOAA

amino-oxyacetic acid (laboratory)

AOAC

Association of Official Agricultural Chemists (agriculture and chemistry)

AOAP

as often as possible

AOAS

American Osteopathic Academy of Sclerotherapy (osteopathic medicine)

AOB

accessory olfactory bulb (otorhinolaryngology)

alcohol on breath (chemical dependency and emergency medicine)

AOC

abridged ocular chart (ophthalmology)

American Ophthalmological Color Chart (ophthalmology)

American Optical Corporation [manufacturer] (ophthalmology)

anodal opening contraction (cardiovascular)

area of concern

A.O.C.

American Optical Corporation [manufacturer] (ophthalmology)

AOCA

American Osteopathic College of Anesthesiologists (anesthesiology and osteopathic medicine)

A.O.C.A.

American Osteopathic College of Anesthesiologists (anesthesiology and osteopathic medicine)

AOCD

American Osteopathic College of Dermatology (dermatology and osteopathic medicine)

A.O.C.D.

American Osteopathic College of Dermatology (dermatology and osteopathic medicine)

AOCl

anodal opening clonus (cardiovascular)

AOCPa

American Osteopathic College of Pathologists (osteopathic medicine and pathology)

A.O.C.Pa.

American Osteopathic College of Pathologists (osteopathic medicine and pathology)

AOCPR
American Osteopathic College of Proctology (gastroenterology and osteopathic medicine)

A.O.C.Pr.
American Osteopathic College of Proctology (gastroenterology and osteopathic medicine)

AOCR
American Osteopathic College of Radiology (osteopathic medicine and radiology)
American Osteopathic College of Rheumatology (osteopathic medicine and rheumatology)

A.O.C.R.
American Osteopathic College of Radiology (osteopathic medicine and radiology)

AOCRM
American Osteopathic College of Rehabilitation (osteopathic medicine and rehabilitation)

AOD
Academy of Operative Dentistry (dentistry)
Administrative Officer of the Day
adult onset diabetes (endocrinology)
arterial occlusive disease (cardiovascular)
auriculo-osteodysplasia (otorhinolaryngology)

AODM
adult onset diabetes mellitus (endocrinology)

AODME
Academy of Osteopathic Directors of Medical Education (education and osteopathic medicine)

AOHA
American Osteopathic Hospital Association (administration and osteopathic medicine)

ao-il
aorta-iliac (cardiovascular)

aortoiliac (cardiovascular)

AOIVM
angiographically occult intracranial vascular malformation (neurosurg)

AOL
acro-osteolysis (orthopedics and podiatry)

AOM
acute otitis media (otorhinolaryngology)
Master of Obstetric Art (education and obstetrics)

AOMA
American Occupational Medical Association (occupational medicine and therapy)

AOO
anodal opening odor (cardiovascular)

AOP
anodal opening picture (cardiovascular)
aortic pressure (cardiovascular)

AoP
left ventricle to aorta pressure gradient (cardiovascular)

AOPA
American Orthotics and Prosthetics Association (orthopedics and rehabilitation)

A.O.P.A.
American Orthotics and Prosthetics Association (orthopedics and rehabilitation)

AORN
Association of Operating Room Nurses (nursing and surgery)

Aort regurg
aortic regurgitation (cardiovascular)

aort regurg
aortic regurgitation (cardiovascular)

aort. regurg.
aortic regurgitation (cardiovascular)

Aort sten
aortic stenosis (cardiovascular)

aort sten
aortic stenosis (cardiovascular)

aort. sten.
aortic stenosis (cardiovascular)

AOS
American Ophthalmological Society
(ophthalmology)
American Orthodontic Society (dentistry)
American Otological Society (otorhinolaryngology)
anodal opening sound (cardiovascular)

A.O.S.
American Otological Society (otorhinolaryngology)

AOSD
adult-onset Still's disease (orthopedics
and rheumatology)

AOSSM
American Orthopedic Society for Sports
Medicine (orthopedics and sports
medicine)

AOT
Association of Occupational Therapists
(occupational therapy)
antiovotransferrin (hematology and laboratory)

A.O.T.
Association of Occupational Therapists
(occupational therapy)

AOTA
American Occupational Therapy Association (occupational therapy)

A.O.T.A.
American Occupational Therapy Association (occupational therapy)

AOTe
anodal opening tetanus (cardiovascular)

AOU
apparent oxygen utilization (cardiovascular and respiratory)

AP
abdominoperineal [resection] (gastroenterology and surgery)
acid phosphatase (endocrinology, gastroenterology, laboratory, oncology,
orthopedics, and urology)
action potential (neurology)
acute proliferation (laboratory)
alkaline phosphatase (gastroenterology,
laboratory, oncology, and orthopedics)
alum-precipitated [referring to vaccines]
(infectious diseases, laboratory, and
pharmacology)
American Pharmacopeia (pharmacology)
aminopeptidase (laboratory)
angina pectoris (cardiovascular)
ante partum [meaning before the onset
of labor] (obstetrics)
antepartum [meaning before childbirth]
(obstetrics)
anterior pituitary [anterior lobe of
pituitary] (endocrinology and neurosurgery)
anteroposterior [projection] (radiology)
anteroposterior (anatomy)
aortic pressure (cardiovascular)
apical pulse (cardiovascular)
apothecary (pharmacology)
appendectomy (gastroenterology and
surgery)
appendicitis (gastroenterology and surgery)
appendix (multiple specialties; primarily
gastroenterology and surgery)
arithmetic progression (laboratory,
mathematics, and statistics)
arterial pressure (cardiovascular)
artificial pneumothorax (respiratory)
associated period
atrium pace (cardiovascular)
axiopulpal (dentistry)

AP-1
protein

Apgar

{not an abbreviation} [The Apgar score is a numerical expression of an infant's condition in the first minutes of life.] (neonatology and pediatrics) {pronounced "ap-gar"}

"ap-gar"

{pronunciation of *APGAR* [adaptability, partnership, growth, affection, and resolve (questionnaire) (psychiatry) and American Pediatric Gross Assessment Record (pediatrics)] and *Apgar* [The Apgar score is a numerical expression of an infant's condition in the first minutes of life. (neonatology and pediatrics)]} {not an abbreviation}

APGL

alkaline phosphatase activity of the granular leukocytes (gastroenterology, hematology, laboratory, oncology, and orthopedics)

APH

antepartum hemorrhage (gynecology and obstetrics)
anterior pituitary hormone (endocrinology and laboratory)
Association of Private Hospitals (administration)

APHA

American Protestant Hospital Association (administration and religion)
American Public Health Association (public health)

A.P.H.A.

American Protestant Hospital Association (administration and religion)
American Public Health Association (public health)

APhA

American Pharmaceutical Association (pharmacology)

A.Ph.A.

American Pharmaceutical Association (pharmacology)

APHP

anti-*Pseudomonas* human plasma (bacteriology and laboratory)

API

Analytical Profile Index (laboratory and microbiology)

APIC

Association for Practitioners in Infection Control (infectious diseases)

A.P.I.M.

Association Professionnele Internationale des Médecins

APIP

additional personal injury protection [insurance]

APKD

adult polycystic kidney disease [also called *adult-onset polycystic kidney disease*] (nephrology)

APL

abductor pollicis longus [muscle] (neurology and orthopedics)
accelerated painless labor (obstetrics)
acute promyelocytic leukemia (hematology and oncology)
anterior pituitary-like [hormone or substance] (endocrinology and laboratory)
chorionic gonadotropin (endocrinology, laboratory, obstetrics, and pharmacology)

A.P.L.

{not an abbreviation} [trademark for preparation of human chorionic gonadotropin] (endocrinology, laboratory, obstetrics, and pharmacology)

AP & Lat.

anteroposterior and lateral [views] (radiology)

A-P & lat.

anteroposterior and lateral [views] (radiology)

APL hormone
anterior pituitary-like hormone (endocrinology and laboratory)

APM
Academy of Parapsychology and Medicine (parapsychology)
Academy of Physical Medicine (physical medicine and rehabilitation)
Academy of Psychosomatic Medicine (psychiatry)
acid-precipitable material (laboratory)
anterior papillary muscle [image on transesophageal echocardiography] (cardiovascular)
aspartame [a sweetening agent] (chemistry and dietary)
Association of Professors of Medicine (education)

A.P.M.
Academy of Physical Medicine (physical medicine and rehabilitation)
Academy of Psychosomatic Medicine (psychiatry)

APMR
Association for Physical and Mental Rehabilitation (physical medicine and rehabilitation)

A.P.M.R.
Association for Physical and Mental Rehabilitation (physical medicine and rehabilitation)

APN
acute pyelonephritis (nephrology and urology)
average peak noise (ecology and industrial medicine)

APO
Adriamycin [doxorubicin], prednisone, and Oncovin [vincristine] (chemotherapy, oncology, and pharmacology)
apomorphine [an emetic] (gastroenterology and pharmacology)

apo E
apolipoprotein E (cardiovascular and laboratory)

"A-poth"
{pronunciation of *apoth* [apothecary]} (pharmacology) {not an abbreviation}

apoth
apothecary (pharmacology) {pronounced "A-poth"}

APP
alum-precipitated protein (laboratory)
alum-precipitated pyridine (laboratory)
avian pancreatic polypeptide (laboratory)

App
appendix (multiple specialties; primarily gastroenterology and surgery)

app
apparent
appendix (multiple specialties; primarily gastroenterology and surgery)

app.
appendix (multiple specialties; primarily gastroenterology and surgery)

APPA
American Psychopathological Association (psychiatry)

appar
apparatus
apparent

APPG
aqueous procaine penicillin G (pharmacology)

appl
appliance
applicable
application
applied

appl.
appliance
applied

applan
applantus [flattened]

applan.
applantus [flattened]

applicand
applicandus [to be applied] (pharmacology)

applicand.
applicandus [to be applied] (pharmacology)

APPR
approaching lactate dehydrogenase [LD] 1:2 flip (cardiovascular and laboratory)

appr
approximate(ly)

appr.
approximate

APPROV
approved

APPROX
approximate(ly)
approximation

approx
approximate(ly)
approximation

Appt
appointment

appt
appointment

appt.
appointment

Appx
appendix (multiple specialties; primarily gastroenterology and surgery)

Appy
appendectomy (gastroenterology and surgery) {pronounced "ap-E"}

appy
appendectomy (gastroenterology and surgery) {pronounced "ap-E"}

APR
abdominoperineal resection (gastroenterology and surgery)
amebic prevalence rate (laboratory)
anterior pituitary resection (endocrinology and surgery)
anatomic porous replacement (orthopedic and surgery)

aprax
apraxia (neurology)

APRL
American Prosthetic Research Laboratory (ophthalmology, orthopedics, and research)

A.P.R.L.
American Prosthetic Research Laboratory (ophthalmology, orthopedics, and research)

APRO
aprobarbital (pharmacology and psychiatry)

AProL
acute progranulocytic leukemia (hematology and oncology)
acute promyelocytic leukemia (hematology and oncology)

APRT
adenine phosphoribosyltransferase (laboratory)

A-PRT
adenine phosphoribusyl-transferase (laboratory)

APS
adenosine phosphosulfate (laboratory)
American Pediatric Society (pediatrics)
American Physiological Society (physiology)
American Proctologic Society (gastroenterology)
American Prosthodontic Society (dentistry)
American Psychological Society (psychology)

American Psychosomatic Society (psychiatry)

A.P.S.
American Pediatric Society (pediatrics)
American Physiological Society (physiology)
American Proctologic Society (gastroenterology)
American Psychological Society (psychology)
American Psychosomatic Society (psychiatry)

APSAC
anisoylated plasminogen streptokinase activator complex (cardiovascular and pharmacology)

APSS
Association for Psychophysiological Study of Sleep (neurology and psychiatry)

APT
alum-precipitated toxoid (immunology, infectious diseases, and pharmacology)

A.P.T.
alum-precipitated toxoid (immunology, infectious diseases, and pharmacology)

APTA
American Physical Therapy Association (physical therapy)

A.P.T.A.
American Physical Therapy Association (physical therapy)

APTC
Army Physical Training Corps (armed forces)

APTD
Aid to Permanently and Totally Disabled (government)

APTT
activated partial thromboplastin time (hematology and laboratory)

aPTT
activated partial thromboplastin time (hematology and laboratory)

APUD
amine precursor uptake and decarboxylation [cells] (endocrinology, laboratory, neurology, and oncology)

APUD-oma
amine precursor uptake and decarboxylation tumor [tumors derived from neural crest] (endocrinology)

APVD
anomalous pulmonary venous drainage (cardiovascular, neonatology, and respiratory)

APVT
Ammons Picture Vocabulary Test (speech and language therapy)

AQ
accomplishment quotient (psychiatry)
achievement quotient (psychiatry)
any quantity

A.Q.
achievement quotient (psychiatry)

Aq
aqua [water]

Aq.
aqua [water]

aq
aqua [water]

aq.
aqua [water]

aq astr
aqua astricta [frozen water]

aq. astr.
aqua astricta [frozen water]

aq bull
aqua bulliens [boiling water]

aq. bull.
aqua bulliens [boiling water]

aq cal
aqua calida [hot water]

aq comm
aqua communis [common water]

aq. comm.
aqua communis [common water]

aq dest
aqua destillata [distilled water]

aq. dest.
aqua destillata [distilled water]

Aq. Dist
distilled water

aq ferv
aqua fervens [hot water]

aq. ferv.
aqua fervens [hot water]

aq fluv
aqua fluvialis [river water]

aq. fluv.
aqua fluvialis [river water]

aq font
aqua fontana [spring water]

aq. font.
aqua fontana [spring water]

aq frig
aqua frigida [cold water]

aq. frig.
aqua frigida [cold water]

aq mar
aqua marina [seawater]

aq. mar.
aqua marina [seawater]

aq niv
aqua nivalis [snow water]

aq. niv.
aqua nivalis [snow water]

aq pluv
aqua pluvialis [rainwater]

aq. pluv.
aqua pluvialis [rainwater]

aq pur
aqua pura [pure water]

aq. pur.
aqua pura [pure water]

aq tep
aqua tepida [lukewarm water, tepid water]

aq. tep.
aqua tepida [lukewarm water, tepid water]

AQS
additional qualifying symptoms

aqu
aqueous

AR
achievement ratio
active resistance [exercise] (rehabilitation)
alarm reaction [also called *fight-or-flight reaction* and *stress reaction*] (psychiatry)
allergic rhinitis (allergy and otorhinolaryngology)
analytical reagent (laboratory)
androgen receptor (endocrinology and laboratory)
aortic regurgitation (cardiovascular)
apical-radial [pulse] (cardiovascular)
Argyll Robertson [pupil] (ophthalmology)
Arkansas [Postal Service state designation]
arsphenamine [obsolete treatment for syphilis] (gynecology, infectious diseases, pharmacology, and urology)

articulare [craniometric point] (radiology)
artificial respiration (respiratory)
artificially ruptured (obstetrics)
at risk
atrophic rhinitis [of swine] (veterinary medicine)
autoradiography (radiology)

A-R
apical-radial [pulse] (cardiovascular)

A/R
apical-radial [pulse] (cardiovascular)

A & R
advised and released

Ar
argon (chemistry, laboratory, laser therapy, and radiology)

ARA
Academy of Rehabilitative Audiometry (otorhinolaryngology)
American Rheumatism Association (rheumatology)
Associate of the Royal Academy

A.R.A.
American Rheumatism Association (rheumatology)

ARA-A
adenine arabinoside [also called *vidarabine*] (chemotherapy, oncology, and pharmacology)

ara-A
adenine arabinoside [also called *vidarabine*] (chemotherapy, oncology, and pharmacology)

ARA-C
cytosine arabinoside [also called *cytarabine* and 1-β-*arabino-furanosylcytosine*] (chemotherapy, oncology, and pharmacology)

Ara-C
cytosine arabinoside [also called *cytarabine* and 1-β-*arabino-furanosylcytosine*] (chemotherapy, oncology, and pharmacology)

ara-C
cytosine arabinoside [also called *cytarabine* and 1-β-*arabino-furanosylcytosine*] (chemotherapy, oncology, and pharmacology)

Ara-C + ADR
Ara-C [*cytarabine*] and Adriamycin [*doxorubicin*] (chemotherapy, oncology, and pharmacology)

Ara-C + DNR + PRED + MP
Ara-C [*cytarabine*], daunorubicin, prednisone, and mercaptopurine (chemotherapy, oncology, and pharmacology)

Ara-C + 6-TG
Ara-C [*cytarabine*] and 6-thioguanine (chemotherapy, oncology, and pharmacology)

ARAS
ascending reticular activating system (neurology)

ARB
any reliable brand (pharmacology)

Arbo
arthropod-borne [virus] (laboratory and respiratory)

ARBOR
arthropod-borne [virus] (laboratory and respiratory)

ARC
accelerating rate calorimeter [for heat measurement] (measurement)
acquired immunodeficiency syndrome [AIDS] related complex (immunology) {pronounced "ark"}
Addiction Research Center [part of National Institute of Mental Health] (chemical dependency and research)
American Red Cross (emergency medicine and hematology)
anomalous retinal correspondence (ophthalmology)
arcuate nucleus [of brain] (neurology)

arr
arrive

ARRC
Associate of the Royal Red Cross (emergency medicine and hematology)

ARRS
American Roentgen Ray Society (radiology)

A.R.R.S.
American Roentgen Ray Society (radiology)

ARRT
American Registered Respiratory Therapist (respiratory)

A.R.R.T.
American Registered Respiratory Therapist (respiratory)
American Registry of Radiologic Technologists (radiology)
American Registry of Radiology Technologists (radiology)

Arry
arrhythmia (cardiovascular)

ARS
adult recovery services (chemical dependency and rehabilitation)
alizarin red [a dye] (laboratory and orthopedics)
American Radium Society (radiology)
American Rhinologic Society (otorhinolaryngology)
antirabies serum (infectious diseases, pharmacology, and toxicology)

A.R.S.
American Radium Society (radiology)
American Rhinologic Society (otorhinolaryngology)

Ars
arsphenamine [obsolete treatment for syphilis] (gynecology, infectious diseases, pharmacology, and urology)

Ars.
arsphenamine [obsolete treatment for syphilis] (gynecology, infectious diseases, pharmacology, and urology)

ARSA
American Reye's Syndrome Association (pediatrics)

ARSC
Associate of the Royal Society of Chemistry (chemistry)

ARSEN
arsenic [a poison] (chemistry, laboratory, and pharmacology)

ARSM
acute respiratory system malfunction (respiratory)

ARSPH
Associate of the Royal Society for the Promotion of Health

ART
absolute retention time
Accredited Record Technician (medical records)
Achilles tendon reflex test (neurology and orthopedics)
acoustic reflex test (neurology and otorhinolaryngology)
arterial (cardiovascular)
automated reagin test (laboratory)

A.R.T.
Accredited Record Technician (medical records)

art
arterial (cardiovascular)
artery (cardiovascular)
articulation (orthopedics and speech and language therapy)
artificial

art.
artery (cardiovascular)
articulation (orthopedics and speech and language therapy)

arthr
athrotomy (orthopedics)

arthro
arthroscopy (orthopedics) {pronounced "are-throw"}

artic
articulation (orthopedics and speech and language therapy) {pronounced "are-tick"}

artif
artificial

art insem
artificial insemination (obstetrics)

art line
arterial line (cardiovascular and surgery)

ARV
acquired immunodeficiency syndrome [AIDS] associated retrovirus (immunology and laboratory)
acquired immunodeficiency syndrome [AIDS] related virus (immunology and laboratory)
anterior right ventricular [wall] (cardiovascular)

AS
above scale (laboratory)
acetylstrophanthidin (cardiovascular and pharmacology)
activated sleep (neurology)
active sleep (neurology)
Adams-Stokes [disease and/or syndrome] (cardiovascular)
alimentary sleep (neurology)
alveolar sac (respiratory)
anal sphincter (gastroenterology and proctology)
androsterone sulfate (laboratory)
ankylosing spondylitis (orthopedics)
antiserum (pharmacology)
antistreptolysin (laboratory)
anxiety state (psychiatry)
aortic sac (cardiovascular)
aortic stenosis (cardiovascular)
aqueous solution (pharmacology)
aqueous suspension (pharmacology)
arteriosclerosis (cardiovascular)

artificial sweetener (dietary)
asymmetric
atherosclerosis (cardiovascular)
audiogenic seizure (neurology)
auris sinistra [left ear] (otorhinolaryngology)

A.S.
aortic stenosis (cardiovascular)
auris sinistra [left ear] (otorhinolaryngology)

A-S
ascendance-submission

As
acetylstrophanthidin (cardiovascular and pharmacology)
arsenic (chemistry, laboratory, and pharmacology)
astigmatism (ophthalmology)

As.
astigmatism (ophthalmology)

A's
amphetamine sulfate [also called *Benzedrine*] (chemical dependency) {slang} {pronounced "az"}

as
auris sinistra [left ear] (otorhinolaryngology)

a.s.
auris sinistra [left ear] (otorhinolaryngology)

ASA
acetylsalicylic acid [aspirin] (pharmacology)
Adams-Stokes attack (cardiovascular)
American Society of Anesthesiologists (anesthesiology)
American Standards Association (measurements)
argininosuccinate (laboratory)
argininosuccinic acid (laboratory)
arylsulfatase A (laboratory)

A.S.A.

American Society of Anesthesiologists (anesthesiology)
American Standards Association (measurements)
American Stomatological Association (dentistry and otorhinolaryngology)
American Surgical Association (surgery)
{not an abbreviation} [trademark for preparation of acetylsalicylic acid (aspirin)] (pharmacology)

ASAA

acquired severe aplastic anemia (hematology)

ASAHP

American Society of Allied Health Professions (allied health)

A.S.A.H.P.

American Society of Allied Health Professionals (allied health)

ASAI

aortic stenosis and aortic insufficiency [murmurs] (cardiovascular)

ASA I

{not an abbreviation} [American Society of Anesthesiologists' patient classification for healthy patient with localized pathology] (anesthesiology)

ASA II

{not an abbreviation} [American Society of Anesthesiologists' patient classification for patient with mild to moderate systemic disease] (anesthesiology)

ASA III

{not an abbreviation} [American Society of Anesthesiologists patient classification for patient with severe systemic disease limiting activity but not incapacitating] (anesthesiology)

ASAIO

American Society for Artificial Internal Organs (research)

A.S.A.I.O.

American Society for Artificial Internal Organs (research)

ASA IV

{not an abbreviation} [American Society of Anesthesiologists patient classification for patient with incapacitating systemic disease] (anesthesiology)

ASAP

American Society for Adolescent Psychology (pediatrics and psychiatry)
as soon as possible

A.S.A.P.

as soon as possible

ASAT

aspartate aminotransferase [also called *aspartate transaminase*; new name for *serum glutamic oxalo-acetic transaminase* (*SGOT*)] (cardiovascular and laboratory)

ASA V

{not an abbreviation} [American Society of Anesthesiologists' patient classification for moribund patient not expected to live] (anesthesiology)

ASB

American Society of Bacteriology (bacteriology and laboratory)
anesthesia standby (anesthesiology)
asymptomatic bacteriuria (bacteriology, laboratory, and urology)

A.S.B.

American Society of Bacteriologists (bacteriology and laboratory)

ASBS

arteriosclerotic brain syndrome (cardiovascular and neurology)

ASC

acetylsulfanilyl chloride (chemistry)
altered state of consciousness (neurology and psychiatry)
ambulatory surgery center (surgery)
American Society of Cytology (laboratory and pathology)
anterior subcapsular cataract (ophthalmology)

ascorbic acid [also called *vitamin C*] (dietary and pharmacology)

A.S.C.
American Society of Cytology (cytology and laboratory)

asc
arteriosclerosis (cardiovascular)
arteriosclerotic (cardiovascular)
ascending

ASCAD
arteriosclerotic coronary artery disease (cardiovascular)

A-scan
{not an abbreviation} [one type of visual display of ultrasonographic echoes] (cardiovascular, obstetrics, and radiology)

ASCH
American Society of Clinical Hypnosis (psychiatry)

A.S.C.H.
American Society of Clinical Hypnosis (psychiatry)

A.S.C.I.
American Society of Clinical Investigation

ASCII
American Standard Code for Informational Interchange (computer science)

Ascit. Fl.
ascitic fluid (cardiovascular, gastroenterology, nephrology, oncology, and respiratory)

ASCL
arteriosclerosis (cardiovascular)

ASCLT
American Society of Clinical Laboratory Technicians (laboratory)

A.S.C.L.T.
American Society of Clinical Laboratory Technicians (laboratory)

ASCMS
American Society of Contemporary Medicine and Surgery

ASCO
American Society of Clinical Oncology (oncology)
American Society of Contemporary Ophthalmology (ophthalmology)

ASCP
American Society of Clinical Pathologists (laboratory and pathology)
American Society of Consulting Pharmacists (pharmacology)

A.S.C.P.
American Society of Clinical Pathologists (laboratory and pathology)

A.S.C.P.C.
American Society of Clinical Pharmacology and Chemotherapy (chemotherapy and pharmacology)

ASCR
American Society of Chiropodical Roentgenology (podiatry and radiology)

ascr
ascriptum [ascribed to] (pharmacology)

ascr.
ascriptum [ascribed to] (pharmacology)

ASCVD
arteriosclerotic cardiovascular disease (cardiovascular)
atherosclerotic cardiovascular disease (cardiovascular)

A.S.C.V.D.
arteriosclerotic cardiovascular disease (cardiovascular)
atherosclerotic cardiovascular disease (cardiovascular)

ASCVRD
arteriosclerotic cardiovascular renal disease (cardiovascular and nephrology)

ASD
aldosterone secretion defect (immunology and laboratory)
atrial septal defect [also called *atrioseptal defect*] (cardiovascular)

ASDA
American Society for Dental Aesthetics (dentistry)
American Student Dental Association (dentistry)

ASDC
American Society of Dentistry for Children (dentistry and pediatrics)
Association of Sleep Disorders Centers (neurology)

ASDH
acute subdural hematoma (neurology)

ASDR
American Society of Dental Radiographers (dentistry and radiology)

ASE
acute stress erosion (gastroenterology)
American Society of Echocardiography (cardiovascular)
axilla, shoulder, elbow [bandage] (orthopedics)

ASECT
American Society of Extra-Corporeal Technology (cardiovascular, hematology, and respiratory)

A.S.E.P.
American Society for Experimental Pathology (pathology)

ASET
American Society of Electroencephalographic Technologists (neurology)

ASF
aniline, formaldehyde, and sulfur [synthetic resin used to mount microscopic slides] (laboratory)

ASG
American Society for Genetics (genetics)
Army Surgeon General (armed forces)

A.S.G.
American Society for Genetics (genetics)

ASGB
Anatomical Society of Great Britain and Ireland (anatomy)

ASGD
American Society of Geriatric Dentistry (dentistry)

ASGE
American Society of Gastrointestinal Endoscopy (gastroenterology)

A.S.G.E.
American Society of Gastrointestinal Endoscopy (gastroenterology)

ASH
American Society for Hematology (hematology)
asymmetrical septal hypertrophy (cardiovascular)

A.S.H.
American Society for Hematology (hematology)

AsH
hypermetropic astigmatism (ophthalmology)

As.H.
hypermetropic astigmatism (ophthalmology)

"ash"
{pronunciation of *IHSS* [idiopathic hypertrophic subaortic stenosis]} (cardiovascular) {not an abbreviation}

ASHA
American School Health Association (administration)
American Social Health Association (administration)
American Speech and Hearing Association (otorhinolaryngology and speech and language therapy)

A.S.H.A.
American School Health Association (administration)
American Speech and Hearing Association (otorhinolaryngology and speech and language therapy)

ASHBM
Associate Scottish Hospital Bureau of Management (administration)

ASHD
arteriosclerotic heart disease (cardiovascular)
atherosclerotic heart disease (cardiovascular)

A.S.H.D.
arteriosclerotic heart disease (cardiovascular)
atherosclerotic heart disease (cardiovascular)

ASHG
American Society for Human Genetics (genetics)

ASHI
Association for the Study of Human Infertility (obstetrics)

A.S.H.I.
Association for the Study of Human Infertility (obstetrics)

ASHN
acute sclerosing hyaline necrosis [of liver] (gastroenterology)

ASHNS
American Society for Head and Neck Surgery (surgery)

ASHP
American Society of Hospital Pharmacists (pharmacology)
American Society for Hospital Planning (administration)

A.S.H.P.
American Society of Hospital Pharmacists (pharmacology)

ASHPA
American Society for Hospital Personnel Administration (administration)

ASIH
absent sick in hospital

ASII
American Science Information Institute (computer science)

A.S.I.I.
American Science Information Institute (computer science)

ASIM
American Society of Internal Medicine (internal medicine)

A.S.I.M.
American Society of Internal Medicine (internal medicine)

ASIS
anterior superior iliac spine [also called *anterosuperior iliac spine*] (orthopedics)

ASK
antistreptokinase (cardiovascular, hematology, and laboratory)

ASL
antistreptolysin [titer] (bacteriology and laboratory)

ASLIB
Association of Special Libraries and Information Bureaux (library science)

ASLM
American Society of Law and Medicine (administration and justice)

ASLO
antistreptolysin-O (bacteriology and laboratory)

ASM
American Society for Microbiology (laboratory and microbiology)

A.S.M.
American Society for Microbiology (laboratory and microbiology)

AsM
myopic astigmatism (ophthalmology)

As.M.
myopic astigmatism (ophthalmology)

ASMA
antismooth muscle antibody (laboratory)

ASME
Association for the Study of Medical Education (education)

A.S.M.E.
Association for the Study of Medical Education (education)

ASMI
anteroseptal myocardial infarction [also called *anterior septal myocardial infarction*] (cardiovascular)

ASMPA
Armed Services Medical Procurement Agency (armed forces)

ASMR
age-standardized mortality ratio (statistics analysis)

ASMT
American Society for Medical Technology
American Society of Medical Technology

A.S.M.T.
American Society of Medical Technology

ASN
alkali-soluble nitrogen (chemistry)
American Society of Nephrology (nephrology)
American Society for Neurochemistry (chemistry and neurology)
Associate in Nursing (education and nursing)

Asn
asparagine (chemistry, laboratory, and pharmacology)

ASO
American Society of Orthodontics (dentistry)
antistreptolysin-O titer (bacteriology and laboratory)
arteriosclerosis obliterans (cardiovascular)

A.S.O.
American Society of Orthodontics (dentistry)

A.S.Oblit.
arteriosclerosis obliterans (cardiovascular)

ASOS
American Society of Oral Surgeons (dentistry)

A.S.O.S.
American Society of Oral Surgeons (dentistry)

ASOT
antistreptolysin-O titer (bacteriology and laboratory)

ASO titer
antistreptolysin-O titer (bacteriology and laboratory)

ASP
acute suppurative parotitis (otorhinolaryngology)
American Society of Parasitologists (laboratory and parasitology)
American Society of Periodontists [previous name of *American Academy of Periodontology (AAP)*] (dentistry)
area systolic pressure (cardiovascular)

A.S.P.
American Society of Parasitologists (laboratory and parasitology)

Asp
aspartic acid (cardiovascular and laboratory)

ASPA
American Society of Physician Analysts
American Society of Podiatric Assistants (podiatry)

ASPER
aspergillosis [a fungal disease] (dermatology, ophthalmology, otorhinolaryngology, and respiratory)

ASPH
Association of Schools of Public Health (education and public health)

ASPM
American Society of Paramedics (emergency medicine)

ASPO
American Society for Psychoprophylaxis in Obstetrics (obstetrics and psychiatry)

ASPP
Association for Sane Psychiatric Practices (psychiatry)

ASPRS
Association of Plastic and Reconstructive Surgeons (plastic surgery)

ASPVD
arteriosclerotic peripheral vascular disease (cardiovascular)

ASR
aldosterone secretion rate (endocrinology and laboratory)
aldosterone secretory rate (endocrinology and laboratory)

ASRT
American Society of Radiologic Technologists (radiology)

A.S.R.T.
American Society of Radiologic Technologists (radiology)

ASS
anterior superior spine [also called *anterosuperior spine*] (orthopedics)

A.S.S.
anterior superior spine [also called *anterosuperior spine*] (orthopedics)

ASSI
Accurate Surgical and Scientific Instruments [Corporation; manufacturer of surgical instruments] (surgery)

Assn
association

Assn.
association

Assoc
associate
association

assocd
associated [with]

ASSR
adult situation stress reaction (psychiatry)

ASST
assistance (rehabilitation)

asst
assistant

asst.
assisted
assistive

AST
angiotensin sensitivity test (cardiovascular and laboratory)
aspartate aminotransferase [also called *aspartate transaminase*; new name for *serum glutamic oxalo-acetic transaminase (SGOT)*] (cardiovascular and laboratory)
Association of Surgical Technologists (surgery)
astemizole [an antihistamine] (allergy,

otorhinolaryngology, pharmacology, and respiratory)
astigmatism (ophthalmology)
audiometry sweep test [British] (otorhinolaryngology)

Ast
astigmatism (ophthalmology)

Ast.
astigmatism (ophthalmology)

ASTA
anti-alpha-staphylolysin (bacteriology and pharmacology)

A.S.T.C.
Association of Science Technology Centers

ASTEC
Association of Science Technology Centers

A sten
aortic stenosis (cardiovascular)

Asth
asthenopia (ophthalmology)

Asth.
asthenopia (ophthalmology)

ASTHO
Association of State and Territorial Health Officials (administration)

A.S.T.H.O.
Association of State and Territorial Health Officials (administration)

ASTI
antispasticity index (neurology)

Astigm
astigmatism (ophthalmology)

ASTM
American Society for Testing and Materials (research)

ASTMH
American Society of Tropical Medicine and Hygiene (tropical medicine)

A.S.T.M.H.
American Society of Tropical Medicine and Hygiene (tropical medicine)

ASTO
antistreptolysin-O (bacteriology and laboratory)

As tol
as tolerated

as tol.
as tolerated

ASTRA-4
{not an abbreviation} [an automated routine analyzer which performs four tests] (laboratory)

ASTZ
antistreptozyme [test] (bacteriology and laboratory)

ASU
acute stroke unit (neurology)
Aeromedical Staging Unit (aerospace medicine)

ASUE
A subgroup [blood type] (hematology and laboratory)

ASUTS
American Society of Ultrasound Technical Specialists (cardiovascular, obstetrics, and radiology)

ASV
anodic stripping voltammetry (cardiovascular)
antisnake venom (pharmacology)
arterio-superficial venous [difference] (cardiovascular)

A-SV
arterio-superficial venous [difference] (cardiovascular)

A/SV
arterio/superficial venous [difference] (cardiovascular)

ASVD
arteriosclerotic vascular disease (cardiovascular)
arteriosclerotic vessel disease (cardiovascular)

ASVO
American Society of Veterinary Ophthalmology (ophthalmology and veterinary medicine)

ASVPP
American Society of Veterinary Physiologists and Pharmacologists (pharmacology and veterinary medicine)

asym
asymmetrical

asym.
asymmetrical

AT
achievement test (psychiatry)
Achilles tendon (neurology and orthopedics)
adenine and thymine (genetics and laboratory)
adjunctive therapy (chemotherapy, oncology, pharmacology, and radiation
therapy)
adjuvant therapy (chemotherapy, oncology, pharmacology, and radiation
therapy)
air temperature
alt Tuberculin [old tuberculin] (infectious diseases, laboratory, pharmacology, and respiratory)
aminotransferase (cardiovascular and
laboratory)
amitriptyline [an antidepressant] (chemical dependency, pharmacology, and
psychiatry)
anaphylatoxin (allergy and laboratory)
antithrombin (hematology, laboratory,
and pharmacology)
antitrypsin (endocrinology, gastroenterology, gynecology, laboratory, obstetrics, oncology, and respiratory)
applanation tonometry (ophthalmology)
ataxia-telangiectasia (endocrinology,
gastroenterology, genetics, immunology, neurology, and ophthalmology)
atraumatic

attenuated
attenuation
cytosine arabinoside and thioguanine
(chemotherapy, oncology, and pharmacology)

A.T.
academically talented (education)
alt Tuberculin [old tuberculin] (infectious diseases, laboratory, pharmacology, and respiratory)

α_1-AT
alpha-1-antitrypsin (endocrinology, gastroenterology, gynecology, laboratory,
obstetrics, oncology, and respiratory)

At
astatine (endocrinology and radiation
therapy)

At.
atrial (cardiovascular)

at
airtight
atom(ic) (chemistry and physics)

ATA
alimentary toxic aleukia (hematology)
American Thyroid Association (endocrinology)
American Tinnitus Association (neurology and otorhinolaryngology)
antithyroglobulin antibody (endocrinology and laboratory)
anti-*Toxoplasma* antibodies (cardiovascular, gastroenterology, laboratory,
neurology, ophthalmology, orthopedics, and respiratory)
atmospheres absolute [hyperbaric oxygen therapy] (barometric medicine,
neurology, and sports medicine)
aurin tricarboxylic acid [a stain; also
called *chrome violet CG*] (chemistry
and laboratory)

ATB
at the time of the bomb [atomic bomb in
Japan]
antibiotic (pharmacology)

ATC
activated thymus cells (endocrinology, hematology, immunology, and laboratory)
all-terrain cycle (emergency medicine and sports medicine)
around the clock

A.T..C.
Certified Athletic Trainer (orthopedics and sports medicine)

ATCC
American Type Culture Collection (laboratory)

ATD
Alzheimer-type dementia (neurology and psychiatry)
anthropomorphic test dummy (research)
antithyroid drug(s) (endocrinology and pharmacology)
asphyxiating thoracic dystrophy (respiratory)
autoimmune thyroid disease (endocrinology and immunology)

ATDC
Association of Thalidomide Damaged Children (genetics and pediatrics)

ATE
adipose tissue extract (laboratory)
patient ate (nursing)

ATEE
N-acetyl-L-tyrosine ethyl ester (chemistry and laboratory)

ATEe
N-acetyl-L-tyrosine ethyl ester (chemistry and laboratory)

At Fib
atrial fibrillation (cardiovascular)

At. Fib.
atrial fibrillation (cardiovascular)

at fib
atrial fibrillation (cardiovascular)

at. fib.
atrial fibrillation (cardiovascular)

ATG
adenine, thymine, guanine (genetics and laboratory)
antihuman thymocyte globulin (endocrinology, hematology, immunology, laboratory, nephrology, and pharmacology)
antithrombocyte globulin (endocrinology, hematology, immunology, and laboratory)
antithymocyte globulin (endocrinology, hematology, immunology, and laboratory)
antithyroglobulin (endocrinology, hematology, immunology, and laboratory)

ATGAM
antithymocyte gamma-globulin (endocrinology, hematology, immunology, and laboratory)

ATH
acetyltyrosine hydrazide (cardiovascular and laboratory)

ATh
Associate in Therapy (education and rehabilitation)

ATHC
allotetrahydrocortisol (chemistry)

ATHR
angina threshold heart rate (cardiovascular)

Athsc
atherosclerosis (cardiovascular)

AT-III
antithrombin III (hematology, laboratory, and pharmacology)

ATL
Achilles tendon lengthening (orthopedics)
adult T-cell leukemia (hematology and oncology)
Advanced Technology Laboratories, Incorporated [manufacturer of real-time

neurosector scanner] (neurology and radiology)
antitension line
atypical lymphocytes (hematology and laboratory)

ATLA
adult T-cell leukemia antigen (hematology, laboratory, and oncology)

ATLS
Advanced Trauma Life Support [Program] (emergency medicine)

ATLV
adult T-cell leukemia virus (hematology, laboratory, and oncology)

atm
atmosphere
atmospheric

atm.
atmosphere

atmos
atmosphere
atmospheric

ATN
acute tubular necrosis (nephrology)

ATNC
atraumatic/normocephalic

aTNM
{not an abbreviation} [autopsy staging of cancer referring to tumor, nodes, and metastases] (oncology and pathology)

at no
atomic number (chemistry)

at. no.
atomic number (chemistry)

ATNR
asymmetrical tonic neck reflex (neurology)

ATP
adenosine triphosphate (laboratory)

ATPase
adenosine triphosphatase (laboratory)

ATPD
ambient temperature and pressure, dry (laboratory and respiratory)

ATPS
ambient temperature and pressure, saturated with water vapor at these conditions (laboratory and respiratory)

ATR
Achilles tendon reflex (neurology and orthopedics)
atrial (cardiovascular)

atr
atrial (cardiovascular)
atrophy

atr.
atrophy

ATR FIB
atrial fibrillation (cardiovascular)

atr. fib.
atrial fibrillation (cardiovascular)

ATS
adjustable thigh antiembolism stockings (cardiovascular)
American Therapeutic Society
American Thoracic Society (cardiovascular and respiratory)
American Trudeau Society
American Trauma Society (emergency medicine)
antitetanic serum [tetanus antitoxin] (infectious diseases, pharmacology, and toxicology)
antitetanus serum (infectious diseases, pharmacology, and toxicology)
antithymocyte serum (endocrinology, hematology, immunology, laboratory, and pharmacology)
anxiety tension state (psychiatry)
arteriosclerosis (cardiovascular)
atherosclerosis (cardiovascular)

A.T.S.
antitetanic serum [tetanus antitoxin] (immunology, pharmacology, and toxicology)
anxiety tension state (psychiatry)
tetanus antitoxin [antitetanic serum] (immunology, pharmacology, and toxicology)

ATT
arginine tolerance test (endocrinology and laboratory)
aspirin tolerance time (laboratory)

att
attending

att.
attending

atto-
{not an abbreviation} [prefix meaning 10^{-18}] (measurement) {pronounced "at-toe"}

"at-toe"
{pronunciation of atto- [prefix for 10^{-18}]} (measurement) {not an abbreviation}

ATTR
see attached report (laboratory)

at. vol.
atomic volume (chemistry and physics)

At. wt.
atomic weight (chemistry and physics)

at wt
atomic weight (chemistry and physics)

at. wt.
atomic weight (chemistry and physics)

ATZ
atypical transformation zone (gynecology)

AU
ad usum [according to custom] (pharmacology)
allergenic units (allergy)
Angstrom unit (chemistry and electricity)

antitoxin unit [diphtheria] (immunology, infectious diseases, laboratory, and respiratory)
astronomical unit (astronomy)
aures unitas [both ears together] (otorhinolaryngology)
auris uterque [each ear] (otorhinolaryngology)
Australia [antigen] (gastroenterology, infectious diseases, laboratory, and pharmacology)

A.U.
Angstrom unit (chemistry and electricity)
antitoxin unit (immunology, infectious diseases, laboratory, and respiratory)
arbitrary units (measurement)
aures unitas [both ears together] (otorhinolaryngology)
auris uterque [each ear] (otorhinolaryngology)
Australia [antigen] (gastroenterology, infectious diseases, laboratory, and pharmacology)
azauridine (chemotherapy, oncology, and pharmacology)

Au
aurum [gold] (chemistry)
Australian antigen (gastroenterology, infectious diseases, laboratory, and pharmacology)

¹⁹⁸Au
radioactive gold (chemistry and radiation therapy)

Au(1)
Australian antigen (gastroenterology, infectious diseases, laboratory, and pharmacology)

a.u.
aures unitas [both ears together] (otorhinolaryngology)
auris uterque [each ear] (otorhinolaryngology)

AUA
American Urological Association (urology)
Association of University Anesthetists (anesthesiology)

A.U.A.
American Urological Association (urology)

AuAg
Australian antigen (gastroenterology, infectious diseases, laboratory, and pharmacology)

Au Ag
Australian antigen (gastroenterology, infectious diseases, laboratory, and pharmacology)

auct
auctorum [of authors]

auct.
auctorum [of authors]

aud
auditory (otorhinolaryngology)

aud.
auditory (otorhinolaryngology)

AUER
Auer [bodies or rods] (hematology, laboratory, and oncology)

aug
augere [increase]

AUHAA
Australia hepatitis–associated antigen (gastroenterology, infectious diseases, laboratory, and pharmacology)

AUL
acute undifferentiated leukemia (hematology and oncology)

AUO
amyloid of unknown origin (cardiovascular, dermatology, gastroenterology, laboratory, nephrology, neurology, oncology, orthopedics, and urology)

AUPHA
Association of University Programs in Health Administration (administration and education)

aur
auris [ear] (otorhinolaryngology)
aurum [gold] (chemistry)

Aur.d.
auris dextra [right ear] (otorhinolaryngology)

aur fib
auricular fibrillation (cardiovascular)

aur. fib.
auricular fibrillation (cardiovascular)

auric
auricular (cardiovascular)

aurin
aurinarium [ear cone] (otorhinolaryngology)

aurist
auristillae [ear drops] (otorhinolaryngology and pharmacology)

Aur.s.
auris sinistra [left ear] (otorhinolaryngology)

Aus
auscultation (cardiovascular and respiratory)

ausc.
auscultation (cardiovascular and respiratory)

AuSH
Australia serum hepatitis [antigen] (gastroenterology, infectious diseases, laboratory, and pharmacology)

AUSPE
audiology and speech pathology (otorhinolaryngology and speech and language therapy)

AVO_2
arteriovenous oxygen difference (laboratory and respiratory)

$A-VO_2$
arteriovenous oxygen difference (laboratory and respiratory)

AVP
Adriamycin, vincristine, and procarbazine (chemotherapy, oncology, and pharmacology)
antiviral protein (laboratory and virology)
8-arginine-vasopressin [also called *arginine vasopressin*] (cardiovascular and pharmacology)

AVP-II
actinomycin D, vincristine, and cisplatin (chemotherapy, oncology, and pharmacology)

AVR
aortic valve replacement (cardiovascular)

aVR
{not an abbreviation} [an augmented unipolar lead in which the positive terminal is on the right arm for an electrocardiogram] (cardiovascular)

aV_R
{not an abbreviation} [an augmented unipolar lead in which the positive terminal is on the right arm for an electrocardiogram] (cardiovascular)

AVRP
atrioventricular refractory period (cardiovascular)

AVS
arteriovenous shunt (cardiovascular)
Association for Voluntary Sterilization (obstetrics)

AVSC
aortic valve cusp separation [on echocardiogram] (cardiovascular)

A-V shunt
arteriovenous shunt (cardiovascular and nephrology)

AVSS
afebrile, vital signs stable

AVT
Allen vision test (ophthalmology)
area ventralis of Tsai [of the brain] (neurology)
8-arginine oxytocin (obstetrics and pharmacology)
arginine vasotocin (cardiovascular, orthopedics, and pharmacology)
atypical ventricular tachycardia (cardiovascular)
Aviation Medicine Technician (aerospace medicine)

AW
above waist (anatomy)
anterior wall [image on transesophageal echocardiography] (cardiovascular)
atomic warfare (armed forces)

A & W
alive and well

A.W.
atomic weight (chemistry and physics)

A/W
alive and well
in accordance with

aw
airways (respiratory)

AWA
American Wrestling Association (sports medicine)
away without authorization

"A-wall"
{pronunciation of *AWOL* and *awol* [absent without leave]} {not an abbreviation}

a waves
{not an abbreviation} [refers to right

atrial contraction waves on phlebogram] (cardiovascular)

AWF
adrenal weight factor (endocrinology and laboratory)

AWH
Association of Western Hospitals (administration)

AWI
anterior wall infarction (cardiovascular)
a walk-in [patient]
authorized walk-in [patient]

AWMI
anterior wall myocardial infarction (cardiovascular)

AWOL
absent without leave {pronounced "A-wall"}

awol
absent without leave {pronounced "A-wall"}

AWP
airway pressure (respiratory)

AWR
aromatic weathering ratio (ecology)

AWRS
antiwhole rabbit serum (immunology and pharmacology)

awu
atomic weight unit (chemistry and physics)

Ax
axillary

ax
axial
axillary
axis

ax.
axilla
axis

AXAF
Advanced X-ray Astrophysics Facility (astrophysics and radiology)

AXF
Advanced X-ray Facility (radiology)

ax grad
axial gradient

ax. grad.
axial gradient

Axis I
{not an abbreviation} [a portion of the psychiatric diagnosis denoting clinical syndromes; conditions not attributable to a mental disorder that are a focus of attention or treatment] (psychiatry)

Axis II
{not an abbreviation} [a portion of the psychiatric diagnosis denoting personality disorders; specific developmental disorders (psychiatry)

Axis III
{not an abbreviation} [a portion of the psychiatric diagnosis denoting physical disorders and conditions] (psychiatry)

Axis IV
{not an abbreviation} [a portion of the psychiatric diagnosis denoting the severity of psychosocial stressors] (psychiatry)

Axis V
{not an abbreviation} [a portion of the psychiatric diagnosis denoting highest level of adaptive functioning in the past year] (psychiatry)

AXM
acetoxycyclohexamine (chemistry)

ayr
{not an abbreviation} [subdetermination of hepatitis B surface antigen

(HB$_s$Ag)] (gastroenterology, infectious diseases, and laboratory)

AXT
alternating exotropia (ophthalmology)

awy1
{not an abbreviation} [subdetermination of hepatitis B surface antigen (HB$_s$Ag)] (gastroenterology, infectious diseases, and laboratory)

awy2
{not an abbreviation} [subdetermination of hepatitis B surface antigen (HB$_s$Ag)] (gastroenterology, infectious diseases, and laboratory)

awy3
{not an abbreviation} [subdetermination of hepatitis B surface antigen (HB$_s$Ag)] (gastroenterology, infectious diseases, and laboratory)

awy4
{not an abbreviation} [subdetermination of hepatitis B surface antigen (HB$_s$Ag)] (gastroenterology, infectious diseases, and laboratory)

AYF
antiyeast factor (laboratory)

AYP
autolysed yeast protein (laboratory)

AZ
Arizona [Postal Service state designation]
Aschheim-Zondek [pregnancy test] (laboratory and obstetrics)

Az
azote [nitrogen] (chemistry)

Az.
azote [nitrogen] (chemistry)

"az"
{pronunciation of *A's* [amphetamine sulfate (also called *Benzedrine*)]} (chemical dependency) {slang} {not an abbreviation}

AZA
azathioprine [an immunosuppressive drug] (nephrology and transplant surgery)

5-AZA
5-azacytidine (chemotherapy, oncology, and pharmacology)

AZA-CR
(chemotherapy)

8-azg.
8-azaguanine [also called *guanazolo*] (chemotherapy, oncology, and pharmacology)

AZQ
aziridinylbenzoquinone (chemotherapy, oncology, and pharmacology)
diaziquone (chemotherapy, oncology, and pharmacology)

AZS
automatic zero set

AZT
Aschheim-Zondek [pregnancy] test (laboratory and obstetrics)
zidovudine [generic name for *Retrovir*; formerly called *azidothymidine*] (chemotherapy, immunology, oncology, and pharmacology)

AZ test
Aschheim-Zondek [pregnancy] test (laboratory and obstetrics)

AZU
6-azauracil (chemotherapy, oncology, and pharmacology)

AzU
6-azauracil (chemotherapy, oncology, and pharmacology)

5-AzU
5-azauracil (chemotherapy, oncology, and pharmacology)

6-AzU
6-azauracil (chemotherapy, oncology, and pharmacology)

AZUR
6-azauridine (chemotherapy, oncology, and pharmacology)

AzUR
6-azauridine (chemotherapy, oncology, and pharmacology)

5-AzUR
5-azauridine (chemotherapy, oncology, and pharmacology)

6-AzUR
6-azauridine (chemotherapy, oncology, and pharmacology)

B

β

beta [second letter of the Greek alphabet]
{not an abbreviation} [symbol indicating second]

B
Bacillus (bacteriology and laboratory)
bacillus (bacteriology and laboratory)
Bacterium (bacteriology and laboratory)
bacterium (bacteriology and laboratory)
Balantidium (gastroenterology, laboratory, and parasitology)
balneum [bath]
band(s)
barometric (laboratory, neurology, respiratory, and sports medicine)
base [as used in chemical formulas] (chemistry and pharmacology)
base [of a prism]
Baumé scale (chemistry, laboratory, and measurement)
bel (audiology, measurement, and physics)
Benoist scale
benzoate (chemistry)
beta (laboratory and radiology)
bicuspid (cardiovascular and dentistry)
bilateral (anatomy)
black
blood (hematology and laboratory)
blue
body [meaning all of the body except the nervous system] (psychiatry)
bone marrow derived [lymphocytes] (hematology and laboratory)
Bordetella (laboratory, parasitology, and respiratory)
boron (chemistry)
Borrelia (bacteriology and laboratory)
both
bound
brother
buccal (dentistry and otorhinolaryngology)
bursa cells [of lymph nodes or thymus]

(hematology, immunology, and laboratory)
gauss (measurement and physics)
magnetic flow density [symbol] (physics)
magnetic induction (physics)

B.
bacillus (bacteriology and laboratory)
balneum [bath]
barometric (laboratory, neurology, respiratory, and sports medicine)
base [as used in chemical formulas] (chemistry and pharmacology)
Baumé scale (chemistry, laboratory, and measurement)
behavior (psychiatry)
Benoist scale
benzoate (chemistry)
bicuspid (cardiovascular and dentistry)
blue
boils at [used with a numeral indicating degrees] (chemistry)
brother
Brucella (laboratory and parasitology)
buccal (dentistry)
Bucky [film in cassette in Potter-Bucky diaphragm] (radiology)
point B [also called *supramentale*; on skull films] (radiology)
tomogram with oscillating Bucky (radiology)
whole blood (hematology and laboratory)
{not an abbreviation} [symbol for gauss] (measurement and physics)

B ♀
black female

B ♂
black male

B₁
thiamine hydrochloride (pharmacology)

B₂
riboflavin (pharmacology)

B4
before [slang]

B₆
pyridoxine hydrochloride (pharmacology)

B₇
biotin (pharmacology)

B₈
adenosine phosphate (pharmacology)

B₁₂
cyanocobalamin (pharmacology)

b
blood [in general in the blood phase] (laboratory and respiratory)
broth (laboratory)

b.
barn
bis [twice, two times]
boils at [used with a numeral indicating degrees] (chemistry)
born

BA
Bachelor of Arts (education)
backache (orthopedics)
bacterial agglutination (bacteriology and laboratory)
balneum arenae [sand bath]
basion [craniometric point] (radiology)
betamethasone acetate [a steroid] (orthopedics, pharmacology, and rheumatology)
benzyladenine (chemistry)
bile acid (gastroenterology and laboratory)
blocking antibody (laboratory)
blood agar (laboratory)
blood alcohol (chemical dependency and laboratory)
bone age (pediatrics and radiology)
boric acid [antiseptic and eye wash] (chemistry, dermatology, ophthalmology, and pharmacology)
Bourns assist

bovine albumin (chemistry, laboratory, and pharmacology)
brachial artery [pressure] (cardiovascular)
breathing apparatus (respiratory)
bronchial asthma (respiratory)
buccoaxial (dentistry)

B.A.
Bachelor of Arts (education)
backache (orthopedics)
bacterial agglutination (bacteriology and laboratory)
balneum arenae [sand bath]
basion [craniometric point] (radiology)
betamethasone acetate [a steroid] (orthopedics, pharmacology, and rheumatology)
blocking antibody (laboratory)
blood alcohol (chemical dependency and laboratory)

B>A
bone greater than air [conduction] (otorhinolaryngology)

B<A
bone less than air [conduction] (otorhinolaryngology)

Ba
barium (chemistry, pharmacology, and radiology)

BAA
benzoyl arginine amide (chemistry)
branched-chain amino acid (laboratory)

BAB
blood agar base (laboratory)

Bab.
Babinski [reflex or sign] (neurology and orthopedics)

BAC
bacteria (bacteriology and laboratory)
bacterial adherent colonies (bacteriology and laboratory)
bacterial antigen complex (bacteriology and laboratory)

benzalkonium chloride [antiseptic and fungicide] (dermatology and pharmacology)

blood alcohol concentration (chemical dependency and laboratory)

British Association of Chemists (chemistry)

bronchoalveolar cells (laboratory and respiratory)

buccoaxiocervical (dentistry)

BACO
bleomycin, Adriamycin, lomustine [CCNU], and vincristine [Oncovin] (chemotherapy, oncology, and pharmacology) {pronounced "bake-oh"}

BACON
bleomycin, Adriamycin, lomustine [CCNU], vincristine [Oncovin], and nitrogen mustard (chemotherapy, oncology, and pharmacology) {pronounced "bake-en"}

BACOP
bleomycin, Adriamycin, cyclophosphamide, vincristine [Oncovin], and prednisone (chemotherapy, oncology, and pharmacology)

BACT
bleomycin, Adriamycin, Cytoxan, tamoxifen (chemotherapy, oncology, pharmacology)

Bact
Bacterium (bacteriology and laboratory)

Bact.
Bacterium (bacteriology and laboratory)

bact
bacteria(l) (bacteriology and laboratory)
bacteriology (bacteriology and laboratory)
bacterium (bacteriology and laboratory)

bact.
bacteria(l) (bacteriology and laboratory)
bacteriology (bacteriology and laboratory)
bacterium (bacteriology and laboratory)

Bacti Lab
bacteriology laboratory (bacteriology and laboratory)

BAD
biological aerosol detection (ecology)
bipolar affective disorder (psychiatry)
British Association of Dermatologists (dermatology)

BAE
bronchial artery embolization (cardiovascular and respiratory)

BaE
barium enema (gastroenterology and radiology)

BAEE
benzoyl arginine ethyl ester [also called *benzylarginine ethyl ester*] (laboratory)

Ba enem
barium enema (gastroenterology and radiology)

BAEP
brain stem auditory evoked potential (neurology)

BAER
brain stem auditory evoked response [waves I-VII] (neurology) {pronounced "bare" or "bear"}

BAERs
brain stem auditory evoked responses [waves I-VII] (neurology) {pronounced "bares" or "bears"}

BAG
buccoaxiogingival (dentistry)

BAGG
buffered azide glucose glycerol [broth] (chemistry and laboratory)

BAIB
beta-aminoisobutyric acid (chemistry)

"bake-en"
{pronunciation of *BACON* [bleomycin, Adriamycin, lomustine (CCNU), vincristine [Oncovin], and nitrogen mustard]} (chemotherapy, oncology, and pharmacology) {not an abbreviation}

"bake-oh"
{pronunciation of *BACO* [bleomycin, Adriamycin, lomustine (CCNU), and vincristine (Oncovin)]} (chemotherapy, oncology, and pharmacology) {not an abbreviation}

Baker-C
Baker/Cummins [company] (pharmacology)

BAL
blood alcohol level (chemical dependency and laboratory)
British anti-Lewisite [also called *dimercaprol*; antidote to metal poisoning] (pharmacology)
bronchoalveolar lavage (respiratory)

bal
balance(d)
balsam (pharmacology)

bal.
balance
balsam (pharmacology)

bal arenae
balneum arenae [sand bath]

bal. arenae
balneum arenae [sand bath]

BALB
binaural alternate loudness balance [test] (otorhinolaryngology)

Balb/c
{not an abbreviation} [Balb/c mice] (laboratory, research, and veterinary medicine)

B-ALL
B-cell acute lymphoblastic leukemia (hematology and oncology)

bal mar
balneum maris [salt water bath, seawater bath]

bal. mar.
balneum maris [salt water bath, seawater bath]

bals
balsamum [balsam] (pharmacology)

bals.
balsamum [balsam] (pharmacology)

bal vap
balneum vapor [steam bath, vapor bath]

bal. vap.
balneum vapor [steam bath, vapor bath]

BAm
mean brachial artery [pressure] (cardiovascular)

BaM
barium meal (gastroenterology, pharmacology, and radiology)

BAMe
benzoyl arginine methyl ester (chemistry)

BAMON
bleomycin, Adriamycin, methotrexate, vincristine [Oncovin], and nitrogen mustard (chemotherapy, oncology, and pharmacology)

BAN
British Association of Neurologists (neurology)

BANDS
band forms [also called *neutrophil bands*] (hematology and laboratory) {pronounced "bandz"}

"bandz"
{pronunciation of *BANDS* [band forms;

also called *neutrophil bands*]} (hematology and laboratory) {not an abbreviation}

B. anthracis
Bacillus anthracis (bacteriology and laboratory)

BAO
Bachelor of the Art of Obstetrics (education and obstetrics)
basal acid output (laboratory)
British Association of Otolaryngologists (otorhinolaryngology)

B.A.O.
Bachelor of the Art of Obstetrics (education and obstetrics)

BAP
bleomycin, Adriamycin, and prednisone (chemotherapy, oncology, and pharmacology)
blood agar plate (laboratory)
bovine albumin in phosphate buffer (chemistry, laboratory, and pharmacology)
brachial artery pressure (cardiovascular)

BAPhysMed
British Association of Physical Medicine (physical medicine)

BAPN
beta-amino-propionitrile fumarate (chemistry)

BAPS
British Association of Paediatric Surgeons (pediatrics and surgery)
British Association of Plastic Surgeons (plastic surgery)

BAPT
British Association of Physical Training (physical therapy)

bar
barometer (measurement)
barometric (neurology, respiratory, and sports medicine)

bar.
barometer (measurement)
barometric (neurology, respiratory, and sports medicine)

μbar
microbar (measurement)

BARB
barbiturate (pharmacology and psychiatry)
barbiturate screen (laboratory)

barb level
barbital level (laboratory and psychiatry)
barbiturate level (laboratory and psychiatry)
phenobarbital level (laboratory and psychiatry)

"bare"
{pronunciation of *BAER* [brain stem auditory evoked response (waves I-VII)]} (neurology) {not an abbreviation}

"bares"
{pronunciation of *BAERs* [brain stem auditory evoked responses (waves I-VII)] (neurology) {not an abbreviation}

bars
parallel bars (orthopedics and physical therapy)

BAS
benzyl analogue of serotonin (genetics, laboratory, nephrology, oncology, and psychiatry)
benzyl antiserotonin (genetics, laboratory, nephrology, oncology, and psychiatry)
Bioanalytical Systems (laboratory)

bas
basophil(s) (hematology and laboratory)

"base-oh"
{pronunciation of *BASO, Baso., baso,* and *baso.* [basophil]} (hematology and laboratory) {not an abbreviation}

BCB
brilliant cresyl blue [stain] (hematology and laboratory)

BC/BS
Blue Cross/Blue Shield (insurance)

BCC
basal cell carcinoma (dermatology, oncology, and pathology)
birth control clinic (obstetrics)

BCCA
basal cell carcinoma (dermatology, oncology, and pathology)

BCCG
British Co-operative Clinical Group

BCCP
biotin carboxyl carrier protein (laboratory)

BCD
basal cell dysplasia (dermatology, oncology, and pathology)
binary-coded decimal (mathematics)
bleomycin, cyclophosphamide, and dactinomycin (chemotherapy, oncology, and pharmacology)

BCE
basal cell epithelioma (dermatology, oncology, and pathology)

B cell
bursa-equivalent lymphocyte [also called *large lymphocyte*] (hematology, immunology, and laboratory)

BCF
basophil chemotactic factor (hematology, immunology, laboratory, and oncology)

BCFP
breast cyst fluid protein (gynecology and laboratory)

BCG
bacille Calmette-Guérin [vaccine for tuberculosis; also called *Bacillius Calmette et Guérin (vaccine)* and *Bacillus Calmette-Guérin (vaccine)*]

(infectious diseases, pharmacology, and respiratory)
ballistocardiogram (cardiovascular)
bicolor guaiac [test] (gastroenterology and laboratory)
bromocresol green (chemistry and laboratory)
bilateral cystograms (radiography)

BCG test
bicolor guaiac test (gastroenterology and laboratory)

BCH
basal cell hyperplasia (dermatology, oncology, and pathology)

BCh
Baccalaureus Chirurgiae [Bachelor of Surgery] (education and surgery)

B.Ch.
Baccalaureus Chirurgiae [Bachelor of Surgery] (education and surgery)

BChD
Bachelor of Dental Surgery (dentistry)

B.Ch.D.
Bachelor of Dental Surgery (dentistry)

BChir
Baccalaureus Chirurgiae [Bachelor of Surgery] (education and surgery)

BChL
bacteriochlorophyll (bacteriology and laboratory)

BCIC
Birth Control Investigation Committee (obstetrics)

B.C.I.C.
Birth Control Investigation Committee (obstetrics)

BCL
basic cycle length

B-CLL
B-cell lymphatic leukemia (hematology and oncology)

BCLS
Basic Cardiac Life Support System (cardiovascular and emergency medicine)

BCM
birth control medication (gynecology, obstetrics, and pharmacology)

bcm
billion cubic meters (measurement)

BCME
bis-chlormethyl ether (chemistry)

BCNU
1,3-bis(2-chlorethyl)-1-nitrosourea [also called *bischloroethylnitrosourea, bis-chloronitrosourea, carmustine,* and *nitrosourea;* also abbreviated *BiCNU*] (chemotherapy, oncology, and pharmacology)

BCOP
carmustine [BCNU], cyclophosphamide, vincristine [Oncovin], and prednisone (chemotherapy, oncology, and pharmacology) [*Note: Not identical to BCVP.*]

BCP
basic calcium phosphate (chemistry, laboratory, and pharmacology)
biochemical profile (laboratory)
birth control pill(s) (gynecology, obstetrics, and pharmacology)
blood pressure cuff (cardiovascular)
Blue Cross Plan (insurance)
bromocresol purple (laboratory)

BCP-D
bromocresol purple desoxycholate [agar] (laboratory)

BCP-D agar
bromocresol purple desoxycholate agar (laboratory)

BCR
bulbocavernosus reflex (neurology and urology)

BCS
battered child syndrome (pediatrics and psychiatry)
blood cell separator (hematology and laboratory)
British Cardiac Society (cardiovascular)
Budd-Chiari syndrome (cardiovascular, gastroenterology, and oncology)

BCSI
breast cancer screening indicator (gynecology and oncology)

BCTF
Breast Cancer Task Force [part of the National Cancer Institute] (gynecology, oncology, and research)

BCUPP
carmustine [BCNU], vinblastine, procarbazine, and prednisone (chemotherapy, oncology, and pharmacology)

BCV
basal cell vigilance

BCVP
carmustine [BCNU], cyclophosphamide, vincristine, and prednisone (chemotherapy, oncology, and pharmacology) [*Note: Not identical to BCOP.*]

BCVPP
carmustine [BCNU], cyclophosphamide, vinblastine, prednisone, and procarbazine (chemotherapy, oncology, and pharmacology)

BCW
biological and chemical warfare (armed forces, biology, and chemistry)

BD
base deficit (laboratory)
base [of prism] down
Batten's disease [also called *juvenile amaurotic familial idiocy*] (genetics, neurology, ophthalmology, and pediatrics)
Becton-Dickinson [spinal needle] (neurology and orthopedics)

behavioral disorder (psychiatry)
belladonna [an anticholinergic and anti-spasmodic drug] (pharmacology)
below diaphragm
Best delay [audiometry] (otorhinolaryn-gology)
bile duct (gastroenterology and surgery)
binocular deprivation (ophthalmology)
birth defect (genetics and neonatology)
Black Death [also called *plague*] (infec-tious diseases)
borderline dull (anatomy, cardiovascu-lar, and respiratory)
bound
brain dead (neurology)
bronchial drainage (respiratory)
buccodistal (dentistry)
bundle

B & D
bondage and discipline (psychiatry)

Bd
board

bd
bis die [twice a day] (pharmacology)

b.d.
bis die [twice a day] (pharmacology)

BDA
British Dental Association (dentistry)

B.D.A.
British Dental Association (dentistry)

BDAC
Bureau of Drug Abuse Control (chemi-cal dependency)

B.D.A.C.
Bureau of Drug Abuse Control (chemi-cal dependency)

BDAE
Boston Diagnostic Aphasia Examination (neurology)

BDB
bis-diazotized-benzidine (chemistry)

BDC
burn-dressing change (burn therapy and dermatology)

Bd. & C.
board and care

BDE
bile duct examination (gastroenterology and surgery)
bile duct exploration (gastroenterology and surgery)

BDentSci
Bachelor of Dental Science [Dublin] (dentistry and education)

BDG
buffered desoxycholate glucose [agar or broth] (laboratory)

BDG agar
buffered desoxycholate glucose agar (laboratory)

BDH
British Drug Houses Limited (pharma-cology)

BDI
Beck Depression Inventory (psychiatry)
Becton Dickinson Diagnostics [manufac-turer] (laboratory and pharmacology)
burn depth indicator [a video camera] (burn therapy and dermatology)

BDIBS
Boston Diagnostic Inventory of Basic Skills (speech and language therapy)

BDI SF
Beck's Depression Index—Short Form (psychiatry)

BDL
below detectable limits (laboratory)
bundle

BDM
border detection method (radiology)

BDOPA
bleomycin, dacarbazine [DTIC], vincristine [Oncovin], prednisone, and Adriamycin (chemotherapy, oncology, and pharmacology)

BDP
beclomethasone diproprionate [a corticosteroid] (pharmacology and respiratory)

BDR
background diabetic retinopathy (endocrinology and ophthalmology)

BDS
Bachelor of Dental Surgery (dentistry and education)
biological detection system (biology and laboratory)

B.D.S.
Bachelor of Dental Surgery (dentistry and education)

bds
bis in die summendus [to be taken twice a day] (pharmacology)

BDSc
Bachelor of Dental Science (dentistry and education)

B.D.Sc.
Bachelor of Dental Science (dentistry and education)

BDTVMI
Beery Developmental Test of Visual-Motor Integration (psychiatry)

BDU
Biomedical Display Unit (laboratory)

BDUR
bromodeoxyuridine (genetics and laboratory)

BE
bacillary emulsion [tuberculin] (infectious diseases, laboratory, pharmacology, and respiratory)
bacterial endocarditis (cardiovascular)
barium enema (gastroenterology and radiology)
base excess (laboratory and respiratory)
below elbow (orthopedics)
bile esculin [a coumarin glycoside] (hematology and pharmacology)
bovine enteritis (gastroenterology)
bread equivalent (dietary)
breast examination (gynecology and obstetrics)
bronchoesophagology (gastroenterology and respiratory)

B.E.
Bacillen emulsion, tuberculin (infectious diseases, laboratory, pharmacology, and respiratory)
barium enema (gastroenterology and radiology)

Be
beryllium (chemistry, dermatology, ophthalmology, and respiratory)

Bé
Baumé [hydrometer scale or specific gravity] (chemistry and laboratory)

b.e.
barium enema (gastroenterology and radiology)

BEAM
brain electrical activity mapping [machine] (neurology)

BEAR
Biological Effects of Atomic Radiation [Committee] (armed forces, chemistry, radiation therapy, and radiology)

"bear"
{pronunciation of *BAER* [brain stem auditory evoked response (waves I-VII)]} (neurology) {not an abbreviation}

"bears"
{pronunciation of *BAERs* [brain stem auditory evoked responses]} (neurology) {not an abbreviation}

BEC
bacterial endocarditis (cardiovascular)

BEE
basal energy expenditure

"bee-mod"
{pronunciation of *B-mod* [behavior modification]} (psychiatry and rehabilitation) {not an abbreviation}

"bee-mode"
{pronunciation of *B-mode* [brightness modulation (a type of ultrasound scanning)]} (cardiovascular, obstetrics, and radiology) {not an abbreviation}

beg
begin

beh
behavior(ism) (psychiatry)

BEI
butanol-extractable iodine (endocrinology and laboratory)

BELB
below elbow (orthopedics)

ben
bene [good, well]

ben.
bene [good, well]

Benz
benzidine (chemistry, laboratory, and oncology)

BEP
brain evoked potential(s) (neurology)
brain stem evoked potential(s) (neurology)

BER
basic electrical rhythm (neurology)

BERA
brain stem evoked response audiometry (neurology and otorhinolaryngology)

BES
balanced electrolyte solution (pharmacology)

BESS
Biomedical Experimental Scientific Satellite (aerospace medicine and research)

bet
between

BETA
beta-streptococcus screen (laboratory)

beta LP
beta-lipoprotein (cardiovascular and laboratory)

BETS
benign epileptiform transients of sleep (neurology)

BEV
baboon endogenous virus (veterinary science)

BeV
billion electron volts (electricity)

beV
billion electron volts (electricity)

Bex
base excess (laboratory)

BF
bentonite flocculation [test] (genetics and laboratory)
black female
blastogenic factor [lymphocyte transforming factor] (hematology and laboratory)
blood flow (cardiovascular)
bone fragment (orthopedics)
bouillon filtre [bouillon filtrate (tuberculin)] (infectious diseases, laboratory, pharmacology, and respiratory)
breakfast fed (dietary and nursing)
buffered (chemistry, laboratory, and pharmacology)

butter fat (dietary)

Deny's tuberculin (infectious diseases, laboratory, pharmacology, and respiratory)

lymphocyte transforming factor [blastogenic factor] (hematology and laboratory)

B/F

bound/free [antibody] (laboratory)

bound/free [antigen] (laboratory)

bF

size of catheter according to French Designation (cardiovascular, surgery, and urology)

BFB

biological feedback (physical therapy, psychiatry, and rehabilitation)

BFC

benign febrile convulsion (neurology)

B fibers

{not an abbreviation} (neurology)

BFL

bird-fancier's lung (respiratory)

BFP

biologic false-positive [reaction] (laboratory)

biologically false positive [reaction] (laboratory)

biologically false positivity (laboratory)

BFR

biological false-positive reaction (laboratory)

biological false-positive reactor (laboratory)

blood flow rate (cardiovascular)

bone formation rate (orthopedics)

BFR sol

buffered Ringer's solution (pharmacology and surgery)

BFT

bentonite flocculation test [for rheumatoid arthritis] (infectious diseases, laboratory, and rheumatology)

BFU-E

burst-forming unit—erythroid (hematology and laboratory)

burst-forming units—erythrocyte (hematology and laboratory)

BFU$_e$

erythroid burst-forming unit (hematology and laboratory)

BFV

bovine feces virus (veterinary medicine)

BG

Bender Gestalt [test] (psychiatry)

bicolor guaiac [test] (gastroenterology and laboratory)

blood glucose (endocrinology and laboratory)

bone graft (orthopedics)

Bordet-Gengou [agar or test] (bacteriology, laboratory, and respiratory)

brilliant green (bacteriology and laboratory)

buccogingival (dentistry)

B-G

Bordet-Gengou [bacillus] (bacteriology, laboratory, and respiratory)

BGC

basal-ganglion calcification (neurology)

blood group class (hematology and laboratory)

BGD

blood group–degrading enzymes (hematology and laboratory)

BGE

butyl glycidyl ether (chemistry)

BGG

bovine gamma-globulin (immunology, laboratory, and pharmacology)

BGGRA

British Gelatine and Glue Research Association (research)

B.I.B.P.D.
brought in by police department (emergency medicine and psychiatry)

BIBRA
British Industrial Biological Research Association (research)

BIC
Biomedical Instrumentation Consultant

bicarb
bicarbonate (laboratory, pharmacology, and respiratory) {pronounced "bicarb"}

"bi-carb"
{pronunciation of *bicarb* [bicarbonate]} (laboratory, pharmacology, and respiratory) {not an abbreviation}

BiCNU
1,3-bis(2-chlorethyl)-1-nitrosourea [also called *bischloroethylnitrosourea*, *bischloronitrosourea*, *carmustine*, and *nitrosourea*; also abbreviated BCNU] (chemotherapy, oncology, and pharmacology)

BID
bis in die [twice a day] (pharmacology)
brought in dead (emergency medicine)

bid
bis in die [twice a day] (pharmacology)

b.i.d.
bis in die [twice a day] (pharmacology)

BIDLB
block in the posteroinferior division of the left branch (cardiovascular)

BIDS
bedtime insulin, daytime sulfonylurea [therapy] (endocrinology and pharmacology)

BIG 6
{not an abbreviation} [analysis of six serum components] (laboratory)

big C
cocaine (chemical dependency) {slang} {pronounced "big-sea"}

"big-E"
{pronunciation of *BIGGY* [bismuth glycine glucose yeast (agar)]} (laboratory) {not an abbreviation}

BIGGY
bismuth glycine glucose yeast [agar] (laboratory) {pronounced "big-E"}

"big-sea"
{pronunciation of *big C* [cocaine]} (chemical dependency) {slang} {not an abbreviation}

BIH
benign intracranial hypertension (cardiovascular and neurology)
bilateral inguinal herniae (gastroenterology and surgery)
bilateral inguinal hernias (gastroenterology and surgery)

bihor
bihorium [during 2 hours]

bihor.
bihorium [during 2 hours]

Bi Isch
between ischial tuberosities (orthopedics)

Bi Isch.
between ischial tuberosities (orthopedics)

BIKE
chemotherapy protocol including:
a. Phase 1: prednisone and vincristine
b. Phase 2: methotrexate followed by 6-mercaptopurine and later followed by cyclophosphamide
(chemotherapy, oncology, and pharmacology)

BIL
bilirubin (gastroenterology, laboratory, and neonatology)

Bil
bilirubin (gastroenterology, laboratory, and neonatology)

bil
bilirubin (gastroenterology, laboratory, and neonatology)

bil.
bilateral (anatomy)

bilat
bilateral (anatomy) {pronounced "bi-latt"}

BILAT SLC
bilateral short-leg casts (orthopedics)

BILAT SXO
bilateral salpingo-oophorectomy (gynecology)

"bi-latt"
{pronunciation of *bilat* [bilateral]} (anatomy) {not an abbreviation}

BILI
bilirubin (gastroenterology, laboratory, and neonatology) {pronounced "bill-E"}

Bili
bilirubin (gastroenterology, laboratory, and neonatology) {pronounced "bill-E"}

bili
bilirubin (gastroenterology, laboratory, and neonatology) {pronounced "bill-E"}

BILI-C
conjugated bilirubin (gastroenterology, laboratory, and neonatology) {pronounced "bill-E-see"}

BILIR
bilirubin (gastroenterology, laboratory, and neonatology)

bilirub
bilirubin (gastroenterology, laboratory, and neonatology) {pronounced "bill-E-rueb"}

"bill-E"
{pronunciation of *BILI*, *Bili*, and *bili* [bilirubin]} (gastroenterology, laboratory, and neonatology) {not an abbreviation}

"bill-E-rueb"
{pronunciation of *bilirub* [bilirubin]} (gastroenterology, laboratory, and neonatology) {not an abbreviation}

"bill-E-see"
{pronunciation of *BILI-C* [conjugated bilirubin]} (gastroenterology, laboratory, and neonatology) {not an abbreviation}

BIMA
bilateral internal mammary arteries (cardiovascular, gynecology, and surgery)

BIN
benign intradermal nevus (dermatology)

bin
bis in nocte [*bis in noctus*, twice a night] (pharmacology)

b.i.n.
bis in nocte [*bis in noctus*, twice a night] (pharmacology)

BioAp
Biological Abstracts

Biochem
biochemical (biology, chemistry, and laboratory) {pronounced "bi-oh-chem"}
biochemistry (biology, chemistry, and laboratory) {pronounced "bi-oh-chem"}

"bi-oh-chem"
{pronunciation of *Biochem* [biochemical and biochemistry]} (biology, chemis-

try, and laboratory) {not an abbreviation}

Biol
biological (biology and laboratory)
biology

biol
biological (biology and laboratory)
biology

Biophys
biophysics (biology, chemistry, laboratory, and physics)

BIP
bacterial intravenous protein (bacteriology and laboratory)
biparietal diameter [of fetal skull] (obstetrics and radiology)
bismuth iodoform paraffin (laboratory, pharmacology, and surgery)
Blue Cross Interim Payment (insurance)

B.I.P.
bismuth iodoform paraffin [paste or Morison's paste] (laboratory, pharmacology, and surgery) {pronounced "bip"}

"bip"
{pronunciation of *B.I.P.* and *bipp* [bismuth iodoform paraffin paste (or Morison's paste)] and *BIPP* [bismuth iodoform paraffin paste and bismuth iodoform petrolatum paste]} (laboratory, pharmacology, and surgery) {not an abbreviation}

BiPD
biparietal diameter (obstetrics)

BIPM
Bureau International des Poids et Mesures [International Bureau of Weight and Measures] (measurement)

B.I.P.M.
Bureau International des Poids et Mesures [International Bureau of Weight and Measures] (measurement)

BIPP
bismuth iodoform paraffin paste (labora-

tory, pharmacology, and surgery) {pronounced "bip"}
bismuth iodoform petrolatum paste (laboratory, pharmacology, and surgery) {pronounced "bip"}

bipp
bismuth iodoform paraffin [paste or Morison's paste] (laboratory, pharmacology, and surgery) {pronounced "bip"}

BIR
backward internal rotation (orthopedics)
basic incidence rate
British Institute of Radiology (radiology)

bis
{not an abbreviation} [Latin word meaning *twice*]

BiSP
between ischial spines (orthopedics)

Bisp.
bispinous diameter (orthopedics)
interspinous diameter (orthopedics)

bisp
bispinous diameter (orthopedics)

BiT
between great trochanters (orthopedics)

BITU
benzyl-thiourea (cardiovascular, endocrinology, and pharmacology)

BIV
bovine immunodeficiency-like virus (immunology, research, and veterinary medicine)

B.I.W.
twice a week (pharmacology)

b.i.w.
twice a week (pharmacology)

BIZ
bizarre

BJ
Bence Jones [protein] (hematology, immunology, laboratory, and oncology)
biceps jerk (neurology and orthopedics)
bone and joint (orthopedics)

B & J
bone and joint (orthopedics)

BJ, BRJ, TJ
biceps jerk, brachioradialis jerk, and triceps jerk (neurology and orthopedics)

BJE
bones, joints, and examination

BJM
bones, joints, and muscles (orthopedics)

BJP
Bence Jones protein (hematology, immunology, laboratory, and oncology)

B J PR
Bence Jones protein (hematology, immunology, laboratory, and oncology)

BJ protein
Bence Jones protein (hematology, immunology, laboratory, and oncology)

BK
below-knee [amputation] (orthopedics)

B/K
below-knee [amputation] (orthopedics)

Bk
berkelium (chemistry)

BKA
below-knee amputation (orthopedics)

bkf
breakfast (dietary and nursing)

bkfst.
breakfast (dietary and nursing)

bkft
breakfast (dietary and nursing)

Bkg
background

BKO
below-knee orthosis (orthopedics)

BKTT
below-knee to toe (neurology and orthopedics)

BKWP
below-knee walking plaster [cast] (orthopedics)

BL
baseline (laboratory)
Bessey-Lowry [unit] (endocrinology, gastroenterology, hematology, laboratory, oncology, orthopedics, and urology)
black light (laboratory)
bleeding (hematology)
blood (hematology and laboratory)
blood loss (hematology and surgery)
bone-marrow-derived lymphocyte (hematology and laboratory)
buccolingual (dentistry)
Burkitt's lymphoma (oncology)

B-L
bursa equivalent lymphocyte (hematology and laboratory)

Bl
black

B-l
bursa equivalent lymphocyte (hematology and laboratory)

bl
black
bleeding (hematology)
blood (hematology and laboratory)
blue

BLAC
bladder urine (laboratory and urology)

BLAD
borderline left axis deviation (cardiovascular)

BLAST
blast cell(s) (hematology and laboratory) {pronounced "blast"}

"blast"
{pronunciation of *BLAST* [blast cell(s)]}
(hematology and laboratory) {not an
abbreviation}

BLASTO
Blastomyces [a fungus] (laboratory)
{pronounced "blast-oh"}

"blast-oh"
{pronunciation of *BLASTO* [Blastomyces
(a fungus)]} (laboratory) {not an ab-
breviation}

BLB
Boothby-Lovelace-Bulbulian [oxygen
mask] (respiratory)

BLB mask
Boothby-Lovelace-Bulbulian mask [for
oxygen administration] (respiratory)

BLB unit
Bessey-Lowry-Brock unit (endocrinology, gastroenterology, hematology,
laboratory, oncology, orthopedics,
and urology)
Boothby, Lovelace, Bulbulian unit (respiratory)

BIC
blood culture (laboratory)

bl cult
blood culture (laboratory)

bl. cult.
blood culture (laboratory)

bld.
blood (hematology and laboratory)

Bld Bk
blood bank (hematology and laboratory)

bld chem
blood chemistry (laboratory)

BLDY
grossly bloody (laboratory)

BLE
both lower extremities (neurology and
orthopedics)

BLEED
bleeding time (hematology and laboratory)

"blee-oh"
{pronunciation of *BLEO* and *Bleo*
[bleomycin sulfate]} (chemotherapy,
oncology, and pharmacology) {not an
abbreviation}

"blee-oh-mop"
{pronunciation of *BLEO-MOPP*
[bleomycin, nitrogen mustard, vincristine (Oncovin), procarbazine, and
prednisone]} (chemotherapy, oncology, and pharmacology) {not an ab-
breviation}

BLEO
bleomycin sulfate (chemotherapy, oncology, and pharmacology) {pro-
nounced "blee-oh"}

Bleo
bleomycin sulfate (chemotherapy, oncology, and pharmacology) {pro-
nounced "blee-oh"}

BLEO-MOPP
bleomycin, nitrogen mustard, vincristine
[Oncovin], procarbazine, and prednisone (chemotherapy, oncology, and
pharmacology) {pronounced "blee-oh-
mop"}

bleph
blepharoplasty (ophthalmology and plastic surgery)

BLE's
both lower extremities (neurology and
orthopedics)

BLESS
bath, laxative, enema, shampoo, and
shower (nursing)

BL-FST
blood-fasting [glucose tolerance test] (endocrinology and laboratory)

BLG
beta-lactoglobulin (dietary, laboratory, and veterinary medicine)

BL GAS
blood gases (laboratory and respiratory)

B lines
{not an abbreviation} [refers to *Kerley's B lines* or *costophrenic septal lines*] (radiology and respiratory)

BLK
black

blk
black
block

BLL
brows, lids, and lashes (anatomy)

BLM
bimolecular liquid membrane
bleomycin sulfate (chemotherapy, oncology, and pharmacology)

BLN
bronchial lymph nodes (respiratory)

BLOBS
bladder obstruction (urology)

BLOT
British Library of Tape [Recordings]

BlP
blood pressure (cardiovascular)

bl. pr.
blood pressure (cardiovascular)

BLROA
British Laryngological, Rhinological, and Otological Association (otorhinolaryngology)

B.L.R.O.A.
British Laryngological, Rhinological, and Otological Association (otorhinolaryngology)

BLS
basic life support (cardiovascular, emergency medicine, and respiratory)
Basic Life Support [Systems] (cardiovascular, emergency medicine, and respiratory)
blood and lymphatic systems (hematology)

BlS
blood sugar (endocrinology and laboratory)

BLT
bilateral tubal ligation (gynecology)
bladder tumor (oncology and urology)
blood-clot lysis time (hematology and laboratory)

BlT
blood type (hematology and laboratory)

BLU
Bessey-Lowry units (endocrinology, gastroenterology, hematology, laboratory, oncology, orthopedics, and urology)

B.L. unit
Bessey-Lowry unit (endocrinology, gastroenterology, hematology, laboratory, oncology, orthopedics, and urology)

BLV
bovine leukemia virus (infectious diseases, laboratory, and veterinary medicine)

B-lymphocyte
"bursa-equivalent" lymphocyte [also called *B-cell*] (hematology and laboratory)

BM
Bachelor of Medicine (education)
basal medium (laboratory)
basal metabolism (laboratory)

basement membrane (endocrinology)
basilar membrane [of cochlear] (otorhinolaryngology)
black male
blind matching (parapsychology)
body mass (anatomy and measurement)
bone marrow (hematology)
bowel movement (gastroenterology)
breast milk (neonatology and obstetrics)
buccal mass (dentistry)
buccomesial (dentistry)
Bureau of Medicine (government)

B.M.
Bachelor of Medicine (education)
balneum maris [seawater bath]
bowel movement (gastroenterology)

bm
balneum maris [seawater bath]

b.m.
balneum maris [seawater bath]

BMA
bone marrow aspirate (hematology and laboratory)
British Medical Association

B.M.A.
British Medical Association

BMB
biomedical belt

BMC
bone marrow cells (hematology and laboratory)

BME
basal medium, Eagle's [diploid cell cultures] (genetics and laboratory)
brief maximal effort (orthopedics and physical therapy)

BMed
Bachelor of Medicine (education)

BMedBiol
Bachelor of Medical Biology (biology and education)

BMedSci
Bachelor of Medical Science (education)

BMG
benign monoclonal gammopathy (immunology)

BMI
body mass index (anatomy and measurement)

BMic
Bachelor of Microbiology (education and microbiology)

BMJ
bones, muscles, and joints (orthopedics)

BMK
birthmark (dermatology)

bmk.
birthmark (dermatology)

BMMP
benign mucous membrane pemphigus (dermatology)

B-mod
behavior modification (psychiatry and rehabilitation) {pronounced "bee-mod"}

B-mode
brightness modulation [a type of ultrasound scanning] (cardiovascular, obstetrics, and radiology) {pronounced "bee-mode"}

BMP
bone marrow pressure (orthopedics and radiology)
bone morphogenic protein (hematology and laboratory)
carmustine [BCNU], methotrexate, and procarbazine (chemotherapy, oncology, and pharmacology)

BMPP
benign mucous membrane pemphigus (dermatology)

BMQA
Board of Medical Quality Assurance

BMR
basal metabolic rate (laboratory)
basic metabolic rate (laboratory)

B.M.R.
basal metabolic rate (laboratory)

BMS
Bachelor of Medical Science (education)
Biomedical Monitoring System (laboratory)
bleomycin sulphate (chemotherapy, oncology, and pharmacology)
Bureau of Medicine and Surgery [Navy] (armed forces)

B.M.S.
Bachelor of Medical Science (education)

BMSA
British Medical Students Association (education)

BMT
Bachelor of Medical Technology (education)
Bailliére's Medical Transparencies (publication)
bilateral myringotomy tubes (otorhinolaryngology)
bone marrow transplant (hematology)
Buschke Memory Test (psychiatry)

BMTU
bone marrow transplant unit (hematology)

BN
brachial neuritis (neurology)

BNA
Basle Nomina Anatomica (anatomy)

BNC
bladder neck contracture (urology)

BNDD
Bureau of Narcotics and Dangerous Drugs (chemical dependency and government)

B.N.D.D.
Bureau of Narcotics and Dangerous Drugs (chemical dependency and government)

BNEd
Bachelor of Nursing Education (education and nursing)

BNEG
B negative [blood type] (hematology and laboratory)

BNF
British National Formulary (pharmacology)

BNG
bromo-naphthyl-beta-galactoside [also called *6-bromo-2-naphthyl-β-galactoside*] (chemistry)

BNGase
bromo-naphthyl-beta-galactosidase [also called *6-bromo-2-naphthyl-β-galactosidase*] (chemistry)

BNL
breast needle location (radiology)

BNMSE
Brief Neuropsychological Mental Status Examination (neurology and psychiatry)

BNO
bladder neck obstruction (urology)
bowels not open (gastroenterology)

BNPA
binasal pharyngeal airway (otorhinolaryngology)

BNR
bladder neck resection (urology)
bladder neck retraction (urology)

BNS
benign nephrosclerosis (nephrology)

BNSc
Bachelor of Nursing Science (education and nursing)

BO
Bachelor of Osteopathy (education and osteopathic medicine)
base [of prism] out
behavior objective (psychiatry)
body odor
Bolton [craniometric point] (radiology)
bowel obstruction (gastroenterology)
bowels open (gastroenterology)
bucco-occlusal (dentistry)

B & O
belladonna and opium [used with paregoric as an antispasmodic and antiperistaltic drug] (gastroenterology and pharmacology)

Bo
bohemium (chemistry)
magnetic induction field (radiology)

bo
bowel (gastroenterology)

BOA
born on arrival (neonatology and obstetrics)
born out of asepsis (neonatology and obstetrics)
British Orthopaedic Association (orthopedics)

B.O.A.
British Orthopaedic Association (orthopedics)

BOB
ball on back

BOBA
beta-oxybutyric acid (chemistry)

BOCG
Brudzinski, Oppenheim, Chaddock, and Gullaird [reflexes and signs] (neurology)

BOD
biochemical oxygen demand (laboratory and respiratory)
biological oxygen demand (laboratory and respiratory)
board of directors
borderline (laboratory)

BodUnit
Bodansky unit (laboratory)

Bod units
Bodansky units (laboratory)

BOE
bilateral otitis externa (otorhinolaryngology)

BOEA
ethyl biscoumacetate (chemistry)

BOH
Board of Health (government)

boil
boiling

bol
bolus [pill] (pharmacology)

bol.
bolus [pill] (pharmacology)

BOLD
bleomycin, vincristine [Oncovin], lomustine, and dacarbazine (chemotherapy, oncology, and pharmacology) {pronounced "bold"}

B.O.L.D.
bleomycin, vincristine [Oncovin], lomustine, and dacarbazine (chemotherapy, oncology, and pharmacology) {pronounced "bold"}

"bold"
{pronunciation of *BOLD* and *B.O.L.D.* [bleomycin, vincristine (Oncovin), lomustine, and dacarbazine]} (chemotherapy, oncology, and pharmacology) {not an abbreviation}

BOM
bilateral otitis media (otorhinolaryngology)

"bom"
{pronunciation of *BOMB* [vincristine, Adriamycin, 6-mercaptopurine, and

prednisone]} (chemotherapy, oncology, and pharmacology) {not an abbreviation}

BOMB
vincristine, Adriamycin, 6-mercaptopurine, and prednisone (chemotherapy, oncology, and pharmacology) {pronounced "bom"}

BONENT
Board of Nephrology Examiners for Nursing and Technology (nephrology and nursing)

BOO
bladder outlet obstruction (urology)

BOP
bleomycin, vincristine, and prednisone (chemotherapy, oncology, and pharmacology) {pronounced "bop"}
Buffalo orphan prototype [referring to viruses] (laboratory)

"bop"
{pronunciation of *BOP* [bleomycin, vincristine, and prednisone]} (chemotherapy, oncology, and pharmacology) {not an abbreviation}

BOPAM
bleomycin, vincristine [Oncovin], prednisone, Adriamycin, nitrogen mustard, and methotrexate (chemotherapy, oncology, and pharmacology) {pronounced "bow-pam"}

BOR
bowels open regularly (gastroenterology)

BORD
borderline (laboratory)

B-O₂S
blood oxygen saturation [on blood gas determinations] (laboratory and respiratory)

BOT
base of tongue (anatomy and otorhinolaryngology)

Bot
botanical (botany)
botany

bot
bottle (chemical dependency and pharmacology)

BOW
bag of waters [also called *amnionic sac*] (obstetrics)

B.O.W.
bag of waters [also called *amnionic sac*] (obstetrics)

"bow-pam"
{pronunciation of *BOPAM* [bleomycin, vincristine (Oncovin), prednisone, Adriamycin, nitrogen mustard, and methotrexate]} (chemotherapy, oncology, and pharmacology) {not an abbreviation}

BP
Bachelor of Pharmacy (education and pharmacology)
back pressure (neurology and orthopedics)
barometric pressure (neurology, respiratory, and sports medicine)
basic protein (laboratory)
bathroom privileges (nursing and rehabilitation)
bedpan (nursing)
behavior pattern (psychiatry)
benzpyrene [also called *3,4-benzpyrene*] (chemistry and laboratory)
benzoyl peroxide (chemistry, dermatology, and pharmacology)
biotic potential
biparietal [diameter of fetal head] (obstetrics and radiology)
birthplace
blood pressure (cardiovascular)
body part (anatomy)
British Pharmacopoeia (pharmacology)
bronchopleural (respiratory)
bronchopulmonary (respiratory)
buccopulpal (dentistry)
bypass (cardiovascular)

Bq.
becquerel (measurement, radiation therapy, and radiology)

BCQ
2,6-dibromoquinonechlorimide [solu-
tion] (chemistry)

BQC sol.
2,6-dibromoquinonechlorimide solution
(chemistry)

BR
bathroom (nursing and rehabilitation)
bed rest (nursing and rehabilitation)
Benzing retrograde
bilirubin (gastroenterology and laboratory)
bridge (dentistry)
British Revision [of Basle Nomina Anatomica (BNA)] (anatomy)
brown

B.R.
bed rest (nursing and rehabilitation)

Br
breech (obstetrics)
bridge (dentistry)
British [referring to nationality]
bromine [a depressant and toxic sub-
stance] (chemistry)
bronchitis (respiratory)
brown
Brucella (bacteriology and laboratory)

Br.
Brucella (bacteriology and laboratory)

br
boiling range (chemistry)
branch
breath (respiratory)
brother

BRA
brain (neurology)

brady
bradycardia (cardiovascular) {pro-
nounced "bray-dee"}

BRAO
branch retinal artery occlusion (ophthalmology)

BRAT
banana, rice cereal, apple sauce, and
crackers [diet] (dietary and pediatrics)
{pronounced "brat"}
banana, rice cereal, apple sauce, and tea
[diet] (dietary and pediatrics) {pro-
nounced "brat"}
banana, rice cereal, apple sauce, and
toast [diet] (dietary and pediatrics)
{pronounced "brat"}

"brat"
{pronunciation of BRAT [banana, rice
cereal, apple sauce, and crackers
(diet); banana, rice cereal, apple
sauce, and tea (diet); and banana, rice
cereal, apple sauce, and toast (diet)]}
(dietary and pediatrics)

BRATT
bananas, rice, apple sauce, tea, and
toast [diet] (dietary and pediatrics)

"bray-dee"
{pronunciation of *brady* [bradycardia]}
(cardiovascular) {not an abbreviation}

BRB
blood-retinal barrier (ophthalmology)

BRBA
Brucella, vitamin K blood agar (bacteriology, hematology, and laboratory)

BRBC
bovine red blood cells (hematology and
laboratory)

BRBNS
blue rubber-bleb nevus syndrome (dermatology)

BRBPR
bright red blood per rectum (gastroenterology)

br bx
breast biopsy (gynecology and surgery)

BRCM
below right costal margin (anatomy)

BRCS
British Red Cross Society (emergency medicine and hematology)

BrDU
5-bromodeoxyuridine (chemotherapy, oncology, pharmacology, and radiation therapy)

BrdU
5-bromodeoxyuridine (chemotherapy, oncology, pharmacology, and radiation therapy)

BrdUrd
5-bromodeoxyuridine (chemotherapy, oncology, pharmacology, and radiation therapy)

B.R.H.
Bureau of Radiological Health (government, radiation therapy, and radiology)

Brhp
bronchophony (respiratory)

BRI
Bio-Research Index (research)

Brit
British [referring to nationality] {pronounced "britt"}

"britt"
{pronunciation of Brit [British (referring to nationality)]} {not an abbreviation}

BRJ
brachioradialis jerk (neurology and orthopedics)

Brkf
breakfast (dietary)

brkf.
breakfast (dietary)

BRL
Beecham Research Laboratories (laboratory and research)
Bethesda Research Laboratories (laboratory and research)
Biometrics Research Laboratory (laboratory and research)

BRM
biological response modifiers (laboratory)
biuret-reactive material (laboratory)

BrM
breast milk (neonatology and obstetrics)

BRN
Board of Registered Nursing (nursing)
brown

BRO
bronchoscopy (respiratory)

BROK
tube broke (laboratory)

Bron
bronchial (respiratory)

bron.
bronchial (respiratory)

bronch
bronchoscopist (respiratory) {pronounced "bronk"}
bronchoscopy (respiratory) {pronounced "bronk"}

broncho
bronchoscopy (respiratory) {pronounced "bronk-O"}

"bronk"
{pronunciation of bronch [bronchoscopist and bronchoscopy]} (respiratory) {not an abbreviation}

"bronk-O"
{pronunciation of broncho [bronchoscopy]} (respiratory) {not an abbreviation}

BRP
bathroom privileges (nursing and rehabilitation)
bilirubin production (gastroenterology
and laboratory)

B.R.P.
bathroom privileges (nursing and rehabilitation)

b.r.p.
bathroom privileges (nursing and rehabilitation)

Br.Rvo
branch retinal vein occlusion (ophthalmology)

BRS
British Roentgen Society (radiology)

B.R.S.
British Roentgen Society (radiology)

BrS
breath sounds (respiratory)

brth.
breath (respiratory)

BRUCL
Brucella agglutinins (bacteriology and
laboratory)

BRW
Brown-Roberts-Wells [computerized tomographic stereotaxic guide] (radiology)

BS
Bachelor of Science (education)
Bachelor of Surgery (education and surgery)
before sleep (pharmacology)
Binet-Simon [test] (psychiatry)
bismuth subsalicylate (gastroenterology,
gynecology, infectious diseases, pharmacology, and urology)
blood sugar (endocrinology and laboratory)
Bloom syndrome (dermatology, genetics, and pediatrics)
Blue Shield (insurance)
bowel sounds (gastroenterology)

breaking strength
breath sounds (respiratory)
British Standard
Bureau of Standards (measurements)

B.S.
Bachelor of Science (education)
Bachelor of Surgery (education and surgery)
blood sugar (endocrinology and laboratory)
bowel sounds (gastroenterology)
breath sounds (respiratory)

B & S
Bartholin's and Skene's [glands] (gynecology)

Bs
breath sounds (respiratory)

bs
bowel sounds (gastroenterology)

b.s.
barium swallow (gastroenterology and
radiology)

BSA
benzenesulfonic acid (chemistry)
Biofeedback Society of America (psychiatry)
bismuth sulfite agar (bacteriology and
laboratory)
bis-trimethylsilylacetamide (chemistry
and laboratory)
Blind Service Association (ophthalmology)
Blue Shield Association (insurance)
body surface area (dermatology and
measurement)
bovine serum albumin (laboratory, nephrology, and pharmacology)

BSAER
brain stem auditory evoked response
(neurology and otorhinolaryngology)

BSAP
brief short-action potential (neurology)

brief, small, abundant potentials (neurology)

BSB
body surface burned (dermatology and measurement)

BSC
bedside commode (nursing and rehabilitation)
Biological Stain Commission (laboratory)
Biomedical Sciences Corps [Air Force] (armed forces)
Biomedical Signal Conditioner (laboratory)

BSc
Bachelor of Science (education)

B.Sc.
Bachelor of Science (education)

B-scan
brightness modulation scan [one type of visual display of ultrasonographic echoes] (cardiovascular, obstetrics, and radiology)

BSCC
British Society of Clinical Cytology (laboratory and pathology)

BSDLB
block in the anterosuperior division of the left branch (cardiovascular)

BSE
bilateral, symmetrical, and equal (neurology, ophthalmology, and orthopedics)
Breast Self Exam (gynecology)
breast self-examination (gynecology)

BSEP
brain stem evoked potentials (neurology)

BSER
brain stem evoked responses (neurology)

BSF
backscatter factor (radiation therapy and radiology)
busulfan (chemotherapy, oncology, and pharmacology)

BSGA
beta-streptococcus group A (bacteriology and laboratory)

BSI
bound serum iron (hematology and laboratory)

BSID
Bayley Scales of Infant Development (psychiatry)
British Standards Institution (measurement)

BSL
benign symmetric lipomatosis (dermatology and surgery)
blood sugar level (endocrinology and laboratory)

BSM
Bachelor of Science in Medicine (education)

BSN
Bachelor of Science in Nursing (education and nursing)
bowel sounds normal (gastroenterology)

BSO
bilateral sagittal osteotomy (neurology and orthopedics)
bilateral salpingo-oophorectomy (gynecology)
bilateral serous otitis (otorhinolaryngology)
British School of Osteopathy (education and osteopathic medicine)

B.S.O.
bilateral salpingo-oophorectomy (gynecology)

BSOM
bilateral serous otitis media (otorhinolaryngology)

BSOT
Bachelor of Science in Occupational Therapy (education and occupational therapy)

BSP
Bromsulphalein [brand name for a preparation of sulfobromophthalein] (gastroenterology, laboratory, and pharmacology)

BSp
bronchospasm (respiratory)

BSPh
Bachelor of Science in Pharmacy (education and pharmacology)

BSPM
body surface potential mapping (dermatology and measurement)

BSR
basal skin resistance (dermatology)
blood sedimentation rate (hematology and laboratory)

BSS
balanced salt solution (pharmacology and surgery)
black silk suture (surgery)
brain stimulation reinforcement (neurology)
buffered saline solution (pharmacology)

BSS
Bachelor of Sanitary Science (education)
balanced salt solution (pharmacology)
buffered salt solution [also called *buffered saline solution*] (pharmacology)
{not an abbreviation} [brand name for a preparation of balanced salt solution] (pharmacology, ophthalmology, and surgery)

BSSG
sitogluside (chemistry)

BST
blood serological test (gynecology, infectious diseases, laboratory, and urology)
brief stimulus therapy (psychiatry and rehabilitation)

BSTFA
bis-trimethylsilyltrifluoroacetamide (chemistry and laboratory)

B.STP
basophilic stippling [on differential] (hematology and laboratory)

BSU
Bartholin's, Skene's, and urethral [glands] (gynecology)

B. subtilis
Bacillus subtilis (bacteriology and laboratory)

BSW
Bachelor of Social Work (education and social work)

BT
Bacillus thuringiensis (bacteriology and laboratory)
bedtime
bitemporal [diameter of fetal head] (obstetrics and radiology)
bituberous (anatomy and pathology)
Blacky Test (psychiatry)
bladder tremor (urology)
bladder tumor (urology)
bleeding time (hematology and laboratory)
blood transfusion (hematology)
blue tetrazolium (chemistry and laboratory)
body temperature
brain tumor (neurology and oncology)
breast tumor (gynecology, oncology, and surgery)
carmustine [BCNU] and triazinate (chemotherapy, oncology, and pharmacology)

BTA
N-benzoyl-l-tyrosine amide (chemistry and laboratory)
Blood Transfusion Association (hematology)

BTB
breakthrough bleeding (gynecology)
bromothymol blue [a pH indicator] (chemistry and laboratory)

BTBC
Boehm Test of Basic Concepts (speech and language therapy)

BTEA
Boston Test for Examining Aphasia (speech and language therapy)

BTFS
breast tumor frozen section (gynecology, oncology, pathology, and surgery)

BTH
butylated hydroxytolulene (chemistry)

BThU
British thermal unit (measurement)

B Th U
British thermal unit (measurement)

BTL
bilateral tubal ligation (gynecology)

BTMD
Batten-Turner muscular dystrophy (neurology)

BTPS
body conditions—body temperature, ambient pressure, and saturated with water vapor at these conditions (laboratory and respiratory)
body temperature, ambient pressure, saturated (laboratory and respiratory)
body temperature, pressure (prevailing atmospheric), and saturation (with water vapor) (laboratory and respiratory)

BTR
Bezold-type reflex [or sign] (otorhinolaryngology)
bladder tumor recheck (urology)

BTS
Blood Transfusion Service (hematology)

BTSG
Brain Tumor Study Group [of the National Cancer Institute] (neurology, oncology, and research)

BTSH
beef thyroid-stimulating hormone (endocrinology and pharmacology)
bovine thyroid-stimulating hormone (endocrinology and pharmacology)
bovine thyrotropin (endocrinology and laboratory)

B-TSH
beef thyroid stimulating hormone (endocrinology and pharmacology)

BTU
British thermal unit (measurement)

B.T.U.
British thermal unit (measurement)

BTX
benzene, toluene, xylene (chemistry)
bungarotoxin [a neurotoxin] (neurology)

BTX-B
brevetoxin-B

BTZ
Butazolidin (orthopedics, pharmacology, and rheumatology)

BTZ alka
Butazolidin alka (orthopedics, pharmacology, and rheumatology)

BU
base [of prism] up
Bodansky unit [of phosphatase activity] (laboratory)

BVX
bacitracin V and X (pharmacology)

BW
bacteriological warfare (armed forces)
below waist
biological warfare (armed forces)
biological weapons (armed forces)
birth weight (neonatology)
bladder washout (urology)
body water
body weight

B-W
Burroughs-Wellcome [pharmaceutical company] (pharmacology)

B & W
Black and White [milk of magnesia and aromatic cascara fluid extract] (chemistry)

BWCS
bagged white cell study (laboratory)

BWD
bacillary white diarrhea [in chicks] (veterinary medicine)

BWFI
bacteriostatic water for injection (pharmacology)

BWRWS
Biological Warfare Rapid Warning System (armed forces)

BWS
battered woman syndrome

BWSV
black widow spider venom (entomology and laboratory)

BWt
birth weight

BX
bacitracin X (pharmacology)
biopsy (surgery)

Bx
biopsy (surgery)

bx
biopsy (surgery)

BX BS
Blue Cross and Blue Shield (insurance)

BYE
Barile-Yaguchi-Eveland [agar, a culture medium] (laboratory)

BYE agar
Barile-Yaguchi-Eveland agar [culture medium] (laboratory)

BYOB
bring your own booze (slang)
bring your own bottle (slang)

BZ
benzodiazepine (pharmacology)
benzoyl (chemistry)

ΦBZ
phenylbutazone (chemistry)

BZDZ
benzodiazepine (pharmacology)

cule of the complement system]
(chemistry)

C-3
third cervical nerve (neurology and orthopedics)
third cervical vertebra (orthopedics)

C4
complement component C4 [also called
complement C4] (laboratory)
fourth cervical nerve (neurology and orthopedics)
fourth cervical vertebra (orthopedics)

C₄
complement component C4 [also called
complement C4] (laboratory)
costa IV [fourth rib] (orthopedics)
fourth cervical nerve (neurology and orthopedics)
fourth cervical vertebra (orthopedics)
{not an abbreviation} [precursor molecule of the complement system]
(chemistry)

C-4
fourth cervical nerve (neurology and orthopedics)
fourth cervical vertebra (orthopedics)

C5
fifth cervical nerve (neurology and orthopedics)
fifth cervical vertebra (orthopedics)

C₅
costa V [fifth rib] (orthopedics)
fifth cervical nerve (neurology and orthopedics)
fifth cervical vertebra (orthopedics)
{not an abbreviation} [precursor molecule of the complement system]
(chemistry)
{not an abbreviation} [a component of
complement] (laboratory)

C-5
fifth cervical nerve (neurology and orthopedics)
fifth cervical vertebra (orthopedics)

C6
sixth cervical nerve (neurology and orthopedics)
sixth cervical vertebra (orthopedics)

C₆
costa VI [sixth rib] (orthopedics)
sixth cervical nerve (neurology and orthopedics)
sixth cervical vertebra (orthopedics)
{not an abbreviation} [precursor molecule of the complement system]
(chemistry)
{not an abbreviation} [a component of
complement] (laboratory)

C-6
hexamethonium (chemistry)
sixth cervical nerve (neurology and orthopedics)
sixth cervical vertebra (orthopedics)

C7
seventh cervical nerve (neurology and
orthopedics)
seventh cervical vertebra (orthopedics)

C₇
costa VII [seventh rib] (orthopedics)
seventh cervical nerve (neurology and
orthopedics)
seventh cervical vertebra (orthopedics)
{not an abbreviation} [precursor molecule of the complement system]
(chemistry)
{not an abbreviation} [a component of
complement] (laboratory)

C-7
seventh cervical nerve (neurology and
orthopedics)
seventh cervical vertebra (orthopedics)

C₈
costa VIII [eighth rib] (orthopedics)
{not an abbreviation} [precursor molecule of the complement system]
(chemistry)
{not an abbreviation} [a component of
complement] (laboratory)

C_9
costa IX [ninth rib] (orthopedics)
{not an abbreviation} [precursor molecule of the complement system] (chemistry)
{not an abbreviation} [a component of complement] (laboratory)

C_{10}
costa X [tenth rib] (orthopedics)

C10
decamethonium (chemistry)

C-10
decamethonium (chemistry)

C_{11}
costa XI [eleventh rib] (orthopedics)

C_{12}
costa XII [twelfth rib] (orthopedics)

^{14}C
radioactive cesium (chemistry)

c
calorie [small calorie] (dietary)
candle
canine [deciduous tooth] (dentistry)
capacity
capillary in the blood phase (laboratory and respiratory)
centi- [prefix indicating 10^{-2}] (measurement) {not an abbreviation}
centum [one hundred]
cibus [meal]
circa [about, approximately]
contact
cubic
cum [with]
curie (radiation therapy and radiology)
cyclic
speed of light (physics)
velocity of light (physics)

c
capillary blood (laboratory) [Note: The abbreviation is subscripted.]

c.
calorie [small calorie] (dietary)
candle
capacity

centi- [prefix for 10^{-2}] (measurement) {not an abbreviation}
centum [one hundred]
cibus [meal]
circa [about, approximately]
contact
cubic
culture [medium] (laboratory)
cum [with]
cup
curie (radiology)
cyclic

$\bar{c}$
cum [with]

$\bar{c}.$
cum [with]

c'
coefficient of partage

$\overset{\prime}{c}$
pulmonary endcapillary in the blood phase (laboratory and respiratory)

μc
microcurie (radiation therapy and radiology)

CA
California [Postal Service state designation]
cancer (oncology)
carbonic anhydrase (chemistry)
carcinoma (oncology)
cardiac arrest (cardiovascular)
carotid artery (cardiovascular)
catecholamine (laboratory)
cathodal (radiology)
cathode (radiology)
cerebral aqueduct (cardiovascular and neurosurgery)
cervicoaxial (dentistry)
Chemical Abstracts (chemistry)
chronological age
coagglutination [test] (laboratory)
Cocaine Anonymous (chemical dependency)
coeliac (celiac) axis (gastroenterology)
cold agglutinin (laboratory)

collagen antigen (laboratory)
commissural-association [zone of brain] (neurosurgery)
common antigen (laboratory)
coronary arrest (cardiovascular)
coronary artery (cardiovascular)
corpora amylacea (anatomy and laboratory)
cortisone acetate (pharmacology)
Council Accepted [American Medical Association]
croup-associated [virus] (infectious diseases and laboratory)
cytosine arabinoside (chemotherapy, oncology, and pharmacology)

CA 125
carbohydrate antigen 125 (laboratory and oncology)

C.A.
Certified Acupuncturist (neurology and orthopedics)

C/A
Clinitest and Acetest (endocrinology, laboratory, and pharmacology)

C & A
Clinitest and Acetest (endocrinology, laboratory, and pharmacology)

Ca
calcium (chemistry, laboratory, and pharmacology)
cancer (oncology)
carcinoma (oncology)
cathodal (radiology)
cathode (radiology)

^{45}Ca
radioactive calcium (chemistry)

ca
candle
circa [about, approximately]

ca.
candle
carcinoma (oncology)
circa [about, approximately]

CAA
constitutional aplastic anemia (hematology)
crystalline amino acids (laboratory)

CAAT
computer-assisted axial tomography (radiology)

CAB
coronary artery bypass (cardiovascular)

"cab-age"
{pronunciation of CABG [coronary artery bypass graft]} (cardiovascular) {not an abbreviation}

CABG
coronary artery bypass graft (cardiovascular) {pronounced "cab-age"}

CABGS
coronary artery bypass graft surgery (cardiovascular)

CaBI
calcium bone index (laboratory)

CABOP
cyclophosphamide, Adriamycin, bleomycin, Oncovin [vincristine], and prednisone (chemotherapy, oncology, and pharmacology)

CA-BOP
cyclophosphamide, Adriamycin, bleomycin, Oncovin [vincristine], and prednisone (chemotherapy, oncology, and pharmacology)

CABP
calcium-binding protein (laboratory)

CaBP
calcium-binding protein (laboratory)

CABS
coronary artery bypass surgery (cardiovascular)

CAC
cardiac-accelerator center (cardiovascular)
cardiac arrest code (cardiovascular)
comprehensive ambulatory care
malignant cell (laboratory and oncology)

CACB
calcium carbonate (laboratory and pharmacology)

CACC
cathodal closure contraction (cardiovascular and radiology)

CaCC
cathodal closure contraction (cardiovascular and radiology)

CACI
computer assisted continuous infusion (pharmacology)

CaCl₂
calcium chloride (pharmacology)

CaCO₃
calcium carbonate (pharmacology)

CACP
cisplatin (chemotherapy, oncology, and pharmacology)

CACX
cancer of the cervix (gynecology and oncology)

CAD
computer-assisted diagnosis (computer science)
computerized-assisted design (computer science)
coronary artery disease (cardiovascular) {pronounced "cad"}
cytosine arabinoside and daunomycin (chemotherapy, oncology, and pharmacology)

C.A.D.
coronary artery disease (cardiovascular)

Cad
cadaver (pathology)

"cad"
{pronunciation of *CAD* [coronary artery disease]} (cardiovascular) {not an abbreviation}

CADI
computer-assisted diabetic instruction [system] (dietary and endocrinology)

CAD-I
Adriamycin, cyclophosphamide, and cisplatin (chemotherapy, oncology, and pharmacology)

CADIC
cyclophosphamide, Adriamycin, and dacarbazine [DTIC] (chemotherapy, oncology, and pharmacology)

CADL
Communication Abilities in Daily Living [test] (speech and language therapy)
Communicative Abilities in Daily Living [test] (speech and language therapy)

CADTe
cathodal duration tetanus (cardiovascular and radiology)

CaDTe
cathodal duration tetanus (cardiovascular and radiology)

CAE
cellulose acetate electrophoresis (laboratory)
contingent after-effects

CaEDTA
calcium disodium ethylenediaminetetraacetate [also called *edathamil calcium disodium*] (chemistry)

caerul
caeruleus [dark blue, dark green]

CAF
cell adhesion factor (laboratory)
citric acid fermenters (chemistry and laboratory)

continuous atrial fibrillation (cardiovascular)

Cooley's Anemia Foundation (hematology)

cyclophosphamide, Adriamycin [doxorubicin], and 5-fluorouracil (chemotherapy, oncology, and pharmacology)

continuous atrial flutter (cardiovascular)

caf
caffeine (chemistry, dietary, laboratory, and pharmacology)

CAFFI
cyclophosphamide, Adriamycin [doxorubicin], and 5-fluorouracil by continuous infusion (chemotherapy, oncology, and pharmacology)

CAFP
cyclophosphamide, Adriamycin, 5-fluorouracil, and prednisone (chemotherapy, oncology, and pharmacology)

CAFT
Clinitron air fluidized therapy (respiratory)

CAFVP
cyclophosphamide, Adriamycin, 5-fluorouracil, vincristine, and prednisone (chemotherapy, oncology, and pharmacology)

CAG
chronic atrophic gastritis (gastroenterology)

CAGB
coronary artery graft bypass (cardiovascular)

CAH
chronic active hepatitis (gastroenterology)

chronic aggressive hepatitis (gastroenterology)

congenital adrenal hyperplasia (endocrinology)

cyanacetic acid hydrazine (chemistry)

CAHD
coronary artery heart disease (cardiovascular)

coronary atherosclerotic heart disease (cardiovascular)

CAHEA
Committee on Allied Health Education and Accreditation (education)

C.A.H.E.A.
Committee on Allied Health Education and Accreditation (education)

CAI
computer-assisted instruction (computer science)

confused artificial insemination (obstetrics)

CA ION
calcium, ionized (chemistry and pharmacology)

CAL
calcium [test] (dentistry)

calculated average life (pharmacology and radiology)

callus (dermatology and orthopedics)

calories (dietary)

chronic airflow limitation (otorhinolaryngology and respiratory)

computer-assisted learning (computer science)

Cal
calcium (chemistry, dietary, laboratory, and pharmacology)

large calorie [kilocalorie in metabolic studies] (dietary and laboratory)

Cal.
large calorie [kilocalorie in metabolic studies] (dietary and laboratory)

cal
caliber (measurement)

small calorie [gram calorie, standard calorie] (dietary and laboratory)

cal.
small calorie [gram calorie, standard calorie] (dietary and laboratory)

CALASP
cytosine arabinoside, vincristine, L-asparaginase, and prednisone (chemotherapy, oncology, and pharmacology)

C_{alb}
albumin clearance (laboratory)

calCd
calculated

CALD
chronic active liver disease (gastroenterology)

calef
calefac [make warm]
calefactus [warmed]

calef.
calefac [make warm]
calefactus [warmed]

CALGB
Cancer and Leukemia Group B (hematology and oncology)

"cal-gee-swab"
{pronunciation of *calgi swab* [calcium alginate swab] (pharmacology and surgery) {not an abbreviation}

calgi swab
calcium alginate swab (pharmacology and surgery) {pronounced "cal-gee-swab"}

calib
calibrated

cALL
common null cell acute lymphoblastic leukemia (hematology and oncology)

CALLA
common acute lymphoblastic leukemia antigen (laboratory)

CAM
cell-associating molecule (laboratory)
chorioallantoic membrane (neonatology and obstetrics)
contralateral axillary metastasis (oncology)
cyclophosphamide, Adriamycin, and methotrexate (chemotherapy, oncology, and pharmacology)

CaM
calmodulin (laboratory)

C_{am}
amylase clearance (laboratory)

CAMAC
computer automated measurement and control (computer science)

CAMB
cyclophosphamide, Adriamycin, methotrexate, and bleomycin (chemotherapy, oncology, and pharmacology)

CAMELEON
cytosine arabinoside, high-dose methotrexate, citrovorum factor, and vincristine (chemotherapy, oncology, and pharmacology)

CAMF
cyclophosphamide, Adriamycin, methotrexate, and fluorouracil (chemotherapy, oncology, and pharmacology)
cyclophosphamide, Adriamycin, methotrexate, and folic acid (chemotherapy, oncology, and pharmacology)

CAMP
Christie, Atkins, Munch-Peterson [test] {pronounced "camp"}
computer-assisted menu planning (dietary) {pronounced "camp"}
cyclophosphamide, Adriamycin [doxorubicin], methotrexate, and procarbazine (chemotherapy, oncology, and pharmacology) {pronounced "camp"}

cAMP
adenosine 3′,5′-cyclic phosphate [also called *cyclic adenosine monophos-*

"carb"
{pronunciation of *CARB* [carbohydrate (dietary and laboratory)] and *carb* [carbonate (chemistry and pharmacology)]} {not an abbreviation}

CARBAM
carbamazepine [Tegretol] (neurology and pharmacology)

carbo
carbohydrate (dietary and laboratory) {pronounced "car-bow"}

"car-bow"
{pronunciation of *carbo* [carbohydrate]} (dietary and laboratory) {not an abbreviation}

CARD
cardiology (cardiovascular)

Card
cardiology (cardiovascular)

card.
cardiology (cardiovascular)

Cardiol
cardiology (cardiovascular)

cardiol.
cardiology (cardiovascular)

CARF
Commission on Accreditation of Rehabilitation Facilities

C.A.R.F.
Commission on Accreditation of Rehabilitation Facilities

C-arm
{not an abbreviation} [fluoroscopy unit] (radiology and surgery)

CAROT
carotene (laboratory)

CART
computer-aided real time transcription (medical records)

CAS
Cancer Attitude Survey (oncology and psychiatry)
cardiac adjustment scale (cardiovascular)
cardiac surgery (cardiovascular)
carotid artery stenosis (cardiovascular)
carotid artery system (cardiovascular)
Center for Alcohol Studies (chemical dependency and research)
cerebral arteriosclerosis (cardiovascular and neurology)
Chemical Abstracts Service (chemistry)
Civil Air Surgeon (aviation medicine)
control adjustment strap
Council of Academic Societies

Cas
casualty

CASA
Computer-Assisted Self Assessment [British] (psychiatry)

casc.
cascara [a cathartic] (pharmacology)

CASHD
coronary arteriosclerotic heart disease (cardiovascular)

CA-SP
calcium urine spot [test] (laboratory)

CAS-REGN
Chemical Abstracts Service Registry Number

CASS
Coronary Artery Surgery Study (cardiovascular, research, and surgery)

CAST
Clearinghouse Announcements in Science and Technology

CASTNO
cast number [in urinalysis] (laboratory, nephrology, and urology)

CAT
cataract (ophthalmology)
catecholamines (laboratory)
Children's Apperception Test (psychiatry)
chloramphenicol acetyltransferase (pharmacology)
chlormerodrin accumulation test (laboratory)
choline acetyltransferase (pharmacology)
classified anaphylatoxin (pharmacology)
college ability test (education)
computed axial tomography (radiology) {pronounced "cat"}
computer-aided transcription (medical records)
computer-assisted tomography (radiology) {pronounced "cat"}
computer of average transients
computerized axial tomography (radiology) {pronounced "cat"}
cytosine arabinoside and thioguanine (chemotherapy, oncology, and pharmacology)
cytosine arabinoside, Adriamycin, and 6-thioguanine (chemotherapy, oncology, and pharmacology)

cat
cataract (ophthalmology)

"cat"
{pronunciation of *CAT* [computed axial tomography, computer-assisted tomography, and computerized axial tomography]} (radiology) {not an abbreviation}

CAT-A-KIT
Catecholamines Radioenzymatic Assay Kit (laboratory)

CATCH
Community Actions to Control High Blood Pressure (cardiovascular)

cat c̄ IL
cataract with intraocular lens (ophthalmology)

Cath
catheter (cardiovascular and urology) {pronounced "cath"}
catheterization (cardiovascular and urology)
Catholic (religion)

cath
cathartic (pharmacology)
catheter (cardiovascular and urology) {pronounced "cath"}
catheterize (cardiovascular and urology)

cath.
catharticus [cathartic] (pharmacology)
catheter (cardiovascular and urology) {pronounced "cath"}
catheterization (cardiovascular and urology)
catheterize (cardiovascular and urology)

"cath"
{pronunciation of *Cath*, *cath*, and *cath.* [catheter]} (cardiovascular and urology) {not an abbreviation}

CATSCAN
computer-assisted tomography scanner (radiology) {pronounced "cat-scan"}
computerized axial tomography scanner (radiology) {pronounced "cat-scan"}

"cat-scan"
{pronunciation of *CATSCAN* [computer-assisted tomography scanner and computerized axial tomography scanner]} (radiology) {not an abbreviation}

Cau
Caucasian (nationality or race)

Cauc
Caucasian (nationality or race)

Cauc.
Caucasian (nationality or race)

Caud
caudal

CAV
congenital absence of vagina (gynecology)
congenital adrenal virilism (endocrinology)
cyclophosphamide, Adriamycin [doxorubicin], and vincristine (chemotherapy, oncology, and pharmacology)

cav
cavity (dentistry)

CAVB
complete atrioventricular block (cardiovascular)

CAVC
common arterioventricular canal (cardiovascular)

CAVD
completion, arithmetic problems, vocabulary, and following directions [a battery of intelligence tests] (psychiatry)

CAVE
CCNU [lomustine], Adriamycin [doxorubicin], and vinblastine (chemotherapy, oncology, and pharmacology)

CAVe
CCNU [lomustine], Adriamycin [doxorubicin], and vinblastine (chemotherapy, oncology, and pharmacology)

CAVH
continuous arteriovenous hemofiltration (nephrology)

CA virus
croup-associated virus (laboratory)

C(a-v)O$_2$
arteriovenous oxygen content difference (laboratory and respiratory)

CAVP
cyclophosphamide, Adriamycin, VM-26, and prednisone (chemotherapy, oncology, and pharmacology)

CAVP-I
cyclophosphamide, Adriamycin, vincristine, and prednisone (chemotherapy, oncology, and pharmacology)

CAVPM
cyclophosphamide, Adriamycin, VP-16, prednisone, and methotrexate (chemotherapy, oncology, and pharmacology)

CAWA
closing abductory wedge osteotomy (orthopedics and podiatry)

CB
carbenicillin (pharmacology)
catheterized bladder (urology)
ceased breathing
cesarean birth (obstetrics)
chair and bed
chest-back
Chirurgiae Baccalaureus [Bachelor of Surgery] (education and surgery)
chronic bronchitis (respiratory)
contrast baths (physical therapy and orthopedics)
code blue [emergency hospital code]

C.B.
Chirurgiae Baccalaureus [Bachelor of Surgery] (education and surgery)

C & B
crown and bridge (dentistry)

CB$_{11}$
phenadoxone hydrochloride [an analgesic and hypnotic] (chemistry and pharmacology)

CB 1348
{not an abbreviation} (chemotherapy, oncology, and pharmacology)

Cb
columbium [now called *niobium*] (chemistry)
complement (laboratory)

cb.
cardboard film holder without intensifying screens (radiology)
plastic film holder without intensifying screens (radiology)

CBA
chronic bronchitis and asthma (respiratory)
chronic bronchitis with asthma (respiratory)

CB agar
chocolate blood agar (laboratory)

CBC
carbenicillin (pharmacology)
complete blood count (laboratory)

C.B.C.
complete blood count (laboratory)

c.b.c.
complete blood count (laboratory)

CBD
closed bladder drainage (urology)
common bile duct (gastroenterology and surgery)

CBDE
common bile duct exploration (GE and surgery)

C.B.E.
Council of Biology Editors (biology and publishing)

CBF
capillary blood flow (cardiovascular)
cerebral blood flow (cardiovascular)
coronary blood flow (cardiovascular)
cortical blood flow (cardiovascular and urology)

CBFS
cerebral blood flow studies (cardiovascular and radiology)

CBFV
cerebral blood flow velocity (cardiovascular)

CBG
capillary blood gas (laboratory)
capillary blood glucose (laboratory)
corticosteroid-binding globulin [also called *transcortin*] (laboratory)
cortisol-binding globulin (laboratory)

CBI
close-binding-intimate (chemistry and laboratory)
continuous bladder irrigation (urology)

CBIP
Canter Background Interference Procedure [for Bender Gestalt test] (psychiatry)

CBIPBG
Canter Background Interference Procedure for Bender Gestalt [test] (psychiatry)

CBL
cord blood leukocytes [referring to umbilical cord] (neonatology, obstetrics, and pediatrics)

Cbl
cobalamin (chemistry and pharmacology)

CBMMP
chronic benign mucous membrane pemphigus (dentistry, dermatology, and otorhinolaryngology)

CBN
chronic benign neutropenia (hematology)
Commission on Biological Nomenclature (biology)

C.B.N.
Commission on Biological Nomenclature (biology)

CBOC
completion bed occupancy care

CBPPA
Cytoxan, bleomycin, procarbazine, pred-

nisone, and Adriamycin (chemotherapy, oncology, and pharmacology)

CBR
carotid bodies resected (cardiovascular)
chemical, biological, and radiological [warfare] (armed forces)
chronic bed rest
complete bed rest
crude birth rate (statistics)

C$_{BR}$
bilirubin clearance (gastroenterology and laboratory)

CBS
chronic brain syndrome (neurology)

C.B.S.
chronic brain syndrome (neurology)

CBV
central blood volume (cardiovascular)
circulating blood volume (cardiovascular)
corrected blood volume (cardiovascular)

CBW
chemical and biological warfare (armed forces)
critical bandwidth [of noise] (otorhinolaryngology)

CBZ
carbamazepine (pharmacology)

CBz
carbobenzoxychloride (chemistry)

CC
calcium cyclamate [also called *cyclamate calcium*; formerly used as a food sweetener] (chemistry)
cardiac catheterization (cardiovascular and radiology)
cardiac cycle (cardiovascular)
cerebral commissure (neurosurgery)
cerebral concussion (neurology)
chief complaint
chondrocalcinosis (orthopedics)
choriocarcinoma (oncology)
chronic complainer
circulatory collapse (cardiovascular)
classical conditioning

clean catch [urine] (laboratory)
clinical course
closing capacity (cardiovascular, laboratory, and respiratory)
coefficient of correlation (physics)
commission-certified [referring to stains] (laboratory)
compound cathartic (pharmacology)
computer-calculated
continuing care
coracoclavicular (orthopedics)
cord compression (neurology and orthopedics)
corpora cardiaca (anatomy)
corpus callosum (neurology)
costochondral (anatomy, cardiovascular, orthopedics, and respiratory)
craniocaudad [view] (radiology)
creatinine clearance (laboratory)
critical care
critical condition
cubic centimeter (measurement)
current complaints

C.C.
chief complaint

C-C
convexoconcave [heart valve] (cardiovascular)

C. C. 914
p-carbamindo-phenyl-bis (carboxymethyl-mercapto)arsine [a thioarsenite] (gastroenterology and pharmacology)

C. C. 1037
p-carbamindo-phenyl-bis (2-carboxyphenyl-mercapto)arsine [a thioarsenite] (laboratory)

Cc
concave

cc
carbon copy to (correspondence and medical records)
chest circumference (neonatology and pediatrics)
condylocephalic
cubic centimeter (measurement)

X   X
STORE: 0583   REG: 01/15   TRAN#: 0588
SALE   02/25/2005   EMP: 00236
****

replacement copies of the original item
Periodicals, newspapers, out-of-print, collectible and pre-owned items
may not be returned
Returned merchandise must be in saleable condition.
****

BORDERS®

Merchandise presented for return, including sale or marked-down items, must be accompanied by the original Borders store receipt. Returns must be completed within 30 days of purchase. The purchase price will be refunded in the medium of purchase (cash, credit card or gift card). Items purchased by check may be returned for cash after 10 business days.

Merchandise unaccompanied by the original Borders store receipt, or presented for return beyond 30 days from date of purchase, must be carried by Borders at the time of the return. The lowest price offered for the item during the 12 month period prior to the return will be refunded via a gift card.

Opened videos, discs, and cassettes may only be exchanged for replacement copies of the original item.
Periodicals, newspapers, out-of-print, collectible and pre-owned items may not be returned.
Returned merchandise must be in saleable condition.

BORDERS®

Merchandise presented for return, including sale or marked-down items, must be accompanied by the original Borders store receipt. Returns must be completed within 30 days of purchase. The purchase price will be refunded in the medium of purchase (cash, credit card or gift card). Items purchased by check may be returned for cash after 10 business days.

Merchandise unaccompanied by the original Borders store receipt, or presented for return beyond 30 days from date of purchase, must be carried by Borders at the time of the return. The lowest price offered for the item during the 12 month period prior to the return will be refunded

with correction (ophthalmology)
with spectacles (ophthalmology)

c̄c̄
with meals (pharmacology)

c̄ c
with correction (ophthalmology)

cc.
cubic centimeter (measurement)

c.c.
cubic centimeter (measurement)

CCA
cephalin cholesterol antigen (laboratory)
chick-cell agglutination [unit] (laboratory)
chimpanzee coryza agent [respiratory syncytial virus] (laboratory and respiratory)
circumflex coronary artery (cardiovascular)
common carotid artery (cardiovascular)

C-C-A
cytidyl-cytidyl-adenyl (chemistry and laboratory)

CCAP
capsule cartilage articular preservation (orthopedics)

CCAT
conglutinating complement absorption test (laboratory)

CCAVV
CCNU [lomustine], cyclophosphamide, Adriamycin, vincristine, and VP-16 (chemotherapy, oncology, and pharmacology)

CCB
calcium channel blocker(s) (pharmacology)

CCBB
Clinical Center Blood Bank (hematology)

CCBV
central circulating blood volume (cardiovascular)

CCC
calcium cyanamide [*carbimide*] citrated (chemistry)
cathodal closure contraction (cardiovascular)
chronic calculous cholecystitis (gastroenterology)
consecutive case conference
county counseling center (psychiatry)
continuing community care (psych)

C.C.C.
Commission on Clinical Chemistry (chemistry)

CC & C
colony count and culture (laboratory)

CCCC
centrifugal countercurrent chromatography (laboratory)

CCCl
cathodal closure clonus (cardiovascular and radiology)

CCCR
closed-chest cardiac resuscitation [also called *closed chest cardiopulmonary resuscitation*] (cardiovascular and respiratory)

CCD
calibration curve data (statistics)
charge-coupled device (scientific photography)

CCDC
Canadian Communicable Disease Center (infectious diseases)

CCDN
Central Council for District Nursing (nursing)

CCE
carboline-carboxylic acid ester (chemistry)
clear-cell carcinoma [of endothelium] (oncology)
clubbing, cyanosis, and edema (cardiovascular)
cyanosis, clubbing, and edema (cardiovascular)

CCF
cardiolipin complement fixation (cardiovascular and laboratory)
cephalin-cholesterol flocculation (laboratory)
compound comminuted fracture (orthopedics)
congestive cardiac failure (cardiovascular)
crystal-induced chemotactic factor (chemistry)

CCFA
cefoxitin cyclosterine fructose agar [medium] (laboratory)

CCFE
cyclophosphamide, cisplatin, fluorouracil, and estramustine (chemotherapy, oncology, and pharmacology)

CCG
cholecystogram (radiology)

CCHD
cyanotic congenital heart disease (cardiovascular)

CCHE
Central Council for Health Education (education)

CCHMS
Central Committee for Hospital Medical Services [British]

CCHP
Consumer Choice Health Plan (insurance)

CCHS
congenital central hypoventilation syndrome (genetics and respiratory)

CCI
chronic coronary insufficiency (cardiovascular)

CCJ
costochondral junction (cardiovascular, orthopedics, and respiratory)

CCK
cholecystokinin (laboratory)

CCK-179
{not an abbreviation} [methanesulfonate salts of equal parts of dihydroergocornine, dihydroergocristine, and dihydroergocryptine] (chemistry)

CCK-OP
cholecystokinin octapeptide (laboratory)

CCK-PZ
cholecystokinin-pancreozymin (laboratory)

CCL
carcinoma cell line (laboratory and oncology)
critical carbohydrate level (dietary and laboratory)

cc/l
cubic centimeter per liter (measurement)

CCM
cyclophosphamide, CCNU [lomustine], and methotrexate (chemotherapy, oncology, and pharmacology)

c. cm.
cubic centimeter (measurement)

CCMA
CCNU [lomustine], cyclophosphamide, methotrexate, and Adriamycin (chemotherapy, oncology, and pharmacology)

CCME
Coordinating Council of Medical Education (education)

CCMS
clean-catch midstream [urine specimen] (laboratory)

CCMSU
clean-catch midstream urine [specimen] (laboratory)

CCMT
catechol-*O*-methyl transferase (laboratory)

CCN
coronary care nursing (cardiovascular)

CCNS
cell cycle nonspecific [antitumor agent] (pharmacology)

C.C.N.S.C.
Cancer Chemotherapy National Service Center (oncology)

CCNU
1(2-chloroethyl)-3-(cyclohexyl)-1-nitrosourea [also called *CEENU, CeeNU,* and *lomustine*] (chemotherapy, oncology, and pharmacology)

CCNU-OP
lomustine [CCNU], Oncovin [vincristine], and prednisone (chemotherapy, oncology, and pharmacology)

CcO₂
oxygen content of pulmonary end-capillary blood (laboratory and respiratory)

CCOB
CCNU [lomustine], cyclophosphamide, Oncovin [vincristine], and bleomycin (chemotherapy, oncology, and pharmacology)

C-collar
cervical collar (neurology and orthopedics)

CCP
ciliocytophthoria (ophthalmology)

CCPD
continuous cyclical peritoneal dialysis (nephrology)
continuous cycling peritoneal dialysis (nephrology)

CCPDS
Centralized Cancer Patient Data System (oncology and research)

CCR
continuous complete remission (oncology)

C$_{CR}$
creatinine clearance (laboratory)

C$_{Cr}$
creatinine clearance (laboratory)

Ccr
creatinine clearance (laboratory)

C$_{cr}$
creatinine clearance (laboratory)

c.cr.
creatinine clearance (laboratory)

CCRN
Critical Care Registered Nurse (nursing)

C.C.R.N.
Critical Care Registered Nurse (nursing)

CCRU
critical care recovery unit

CCS
casualty clearing station
cell-cycle-specific [antitumor agent]
Clinical Sleep Society (neurology)
concentration camp syndrome (psychiatry)
Crippled Children's Society (pediatrics)

CC & S
cornea, conjunctiva, and sclera (ophthalmology)

CCT
chocolate-coated tablet (pharmacology)
clear, creamy layer at top (laboratory)
coated compressed tablet (pharmacology)
combined cortical thickness (radiology)
composite cyclic therapy
congenitally corrected transposition [of the great vessels] (cardiovascular)
controlled cord traction
coronary care team (cardiovascular)
cranial computerized tomography (radiology)

CCTe
cathodal closure tetanus (cardiovascular and radiology)

CCTGA
congenitally corrected transposition of the great arteries (cardiovascular)

CCT in PET
crude coal tar in petroleum (pharmacology)

C.C.T.P.
Coronary Care Training Project (cardiovascular)

CCTV
closed circuit television

CCU
cardiac care unit (cardiovascular)
Cherry-Crandall units
color changing unit(s)
community care unit
coronary care unit (cardiovascular)
critical care unit

CCUP
colpocystourethropexy (gynecology and urology)

CCV
CCNU [lomustine], cyclophosphamide, and vincristine (chemotherapy, oncology, and pharmacology)
conductivity cell volume (laboratory)

CCVB
CCNU [lomustine], cyclophosphamide, vincristine, and bleomycin (chemotherapy, oncology, and pharmacology)

CCVPP
cyclophosphamide, CCNU [lomustine], vinblastine, procarbazine, and prednisone (chemotherapy, oncology, and pharmacology)

CCVV
cyclophosphamide, CCNU [lomustine], VP-16, and vincristine (chemotherapy, oncology, and pharmacology)

CCVVP
cyclophosphamide, CCNU [lomustine], VP-16, vincristine, and cisplatin (chemotherapy, oncology, and pharmacology)

CCW
counterclockwise

CCX
complications

CD
cadaver donor (transplantation surgery)
canine distemper (infectious diseases and veterinary medicine)
carbonate dehydratase (chemistry)
cardiac disease (cardiovascular)
cardiac dullness (cardiovascular)
cardiovascular disease (cardiovascular)
Carrel-Dakin [fluid] (pharmacology)
caudal
cesarean-delivered (obstetrics)
cesarean delivery (obstetrics)
channel down (laboratory)
circular dichroism (physics)
civil defense (government)
colla dextra [with the right hand]
combination drug (pharmacology)
common duct (gastroenterology)
communicable disease (infectious diseases)
compact disk [player] (electronics)
completely denatured (chemistry)
conjugata diagonalis [diagonal conju-

gate diameter of the pelvic inlet] (obstetrics)
consanguineous donor (obstetrics)
contact dermatitis (allergy and dermatology)
contagious disease (infectious diseases)
continuous drainage (surgery)
control diet (dietary)
convulsive disorder (neurology)
convulsive dose (pharmacology)
Crohn's disease (gastroenterology)
curative dose (chemotherapy and radiation therapy)
cutdown (cardiovascular and surgery)
cystic duct (gastroenterology)

C.D.
conjugata diagonalis [diagonal conjugate] (obstetrics)
curative doses (pharmacology)

CD$_{50}$
median curative dose (chemotherapy and radiation therapy)

C.D.$_{50}$
median curative dose (chemotherapy and radiation therapy)

C/D
cigarettes per day
cup to disk [ratio] (ophthalmology)

C & D
curettage and desiccation (gynecology)
cystoscopy and dilatation (urology)

Cd
cadmium (chemistry)
caudal (orthopedics)
coccygeal (orthopedics)
drug coefficient (pharmacology)

^{115}Cd
radioactive cadmium (chemistry)

cd
candela (measurement and physics)

CDA
chenodeoxycholic acid [also called *chenodiol*] (chemistry)
completely denatured alcohol (chemistry and pharmacology)

congenital dyserythropoietic anemia (hematology and oncology)

CDAA
chlorodiallylacetamide (chemistry)

CDAI
Crohn's Disease Activity Index (gastroenterology)

CDB
cough, deep breath (respiratory)

C & DB
cough and deep breath (respiratory)
cough and deep breathe (respiratory)

CDC
calculated date of confinement (obstetrics)
Cancer Detection Center (oncology)
cell division cycle (laboratory)
Centers for Disease Control [formerly called *Communicable Disease Center*] (government and infectious diseases)
chenodeoxycholate (chemistry)
chenodeoxycholic acid (chemistry)

C.D.C.
Centers for Disease Control [formerly called *Communicable Disease Center*] (government and infectious diseases)

CD-C
controlled drinker—control (rehabilitation)

CDCA
chenodeoxycholic acid [also called *chenodiol*; used to dissolve gallstones] (chemistry, gastroenterology, and pharmacology)

CDD
certificate of disability for discharge
chronic disabling dermatosis (dermatology)

cystic fibrosis (respiratory)
{not an abbreviation} [chest and left leg electrode placement for an electrocardiogram] (cardiovascular)

C.F.
carbolfuchsin [stain] (laboratory)
citrovorum factor (laboratory)
count fingers (neurology and ophthalmology)

C & F
curettage and electrodesiccation [fulguration] (surgery)

Cf
californium (chemistry)
iron carrier (laboratory)

Cf.
carrier of ferrum [iron] (laboratory)

cf
compare
confer [bring together, confer with, refer to]
counting fingers (neurology and ophthalmology)
cystic fibrosis (respiratory)

cf.
compare
confer [bring together, confer with, refer to]

c.f.
count fingers (neurology and ophthalmology)
counting finger (neurology and ophthalmology)

c/f
colored female (nationality or race)

CFA
common femoral artery (cardiovascular)
complement-fixing antibody (laboratory)
complete Freund adjuvant (immunology, infectious diseases, and pharmacology)

CFAC
complement-fixing antibody consumption (laboratory)

C factor
{not an abbreviation} (laboratory)

C-factor
cleverness factor (psychiatry)

CFCCT
Committee for Freedom of Choice in Cancer Therapy (oncology)

CFD
Concern for the Dying (psychiatry)

CFF
critical flicker frequency [test] (cardiovascular)
critical flicker fusion [test] (cardiovascular)
critical fusion frequency [test]
Cystic Fibrosis Foundation (respiratory)

c.f.f.
critical fusion frequency [flicker fusion threshold] (cardiovascular)

Cf-Fe
carrier-bound iron (laboratory)

CFH
Council on Family Health

CFI
chemotactic factor inactivator (laboratory)
complement-fixation inhibition [test] (laboratory)

C fibers
{not an abbreviation} (neurology)

CFM
chlorofluoromethane [also called *fluorocarbon*] (chemistry)
close-fitting mask (respiratory)

cfm
cubic feet per minute (measurement)

CFMA
Council for Medical Affairs

CFMG
Commission on Foreign Medical Graduates

CFP
cerebrospinal fluid protein (laboratory and neurology)
chronic false-positive (laboratory)
cyclophosphamide, 5-fluorouracil, and prednisone (chemotherapy, oncology, and pharmacology)
cystic fibrosis of the pancreas (gastroenterology)
cystic fibrosis protein (laboratory)

CFR
case-fatality ratio (statistics)
citrovorum-factor rescue (laboratory)

CFS
cancer family syndrome (oncology)
contoured femoral stem [total hip prosthesis] (orthopedics)
Cystic Fibrosis Society (respiratory)
{not an abbreviation} [brand name for a total hip prosthesis] (orthopedics)
contoured femoral stem (orthopedics and surgery)

cfs
cubic feet per second (measurement)

CFSE
crystal field stabilization energy (physics)

CFSTI
Clearinghouse for Federal Scientific and Technical Information

C.F.S.T.I.
Clearinghouse for Federal Scientific and Technical Information

CFT
clinical full-time
complement-fixation test (laboratory)

C.F.T.
complement-fixation test (laboratory)

CF test
complement-fixation test (laboratory)

CFU
colony-forming units (laboratory)
color-forming units

CFU-C
colony-forming unit—culture (laboratory)

CFU-E
colony-forming unit—erythroid (laboratory)

CFU$_{EOS}$
colony-forming unit—eosinophil (laboratory)

CFU-GM
colony-forming unit—granulocyte macrophage (laboratory)

CFU-L
colony-forming unit—lymphoid (laboratory)

CFU-M
colony-forming unit—megakaryocyte (laboratory)

CFU$_{MEG}$
colony-forming unit—megakaryocyte (laboratory)

CFU$_{-mL}$
colony-forming unit per milliliter (laboratory)

CFU$_{NM}$
colony-forming unit—neutrophil-monocyte (laboratory)

CFU-S
colony-forming unit—spleen [hematopoietic] (laboratory)

CFWM
cancer-free white mouse (laboratory)
Carworth Farm mice [Webster strain] (research)

CFX
circumflex [coronary artery] (cardiovascular)

CG
Cardio-Green [trademark for preparation of indocyanine green dye] (cardiovascular and gastroenterology)
choking gas [phosgene] (chemistry)
cholecystogram (radiology)
chorionic gonadotropin (laboratory)
chronic glomerulonephritis (nephrology)
colloidal gold (chemotherapy, oncology, and pharmacology)
control group (research)
cryoglobulin (laboratory)
cystine guanine (laboratory)
{not an abbreviation} [trademark for preparation of indocyanine green dye] (cardiovascular and gastroenterology)

cg
center of gravity
centigram (measurement)
chemoglobulin (laboratory)

cg.
centigram (measurement)

CGB
chronic gastrointestinal [tract] bleeding (gastroenterology)

CGD
chronic granulomatous disease (respiratory)
commissural gastric driver (gastroenterology)

CGFNS
Commission on Graduates of Foreign Nursing Schools (nursing)

CGH
chorionic gonadotropic hormone (endocrinology and laboratory)

CGI
carbimazole (endocrinology and pharmacology)
clinical global impression
Clinical Global Impression [scale]

CGL
chronic granulocytic leukemia (hematology and oncology)
correction with glasses (ophthalmology)

c. gl.
correction with glasses (ophthalmology)

CGM
central gray matter [of spinal cord] (neurology)

cgm
centigram (measurement)

cgm.
centigram (measurement)

cGMP
cyclic guanosine monophosphate (chemistry)

CGN
chronic glomerulonephritis (nephrology)

CGNB
composite ganglioneuroblastoma (neurology)

CG/OQ
cerebral glucose oxygen quotient (neurology)

CGP
N-carbobenzoyl-glycyl-L-phenylalanine (chemistry)
choline glycerophosphatide (chemistry)
chorionic growth hormone prolactin (endocrinology and laboratory)
circulating granulocyte pool (laboratory)

CGRN
coarsely granular (laboratory)

CGS
catgut suture (surgery)

C.G.S.
centimeter-gram-second [system] (measurement)

cgs
centimeter-gram-second [system] (measurement)

c.g.s.
centimeter-gram-second [system] (measurement)

cgs system
centimeter-gram-second system (measurement)

CGS unit
centimeter-gram-second unit (measurement)

CGT
N-carbobenzoyl-a-glutamyl-L-tyrosine (chemistry)
chorionic gonadotropin (endocrinology and laboratory)

CGTT
cortisol glucose tolerance test (laboratory)
cortisone glucose tolerance test (laboratory)

cGy
centigray [new name for *rad*] (radiation therapy and radiology)

CH
Certified Herbalist
chest
chief
child
chirurgiae [surgery]
cholesterol (laboratory)
Christchurch chromosome (genetics and laboratory)
chronic
cluster headache (neurology)
convalescent hospital
crown-heel [length of fetus/infant] (neonatology and radiology)
wheelchair

C.H.
Community Health
crown-heel [length of fetus/infant] (neonatology and radiology)

C & H
cocaine and heroin (chemical dependency and pharmacology)

CH$_{50}$
total hemolytic complement (hematology and laboratory)

C'H$_{50}$
total hemolytic complement (hematology and laboratory)

Ch
chapter
check
chest
Chido [antibodies] (laboratory)
chief
child
choline (laboratory and pharmacology)

Ch'
Christchurch chromosome (genetics and laboratory)

Ch^1
Christchurch chromosome (genetics and laboratory)

cH
hydrogen ion concentration (chemistry)

ch
chronic

ch.
chest
chief
child
choline (laboratory and pharmacology)

μc.h.
microcurie-hour (measurement, radiation therapy, and radiology)

CHA
Catholic Hospital Association [of the United States]
chronic hemolytic anemia (hematology)
congenital hypoplastic anemia (hematology)

cyclohexyladenosine (chemistry)
cyclohexylamine (chemistry)

C.H.A.
Catholic Hospital Association

ChA
choline acetylase [also called *choline acetyltransferase*] (laboratory and neurology)

CHAD
cyclophosphamide, Adriamycin, cisplatin, and hexamethylmelamine (chemotherapy, oncology, and pharmacology)

CHAI
continuous hepatic artery infusion

CHAMPUS
Office of Civilian Health and Medical Programs of the Uniformed Services (armed forces, government, and insurance) {pronounced "cham-pus"}

C.H.A.M.P.U.S.
Office of Civilian Health and Medical Programs of the Uniformed Services (armed forces, government, and insurance) {pronounced "cham-pus"}

"cham-pus"
{pronunciation of *CHAMPUS* and *C.H.A.M.P.U.S.* [Office of Civilian Health and Medical Programs of the Uniformed Services]} (armed forces, government, and insurance) {not an abbreviation}

CHANCE
Coalition for Handicapped Children's Education (education)

CHAP
Certified Hospital Admission Program

chap
chapter

CHAP-S
cyclophosphamide, hexamethylmelamine, Adriamycin, and cisplatin

(chemotherapy, oncology, and pharmacology)

chart
charta [paper]

chart.
charta [paper]

chart bib
charta bibula [blotting paper]

chart cerat
charta cerata [waxed paper]

CHB
complete heart block (cardiovascular)

ChB
Chirurgiae Baccalaureus [Bachelor of Surgery] (education)

Ch.B.
Chirurgiae Baccalaureus [Bachelor of Surgery] (education)

CHBA
congenital Heinz body hemolytic anemia (hematology)

CHC
community health center
Community Health Computing
community health council

CHCA
Corresponding Health Care Associates

CH₃-CCNU
semustine (chemotherapy, oncology, and pharmacology)

CHCP
Correctional Health Care Program

CHD
Chediak-Higashi disease (genetics)
childhood disease(s) (pediatrics)
common hepatic duct (gastroenterology)

congenital heart disease (cardiovascular, neonatology, and pediatrics)
congestive heart disease (cardiovascular)
coronary heart disease (cardiovascular)
cyclophosphamide, hexamethylmelamine, and cisplatin (chemotherapy, oncology, and pharmacology)

ChD
Chirurgiae Doctor [Doctor of Surgery] (education)

Ch.D.
Chirurgiae Doctor [Doctor of Surgery] (education)

CHD-R
cyclophosphamide, hexamethylmelamine, and cisplatin plus radiotherapy (chemotherapy, oncology, pharmacology, and radiation therapy)

ChE
cholinesterase (laboratory)

CHEC
Community Hypertension Evaluation Clinic (cardiovascular)

CHEF
Chinese hamster embryo fibroblast(s) (laboratory)

CHEM
chemistry {pronounced "kem"}

Chem.
chemotherapy

chem
chemical (chemistry)
chemistry {pronounced "kem"}

chem.
chemistry {pronounced "kem"}

chemo.
chemotherapy {pronounced "khem-o"}

CHF
chick heart fibroblast (laboratory)
chronic heart failure (cardiovascular)
congestive heart failure (cardiovascular)

Crimean hemorrhagic fever [also called *Congo-Crimean hemorrhagic fever*] (hematology)

C.H.F.
congestive heart failure (cardiovascular)

CHFV
combined high frequency of ventilation (respiratory)

CHG
change

chg
change
charge

Ch GN
chronic glomerulonephritis (nephrology)

CHH
cartilage-hair hypoplasia (genetics)

CHI
closed head injury (emergency medicine and neurology)
creatinine height index (laboratory)

CHINS
child in need of service [petition] (pediatrics and social services)
children in need of service (pediatrics and social service)

CHIP
Comprehensive Health Insurance Plan (insurance)

Chir Doct
Chirurgiae Doctor [Doctor of Surgery] (education)

Chir. Doct.
Chirurgiae Doctor [Doctor of Surgery] (education)

CHL
chlorambucil (chemotherapy, oncology, and pharmacology)
chloramphenicol (pharmacology)

Chl
chloroform (pharmacology)

Chl.
chloroform (pharmacology)

CHLA
cyclohexyl linoleic acid (chemistry)

Chlb
chlorobutanol (pharmacology)

CHL + PRED
chlorambucil and prednisone (chemotherapy, oncology, and pharmacology)

ChM
Chirurgiae Magister [Master of Surgery]

Ch.M.
Chirurgiae Magister [Master of Surgery]

CHN
carbon, hydrogen, nitrogen (chemistry)
central hemorrhagic necrosis (hematology)
Child Neurology (neurology and pediatrics)

CHO
carbohydrate (chemistry, dietary, and laboratory)
cyclophosphamide, Adriamycin, and Oncovin (vincristine) (chemotherapy, oncology, and pharmacology)

Cho
choline (laboratory and pharmacology)

CHOB
cyclophosphamide, hydroxydaunorubicin [Adriamycin or doxorubicin], Oncovin (vincristine), and bleomycin (chemotherapy, oncology, and pharmacology)

Chol
cholesterol (dietary and laboratory)

chol
cholesterol (dietary and laboratory)

chol.
cholesterol (dietary and laboratory)

c̄ hold
withhold

CHOL E
cholesterol esters (laboratory)

chole
cholecystectomy (gastroenterology and surgery)

chol est
cholesterol esters (laboratory)

chol. est.
cholesterol esters (laboratory)

CHOP
cyclophosphamide (Cytoxan), hydroxydaunorubicin [doxorubicin or Adriamycin], vincristine [Oncovin], and prednisone (chemotherapy, oncology, and pharmacology) {pronounced "chop"}

"chop"
{pronunciation of *CHOP* [cyclophosphamide (Cytoxan), hydroxydaunorubicin (doxorubicin or Adriamycin), vincristine (Oncovin), and prednisone]} (chemotherapy, oncology, and pharmacology) {not an abbreviation}

CHOPBLEO
cyclophosphamide, hydroxydaunorubicin [doxorubicin or Adriamycin], vincristine [Oncovin], prednisone, and bleomycin (chemotherapy, oncology, and pharmacology)

CHOR
cyclophosphamide, hydroxydaunorubicin [doxorubicin or Adriamycin], vincristine, and radiotherapy (chemotherapy, oncology, pharmacology, and radiation therapy)

CHP
child psychiatry (pediatrics and psychiatry)
comprehensive health planning

ChP
Chest Physician (cardiovascular and respiratory)

CHPI
{not an abbreviation} [see *HPI* (see history of present illness)]

chpx.
chickenpox (infectious diseases and pediatrics)

CHR
cercarienhüllenreaktion (laboratory)

Chr
Chromobacterium (laboratory)

Chr.
Chromobacterium (laboratory)

μC hr.
microcurie-hour (measurement, radiation therapy, and radiology)

chr
chronic

chr.
chronic

c hr
candle hour (measurement)

c-hr.
curie-hour (measurement and radiology)

ChrBrSyn
chronic brain syndrome (neurology)

Chr. Etoh.
chronic ethanolism [also called *chronic alcoholism*] (chemical dependency)

chr etoh
chronic ethanolism [also called *chronic alcoholism*] (chemical dependency)

Chron
chronic
chronological

chron.
chronological

CHRS
congenital hereditary retinoschisis (ophthalmology)
cerebrohepatorenal syndrome (genetics, neurology, urology)

CHS
Chediak-Higashi syndrome (genetics)
cholinesterase (chemistry and laboratory)
compression hip screw [system] (orthopedics)

CHSD
Children's Health Services Division (pediatrics)

CHSS
Cooperative Health Statistics System (statistics)

CHT
closed head trauma (emergency medicine)

ChTg
chymotrypsinogen (laboratory)

ChTK
chicken thymidine kinase (laboratory)

CHU
closed head unit (neurology)

CHVP
cyclophosphamide, hydroxydaunorubicin [doxorubicin or Adriamycin], VM-26, and prednisone (chemotherapy, oncology, and pharmacology)

CI
cardiac index (cardiovascular)
cardiac insufficiency (cardiovascular)
cephalic index [on ultrasound] (obstetrics and radiology)
cerebral infarction (neurology)
cesium implant (oncology and radiation therapy)
chemotherapeutic index (chemotherapy)
clinical investigation

clonus index (neurology)
cochlear implant (otorhinolaryngology)
coefficient of intelligence (psychiatry)
colloidal iron (chemistry)
color index (hematology and laboratory)
complete iridectomy (ophthalmology)
confidence interval (statistic analysis)
contamination index (laboratory)
coronary insufficiency (cardiovascular)
corrected count increment (laboratory)
crystalline insulin (endocrinology and
　pharmacology)
cytotoxic index (pharmacology and radi-
　ation therapy)
first cranial nerve (neurology)

C.I.
color index (hematology and laboratory)
Colour Index [used in the dye industry]
　(manufacturing)

C_I
first cranial nerve (neurology)

Ci
curie(s) [per International Commission
　on Radiological Units and Measure-
　ments] (measurement, radiation ther-
　apy, and radiology)

ci
curie(s) (measurement, radiation ther-
　apy, and radiology)

CIA
CCNU [lomustine or CeeNU], isophos-
　phamide, and Adriamycin (chemo-
　therapy, oncology, and pharmacology)
Central Intelligence Agency (govern-
　ment)
chronic idiopathic anhidrosis (internal
　medicine)
chymotrypsin inhibitor activity (labora-
　tory)

CIAED
collagen-induced autoimmune ear dis-
　ease (immunology and otorhinolaryn-
　gology)

CIB
Carnation Instant Breakfast (dietary)
cytomegalic inclusion bodies (labora-
　tory)

cib
cibus [food]

cib.
cibus [food]

CIBA's
glutethimide [also called Doriden]
　(chemical dependency) {slang from
　manufacturer's name, Ciba Pharma-
　ceutical} {pronounced "sea-bahz"}

CIBD
chronic inflammatory bowel disease
　(gastroenterology)

CIBHA
congenital inclusion body hemolytic
　anemia (hematology)

CIC
cardiac inhibitory center (cardiovascu-
　lar)
circulating immune complexes (immu-
　nology and laboratory)

CICE
combined intracapsular cataract extrac-
　tion (ophthalmology)

CICS
Adriamycin, VM-26, cyclophosphamide,
　and prednisone (chemotherapy, oncol-
　ogy, and pharmacology)

CICU
cardiac intensive care unit (cardiovascu-
　lar)
cardiovascular inpatient care unit (car-
　diovascular)
coronary intensive care unit (cardiovas-
　cular)

CID
chick infective dose (laboratory)
cytomegalic inclusion disease (dermatol-
　ogy, gastroenterology, genetics, neu-
　rology, ophthalmology, otorhinolaryn-
　gology, and respiratory)

CIDP
chronic inflammatory demyelinating
polyradiculoneuropathy (neurology)

CIDS
cellular immunity deficiency syndrome
(immunology)
cellular immunodeficiency syndrome
(immunology)
continuous insulin delivery system (endocrinology and pharmacology)

CIE
countercurrent immunoelectrophoresis
(laboratory)

CIEP
counterimmunoelectrophoresis (laboratory)

CIF
cartilage induction factor (laboratory)
cloning inhibiting factor (laboratory)

CIFC
Council for the Investigation of Fertility
Control (obstetrics)

cIgM
cytoplasmic immunoglobulin M (laboratory)

CIH
carbohydrate-induced hyperglycer-
idemia (endocrinology)
Certificate in Industrial Health
Children in Hospitals (pediatrics)

Ci-hr.
curie-hour (measurement and radiology)

CII
controlled substance, class two (pharmacology)
second cranial nerve (neurology)

C$_{II}$
second cranial nerve (neurology)

CIII
third cranial nerve (neurology)

CIIS
Cattell Infant Intelligence Scale (pediatrics and psychiatry)

C.I.L.
Center for Independent Living (rehabilitation)

CIM
cortically induced movement (neurology)
Cumulated Index Medicus

CIN
cervical intraepithelial neoplasia [or
neoplasm] (gynecology and laboratory)
chronic interstitial nephritis (nephrology)

C$_{in}$
inulin clearance (laboratory)

CIOMS
Council for International Organizations
of Medical Sciences

C.I.O.M.S.
Council for International Organizations
of Medical Sciences

cir
circular

Circ
circuit
circular
circulatory
circumcised (urology)
circumcision (urology) {pronounced
"cirk" or "serk"}
circumference

circ
circumcision (urology) {pronounced
"cirk" or "serk"}

circ.
circulation
circumcision (urology) {pronounced
"cirk" or "serk"}

circum
circumcision (urology)

"cirk"
{pronunciation of *circ* [circumcision]}
    (surgery and urology) {not an abbreviation}

CIRM
Centro Internazionale Radio-Medico (radiology)

CIS
Cancer Information Service (oncology)
carcinoma in situ (oncology)
central inhibitory state (neurology)
Chemical Information System (chemistry)

CISCA
cisplatin, Cytoxan [cyclophosphamide],
    and Adriamycin [doxorubicin] (chemotherapy, oncology, and pharmacology)

cis-DDP
diamminedichloroplatinum [also called
    cisplatin] (chemotherapy, oncology,
    and pharmacology)

CIT
combined intermittent therapy
counselor-in-training (Girl Scouts)

cit
citrate (chemistry)

cit.
citrate (chemistry)

cito disp
cito dispensetur [dispense quickly]
    (pharmacology)

cito disp.
cito dispensetur [dispense quickly]
    (pharmacology)

CIU
chronic idiopathic urticaria (dermatology)

CIV
fourth cranial nerve (neurology)

CIX
ninth cranial nerve (neurology)

CIXU
constant infusion excretory urogram (radiology and urology)

CJD
Creutzfeldt-Jakob disease (neurology)

CJR
centric jaw relationship (dentistry and
    otorhinolaryngology)

CK
check
choline kinase (laboratory)
creatine kinase (laboratory)
cyanogen chloride [a fumigating gas]
    (chemistry)
cytokinin (laboratory)

CK$_1$
{not an abbreviation} [an isoenzyme of
    creatine kinase] (laboratory)

CK$_2$
{not an abbreviation} [an isoenzyme of
    creatine kinase] (laboratory)

CK$_3$
{not an abbreviation} [an isoenzyme of
    creatine kinase] (laboratory)

ck
check(ed)

ck.
check

CKC
cold knife conization (gynecology)

CK-MB
{not an abbreviation} [a creatine kinase isoenzyme] (laboratory)

CL
cholesterol-lecithin [test] (laboratory)
chronic leukemia (hematology and oncology)
clinical laboratory (laboratory)
corpus luteum (gynecology)
critical list
lung compliance (respiratory)
{not an abbreviation} [chest and left arm electrode placement for an electrocardiogram] (cardiovascular)

CL1
Papanicolaou class I (gynecology, laboratory, and pathology)

CL2
Papanicolaou class II (gynecology, laboratory, and pathology)

CL3
Papanicolaou class III (gynecology, laboratory, and pathology)

CL4
Papanicolaou class IV (gynecology, laboratory, and pathology)

CL5
Papanicolaou class V (gynecology, laboratory, and pathology)

Cl
chloride (chemistry)
chlorine (chemistry and laboratory)
clavicle (orthopedics)
clinic
Clostridium (laboratory)
closure
colistin [an antibiotic] (pharmacology)

cl
centiliter (measurement)
clear (laboratory)

cl.
centiliter (measurement)
cloudy (laboratory)

CLA
cervicolinguoaxial (dentistry)
community living arrangements
cyclic lysine anhydride (chemistry)

C.L.A.
Certified Laboratory Assistant (laboratory)

C.L.A.(ASCP)
Clinical Laboratory Assistant (American Society of Clinical Pathologists) (laboratory)

ClAc
chloroacetyl (chemistry)

C lam
cervical laminectomy (neurology and orthopedics) {pronounced "see lam"}

CLAS
congenital localized absence of skin (genetics and neonatology)

class
classification

Clav
clavicle (orthopedics)

CLB
chlorambucil (chemotherapy, oncology, and pharmacology)

CLBBB
complete left bundle-branch block (cardiovascular)

CL. botulinum
Clostridium botulinum (bacteriology and laboratory)

CLC
cork leather and celastic [orthotic] (orthopedics)

CL/CP
cleft lip and cleft palate (neonatology
and plastic surgery)

CLD
chronic liver disease (gastroenterology)
chronic lung disease (respiratory)

CLDY
cloudy (laboratory)

cldy
cloudy (laboratory)

cldy.
cloudy (laboratory)

CLE
centrilobular emphysema (respiratory)

CLED
cystine-lactose electrolyte deficient (laboratory)

CLER
clear (laboratory)

CLF
cholesterol-lecithin flocculation (laboratory)

CLH
chronic lobular hepatitis (gastroenterology)

Clin
clinic
clinical

clin.
clinic
clinical

clini
Clinitest (endocrinology and laboratory)

Clin path
clinical pathology

Clin proc
clinical procedure(s)

CLIP
corticotropin-like intermediate lobe
peptide (laboratory)

CLL
cholesterol-lowering lipid (laboratory)
chronic lymphatic leukemia (hematology and oncology)
chronic lymphocytic leukemia (hematology and oncology)

CLLE
columnar-lined lower esophagus (gastroenterology)

cl liq
clear liquid (dietary)

CL LYS
clot lysis (hematology)

C.L.M.A.
Clinical Laboratory Management Association (laboratory)

CLML
Current List of Medical Literature (publishing)

CLMN
complete lower motor neuron [lesion]
(neurology)

CLMP
clumped (laboratory)

CLO
close
cod liver oil (pharmacology)

Clon
Clonorchis [a liver fluke] (gastroenterology and laboratory)

CLOT R
clot retraction (hematology)

CL & P
cleft lip and palate (neonatology and
plastic surgery)

CIP
clinical pathology

cl pal
cleft palate (genetics and otorhinolaryngology)

CLR
chloride test (dentistry)

C.L.S.
Clinical Laboratory Scientist (laboratory)

CLSL
chronic lymphosarcoma [cell] leukemia (hematology and oncology)

CLT
chronic lymphocytic thyroiditis (endocrinology)
clot-lysis time (laboratory)
clotted (laboratory)
total lung compliance (respiratory)

CL VOID
clean voided [specimen] (laboratory)

Clysis
hypodermoclysis [fluid replacement] (pharmacology)

clysis
hypodermoclysis [fluid replacement] (pharmacology)

CM
California mastitis [test] (gynecology)
capreomycin (pharmacology)
carboxymethyl cellulose (chemistry)
cardiac monitor (cardiovascular)
cardiomyopathy (cardiovascular)
Caucasian male (race)
centimeter (measurement)
Chick-Martin [coefficient or method] (ecology and laboratory)
Chirurgiae Magister [Master in Surgery] (education)
chloroquine-mepacrine (pharmacology)
chondromalacia (orthopedics)
chopped meat [medium] (laboratory)
circular muscle (orthopedics)
cochlear microphonic(s) (otorhinolaryngology)

common migraine (neurology)
complete medium (laboratory and microbiology)
complications
congenital malformation (genetics and neonatology)
congestive myocardiopathy (cardiovascular)
continuous murmur (cardiovascular)
contrast media (radiology)
copulatory mechanism (gynecology, obstetrics, and urology)
costal margin (anatomy)
cow's milk (dietary)
culture media (laboratory)

C.M.
Chirurgiae Magister [Master in Surgery] (education)

C & M
cocaine and morphine mixed (pharmacology)

Cm
capreomycin [an antibiotic] (pharmacology)
curium (chemistry)

C_m
maximum clearance [referring to urea clearance] (laboratory)

cm
centimeter (measurement)
costal margin (anatomy)
cras mane [tomorrow morning]

cm.
centimeter (measurement)

c.m.
costal margin (anatomy)
cras mane [tomorrow morning] (pharmacology)

cm²
square centimeter (measurement)

cm³
cubic centimeter (measurement)

CMA
Canadian Medical Association
Certified Medical Assistant

C.M.A.
Canadian Medical Association
Certified Medical Assistant

CMB
carbolic methylene blue [an indicator and stain] (chemistry, hematology, laboratory, and pharmacology)
Central Midwives' Board (nursing)
p-chloromercuribenzoate (chemistry and laboratory)

CMBBT
cervical mucous basal body temperature (gynecology and obstetrics)

CMC
carboxymethyl cellulose (chemistry)
carpometacarpal (orthopedics and podiatry)
cell-mediated cytolysis (laboratory)
chloramphenicol (pharmacology)
chronic mucocutaneous moniliasis (dermatology, gynecology, otorhinolaryngology, and respiratory)
Consolidated Midland Corporation (pharmacology)
cyclophosphamide, methotrexate, and CCNU [CeeNU or lomustine] (chemotherapy, oncology, and pharmacology)

cmc.
critical micelle concentration (laboratory)

CM-cellulose
carboxymethylcellulose (chemistry)

CMC-high dose
cyclophosphamide, methotrexate, and CCNU [CeeNU or lomustine] (chemotherapy, oncology, and pharmacology)

CMD
childhood muscular dystrophy (neurology and pediatrics)
count median diameter [of particles] (chemistry, laboratory, and physics)

CME
continuing medical education (education)
crude marijuana extract (chemical dependency, chemistry, laboratory, and pharmacology)
cystic macular edema (ophthalmology)
cystoid macular edema (ophthalmology)

CME(AMA)
Council on Medical Education of the American Medical Association (education)

CMF
chondromyxoid fibroma (neurology and orthopedics)
Christian Medical Fellowship [British]
cortical magnification factor
cyclophosphamide [Cytoxan], methotrexate, and 5-fluorouracil (chemotherapy, oncology, and pharmacology)

CMF-BLEO
cyclophosphamide [Cytoxan], methotrexate, 5-fluorouracil, and bleomycin (chemotherapy, oncology, and pharmacology)

CMF-FLU
cyclophosphamide [Cytoxan], methotrexate, 5-fluorouracil, and fluoxymesterone (chemotherapy, oncology, and pharmacology)

CMFH
cyclophosphamide [Cytoxan], methotrexate, 5-fluorouracil, and hydroxyurea (chemotherapy, oncology, and pharmacology)

CMFP
cyclophosphamide [Cytoxan], methotrexate, 5-fluorouracil, and prednisone (chemotherapy, oncology, and pharmacology)

CMFVP
cyclophosphamide, methotrexate, 5-fluorouracil, vincristine, and prednisone [also called *Cooper's Regimen*] (che-

motherapy, oncology, and pharmacology)

CMFP-VA
cyclophosphamide, methotrexate, 5-fluorouracil, prednisone, vincristine, and Adriamycin (chemotherapy, oncology, and pharmacology)

CMF-TAM
cyclophosphamide [Cytoxan], methotrexate, 5-fluorouracil, and tamoxifen (chemotherapy, oncology, and pharmacology)

CMFV
cyclophosphamide [Cytoxan], methotrexate, 5-fluorouracil, and vincristine (chemotherapy, oncology, and pharmacology)

CMFVP
cyclophosphamide [Cytoxan], methotrexate, 5-fluorouracil, vincristine, and prednisone (chemotherapy, oncology, and pharmacology)

CMG
chopped meat glucose [agar] (laboratory)
cystometrogram (radiology and urology)

CMGN
chronic membranous glomerulonephritis (nephrology)

CMH
congenital malformation of heart (cardiovascular)

CMHC
community mental health center (psychiatry)

CMHN
Community Mental Health Nurse (psychiatry)

CmH₂O
centimeters of water [cuff pressure (blood pressure cuff or tourniquet)] (measurement, cardiovascular, and surgery)

CMI
carbohydrate metabolism index (laboratory)
cell-mediated immunity (laboratory)
chronic mesenteric ischemia (gastroenterology)
Commonwealth Mycological Institute
Cornell Medical Index

CMID
cytomegalic inclusion disease (dermatology, gastroenterology, genetics, neurology, ophthalmology, otorhinolaryngology, and respiratory)

c/min
cycles per minute (measurement)

c./min.
cycles per minute (measurement)

CMIT
Current Medical Information and Technology

CMJ
carpometacarpal joint (orthopedics)
Committee on Medical Journalism (publishing)

CMK
chloromethyl ketone (laboratory)
congenital multicystic kidney (nephrology)

CML
cell-mediated lympholysis [also called *cell-mediated lymphocytolysis*] (laboratory)
chronic myelocytic leukemia (hematology and oncology)
chronic myelogenous leukemia (hematology and oncology)

CMM
cutaneous malignant melanoma (oncology)

cmm
cubic millimeter (measurement)

c.mm.
cubic millimeter (measurement)

c.mm./s.
cubic millimeters per second (measurement)

CMMT
Columbia Mental Maturity Test (psychiatry)

CMN
cystic medial necrosis [of aorta] (cardiovascular)

CMN-AA
cystic medial necrosis of the ascending aorta (cardiovascular)

CMO
cardiac minute output (cardiovascular)
Chief Medical Officer (administration and armed forces)
comfort measures only [meaning no heroic or resuscitative measures are to be used] (cardiovascular and respiratory)
corticosterone methyl oxidase (laboratory)

C.M.O.
Chief Medical Officer (administration and armed forces)

cMo.
centimorgan (measurement)

CMoL
chronic monoblastic leukemia (hematology and oncology)
chronic monocytic leukemia (hematology and oncology)

C-MOPP
cyclophosphamide, nitrogen mustard, vincristine [Oncovin], procarbazine, and prednisone (chemotherapy, oncology, and pharmacology)

"C" MOPP
cyclophosphamide, Oncovin [vincristine], procarbazine, and prednisone [also called COPP] (chemotherapy, oncology, and pharmacology)

CMOR
craniomandibular orthopedic repositioning device (dentistry, oral surgery, and orthopedics)

CMOS
complementary metal oxide semiconductor [logic] (computer science)

CMP
cardiomyopathy (cardiovascular)
CCNU [CeeNU or lomustine], methotrexate, and procarbazine (chemotherapy, oncology, and pharmacology)
chondromalacia patellae (orthopedics)
Competitive Medical Plans (insurance)
Comprehensive Medical Plan (insurance)
cytidine monophosphate (chemistry)
cytidine-5'-phosphate (chemistry)

cmp'd.
compound (chemistry and laboratory)

CMPF
cyclophosphamide, methotrexate, prednisone, and 5-fluorouracil (chemotherapy, oncology, and pharmacology)

CMP-FX
complement fixation (laboratory)

CMR
cerebral metabolic rate (laboratory)
crude mortality ratio (chemotherapy, radiation therapy, and statistics)

C.M.R.
cerebral metabolic rate (laboratory)
Certified Medical Representative

CMRG
cerebral metabolic rate of glucose (laboratory)

CMRNG
chromosomally resistant *Neisseria gonorrhoeae* (laboratory)

CMRO
cerebral metabolic rate of oxygen (laboratory)

CMRO$_2$
cerebral metabolic rate for oxygen (laboratory)

CMRR
common mode rejection ratio [of amplifiers]

CMS
central material section
central material supply
cervical mucous solution (gynecology)
Christian Medical Society
chromosome modification site (genetics and laboratory)
circulation, motion, and sensation (orthopedics and physical therapy)
circulation, muscle sensation (orthopedics and physical therapy)
circulatory, musculatory, and sensory (orthopedics and physical therapy)
click murmur syndrome (cardiovascular)
Clyde Mood Scale (psychiatry)
Conflict Management Survey (psychiatry)
conversational monitor system (computer science)

cms
cras mane sumendus [to be taken tomorrow morning] (pharmacology)

c.m.s.
cras mane sumendus [to be taken tomorrow morning] (pharmacology)

cm/s
centimeter per second (measurement)

CMSS
circulation, motor ability, sensation, and swelling (orthopedics and physical therapy)
Council of Medical Specialty Societies

CMSUA
clean midstream urinalysis (laboratory)

CMT
California mastitis test (gynecology and laboratory)
catechol-*O*-methyl transferase (laboratory)
Certified Medical Transcriptionist (medical records)
cervical motion tenderness
Council on Medical Television
current medical terminology

C.M.T.
Certified Medical Transcriptionist (medical records)

CMU
chlorophenyldimethylurea (chemistry)

CMV
cool mist vaporizer (respiratory)
continuous mechanical ventilation (respiratory)
controlled mechanical ventilation (respiratory)
cytomegalovirus (laboratory)

CN
caudate nucleus (neurology)
cellulose nitrate (chemistry)
charge nurse (nursing)
child nutrition (dietary)
chloroacetophenone (chemistry)
clinical nursing (nursing)
cochlear nucleus [of brain] (neurology)
cranial nerve(s) (neurology)
cyanide anion (chemistry)
cyanogen radical (chemistry)

C.N.
cras nocte [tomorrow night] (pharmacology)

C/N
carbon to nitrogen [ratio] (chemistry and laboratory)

Cn
cyanide (chemistry and pharmacology)

c.n.
cras nocte [tomorrow night] (pharmacology)

CNA
chart not available
Canadian Nurses' Association (nursing)

C.N.A.
Canadian Nurses' Association (nursing)

CNB
cutting needle biopsy (surgery)

CNC
clear, no creamy layer (laboratory)

C.N.C.
Critical Nursing Conference (nursing)

CNE
chronic nervous exhaustion (neurology and psychiatry)

CNF
cyclophosphamide, mitoxantrone, and fluorouracil (chemotherapy, oncology, and pharmacology)

CNH
central neurogenic hyperpnea (neurology and respiratory)
community nursing home
contract nursing home

CNHD
congenital nonspherocytic hemolytic disease (hematology and oncology)

C.N.H.I.
Committee for National Health Insurance (insurance)

CN II-XII
cranial nerves II through XII (neurology and orthopedics)

CNL
cardiolipin natural lecithin (laboratory)

CNM
Certified Nurse-Midwife (obstetrics)

C.N.M.
Certified Nurse-Midwife (obstetrics)

CNMT
Certified Nuclear Medicine Technologist (radiology)

C.N.M.T.
Certified Nuclear Medicine Technologist (radiology)

CNP
continuous negative pressure

CNR
Civil Nursing Reserve (nursing)
Council of National Representatives [of International Council of Nurses] (nursing)

CNS
central nervous system (neurology)
Chief, Nursing Services (nursing)
clinical nurse specialist (nursing)
sulfocyanate (chemistry)

C.N.S.
central nervous system (neurology)

cns
cras nocte sumendus [to be taken tomorrow night] (pharmacology)

c.n.s.
cras nocte sumendus [to be taken tomorrow night] (pharmacology)

CNSHA
congenital nonspherocytic hemolytic leukemia (hematology and oncology)

CNT
could not test (laboratory)

CNV
colistimethate, nystatin, vancomycin (pharmacology)
conative negative variation
contigent negative variation

CO

carbon monoxide (chemistry, laboratory, and respiratory)
cardiac output (cardiovascular)
castor oil (pharmacology)
casualty officer (armed forces and emergency medicine)
centric occlusion (cardiovascular)
cervicoaxial (dentistry)
choline oxidase (chemistry and laboratory)
coenzyme (laboratory)
Colorado [Postal Service state designa-
tion]
compound
corneal opacity (ophthalmology)
corpus [referring to uterus] (gynecology
and obstetrics)
crossover(s) (genetics)

C/O

care of
check out
complained of
complains of
complaints
in care of [Postal Service]
under care of

C.O.

cardiac output (cardiovascular)

CO₂

carbon dioxide (chemistry, laboratory,
and respiratory)

Co

cobalt (chemistry, radiation therapy,
and radiology)
coenzyme (laboratory)

⁶⁰Co

radioactive cobalt (chemistry, radiation
therapy, and radiology)

co

company
compositus [compound] (pharmacology)
compounded

co.

company
compositus [compound] (pharmacology)
compounded

c/o

complaint of
in care of [Postal Service]

C.O.A.

Canadian Orthopaedic Association (orthopedics)

CoA

coarctation of the aorta (cardiovascular,
neonatology, and pediatrics)
coenzyme A (laboratory)

COAD

chronic obstructive airway disease (respiratory)
chronic obstructive arterial disease (cardiovascular)

COAG

chronic open-angle glaucoma (ophthalmology)

coag

coagulation (hematology and laboratory) {pronounced "co-ag"}
coagulate (hematology and laboratory)
{pronounced "co-ag"}

coag.

coagulation (hematology and laboratory) {pronounced "co-ag"}
coagulate (hematology and laboratory)
{pronounced "co-ag"}

"co-ag"

{pronunciation of coag and coag. [coagu-
lation and coagulate]} (hematology
and laboratory) {not an abbreviation}

COAG PD

coagulation profile—diagnosis (hematology and laboratory)

COAG PP

coagulation profile—presurgery (hematology and laboratory)

COAP

cyclophosphamide, vincristine, cytara-

bine [cytosine arabinoside], and prednisone (chemotherapy, oncology, and
pharmacology)

COAP-BLEO
cyclophosphamide, vincristine, cytarabine [cytosine arabinoside], prednisone, and bleomycin (chemotherapy,
oncology, and pharmacology)

coarc
coarctation [of aorta] (cardiovascular,
neonatology, and pediatrics) {pro-
nounced "co-ark"}

"co-ark"
{pronunciation of *coarc* [coarctation (of
aorta)]} (cardiovascular, neonatology,
and pediatrics) {not an abbreviation}

COB
cisplatin, Oncovin [vincristine], and
bleomycin (chemotherapy, oncology,
and pharmacology)

$^{60}CoB_{12}$
radioactive cobalt-labeled cyanobalamin
(chemistry and radiology)

"co-ball"
{pronunciation of *COBOL* [common
business oriented language (computer
language)} (computer science) {not an
abbreviation}

COBOL
common business oriented language
[computer language] (computer science) {pronounced "co-ball"}

COBS
cesarean-obtained barrier-sustained (obstetrics)

COBT
chronic obstruction of biliary tract (gastroenterology)

COC
cathodal opening clonus (cardiovascular)
cathodal opening contraction (cardiovascular)
coccygeal (orthopedics)

combination-type oral contraceptive
(gynecology and pharmacology)

COCAIN
cocaine (anesthesiology, chemical dependency, laboratory, and pharmacology)

cocci
coccidioidomycosis (laboratory) {pro-
nounced "cock-see" or "kok-see}

coch
cochlear [a spoonful, by spoonfuls,
cochleare, cochleatum] (pharmacology)

coch amp
cochleare amplum [a heaping spoonful]
(pharmacology)

cochl.
cochleare [a spoonful] (pharmacology)

cochl. amp.
cochleare amplum [a heaping spoonful]
(pharmacology)

cochleat
cochlear [a spoonful, by spoonfuls,
cochleare, cochleatum] (pharmacology)

cochl. mag.
cochleare magnum [a tablespoonful]
(pharmacology)

cochl. med.
cochleare medium [a dessert spoonful]
(pharmacology)

cochl. parv.
cochleare parvum [a teaspoonful]
(pharmacology)

coch mag
cochleare magnum [a tablespoonful]
(pharmacology)

---

coch med
cochleare medium [a dessert spoonful] (pharmacology)

coch parv
cochleare parvum [a teaspoonful] (pharmacology)

COCI
Consortium on Chemical Information [British] (chemistry)

"cock-see"
{pronunciation of *cocci* [coccidioidomycosis]} (laboratory) {not an abbreviation}

COCL
cathodal opening clonus (cardiovascular)

COCl
cathodal opening clonus (cardiovascular)

coct.
coctio [boiling] (pharmacology)

COD
cause of death
chemical oxygen demand (chemistry)
codeine (pharmacology)
condition on discharge
Council of Deans (education)

cod
codeine (pharmacology)

cod.
codeine (pharmacology)

code 2
{not an abbreviation} [refers to code for urgent transport without lights and siren] (emergency medicine)

code 3
{not an abbreviation} [refers to code for emergency transport with lights and siren] (emergency medicine)

CODEIN
codeine (pharmacology)

COEAMRA
Council on Education of the American Medical Record Association (education and medical records)

coeff
coefficient (mathematics)

COEPS
cortically originating extrapyramidal symptoms (neurology)
cortically originating extrapyramidal system (neurology)

CoF
cobra factor (laboratory)
cofactor (laboratory)

C of A
coarctation of the aorta (cardiovascular, neonatology, and pediatrics)

COG
Central Oncology Group (oncology)
cognitive [function tests] (neurology and psychiatry)

COGTT
cortisone-primed oral glucose tolerance test (endocrinology and laboratory)

COH
carbohydrate (dietary and laboratory)

COHB
carboxyhemoglobin [also called *carbonmonoxyhemoglobin*] (hematology and laboratory)

COHb
carboxyhemoglobin [also called *carbonmonoxyhemoglobin*] (hematology and laboratory)

CoI
coenzyme I [nicotinamide adenine dinucleotide; also called *diphosphopyridine nucleotide* (*DPN*)] (laboratory)

Co I
coenzyme I [nicotinamide adenine dinu-
cleotide] also called *diphosphopyridine nucleotide (DPN)*] (laboratory)

CoII
coenzyme II [nicotinamide adenine dinucleotide phosphate; also called *triphosphopyridine nucleotide (TPN)*]
(laboratory)

Co II
coenzyme II [nicotinamide adenine dinucleotide phosphate; also called *triphosphopyridine nucleotide (TPN)*]
(laboratory)

Coke
Coca-Cola [trademark name] {not an ab-
breviation}
cocaine (chemical dependency and
pharmacology)

Col
colony [or colonies] (bacteriology and
laboratory)

col
cola [strain] (pharmacology)
colony [or colonies] (bacteriology and
laboratory)
colored
column

col.
cola [strain] (pharmacology)
colony (bacteriology and laboratory)
colored
column

colat
colatus [strained] (pharmacology)

colat.
colatus [strained] (pharmacology)

COLD
chronic obstructive lung disease [Do not
confuse with the *common cold*] (respiratory) {pronounced "cold"}

"cold"
{pronunciation of *COLD* [chronic ob-

structive lung disease]} (respiratory)
{not an abbreviation}

COLD A
cold agglutinin titer (laboratory)

COLDAG
cold agglutinins (laboratory) {pro-
nounced "cold-ag"}

"cold-ag"
{pronunciation of *COLDAG* [cold agglu-
tinins]} (laboratory) {not an abbrevia-
tion}

colen
colentur [let them be strained] (pharmacology)

colet
coletur [let it be strained] (pharmacology)

colet.
coletur [let it be strained] (pharmacology)

coll
collect(ion)
college (education)
colloidal (chemistry, laboratory, and
pharmacology)
collyrium [eyewash] (pharmacology)
colorless (laboratory)

coll.
collyrium [eyewash] (pharmacology)

colat
collateral

collun
collunarium [nose wash] (pharmacology)

collun.
collunarium [nose wash] (pharmacology)

collut
collutorium [mouthwash] (pharmacology)

collut.
collutorium [mouthwash] (pharmacology)

coll vol
collective volume

collyr
collyrium [eyewash] (pharmacology)

collyr.
collyrium [eyewash] (pharmacology)

col/ml
colonies per milliliter (laboratory and measurement)

color.
coloretur [let it be colored] (pharmacology)
colorimetry [including spectrophotometry and photometry] (chemistry and laboratory)

colpo
colposcopy (gynecology)

COM
College of Osteopathic Medicine (osteopathic medicine)
cyclophosphamide, Oncovin [vincristine], and MeCCNU [methyl-CCNU or semustine] (chemotherapy, oncology, and pharmacology)

C.O.M.
College of Osteopathic Medicine (osteopathic medicine)

COM3
coma level greater than 400 milligrams per liter (laboratory, pharmacology, and radiology)

COMA-A
cyclophosphamide, Oncovin [vincristine], methotrexate, Adriamycin, citrovorum factor, and cytosine arabinoside [ara-C or cytarabine] (chemotherapy, oncology, and pharmacology)

COMB
cyclophosphamide, Oncovin [vincristine], MeCCNU [methyl-CCNU or se-mustine], and bleomycin (chemotherapy, oncology, and pharmacology)

COMBAP
Cytoxan [cyclophosphamide], Oncovin [vincristine], methotrexate, bleomycin, Adriamycin, and prednisone (chemotherapy, oncology, and pharmacology)

COMe
Cytoxan [cyclophosphamide], Oncovin [vincristine], and methotrexate (chemotherapy, oncology, and pharmacology)

COMF
cyclophosphamide, Oncovin [vincristine], methotrexate, and 5-fluorouracil (chemotherapy, oncology, and pharmacology)

com fix
complement fixation (laboratory)

COMLA
cyclophosphamide [Cytoxan], Oncovin [vincristine], methotrexate, ara-C [cytarabine] (chemotherapy, oncology, and pharmacology)

commun dis
communicable disease (infectious diseases)

COMP
complications
compound
cyclophosphamide, Oncovin [vincristine], methotrexate, and procarbazine (chemotherapy, oncology, and pharmacology)

comp
compare
compensated
complaint
composition
compositus [compound, compounded of] (pharmacology)

comp.
compare
compensated
complaint
composition
compositus [compound] (pharmacology)

Comp A
compound A [also called *11-dehy-drocorticosterone*] (pharmacology)

Comp B
compound B [also called *corticosterone*] (pharmacology)

Comp case
compensation case [referring to Worker's Compensation]

compd
compound

Comp E
compound E [also called *cortisone*] (pharmacology)

Comp F
compound F [also called *cortisol* or *hydrocortisone*] (pharmacology)

compl
completed
complement (laboratory)
complications

COMPLEX
Committee on Lunar and Planetary Exploration (aerospace science)

Complic
complications

compn
composition

COMPS
compound S [also called *11-deoxycortisol*] (pharmacology)

COMT
catechol-*O*-methyl transferase (chemistry and laboratory)
Certified Ophthalmic Medical Assistant (ophthalmology)

COMTRAC
computer-based case tracing (computer science and medical records)

CON
certificate of need

con
contra [against]

con.
contra [against]

CON A
concanavalin A (laboratory)

ConA
concanavalin A (laboratory)

CONC
concentrated
concentration

conc
concentrated
concentration

conc.
concentrated
concentration

concentr
concentrated

concis
concisus [cut]

concis.
concisus [cut]

cond
condensed
condition(s)
conditional
conductivity

cond.
condensed
condition(s)
conditional
conductivity

cond ref
conditioned reflex (neurology and psychiatry)

cond resp
conditioned response (neurology and
psychiatry)

cone
conization [of cervix] (gynecology) {pro-
nounced "cone"}

"cone"
{pronunciation of *cone* [conization (of
cervix)]} (gynecology) {not an abbrevi-
ation}

conf
confectio [confection]
conference
confirmed (laboratory)

conf.
confectio [confection]
conference

config.
configuration

CONG
congenital
congius [gallon]

cong
congenital (genetics)
congius [gallon] (measurement)

cong.
congius [gallon] (measurement)

congen
congenital (genetics) {pronounced "con-
gen"}

"con-gen"
{pronunciation of *congen* [congenital]}
(genetics) {not an abbreviation}

CO(NH₂)₂
urea (chemistry and laboratory)

coniz
conization (gynecology)

conj
conjunctiva (ophthalmology)

conjunc
conjunctiva (ophthalmology)

CONPADRI I
cyclophosphamide, vincristine, doxorubicin, and melphalan (chemotherapy,
oncology, and pharmacology)

CONPADRI II
cyclophosphamide, vincristine, doxorubicin, melphalan, and high dose methotrexate (chemotherapy, oncology,
and pharmacology)

CONPADRI III
cyclophosphamide, vincristine, doxorubicin, melphalan, and intensified
doxorubicin (chemotherapy, oncology, and pharmacology)

CONPADRI-V
cyclophosphamide, vincristine, melphalan, Adriamycin, and methotrexate
(chemotherapy, oncology, and pharmacology)

Cons
consultant
consultation
consulting

cons
conserva [keep]
consonans [tinkling]

cons.
conserva [keep]

consperg
consperge [dust, sprinkle] (pharmacology)

const
constant

constit
constituent
constitution(al)

CONT
continuous

CON'T
continue(d)

cont
containing
contents
continue(d)
continuously
contra [against]
contusus [bruised]

cont.
containing
contents
continue(d)
continuously
contra [against]
contusus [bruised]

contag
contagious (infectious diseases)

conter
contere [rub together]

contg
containing

contin
continuetur [let it be continued] (pharmacology)

contin.
continue
continued
continuetur [let it be continued] (pharmacology)

contr
contraction (neurology, obstetrics, and orthopedics)

contra
contraindicated

contra.
contraindicated

contralat
contralateral

contralat.
contralateral

cont rem
continuetur remedium [let the medicine be continued] (pharmacology)

cont. rem.
continuetur remedium [let the medicine be continued] (pharmacology)

contrit
contritus [broken, ground] (pharmacology)

CONTRL
control

contus
contusus [bruised]

contus.
contusus [bruised]

conv
convalescence
convalescent

conv.
convalescent
conventional [rat] (laboratory)

CONVAL
convalescent [specimen] (laboratory)

Conv. Hosp.
convalescent hospital

conv strab
convergent strabismus (ophthalmology)

COOD
chronic obstructive outflow disease (respiratory)

co-op
cooperative

COORD
coordination (neurology)

coord
coordination (neurology)

"coo-sah"
{pronunciation of *CUSA* [Cavitron Ultrasonic Surgical Aspirator]} (neurosurgery and ophthalmology) {not an abbreviation}

COP
change of plaster (orthopedics)
cicatricial ocular pemphigoid (ophthalmology)
colloid(al) osmotic pressure (laboratory)
cyclophosphamide [Cytoxan], Oncovin [vincristine], and prednisolone (chemotherapy, oncology, and pharmacology)
cyclophosphamide [Cytoxan], Oncovin [vincristine], and prednisone (chemotherapy, oncology, and pharmacology)

"cop"
{pronunciation of *COPP* (cyclophosphamide [Cytoxan], Oncovin [vincristine], procarbazine, and prednisone)} (chemotherapy, oncology, and pharmacology) {not an abbreviation}

COPA
Council on Postsecondary Accreditation (education)
cyclophosphamide [Cytoxan], Oncovin [vincristine], Adriamycin, and prednisone (chemotherapy, oncology, and pharmacology)

COPAC
CCNU [CeeNU or lomustine], Oncovin [vincristine], prednisone, Adriamycin, and cyclophosphamide [Cytoxan] (chemotherapy, oncology, and pharmacology)

COPB
cyclophosphamide [Cytoxan], Oncovin [vincristine], prednisone, and bleomycin (chemotherapy, oncology, and pharmacology)

COP-BLAM
cyclophosphamide [Cytoxan], Oncovin [vincristine], prednisone, procarbazine, bleomycin, and Adriamycin

(chemotherapy, oncology, and pharmacology)

COPC
Community Oriented Primary Care

COPD
chronic obstructive pulmonary disease (respiratory)

C.O.P.D.
chronic obstructive pulmonary disease (respiratory)

COPE
chronic obstructive pulmonary emphysema (respiratory)

C.O.P.E.
Committee on Political Education (education)

COPI
California Occupational Preference Inventory (psychiatry)

COPP
cyclophosphamide [Cytoxan], Oncovin [vincristine], procarbazine, and prednisone (chemotherapy, oncology, and pharmacology) {pronounced "cop}

COPRO
coproporphyrin (laboratory)

COQ
coenzyme Q [ubiquinone] (laboratory)

coq
coque [boil] (pharmacology)

coq.
coque [boil] (pharmacology)

coq in sa
coque in sufficiente aqua [boil in sufficient water] (pharmacology)

coq. in s. a.
coque in sufficiente aqua [boil in sufficient water] (pharmacology)

C.P.
candlepower (electricity and measurement)
cerebral palsy (genetics and neurology)
chemically pure (chemistry)

C/P
cholesterol-phospholipid [ratio] (laboratory)

C & P
compensation and pension (armed
forces and government)
cystoscopy and pyelography (radiology
and urology)

Cp
chickenpox (infectious diseases and pediatrics)

C$_p$
phosphate clearance (laboratory)

cP
centipoise (measurement)

cp
candlepower (electricity and measurement)
centipoise (measurement)
compare

c.p.
candlepower (electricity and measurement)

CPA
Canadian Psychiatric Association (psychiatry)
cardiopulmonary arrest (cardiovascular
and respiratory)
Caribbean Psychiatric Association (psychiatry)
carotid phonoangiography (cardiovascular and radiology)
carotid photoangiography (cardiovascular and radiology)
cerebellar pontine angle (neurology)
chlorophenylalanine (chemistry and laboratory)
circulating platelet aggregate (hematology and laboratory)
costophrenic angle (anatomy)

Council on Postsecondary Accreditation
(education)
cyclophosphamide (chemotherapy, oncology, and pharmacology)

CPAF
chlorpropamide-alcohol flush(ing) (endocrinology)

Cpah
p-aminohippuric acid clearance (laboratory)

C$_{pah}$
para-aminohippurate clearance (laboratory)

CPAP
constant positive air pressure (respiratory)
continuous positive air pressure (respiratory) {pronounced "see-pap"}
continuous positive airway pressure
(respiratory) {pronounced "see-pap"}

C-PAP
continuous positive air pressure (respiratory) {pronounced "see-pap"}
continuous positive airway pressure (respiratory) {pronounced "see-pap"}

C.P.A.P.
continuous positive air pressure (respiratory) {pronounced "see-pap"}
continuous positive airway pressure
(respiratory) {pronounced "see-pap"}

C-Parvum
Corynebacterium parvum [used in che-
motherapy] (chemotherapy, oncology,
and pharmacology)

CPB
cardiopulmonary bypass (cardiovascular
and respiratory)
cetyl pyridinium bromide (chemistry)
competitive protein binding (laboratory)

CPBA
competitive protein-binding analysis
  (laboratory)
competitive protein-binding assay (laboratory)

CPC
cerebral palsy clinic (neurology)
cetylpyridinium chloride (chemistry)
chronic passive congestion (cardiovascular and respiratory)
circumferential pneumatic compression
  (surgery)
clinical pathological conference (pathology)
clinical pathology conference (pathology)
clinicopathological conference (pathology)

cpc
chronic passive congestion (cardiovascular and respiratory)

CPCL
congenital pulmonary cystic lymphangi-
  ectasis (respiratory)

CPCP
chronic progressive coccidioidal pneumonitis (respiratory)

CPCR
cardiopulmonary-cerebral resuscitation
  (cardiovascular, emergency medicine,
  and respiratory)

CPD
cephalopelvic disproportion (obstetrics)
chorioretinopathy and pituitary dysfunction [syndrome] (endocrinology and
  ophthalmology)
citrate-phosphate-dextrose (chemistry)
compound
contact potential difference
contagious pustular dermatitis (dermatology)
cyclopentadiene (chemistry)

cpd
compound

cpd.
compound

CPDA-1
citrate-phosphate-dextrose-adenine
  (chemistry)

CPDD
calcium pyrophosphate deposition disease (rheumatology)
cis-platinumdiamminedichloride [also
  called *cisplatin* and *Platinol*] (chemotherapy, oncology, and pharmacology)

CPE
cardiogenic pulmonary edema (cardiovascular and respiratory)
chronic pulmonary emphysema (respiratory)
cis-platinumdiamminedichloride [also
  called *cisplatin* and *Platinol*] (chemotherapy, oncology, and pharmacology)
compensation, pension, and education
corona-penetrating enzyme (laboratory)
cytopathic effect (chemistry, chemotherapy, laboratory, pharmacology, radiation therapy, and radiology)
cytopathogenic effect(s) (chemistry,
  chemotherapy, laboratory, pharmacology, radiation therapy, and radiology)

C.Ped.
Certified Pedorthist (orthopedics)

C.P.E.H.S.
Consumer Protection and Environmental
  Health Service (ecology and govern-
  ment)

C peptide
{not an abbreviation} [an amino acid
  residue] (endocrinology and laboratory)

CPF
clot-promoting factor (hematology and
  laboratory)

CPG
capillary blood gases (laboratory and
  respiratory)

CPGN
chronic progressive glomerulonephritis (nephrology)

CPH
Certificate in Public Health
chronic persistent hepatitis (gastroenterology)

C.P.H.
Certificate in Public Health

CPH 5
Cutter protein hydrolysate five percent (5%) in water (pharmacology)

CPHA
Committee on Professional and Hospital Activities

C.P.H.A.
Committee on Professional and Hospital Activities

CPHE
crew personal hygiene equipment (armed forces)

CPI
California Psychological Inventory (psychiatry)
Cancer Potential Index [for environmental monitoring] (ecology and oncology)
constitutionally psychopathia inferior (psychiatry)
constitutional psychopathic inferiority (psychiatry)
coronary prognostic index (cardiovascular)

CPIB
chlorophenoxyisobutyrate (chemistry)

CPID
chronic pelvic inflammatory disease (gynecology)

CPIP
common peak developed isovolumic pressure (cardiovascular)

CPK
creatine phosphokinase (cardiovascular, chemistry, and laboratory)

CPK BB
creatine phosphokinase BB [isoenzyme] (cardiovascular and laboratory)

CPKD
childhood polycystic kidney disease (nephrology)

CPKI
creatine phosphokinase isoenzymes (cardiovascular and laboratory)

CPKISO
creatine phosphokinase isoenzymes (cardiovascular and laboratory)

CPK MB
creatine phosphokinase MB [isoenzyme] (cardiovascular and laboratory)

CPK MM
creatine phosphokinase MM [isoenzyme] (cardiovascular and laboratory)

CPL
criminal procedure law

cpl
complete

CPLM
cysteine-peptone-liver infusion media (laboratory)

CPM
central pontine myelinolysis (neurology)
chlorpheniramine maleate (pharmacology)
continue present management
continuous passive motion [machine] (physical therapy and orthopedics)
counts per minute (measurement)
cycles per minute (measurement)
cyclophosphamide (chemotherapy, oncology, and pharmacology)

c.p.m.
counts per minute (measurement)
cycles per minute (measurement)

CPmax
peak serum concentration (laboratory)

CPmin
trough serum concentration (laboratory)

CPN
chronic pyelonephritis (nephrology)

CPOB
cyclophosphamide, prednisone, Oncovin [vincristine], and bleomycin (chemotherapy, oncology, and pharmacology)

CPP
carboxy terminus of propressophysin (laboratory)
cerebral perfusion pressure (cardiovascular)
cryoprecipitate (laboratory)
cyclopentenophenanthrene (chemistry)

CPPB
constant positive-pressure breathing (respiratory)
continuous positive-pressure breathing (respiratory)

CPPD
calcium pyrophosphate deposition disease (rheumatology)
calcium pyrophosphate dihydrate (chemistry and laboratory)

CPPV
continuous positive-pressure ventilation (respiratory)

CPR
cardiac pulmonary reserve (cardiovascular and respiratory)
cardiopulmonary resuscitation (cardiovascular and respiratory)
centripetal rub (cardiovascular)
cerebral cortex perfusion rate (cardiovascular and neurology)
chlorophenyl red (chemistry)
cortisol production rate (laboratory)

C.P.R.
cardiopulmonary resuscitation (cardiovascular and respiratory)

CPRCASC
Cytotechnology Programs Review Committee of the American Society of Cytology (cytology, laboratory, and pathology)

CPRD
Committee on Prosthetics Research and Development (orthopedics)

CPS
chloroquine, pyrimethamine, and sulfisoxazole (pharmacology)
clinical performance score
complex partial seizure (neurology)
constitutional psychopathic state (psychiatry)
C-polysaccharide (chemistry and laboratory)
cumulative probability of success (statistics)

cps
cycles per second (measurement)

cps.
counts per second (measurement)
cycles per second (measurement)

c.p.s.
cycles per second (measurement)

CPT
carotid pulse tracing (cardiovascular)
chest physiotherapy (respiratory)
ciliary particle transport [activity]
clinical pharmacokinetics team (pharmacology)
cold pressor test (cardiovascular)
cold pressure test (cardiovascular)
combining power test (laboratory)
concentration performance test
continuous performance task (psychiatry)
Continuous Performance Test (psychiatry)
Continuous Primary Tests (psychiatry)

Current Procedural Terminology [of the American Medical Association]

CPTH
chronic post-traumatic headache (neurology)
C-terminal parathyroid hormone (endocrinology and laboratory)

CPU
central processing unit (computer science)

CPUE
chest pain of unknown etiology (cardiovascular)

CPX
complete physical examination

CPZ
chlorpromazine [Thorazine] (pharmacology and psychiatry)
Compazine [prochlorperazine] (gastroenterology and pharmacology)

CQ
chloroquine (pharmacology)
chloroquine-quinine (pharmacology)
circadian quotient
conceptual quotient

C1q
{not an abbreviation} [a protein of the complement system] (laboratory)

CQM
chloroquine mustard (chemistry)

C.Q.U.C.C.
Commission on Quantities and Units in Clinical Chemistry (chemistry)

CR
calculus removal (orthopedics and podiatry)
cardiac rehabilitation (cardiovascular and rehabilitation)
cardiorespiratory (cardiovascular and respiratory)
cartilage residue (orthopedics)
centric relation [also called *centric jaw relation*] (dentistry and otorhinolaryngology)

chest roentgenogram (cardiovascular, radiology, and respiratory)
clinical record (medical records)
clinical research (research)
closed reduction (orthopedics)
clot retraction (cardiovascular and hematology)
coefficient of fat retention (laboratory)
colon resection (gastroenterology and surgery)
complement receptor (laboratory)
complete remission
complete response
conditioned reflex (neurology and psychiatry)
conditioned response (neurology and psychiatry)
controlled reflex (neurology and psychiatry)
controlled release (neurology and psychiatry)
controlled response (neurology and psychiatry)
conversion ratio (endocrinology and laboratory)
creatinine (laboratory)
cresyl red (chemistry)
critical ratio
crown-rump [measurement] (embryology, obstetrics, and radiology)
{not an abbreviation} [chest and right arm electrode placement for an electrocardiogram] (cardiovascular)

C.R.
crown-rump [measurement] (embryology, obstetrics, and radiology)

C & R
convalescent and rehabilitation (rehabilitation)

CR$_1$
first cranial nerve (neurology)

CR$_2$
second cranial nerve (neurology)

Cr
chromium (chemistry)
cranial (anatomy)

cream (pharmacology)
creatinine (laboratory)
crown (anatomy and dentistry)

Cr^{51}
radioactive sodium chromate (chemistry)

^{51}Cr
radioactive sodium chromate (chemistry)

cr
cras [tomorrow]
crown (anatomy and dentistry)

cr.
cras [tomorrow]

CRA
central retinal artery (cardiovascular and ophthalmology)
Chinese restaurant asthma (allergy and respiratory)

CRAB
Chief's Review and Advisory Board

CRABP
cellular retinoic acid-binding protein (laboratory)

cran.
cranial (anatomy)

CRAO
central retinal artery occlusion (cardiovascular and ophthalmology)

crast
crastinus [for tomorrow] (pharmacology)

crast.
crastinus [for tomorrow] (pharmacology)

CRB
chemical, radiological, and biological [warfare] (armed forces)
Curriculum Review Board of the American Association of Medical Assistants (education)

CRBBB
complete right bundle-branch block (cardiovascular)

Cr & Br
crown and bridge (dentistry)

CRC
calomel, rhubarb, colocynth [a cathartic] (gastroenterology and pharmacology)
cardiac reconditioning center (cardiovascular and rehabilitation)
cardiovascular reflex conditioning (cardiovascular)
Clinical Research Centre [of Medical Research Council] (research)
colorectal cancer (gastroenterology and oncology)
Crisis Resolution Center (psychiatry)

CrCl
creatinine clearance (laboratory)

CRCS
cardiovascular reflex conditioning system (cardiovascular)

CRD
chronic renal disease (nephrology)
chronic respiratory disease (respiratory)
complete reaction of degeneration (chemistry and laboratory)
crown-rump distance [of fetus] (embryology, obstetrics, and radiology)

C.R.D.
chronic respiratory disease [of poultry] (respiratory and veterinary medicine)

CRE
cumulative radiation effect (radiation therapy and radiology)

CREA
creatinine (laboratory)

CREA-S
creatinine urine spot [test] (laboratory)

creat.
creatine (laboratory)

CREA-U
creatinine urine [test] (laboratory)
creatinine (laboratory)

CREN
crenated [red blood cells] (hematology
and laboratory)

CRENA
crenated [red blood cells] (hematology
and laboratory)

CRENA%
percent of crenated [red blood cells on
differential count] (hematology and
laboratory)

crep
crepitus [crepitation] (orthopedics and
respiratory)

crep.
crepitus [crepitation] (orthopedics and
respiratory)

creps
crepitations (orthopedics and respiratory) {pronounced "crepz"}

"crepz"
{pronunciation of *creps* [crepitations]}
(orthopedics and respiratory) {not an
abbreviation}

CREST
calcinosis, Raynaud's phenomenon,
esophageal dysmotility [or dys-
function], sclerodactyly, and telangiectasia [syndrome] (rheumatology)
{pronounced "crest"}

"crest"
{pronunciation of *CREST* [calcinosis,
Raynaud's phenomenon, esophageal
dysmotility (or dysfunction), sclerodactyly, and telangiectasia (syndrome)]} (rheumatology) (not an abbreviation)

CRF
chronic renal failure (nephrology)

chronic respiratory failure (respiratory)
coagulase-reacting factor (laboratory)
corticotropin-releasing factor [also
called *corticotrophin-regulating factor*] (laboratory)

CRG
cardiorespirogram (cardiovascular and
respiratory)

CRH
corticotropin-releasing hormone (laboratory)

CRHL
Collaborative Radiological Health Laboratory (laboratory, radiology, and research)

CRI
chemical rust-inhibiting [germicide]
(chemistry)
chronic renal insufficiency (nephrology)
cold running intelligibility [referring to a
test for hearing continuous speech]
(otorhinolaryngology)
concentrated rust inhibitor (chemistry)
cross-reactive idiotype (genetics and
laboratory)

Cr$_I$
first cranial nerve (neurology)

CRIE
crossed radioimmunoelectrophoresis
(laboratory)

Cr$_{II}$
second cranial nerve (neurology)

Cr$_{III}$
third cranial nerve (neurology)

Crit
hematocrit (hematology and laboratory)
{pronounced "crit" or "krit"}

crit.
hematocrit (hematology and laboratory)
{pronounced "krit"}

"crit"
{pronunciation of *Crit* and *crit*. [hematocrit]} (hematology and laboratory) {not an abbreviation}

Cr$_{IV}$
fourth cranial nerve (neurology)

Cr$_{IX}$
ninth cranial nerve (neurology)

CRL
Certified Record Librarian (medical records)
complement receptor lymphocyte (laboratory)
crown-rump length (embryology, obstetrics, and radiology)

CRM
Certified Reference Materials (publishing)
cross-reacting material (laboratory)

C.R.M.
Certified Reference Materials (publishing)

CRN
complement-requiring neutralizing (laboratory)

CrN
cranial nerves (neurology)

Cr.N.
cranial nerves (neurology)

CRNA
Certified Registered Nurse Anesthetist (anesthesiology and nursing)

C.R.N.A.
Certified Registered Nurse Anesthetist (anesthesiology and nursing)

cRNA
chromosomal ribonucleic acid (genetics and laboratory)

CRNI
Certified Registered Nurse Intravenous (nursing)

cr nn
cranial nerves (neurology)

CRNP
Certified Registered Nurse Practitioner (nursing)

cr. ns.
cranial nerves (neurology)

CRO
cathode ray oscillograph (cardiovascular and radiology)
cathode ray oscilloscope (cardiovascular and radiology)
centric relation occlusion (dentistry and otorhinolaryngology)

CROP
cyclophosphamide, rubidazone, Oncovin [vincristine], and prednisone (chemotherapy, oncology, and pharmacology)

CROPAM
cyclophosphamide, rubidazone, Oncovin [vincristine], prednisone, L-asparaginase, and methotrexate (chemotherapy, oncology, and pharmacology)

CROS
contralateral routing of signal (neurology)
contralateral routing of signs (neurology)

CRP
C-reactive protein {*C* is not an abbreviation} (laboratory)

CrP
creatine phosphate [also called *phosphocreatine*] (laboratory)

Cr. P.
creatine phosphate [also called *phosphocreatine*] (laboratory)

CRPA
C-reactive protein antiserum {*C* is not an abbreviation} (laboratory)

CRPF
chloroquine-resistant *Plasmodium falciparum* (laboratory)

CRRT
Certified Respiratory Therapy Technician (respiratory)

CRS
central supply room
Chinese restaurant syndrome (allergy)
colon-rectal surgery (gastroenterology and surgery)
colorectal surgery (gastroenterology and surgery)
congenital rubella syndrome (infectious diseases, neonatology, and pediatrics)

CRST
calcification, Raynaud's phenomenon, scleroderma, and telangiectasia [syndrome] (rheumatology)
calcinosis cutis, Raynaud's phenomenon, sclerodactyly, and telangiectasia [syndrome] (rheumatology)
calcinosis, Raynaud's phenomenon, scleroderma, and telangiectasia [syndrome] (rheumatology)

CRT
cardiac resuscitation team (cardiovascular)
cathode ray tube (radiology)
central reaction time (neurology)
complex reaction timer (neurology)
copper reduction test (chemistry)
corrected retention time

CRTP
Consciousness Research and Training Project (psychiatry and research)

Cr Tr
crutch training (orthopedics, physical therapy, and rehabilitation)

CRTT
Certified Respiratory Therapy Technician (respiratory)

C.R.T.T.
Certified Respiratory Therapy Technician (respiratory)

CRTX
cast removed, take to x-ray (orthopedics)

CRU
clinical research unit (research)
Crisis Resolution Center (psychiatry)

CRV
central retinal vein (cardiovascular and ophthalmology)

Cr_V
fifth cranial nerve (neurology)

Cr_{VI}
sixth cranial nerve (neurology)

Cr_{VII}
seventh cranial nerve (neurology)

Cr_{VIII}
eighth cranial nerve (neurology)

CRVO
central retinal vein occlusion (cardiovascular and ophthalmology)

CRVS
California Relative Value Studies (statistics)

Cr_X
tenth cranial nerve (neurology)

Cr_{XI}
eleventh cranial nerve (neurology)

Cr_{XII}
twelfth cranial nerve (neurology)

CRY-AB
cryptococcal antibody (laboratory)

CRY-AG
cryptococcal antigen (laboratory)

CRY N
crystal number [on urinalysis] (laboratory, nephrology, and urology)

CRYO
cryoglobulin (laboratory) {pronounced "cry-oh"}

cryo
cryosurgery (surgery) {pronounced "cry-oh"}
cryotherapy (surgery) {pronounced "cry-oh"}

"cry-oh"
{pronunciation of CRYO [cryoglobulin (laboratory)] and cryo [cryosurgery and cryotherapy (surgery)]} {not an abbreviation}

CRYPTO
cryptococcus (laboratory) {pronounced "cryp-toe" or "crypt-oh"}

"cryp-toe"
{pronunciation of CRYPTO [cryptococcus]} (laboratory) {not an abbreviation}

"crypt-oh"
{pronunciation of CRYPTO [cryptococcus]} (laboratory) {not an abbreviation}

crys
crystalline (laboratory)
crystallinized (laboratory)

crys.
crystal (laboratory)

CRYST
crystal examination screen (laboratory, nephrology, and urology)

cryst
crystalline (laboratory)
crystallinized (laboratory)

CS
calf serum (laboratory)
carcinoid syndrome (oncology)
cardiogenic shock (cardiovascular)
carotid sheath (cardiovascular)
carotid sinus (cardiovascular)
cat scratch [disease] (infectious diseases)
celiac sprue

central service
central supply
cerebrospinal (laboratory and neurology)
cervical spine (neurology and orthopedics)
cervical stimulation
cesarean section (obstetrics)
chemical sympathectomy (neurology)
chest strap
chief of staff (administration)
chondroitin sulfate (chemistry)
chorionic somatomammotropin (laboratory)
Christian Scientist (religion)
chronic schizophrenia (psychiatry)
Church of Scotland (religion)
cigarette smoke (cardiovascular and respiratory)
cigarette smoker (cardiovascular and respiratory)
citrate synthase (laboratory)
clinical stage
clinical state
Cockayne's syndrome (genetics)
colla sinistra [with the left hand]
Collet-Sicard [syndrome] (otorhinolaryngology and neurology)
completed stroke (neurology)
completed suicide (psychiatry)
concentrated strength [of solutions] (chemistry and pharmacology)
conditioned stimulus (neurology and psychiatry)
congenital syphilis (gynecology, infectious diseases, neonatology, and urology)
conjunctiva-sclera (ophthalmology)
conjunctival secretions (ophthalmology)
conscious (neurology and psychiatry)
consciousness (neurology and psychiatry)
contact sensitivity (allergy and dermatology)
continue same [treatment]
continuing smoker (cardiovascular and respiratory)
continuous stripping (surgery)
convalescent status
coronary sclerosis (cardiovascular)
coronary sinus (cardiovascular)

CSN
carotid sinus nerve (neurology)

CSOM
chronic serous otitis media (otorhinolaryngology)
chronic suppurative otitis media (otorhinolaryngology)

CSP
cavum septum pellucidum
cellulose sodium phosphate (chemistry)
Chartered Society of Physiotherapy (rehabilitation)
Cooperative Statistical Program [for intrauterine death data] (neonatology,
obstetrics, and statistics)
criminal sexual psychopath (psychiatry)

CSPI
Center for Science in the Public Interest

C/spine
cervical spine (neurology and orthopedics)

C-spine
cervical spine (neurology and orthopedics)

CSR
central supply room
Cheyne-Stokes respiration (respiratory)
corrected sedimentation rate (laboratory)
corrective septorhinoplasty (otorhinolaryngology)
cortical secretion rate [of adrenal
glands] (endocrinology and laboratory)
cortisol secretion rate (endocrinology
and laboratory)

CSS
carotid sinus stimulation (cardiovascular)
Central Sterile Supply
chewing, sucking, swallowing (neurology)
chronic subclinical scurvy [syndrome]
(dentistry, dietary, hematology, and
orthopedics)

CSSD
central sterile supply department

CST
cardiac stress test (cardiovascular)
cavernous sinus thrombosis (cardiovascular)
Certified Surgical Technologist (surgery)
contraction stress test (obstetrics)
convulsive shock therapy (psychiatry)
cosyntropin stimulation test (endocrinology and laboratory)

Cst
static compliance (laboratory and respiratory)

cSt.
centistoke (measurement)

C Stat
static lung compliance (respiratory)

Cstat
static lung compliance (respiratory)

CSTI
Clearinghouse for Scientific and Technical Information

CStJ
Commander, Order of Saint John of Jerusalem

CSU
cardiac surveillance unit (cardiovascular)
cardiovascular surgery unit (cardiovascular)
catheter specimen of urine (laboratory)
Central Statistical Unit [of the Venereal
Disease Research Laboratory] (infectious diseases, gynecology, laboratory,
research, statistics, and urology)

C.S.W.
Certified Social Worker (social work)

CT
calcitonin (laboratory)
cardiothoracic [ratio] (cardiovascular)

Cardiovascular Technologist (cardiovascular)
carotid tracing (cardiovascular)
carpal tunnel (neurology and orthopedics)
cellular therapy
cerebral thrombosis (cardiovascular and neurology)
cervical traction (neurology, orthopedics, and physical therapy)
chest tube (cardiovascular, respiratory, and surgery)
chlorothiazide (pharmacology)
cholera toxin (infectious diseases and pharmacology)
chymotrypsin (gastroenterology, laboratory, and pharmacology)
circulating time (cardiovascular and hematology)
circulation time (cardiovascular and hematology)
classic technique (surgery)
clotting time (hematology and laboratory)
coagulation time (hematology and laboratory)
coated tablet (pharmacology)
collecting tubule (nephrology)
compressed tablet (pharmacology)
computed tomography (radiology)
computerized tomography (radiology)
Connecticut [Postal Service state designation]
connective tissue (orthopedics and rheumatology)
continue treatment
continuous-flow tub (rehabilitation)
contraceptive technique(s) (gynecology, obstetrics, and urology)
contraction time (obstetrics)
controlled temperature (laboratory and pharmacology)
Coombs' test (hematology and laboratory)
corneal thickness (ophthalmology)
corneal transplant (ophthalmology)
coronary thrombosis (cardiovascular)
corrected transposition (cardiovascular)
corrective therapist (rehabilitation)
corrective therapy
crest time
cystine-tellurite [medium] (laboratory)
Cytotechnologist (laboratory and pathology)

C.T.
corrective therapy (rehabilitation)

C$_{T-1824}$
clearance of Evans blue [T-1824] (laboratory)

Ct
Ctenocephalides [a genus of fleas] (entomology)

ct
count (laboratory)

CTA
Canadian Tuberculosis Association (infectious diseases and respiratory)
chromotropic acid (chemistry)
clear to auscultation (respiratory)
computerized tomoangiography (radiology)
cyanotrimethyl-androsterone (endocrinology and laboratory)
cyproterone acetate (chemistry)
cystine trypticase agar (laboratory)
cytotoxic assay (laboratory)

C.T.A.
Canadian Tuberculosis Association (infectious diseases and respiratory)
Committee on Thrombolytic Agents [units] (hematology)

CTa
catamenia [menses] (gynecology)

Cta
catamenia [menses] (gynecology)

CTAB
cetyltrimethylammonium bromide (chemistry)

CTAC
Cancer Treatment Advisory Committee (chemotherapy, oncology, and radiation therapy)
Carrow Test for Auditory Comprehension (speech and language pathology)

⁶⁴Cu
radioactive copper (chemistry)

⁶⁵Cu
radioactive copper (chemistry)

cu
cubic (measurement)

cu.
cubic (measurement)

CuB
copper band (dentistry)

CUC
chronic ulcerative colitis (gastroenterology)

¹⁴C-UCBR
carbon-14-labeled unconjugated bilirubin (radiology)

cu cm
cubic centimeter (measurement)

cu. cm.
cubic centimeter (measurement)

CUD
cause undetermined

cu ft
cubic foot (measurement)

cu. ft.
cubic foot (measurement)

CUG
cystidine-uridine-guanidine (chemistry and laboratory)
cystourethrogram (radiology and urology)

cu in
cubic inch (measurement)

cu. in.
cubic inch (measurement)

cuj
cujus [of any, of which]

cuj.
cujus [of any, of which]

cuj lib
cujus libet [of any you desire, of whatever you please]

cuj. lib.
cujus libet [of any you desire, of whatever you please]

cult
culture (bacteriology and laboratory)

cu m
cubic meter (measurement)

cu. m.
cubic meter (measurement)

cu mm
cubic millimeter (measurement)

cu. mm.
cubic millimeter (measurement)

CUMITECH
Cumulative Techniques and Procedures in Clinical Microbiology (laboratory and microbiology)

cu mu
cubic micrometer (measurement)

CUP
Care Unit Program (chemical dependency)

cur
curative
current

curat
curatio [dressing]

curat.
curatio [dressing]

CURN
Conduct and Utilization of Research in Nursing (nursing and research)

CUS

chronic undifferentiated schizophrenia (psychiatry)

CUSA

Cavitron Ultrasonic Surgical Aspirator (neurosurgery and ophthalmology) {pronounced "coo-sah" or "koo-sah"}

cusp.

cuspid (dentistry)

CUX

checkup x-ray (radiology)

CV

cardiovascular (cardiovascular)
cell volume (laboratory)
central venous (cardiovascular)
cerebrovascular (cardiovascular and neurology)
cervical vertebra (neurology and orthopedics)
closed vitrectomy (ophthalmology)
closing volume (laboratory and respiratory)
coefficient of variation (mathematics)
color vision (ophthalmology)
concentrated volume [solutions]
conjugata vera [conjugate diameter of pelvic inlet] (obstetrics)
conversational voice (otorhinolaryngology and speech therapy)
corpuscular volume (hematology and laboratory)
costovertebral [angle] (anatomy)
cras vespere [tomorrow evening] (pharmacology)
cresyl violet [a dye] (laboratory and pathology)
crystal violet [also called *gentian violet*] (pharmacology)
cyclophosphamide and VP-16 (chemotherapy, oncology, and pharmacology)
fifth cranial nerve (neurology)

Cv

specific heat at constant volume (chemistry)

cv

cardiovascular (cardiovascular)

c.v.

conjugata vera [true conjugate diameter of pelvic inlet] (obstetrics)
cras vespere [tomorrow evening] (pharmacology)

CVA

cardiovascular accident (cardiovascular)
cerebrovascular accident [also called *cerebral vascular accident* or *stroke*] (cardiovascular and neurology)
costovertebral angle (anatomy)
cyclophosphamide, vincristine, and Adriamycin (chemotherapy, oncology, and pharmacology)

C.V.A.

cerebrovascular accident [also called *cerebral vascular accident* or *stroke*] (neurology)

Cva

costovertebral angle (anatomy)

cva

costovertebral angle (anatomy)

C-Vasc

cerebral vascular profile study (cardiovascular and neurology)

CVAT

costovertebral angle tenderness (nephrology and urology)

CVB

CCNU [CeeNU or lomustine], vinblastine, and bleomycin (chemotherapy, oncology, and pharmacology)

CVC

central venous catheter (cardiovascular)
convalescent camp (rehabilitation)

CVCT

cardiovascular computerized tomography [scanner] (cardiovascular)

CVD

cardiovascular disease (cardiovascular)

childbirth without pain (obstetrics)
coal workers' pneumoconiosis (respiratory)

C.W.P.
centimeters of water pressure (measurement)

CWPEA
Childbirth Without Pain Education Association (obstetrics)

CWS
Child Welfare Service (social services)
cold-water soluble
cotton-wool spots (ophthalmology)

CWT
cold water treatment

Cwt.
hundredweight (measurement)

cwt.
hundredweight (measurement)

CX
cervix (gynecology and obstetrics)
chest x-ray (cardiovascular, radiology, and respiratory)
cyclophosphamide [Cytoxan] (chemotherapy, oncology, and pharmacology)
tenth cranial nerve (neurology)

Cx
cancel
cervix (gynecology and obstetrics)
chest x-ray (cardiovascular, radiology, and respiratory)
clearance (laboratory and physiology)
convex
culture (laboratory)

cx
cylinder axis (ophthalmology)

CXI
eleventh cranial nerve (neurology)

CXII
twelfth cranial nerve (neurology)

CxMT
cervical motion tenderness (gynecology)

CXR
chest roentgenogram [chest x-ray] (cardiovascular, radiology, and respiratory)

CY
calendar year

Cy
cyanogen (chemistry)
cyclonium (chemistry)

cy.
copy

CYA
cyclosporine (pharmacology)

CyA
cyclosporine (pharmacology)

cyath
cyathus [a glass, a glassful] (pharmacology)

cyath.
cyathus [a glass, a glassful] (pharmacology)

cyath vin
cyathus vinarius [a wineglass]

cyborg
cybernetic organism (computer sciences and research) {pronounced "sighborg"}

CYC
cyclophosphamide (chemotherapy, oncology, and pharmacology)

cyc
cyclazocine (chemical dependency and pharmacology)
cycle
cyclotron (physics)

cyclic AMP
cyclic adenosine monophosphate (chemistry)

cyclic GMP
cyclic guanosine monophosphate (chemistry)

Cyclo.
cyclophosphamide (chemotherapy, oncology, and pharmacology)
cyclopropane (chemistry)

Cyclo C
cyclocytidine hydrochloric acid (chemistry and laboratory)

CYE
charcoal yeast extract [medium] (laboratory)

CYFL
cyst fluid (laboratory)

CYL
casein yeast lactate [media] (laboratory)

cyl
cylinder
cylindrical lens (ophthalmology)

cyl.
cylinder
cylindrical lens (ophthalmology)

CYN
cyanide [a poison] (chemistry, laboratory, and pharmacology)

CYS
cystoscopy (urology)

Cys
cysteine (chemistry and laboratory)
cystine (chemistry and laboratory)

Cys.
cysteine (chemistry and laboratory)
cystine (chemistry and laboratory)

Cys-Cys
cystine (chemistry and laboratory)

Cys-cys
cystine (chemistry and laboratory)

cys.
cysteine (chemistry and laboratory)

CYSTIN
cystine [in urine] (chemistry and laboratory)

CYSTO
cystogram (urology) {pronounced "sistow"}
cystoscopy (urology) {pronounced "sistow"}

cysto
cystoscopic [examination] (urology) {pronounced "sis-tow"}
cystoscopy (urology) {pronounced "sistow"}

CYT
cyclophosphamide (chemotherapy and pharmacology)

cytol
cytological (laboratory)
cytology (laboratory)

CYTOMG
cytomegalovirus (laboratory)

cyt sys
cytochrome system (laboratory)

CY-VA-DACT
cyclophosphamide, vincristine, Adriamycin, and actinomycin D (chemotherapy, oncology, and pharmacology) {pronounced "sigh-vay-dact"}

CYVADIC
cyclophosphamide [Cytoxan], vincristine [Oncovin], Adriamycin [doxorubicin], and dacarbazine [DTIC] (chemotherapy, oncology, and pharmacology) {pronounced "sigh-vay-dick"}

CY-VA-DIC
cyclophosphamide [Cytoxan], vincristine [Oncovin], Adriamycin [doxorubicin], and dacarbazine [DTIC] (chemotherapy, oncology, and pharmacology) {pronounced "sigh-vay-dick"}

D$_6$
sixth dorsal nerve (neurology and ortho-
    pedics)
sixth dorsal vertebra (orthopedics)

D7
seventh dorsal vertebra (orthopedics)

D$_7$
seventh dorsal nerve (neurology and or-
    thopedics)
seventh dorsal vertebra (orthopedics)

D8
eighth dorsal vertebra (orthopedics)

D$_8$
eighth dorsal nerve (neurology and or-
    thopedics)
eighth dorsal vertebra (orthopedics)

D9
ninth dorsal vertebra (orthopedics)

D$_9$
ninth dorsal nerve (neurology and ortho-
    pedics)
ninth dorsal vertebra (orthopedics)

D10
tenth dorsal vertebra (orthopedics)

D$_{10}$
tenth dorsal nerve (neurology and ortho-
    pedics)
tenth dorsal vertebra (orthopedics)

D11
eleventh dorsal vertebra (orthopedics)

D$_{11}$
eleventh dorsal nerve (neurology and or-
    thopedics)
eleventh dorsal vertebra (orthopedics)

D12
twelfth dorsal vertebra (orthopedics)

D$_{12}$
twelfth dorsal nerve (neurology and or-
    thopedics)
twelfth dorsal vertebra (orthopedics)

17-D
{not an abbreviation} [a modified yellow
    fever virus] (infectious diseases, labo-
    ratory, research, and virology)

D 860
tolbutamide (endocrinology and phar-
    macology)

d
day
dead
deceased
deci- [prefix for 10^{-1}] (measurement)
    {not an abbreviation}
density
deoxyribose (genetics and laboratory)
dexter [right]
dextra [right]
dextrorotary
diameter (measurement)
diastolic (cardiovascular)
distal
died
dies [day]
diopter (measurement and ophthalmol-
    ogy)
distal
diurnal
dorsal
dosis [dose] (pharmacology)
doubtful
duration
dyne (measurement and physics)
relative to rotation of a beam of polar-
    ized light
{not an abbreviation} [atomic orbital
    with angular momentum quantum
    number 2] (physics)
{not an abbreviation} [prefix meaning
    deci- (10^{-1})] (measurement)

d.
dare [to give] (pharmacology)
day
detur [let it be given] (pharmacology)
dies [day]
dosis [dose] (pharmacology)

d-
dextro- [chemical symbol meaning to the right or clockwise] (chemistry)

DA
daunomycin and cytosine arabinoside (chemotherapy, oncology, and pharmacology)
decubitus angina (cardiovascular)
degenerative arthritis (orthopedics)
delayed action (pharmacology)
dental assistant (dentistry)
developmental age (pediatrics and psychiatry)
diphenylchlorarsine [also called *sneezing gas*] (armed forces and chemistry)
Diploma in Anaesthetics (anesthesiology)
direct admission
direct agglutination (laboratory)
disability assistance
disaggregated (laboratory)
District Administrator (administration)
District Attorney (law)
dopamine (pharmacology)
dopaminergic (pharmacology)
drug addict (chemical dependency)
ductus arteriosus (cardiovascular)

D.A.
developmental age (pediatrics and psychiatry)
District Attorney (law)

D/A
discharge and advise

D-A
donor-acceptor

d/A
day of admission

da
daughter
day
{not an abbreviation} [prefix for *deca-* (10^1)] (measurement)

DAB
dimethylaminoazobenzene (chemistry)
dysrhythmic aggressive behavior (psychiatry)

DAC
digital-to-analog converter (computer science, radiology)
Disaster Assistance Center (government)
Disablement Advisory Committee [British]
Division of Ambulatory Care

DACA
Drug Abuse Control Amendments (chemical dependency)

DACT
dactinomycin [also called *actinomycin D*] (chemotherapy, oncology, and pharmacology)

Dact
dactinomycin [also called *actinomycin D*] (chemotherapy, oncology, and pharmacology)

DAD
dispense as directed (pharmacology)
drug administration device (pharmacology)
father

DADAVS
Deputy Assistant Director Army Veterinary Services (armed forces and veterinary medicine)

DADDS
diacetyl diaminodiphenylsulfone [also called *acedapsone*] (pharmacology)

DADLE
D-Ala, D-Leu encephalin

DADMS
Deputy Assistant Director of Medical Services (armed forces)

DADPS
diphenylsulfone [also called *dapsone*] (pharmacology)

DADS
Director of Army Dental Service (armed forces and dentistry)

DAE
diphenylanthracene endoperoxide [a dye] (chemistry and laboratory)
diving air embolism (cardiovascular, respiratory, and sports medicine)

DAF
delayed auditory feedback (otorhinolaryngology)
Draw-A-Family [test] (psychiatry)

DAG
dianhydrogalacitol (chemistry, chemotherapy, oncology, and pharmacology)

DAGT
direct antiglobulin test (laboratory)

DAH
disordered action of the heart (cardiovascular)

D.A.H.
disordered action of the heart (cardiovascular)

DAHEA
Department of Allied Health Education and Accreditation [of the American Medical Association]

DAHM
Division of Allied Health Manpower

"dah-sah"
{pronunciation of *DASA* [distal articular set angle]} (podiatry and orthopedics) {not an abbreviation}

DAI
diffuse axonal injury (neurology)

DAL
drug analysis laboratory (laboratory)

DALA
delta-aminolevulinic acid (chemistry)

DALE
Drug Abuse Law Enforcement (chemical dependency and law)

DAM
degraded amyloid (laboratory)
diacetyl monoxine (chemistry)
diacetylmonoxine (chemistry)
diacetylmorphine (chemistry)
Dictionary of Abbreviations in Medicine (reference)

dam
decameter (measurement)

dAMP
deoxyadenosine monophosphate (chemistry)
deoxyadenosine-5'-phosphate (chemistry)

DANA
drug-induced antinuclear antibodies (laboratory)

dand
dandus [to be given] (pharmacology)

DANS
1-methylaminonaphthalene-5-sulphonyl chloride (chemistry)

DAO
diamine oxidase (chemistry)
duly authorized officer

DAP
diaminopimelic acid
dihydroxyacetone phosphate (chemistry)
direct [latex] agglutination pregnancy [test] (laboratory and obstetrics)
Director of Army Psychiatry [British] (armed forces and psychiatry)
Draw-A-Person [test] (psychiatry)

DAP & E
Diploma of Applied Parasitology and Entomology (education)

DAP I
diahydrogalactitol, Adriamycin, and cisplatin (chemotherapy, oncology, and
pharmacology)

DAP II
diahydrogalactitol, Adriamycin, and
high dose cisplatin (chemotherapy,
oncology, and pharmacology)

DAPRU
drug abuse prevention resource unit
(chemical dependency)

DAPST
Denver Auditory Phoneme Sequencing
Test (speech and language therapy)

DAPT
direct agglutination pregnancy test (laboratory and obstetrics)

Dapt
Daptazole (pharmacology)

DARTS
Drug and Alcohol Rehabilitation Testing
System (chemical dependency) {pro-
nounced "dartz"}

"dartz"
{pronunciation of *DARTS* [Drug and Alcohol Rehabilitation Testing System]}
(chemical dependency) {not an abbre-
viation}

DAS
data acquisition system (radiology)
dextroamphetamine sulfate (chemistry)

DASA
distal articular set angle (orthopedics
and podiatry) {pronounced "dah-sah"}

DASH
Distress Alarm for the Severely Handicapped [British] (rehabilitation)

DASI
Developmental Activities Screening Inventory (speech and language therapy)

DAT
daunorubicin, cytarabine [ARA-C], and
thioguanine (chemotherapy, oncology,
and pharmacology)
delayed action tablet (pharmacology)
dementia of the Alzheimer's type (neurology and psychiatry)
Dental Admission Test (dentistry)
diet as tolerated (dietary)
differential agglutination titer (laboratory)
differential antibody titer (laboratory)
differential aptitude test (psychiatry)
diphtheria antitoxin (pharmacology)
direct agglutination test (laboratory)
Disaster Action Team [of the Red Cross]

dau
daughter

Daun
daunorubicin (chemotherapy, oncology,
and pharmacology)

DAV
Disabled American Veterans {pro-
nounced "dave"}

"dave"
{pronunciation of *DAV* [Disabled American Veterans]} {not an abbreviation}

DAV & RS
Director of Army Veterinary and Re-
mount Services (armed forces and
veterinary medicine)

DAvMed
Diploma in Aviation Medicine (education)

DAW
dispense as written (pharmacology)

DAyM
Doctor of Ayurvedic Medicine [refers to
use of treatment with Indian herbs
and plants] (education)

DB
Baudelocque's diameter [external conju-

DCAMP
dibutyryl cyclic adenosine monophosphate (laboratory)

dCAMP
dibutyryl cyclic adenosine monophosphate (laboratory)

DC & B
dilation, curettage, and biopsy (gynecology)

DCC
day care center
Disaster Control Center (government)

DCc
double concave

D.Cc.
double concave

DCCMP
daunomycin, cyclocytidine, 6-mercaptopurine, and prednisolone (chemotherapy, oncology, and pharmacology)

DC$_{co}$
diffusing capacity for carbon dioxide (laboratory and respiratory)

DCD
Diploma in Chest Diseases [British] (education)

DCE
dichloroethylene (chemistry)

DCF
deoxycoformycin
direct centrifugal flotation [method; also called *Lane method*] (gastroenterology and laboratory)

D.C.F.
direct centrifugal flotation [method; also called *Lane method*] (gastroenterology and laboratory)

DCFM
Doppler color flow mapping (cardiovascular)

D.C.F. method
direct centrifugal flotation method [also called *Lane method*] (laboratory)

DCG
deoxycorticosterone glucoside (chemistry)
disodium cromoglycate (chemistry)

DCH
delayed cutaneous hypersensitivity (hematology)
Diploma in Child Health (education)

D.C.H.
Diploma in Child Health (education)

DCh
Doctor Chirurgiae [Doctor of Surgery]

D.Ch.
Doctor Chirurgiae [Doctor of Surgery]

DCHFB
dichlorohexafluorobutane (chemistry)

DCHN
dicyclohexaylamine nitrite (chemistry)

DChO
Doctor of Ophthalmic Surgery [British] (education)

DCI
dichloroisoproterenol [also called *dichloroisoprenaline*] (cardiovascular and pharmacology)

DCL
digital counter/locator [on dictating and transcribing equipment] (medical transcription)

DCLS
deoxycholate citrate lactose saccharose [agar] (laboratory)

DCLS agar
deoxycholate citrate lactose saccharose agar (laboratory)

DCM
dichloromethane (chemistry)
dichloromethotrexate (chemotherapy, oncology, and pharmacology)
Doctor of Comparative Medicine

DCMP
daunomycin, cytosine arabinoside, 6-mercaptopurine, and prednisolone (chemotherapy, oncology, and pharmacology)

dCMP
deoxycytidine monophosphate (chemistry)
deoxycytidine-5'-phosphate (chemistry)

DCMT
Doctor of Clinical Medicine of the Tropics [British]

DCMXT
dichloromethotrexate (chemotherapy, oncology, and pharmacology)

DCN
delayed conditional necrosis (psychiatry)
dorsal cutaneous nerve (neurology)

DCNU
chlorozotocin (chemistry)

DCO
diffusing capacity of carbon monoxide (laboratory and respiratory)
Diploma of the College of Optics [British] (education and ophthalmology)

D$_{CO}$
pulmonary diffusion capacity for carbon monoxide (laboratory and respiratory)

DCOG
Diploma of the College of Obstetricians and Gynaecologists [British] (education, gynecology, and obstetrics)

D.C.O.G.
Diploma of the College of Obstetricians and Gynaecologists [British] (education, gynecology, and obstetrics)

DCOME
Dworkin/Culatta Oral Mechanism Examination (speech and language therapy)

DCP
decentralized pharmacy (pharmacology)
dicalcium phosphate [also called *calcium phosphate, dibasic*] (chemistry)
Diploma in Clinical Pathology (education)
Diploma in Clinical Psychology (education)
District Community Physician
dynamic compression plate (orthopedics)

DCR
dacryocystorhinostomy (otorhinolaryngology)
delayed cutaneous reaction (dermatology)
direct cortical response (neurology)

DCS
dense canalicular system (ophthalmology)
Doctors of Christian Science (religion)
dorsal column stimulator (neurology and orthopedics)

DCSA
double contrast shoulder arthrography (orthopedics and radiology)

DCT
deep chest therapy (respiratory)
diastolic control team (cardiovascular)
direct [antiglobulin] Coombs' test (laboratory)
distal convoluted tubule [of kidney] (nephrology)

DCTM
delay computer tomographic myelography (radiology)

DCTMA
deoxycorticosterone trimethylacetate (chemistry)

DCTPA
deoxycorticosterone triphenylacetate (chemistry)

DCU
dichloral urea (laboratory)

DCV
dacarbazine [DTIC], lomustine [CCNU or CeeNU], and vincristine (chemotherapy, oncology, and pharmacology)

DCVO
Deputy Chief Veterinary Officer (veterinary medicine)

DCx
double convex

D.Cx.
double convex

DD
dangerous drug (pharmacology)
de die [daily] (pharmacology)
degenerative disease
dependent drainage (surgery)
developmental disability (neurology and psychiatry)
died of the disease
differential diagnosis
disc diameter (ophthalmology)
discharged dead
disk diameter (ophthalmology)
double diffusion [test] (laboratory)
down drain (surgery)
dry dressing (surgery)
Duchenne's dystrophy (cardiovascular, genetics, neurology, orthopedics, and respiratory)

D.D.
developmental disability (genetics and pediatrics)

D & D
diarrhea and dehydration (gastroenterology)

D/D
differential diagnosis

d/D
day of discharge

d.d.
detur ad [let it be given to] (pharmacology)

DDA
Dangerous Drugs Act (pharmacology)
dideoxyadenosine (genetics and laboratory)

DDAVP
1-deamino-(8-D-arginine)-vasopressin [also called desmopressin acetate] (endocrinology, hematology, and pharmacology)
{not an abbreviation} [trademark for desmopressin acetate] (pharmacology)

DDC
dangerous drug cabinet (pharmacology)
diethyldithiocarbamate [also called diethyldithiocarbamic acid; an herbicide] (chemistry)
dihydrocollidine (chemistry)
direct display console (computer science)

D.D.C.
Developmental Disability Council (genetics and pediatrics)

DDD
degenerative disc [or disk] disease (neurology and orthopedics)
dense deposit disease (nephrology)
dichlorodiphenyldichloroethane (chemistry)
dihydroxydinaphthyl disulfide (chemistry)
three dimensional

DDE
dichlorodiphenyldichloroethylene (chemistry)

DDG
deoxy-D-glucose (chemistry)

DDH
Diploma in Dental Health [British] (education)

D.D.H.
Division of Dental Health (dentistry)

DDI
dressing dry and intact

DDIB
Disease Detection Information Bureau (government)

dd in d
de die in diem [from day to day]

dd. in d.
de die in diem [from day to day]

DM
Diploma in Dermatological Medicine (education)
Doctor of Dental Medicine (dentistry)

DDMS
Deputy Directory of Medical Services (armed forces)

DDO
Diploma in Dental Orthopaedics (education)

DDP
cisplatin (chemotherapy, oncology, and pharmacology)

DDR
Diploma in Diagnostic Radiology (education and radiology)

DDRB
Doctors' and Dentists' Review Body [British]

DDS
Demos Dropout Scale (psychiatry)
dialysis disequilibrium syndrome (nephrology)
diaminodiphenylsulfone [also called *dapsone* and *4,4-diaminodiphenylsulfone*] (chemistry)
Director of Dental Services (dentistry)
Doctor of Dental Science (dentistry and education)
Doctor of Dental Surgery (dentistry and education)

dystrophy-dystocia syndrome (obstetrics)

D.D.S.
Doctor of Dental Surgery (dentistry and education)

DDS4,4'
diaminodiphenylsulfone [also called *dapsone* and *4,4-diaminodiphenylsulfone*; an antibacterial and leprostatic] (infectious diseases and pharmacology)

DDSc
Doctor of Dental Science (dentistry and education)

D.D.Sc.
Doctor of Dental Science (dentistry and education)

DDSO
4,4'-diaminodiphenylsulfoxide [also called *dapsone*; an antibacterial and leprostatic] (infectious diseases and pharmacology)

DDST
Denver Developmental Screening Test (psychiatry)

DDT
dichlorodiphenyltrichloroethane [also called *chlorophenothane*; an insecticide] (chemistry)
ductus deferens tumor (urology)

DDVP
dichlorvos [also called *2,2-dichlorovinyl dimethyl phosphate*] (chemistry)

DDx
differential diagnosis

DE
Delaware [Postal Service state designation]
dentistry
deprived eye (ophthalmology)
digestive energy (laboratory)

dose equivalent (radiology)
dream elements (psychiatry)
drug evaluation (pharmacology)
duration of ejection

D & E
diet and elimination (dietary and gastroenterology)
diet and excretion (dietary and gastroenterology)
dilatation and evacuation (gynecology
   and obstetrics)

DEA
dehydroepiandrosterone (endocrinology
   and laboratory)
diethanolamine (chemistry)
Drug Enforcement Administration
   (chemical dependency and law)

DEAE
diethylaminoethanol (chemistry)
diethylaminoethyl (chemistry)
diethylaminoethylcellulose (chemistry)

DEAE-D
diethylaminoethyl dextran (chemistry)

dearg pil
deargentur pilulae [let the pills be sil-
   vered] {obsolete} (pharmacology)

dearg. pil.
deargentur pilulae [let the pills be sil-
   vered] {obsolete} (pharmacology)

deaug pil
deaurentur pilulae [let the pills be
   gilded] {obsolete} (pharmacology)

deaug. pil.
deaurentur pilulae [let the pills be
   gilded] {obsolete} (pharmacology)

DEB
diethylbutanediol (chemistry)
Division of Environmental Biology (biology and ecology)

DEBA
diethylbarbituric acid (chemistry)

deb
debridement (surgery)

DEBRA
Dystrophic Epidermolysis Bullosa Research Association (dermatology, genetics, and research)

deb spis
debita spissitudine [of the proper con-
   sistency] (pharmacology)

deb. spis.
debita spissitudine [of the proper con-
   sistency] (pharmacology)

DEC
decrease
diethylcarbamazine (chemistry)
dynamic environmental conditioning
   [cycle]

dec
decanta [pour off] (pharmacology)
deceased
deciduous
decompose
decrease

dec.
decanta [pour off] (pharmacology)
deceased
deciduous
decompose
decrease

deca-
{not an abbreviation} [prefix for 10^1]
   (measurement) {pronounced "deck-
   ah"}

decd
deceased

deci-
{not an abbreviation} [prefix for 10^{-1}]
   (measurement) {pronounced "des-E"}

decid
deciduous

"deck-ah"
{pronunciation of *deca-* [prefix for 10^1]}
   (measurement) {not an abbreviation}

DECO
decreasing consumption of oxygen (laboratory and respiratory)

decoct
decoctum [a decoction] (pharmacology)

decoct.
decoctum [a decoction] (pharmacology)

decomp
decompose
decomposition

dec (R)
decrease, relative

decr
decrease(d)

decr.
decrease(d)

DECS
deceased

DECUB
decubitus [lying down position]

decub
decubitus [lying down position]

DED
date of expected delivery (obstetrics)
delayed erythema dose (radiation therapy)

de d in d
de die in diem [from day to day]

de d. in d.
de die in diem [from day to day]

DEEG
depth electroencephalogram (neurology)
depth electroencephalography (neurology)
depth electrography (neurology)

"dee-mardz"
{pronunciation of *DMARD's* [disease-modifying antirheumatic drugs]}

(pharmacology and rheumatology) {not an abbreviation}

DEET
diethyltoluamide (pharmacology)

DEF
decayed, extracted, or filled [teeth] (dentistry)
{not an abbreviation} [an expression of dental caries experience in the deciduous teeth, *D* representing the number of teeth indicated for filling, *E* the number indicated for extraction, and *F* the number of filled teeth] (dentistry)

def
defecation (gastroenterology)
deficiency
deficient
define
definition

def.
defecation (gastroenterology)
deficiency

defib
defibrillate (cardiovascular) {pronounced "de-fib"}
defibrillation (cardiovascular) {pronounced "de-fib"}

"de-fib"
{pronunciation of *defib* [defibrillate and defibrillation]} (cardiovascular) {not an abbreviation}

defic
deficiency
deficit

deform
deformity

Deg.
degeneration
degree

det.
detur [let it be given] (pharmacology)

determin
determination

det in dup
detur in duplo [let twice as much be given] (pharmacology)

det. in dup.
detur in duplo [let twice as much be given] (pharmacology)

det in 2 plo
detur in duplo [let twice as much be given] (pharmacology)

det. in 2 plo
detur in duplo [let twice as much be given] (pharmacology)

detn
detention

detox
detoxification (chemical dependency)
detoxify (chemical dependency)

detox unit
detoxification unit (chemical dependency)

d et s
detur et signetur [let it be given and labeled] (pharmacology)

d. et s.
detur et signetur [let it be given and labeled] (pharmacology)

DEV
development
deviation
duck egg vaccine (pharmacology)
duck egg virus (laboratory)
duck embryo vaccine (pharmacology)
duck embryo virus (laboratory)

Dev
develop
development

dev
deviation

devel
develop
development(al)

DEVR
dominant exudative vitreoretinopathy (ophthalmology)

dex
dexter [right]
dextrose (pharmacology)
Dextro-Stix (endocrinology and pharmacology)

DF
decapacitation factor [referring to sperm] (laboratory and urology)
decayed and filled (dentistry)
deferoxamine mesylate (pharmacology)
deficiency factor
degree of freedom [of movement]
Dermatology Foundation (dermatology)
desferrioxamine [also called *deferoxamine*] (pharmacology)
diabetic father (endocrinology)
dietary fiber (dietary)
discriminant function
disseminated foci (oncology)
distribution factor (radiology)
dorsiflexion (orthopedics)

df.
degrees of freedom

DFA
diet for age (dietary and pediatrics)
direct fluorescent antibody [test] (laboratory)

DFB
dinitrofluorobenzene (immunology and laboratory)
dysfunctional uterine bleeding (gynecology)

DFC
dry-filled capsules (pharmacology)

DFD
defined formula diets (dietary)
di-isopropyl phosphorofluoridate (chemistry)

DFDD
difluoro-diphenyl-dichloroethane (chemistry)

DFDT
difluoro-diphenyl-trichloroethane [an insecticide; trade name *GIX*] (chemistry)

DFE
distal femoral epiphysis (orthopedics)

DFHom
Diploma of the Faculty of Homoeopathy (education)

DFI
disease-free intervals

DFL
Doctor of Family Life (education)

DFMC
daily fetal movement count (obstetrics)

DFMO
difluoromethyl ornithine (chemistry)

DFMR
daily fetal movements record (obstetrics)

DFO
deferoxamine (pharmacology)
District Finance Officer (business)

DFOM
deferoxamine (pharmacology)

DFP
diastolic filling period (cardiovascular)
di-isopropyl fluorophosphate [also called *dyflos* and *isoflurophate*] (chemistry)

DFP^{32}
di-isopropylfluorophosphate (chemistry)

DF^{32}P
di-isopropylfluorophosphate (chemistry)

DFR
diabetic floor routine (endocrinology)

DFSP
dermatofibrosarcoma protuberans (oncology)

DFU
dead fetus in utero (obstetrics)
dead fetus in uterus (obstetrics)
dideoxyfluorouridine (chemistry)

DG
deoxy-D-glucose (chemistry)
deoxyglucose (chemistry)
diagnosis
diastolic gallop (cardiovascular)
diglyceride (chemistry)
distogingival (dentistry)

2DG
2-deoxy-D-glucose (chemistry)

Dg
diagnosis

dG
deoxyguanylate (genetics and laboratory)

dg
decigram (measurement)

dg.
decigram (measurement)

DGE
density gradient electrophoresis (laboratory)

DGI
disseminated gonococcal infection (gynecology, infectious diseases, obstetrics, and urology)

DGM
ductal glandular mastectomy (surgery)

dgm
decigram (measurement)

DHSS
Department of Health and Social Security [United Kingdom] (government)
dihydrostreptomycin sulfate (pharmacology)

DHT
dihydrotachysterol [also called *AT-10*] (chemistry)
4-dihydrotestosterone [also called *stanolone*] (laboratory)
dihydrothymine (laboratory)
(1,2-dihydroxy-3-propyl)theo-phylline (pharmacology)

DHTB
dihydroteleocidin B (pharmacology)

DHTP
dihydrotestosterone proprionate (pharmacology)

D.Hy.
Doctor of Hygiene (education)

DHyg
Doctor of Hygiene (education)

DHZ
dihydralazine (pharmacology)

DI
defective-interfering
deterioration index
detrusor instability (urology)
diabetes insipidus (endocrinology)
diagnostic imaging (radiology)
distoincisal (dentistry)
double indemnity (insurance)
drug information (pharmacology)
drug interactions (pharmacology)
dyskaryosis index (laboratory and pathology)
dyspnea index (respiratory)

D$_I$
insulin dialysance (endocrinology)

Di
didymium (chemistry)

DIA
Drug Information Association (pharmacology)

dia
diathermy (physical therapy)

diab
diabetic (endocrinology)

diab.
diabetic (endocrinology)

DIAC
di-iodothyroacetic acid (chemistry)

diag
diagnosis
diagnostic
diagonal
diagram

diag.
diagnosis

Diam
diameter

diam
diameter

diam.
diameter

diaph.
diaphragm
diaphragmatic (gastroenterology and respiratory)

dias
diastolic (cardiovascular)

dias.
diastolic (cardiovascular)

Diast.
diastolic (cardiovascular)

diath
diathermy (physical therapy)

Diath SW
diathermy short wave (physical therapy)

DIB
butyl di-iodohydroxybenzoate (chemistry)
disability insurance benefits (insurance)

DIC
5-(3,3dimethyl-1-triazeno)imidazole-4-carboxamide [also called *dacarbazine*] (chemotherapy, oncology, and pharmacology)
different interference contrast [microscope] (laboratory)
differential interference contrast [microscope] (laboratory)
diffuse intravascular coagulation (hematology)
diffuse intravascular coagulopathy (hematology)
dimethyl imidazole carboxamide (chemotherapy, oncology, and pharmacology)
disseminated intravascular coagulation (hematology)
disseminated intravascular coagulopathy (hematology)
Drug Information Center (pharmacology)

D.I.C.
disseminated intravascular coagulopathy (hematology)

dic.
dicentric

dick
ethyldichloroarsine (chemistry)

dict
dictionary

DID
dead of intercurrent disease

DIE
died in emergency department
died in emergency room
direct injection enthalpimetry (physical medicine)

dieb alt
diebus alternis [on alternate days] (pharmacology)

dieb. alt.
diebus alternis [on alternate days] (pharmacology)

dieb tert
diebus tertius [every third day] (pharmacology)

dieb. tert.
diebus tertius [every third day] (pharmacology)

DIEDA
diethyl-iminodiacetic acid

Diet. Tech.
Dietetic Technician (dietary)

"die-ver-tick"
{pronunciation of *divertic* [diverticulum]} {not an abbreviation}

DIFF
differential [blood count] (laboratory) {pronounced "diff"}

diff
difference
different
differential {pronounced "diff"}
differential [blood count] (laboratory) {pronounced "diff"}
difficult

"diff"
{pronunciation of *DIFF* and *diff* [differential and differential (blood count)]} (laboratory) {not an abbreviation}

diff diag
differential diagnosis

DIFP
di-isopropyl fluorophosphonate (chemistry)

DIG
digoxin (cardiovascular and pharmacology)

D#IG

\# percent dextrose in Isolyte G [*Note:*
The number sign would be replaced
with the correct percentage given.]
(pharmacology)

Dig

digeratur [let it be digested] (pharmacology)

dig

digitalis {pronounced "deg"} (cardiovascular and pharmacology)
digitoxin {pronounced "deg"} (pharmacology)
digoxin {pronounced "deg"} (cardiovascular and pharmacology)

dig.

digeratur [let it be digested] (pharmacology)

digit

{not an abbreviation} [First digit of hand
is the thumb, second digit the index
finger, third digit the long finger,
fourth digit the ring finger, and fifth
digit the little finger] (neurology and
orthopedics)

DIGOXN

digoxin (cardiovascular and pharmacology)

dig tox

digitalis toxicity (cardiovascular, emergency medicine, and pharmacology)
{pronounced "deg-tox"}

DIH

Diploma in Industrial Health (education)

D#IH

\# percent dextrose in Isolyte H [*Note:*
The number sign would be replaced
with the correct percentage given.]
(pharmacology)

DIHPPA

di-iodohydroxyphenylpyruvic acid (laboratory)

DIJOA

dominantly inherited juvenile optic atrophy (genetics and ophthalmology)

dil

dilue [dilute, dissolve] (pharmacology)
dilutus [diluted] (pharmacology)

dil.

dilue [dilute, dissolve] (pharmacology)

DILAN

Dilantin (neurology and pharmacology)

dilat

dilatation
dilated

DILD

diffuse infiltrative lung disease (respiratory)

dild

diluted

DILE

drug-induced lupus erythematosus
(rheumatology)

"dill"

{pronunciation of *dl* [deciliter]} (measurement) {not an abbreviation}

diln

dilution

DILS

dilutions

diluc

diluculo [at daybreak] (pharmacology)

diluc.

diluculo [at daybreak] (pharmacology)

dilut

dilutus [diluted] (pharmacology)

dilut.

dilutus [diluted] (pharmacology)

DIM
diminish
divalent ion metabolism (laboratory)

dim
dimidius [one-half] (pharmacology)
diminish
diminutive
diminutus [diminished]

dim.
dimidius [one-half] (pharmacology)
diminutus [diminished]

D.I.M.E.
Division of International Medical Education (education)

DIMOAD
diabetes insipidus, diabetes mellitus, optic atrophy, and deafness [syndrome] (endocrinology, ophthalmology, and otorhinolaryngology)

d in p aeq
divide in partes aequales [divide into equal parts] (pharmacology)

d. in p. aeq.
divide in partes aequales [divide into equal parts] (pharmacology)

DIP
desquamative interstitial pneumonia (respiratory)
desquamative interstitial pneumonitis (respiratory)
di-isopropyl phosphate (chemistry)
distal interphalangeal [joint] (orthopedics and podiatry)
drip infusion pyelogram (radiology and nephrology)
dual in-line package

D.I.P.
distal interphalangeal [joint] (orthopedics and podiatry)

D#IP
percent dextrose in Isolyte P [*Note: The number sign would be replaced with the correct percentage given.*] (pharmacology)

Dip
diploma (education)
diplomate

DIPA
disiopropylamine (laboratory)

DipAmerBdP & N
Diplomate, American Board of Psychiatry and Neurology (neurology and psychiatry)

DipBact
Diploma in Bacteriology (education)

DipChem
Diploma in Chemistry [British] (education)

DipClinPath
Diploma in Clinical Pathology [British] (education)

diph
diphtheria (infectious diseases)

diph.
diphtheria (infectious diseases)

Diph. Tet.
diphtheria-tetanus [toxoid] (infectious diseases, pharmacology, and respiratory)

diph-tet
diphtheria-tetanus (infectious diseases)

diph-tox
diphtheria toxoid (plain) (infectious diseases and pharmacology)

diph-tox AP
diphtheria toxoid (alum precipitated) (infectious diseases and pharmacology)

DIPJ
distal interphalangeal joint (orthopedics and podiatry)

DipMicrobiol
Diploma in Microbiology (education)

DipSocMed
Diploma in Social Medicine [British] (education)

Dir
director

dir
directione [directions]

dir.
directione [directions]

dir prop
directione propria [with a proper direction, with the proper directions] (pharmacology)

dir. prop.
directione propria [with a proper direction, with the proper directions] (pharmacology)

DIS
Diagnostic Interview Scheduled [questionnaire]

Dis
disease

dis
disability
disabled
disease
dislocation
distance

dis.
disability
disabled
disease
dislocation
distance

DISC
discharge(d)

disc
discontinue

disc.
discontinue

disch
discharge(d)

disch.
discharge(d)

DISH
diffuse idiopathic skeletal hyperostosis (orthopedics) {pronounced "dish"}
disseminated idiopathic skeletal hyperostosis (orthopedics) {pronounced "dish"}

"dish"
{pronunciation of *DISH* [diffuse idiopathic skeletal hyperostosis and disseminated idiopathic skeletal hyperostosis]} (orthopedics) {not an abbreviation}

DISI
dorsal intercalary segment instability (orthopedics)

Disl
dislocation (orthopedics)

disloc
dislocation (orthopedics)

disod
disodium (chemistry)

disp
dispensa [to dispense] (pharmacology)
dispensary (pharmacology)
dispense (pharmacology)

disp.
dispensare [to dispense] (pharmacology)
dispensatory

dispo
disposition {pronounced "dis-poe"} {not an abbreviation}

"dis-poe"
{pronunciation of *dispo* [disposition]}
{not an abbreviation}

diss
dissolve(d)

dissem
disseminated

dist
distal
distance
distilla [distill] (pharmacology)
distilled (pharmacology)

dist.
distance
distilla [distill] (pharmacology)
distilled (pharmacology)

dist f
distinguished from

dist H₂0
distilled water (pharmacology)

distn
distillation

DIT
diiodotyrosine (endocrinology and laboratory)

DIV
double-inlet ventricle (cardiovascular)

div
divergence
divide
divido [to divide] (pharmacology)
division
divorced

div.
divide
divido [to divide] (pharmacology)
division

DIVA
digital intravenous angiography (cardiovascular and radiology)

divertic
diverticulum {pronounced "die-vertick"}

div in par aeq
dividatur in partes aequales [divide into equal parts] (pharmacology)

div. in par. aeq.
dividatur in partes aequales [divide into equal parts] (pharmacology)

DJD
degenerative joint disease (orthopedics)

D.J.D.
degenerative joint disease (orthopedics)

DK
dark
decay
diseased kidney (nephrology)
dog kidney (laboratory and research)

Dk
diffusion coefficient [or permeability constant] as described by Krogh (laboratory and respiratory)

dk
dark
deka- [prefix for 10] (measurement)

DKA
diabetic ketoacidosis (endocrinology)

DKB
deep knee bends (orthopedics and physical therapy)

dkg
decagram (measurement)

dkg.
decagram (measurement)

dkm
decameter (measurement)

dkm.
decameter (measurement)

dimethylamine (laboratory)
dimethylarginine (laboratory)
direct memory access (computer science)

DMAB
dimethylaminobenzaldehyde (chemistry and laboratory)

DMAC
N,*N*-dimethylacetamide (chemistry and pharmacology)

DMARD's
disease-modifying antirheumatic drugs (pharmacology and rheumatology) {pronounced "dee-mardz"}

DMBA
7,12-dimethylbenz[a]-antracene [also called *dimethylbenzantracene*] (chemistry)

DMC
demeclocycline [also called *demethylchlortetracycline*] (pharmacology)
dimite(1,1-bis-[*p*-chloro-phenyl] ethanol (chemistry)
di(*p*-chlorophenyl) methylcarbinol [also called *avantin, dichlorodiphenyl methyl carbinol, dimethylcarbinol,* and *isopropanol*] (chemistry)
direct microscopic count (laboratory)

DMCC
direct microscopic clump count (laboratory)

DMCM
dimethoxyethylcarboline carboxylate (chemistry)

DMCT
dimethylchlortetracycline (pharmacology)

DMCTC
dimethylchlortetracycline (pharmacology)

DMD
Doctor of Dental Medicine (dentistry and education)

Duchenne's muscular dystrophy (neurology)

D.M.D.
Doctor of Dental Medicine (dentistry and education)

DMDT
dimethoxydiphenyl trichloroethane (chemistry)
methoxychlor [also called *Marlate*; an insecticide] (chemistry)

DME
dextromethorphan (pharmacology and respiratory)
dimethyl ether (chemistry)
Director of Medical Education (education)
Dulbecco's modified Eagle's [medium] (laboratory)
durable medical equipment (physical therapy and rehabilitation)

D.M.E.
Director of Medical Education (administration and education)

DMF
decayed, missing, or filled [teeth] (dentistry)
{not an abbreviation} [expression of accumulated dental caries in permanent teeth, D indicating the number of carious teeth, M the number of missing teeth, and F the number of filled teeth] (dentistry)
N,*N*-dimethylformamide (chemistry)

DMFT
decayed, missing, and filled permanent teeth (dentistry)

DMGBL
dimethyl-gamma-butyrolacton (chemistry)

DMH
Department of Mental Health (psychiatry)

Department of Mental Hygiene (psychiatry)

D.M.H.
Department of Mental Health (psychiatry)

DMHS
Director of Medical and Health Services (administration)

DMI
desipramine (pharmacology)
Diagnostic Medical Instruments [equipment] (laboratory and manufacturing)
diaphragmatic myocardial infarct (cardiovascular)

DMJ
Diploma in Medical Jurisprudence (education and law)

DMKA
diabetes mellitus ketoacidosis (endocrinology)

DML
diffuse mixed lymphoma (oncology)

DMM
dimethylmyleran (chemistry)

DMN
dimethylnitrosamine (chemistry)
dorsal motor nucleus [of the vagus] (gastroenterology and neurology)

DMO
dimethadone (pharmacology)
5,5-dimethyl-2,4-oxazolidinedione [also called *5,5-dimethyloxazolidine-2,4-dione*] (chemistry)
District Medical Officer
Divisional Medical Officer

DMOOC
diabetes mellitus out of control (endocrinology)

DMP
dimethylphthalate (chemistry)

DMPA
depomedroxyprogesterone acetate (chemistry)

DMPE
3,4-dimethoxyphenylethylamine [also called *dimethoxyphenyl-ethylamine*] (chemistry)

DMPP
dimethylphenylpiperazinium (chemistry)
1,1-dimethyl-4-phenylpiperazinium iodide (chemistry)

DMR
Diploma in Medical Radiology (education and radiology)
Directorate of Medical Research [Army] (armed forces and research)

D.M.R.
Diploma in Medical Radiology (education and radiology)

DMRD
Diploma in Medical Radio-Diagnosis [British] (education and radiology)

D.M.R.D.
Diploma in Medical Radio-Diagnosis [British] (education and radiology)

DMRE
Diploma in Medical Radiology and Electrology (education and radiology)

DMRT
Diploma in Medical Radio-Therapy [British] (education, radiation therapy, and radiology)

D.M.R.T.
Diploma in Medical Radio-Therapy [British] (education, radiation therapy, and radiology)

DMS
Department of Medicine and Surgery
dermatomyositis (dermatology)

Diagnostic Medical Sonographer (cardiovascular, obstetrics, and radiology)
dimethyl sulfoxide (chemistry)
Director of Medical Services (armed forces)
District Management Team [British]
Doctor of Medical Science (education)

D.M.S.
Department of Medicine and Surgery

DMSA
2,3-dimercaptosuccinic acid [scanning and toxicity of lead poisoning in children] (pediatrics, pharmacology, and radiology)

DMSLT
daytime multiple sleep latency test (neurology)

DMSO
dimethyl sulfoxide (pharmacology)

DMSS
Director of Medical and Sanitary Services

DMT
dimethyltryptamine [a hallucinogen; also called *N,N-dimethyltryptamine*] (chemical dependency and chemistry)
Doctor of Medical Technology (education)

DMU
dimethanolurea (laboratory, nephrology, and urology)
dimethyluracil (laboratory, nephrology, and urology)

DMV
Department of Motor Vehicles (government)
Doctor of Veterinary Medicine (education and veterinary medicine)

DMX
diathermy, massage, and exercise (physical therapy)

DMZ
demilitarized zone (armed forces)

DN
dextrose-nitrogen [ratio] (laboratory)
dibucaine number (laboratory)
dicrotic notch (cardiovascular)
Diploma in Nursing (education and nursing)
Diploma in Nutrition (dietary and education)
District Nurse (nursing)
Doctor of Nursing (education and nursing)
down

D.N.
dibucaine number (laboratory)

D/N
dextrose-nitrogen [ratio in urine] (laboratory)

Dn.
dekanem (measurement)

dn
decinem (measurement)

dn.
decinem (measurement)

DNA
deoxyribonucleic acid [also called *desoxyribonucleic acid*] (genetics, laboratory, and oncology)
does not apply

DNA-P
deoxyribonucleic acid-phosphorus (genetics and laboratory)

DNase
deoxyribonuclease [also called *desoxyribonuclease*] (genetics and laboratory)

DNB
dinitrobenzene (chemistry)
Diplomate of the National Board [of Medical Examiners]

D.N.B.
dinitrochlorobenzene (chemistry)

Diplomate of the National Board [of Medical Examiners]

DNBP
dinitrobutyphenol (chemistry)

DNC
did not come
dinitrocarbanilide (chemistry)
Disaster Nursing Chairman (nursing)

DNCB
dinitrochlorobenzene (chemistry)

DND
died a natural death

DNE
Director of Nursing Education (education and nursing)
Doctor of Nursing Education (education and nursing)
group D nonenterococcal streptococcus (laboratory)

DNFB
dinitrofluorobenzene (chemistry)

DNI
do not intubate (respiratory)

DNKA
did not keep appointment

DNL
Director of Naval Laboratories (armed forces and laboratory)

DNO
District Nursing Officer (nursing)

DNOC
dinitro-orthocresol [also called *dinitro-o-cresol*] (chemistry)

DNP
deoxyribonucleoprotein (genetics and laboratory)
dinitrophenol (chemistry)
2-4-dinitrophenyl group (chemistry)
do not publish

DNPH
dinitrophenylhydrazine (chemistry)

DNPM
dinitrophenylmorphine (chemistry)

DNR
daunorubicin [also called *daunomycin*] (chemotherapy, oncology, and pharmacology)
do not report
do not resuscitate (cardiovascular and respiratory)

DNS
deviated nasal septum (otorhinolaryngology)
diaphragm nerve stimulation (neurology and respiratory)
did not show
do not show
dysplastic nevus syndrome (dermatology)

D5-½NS
dextrose five percent [5%] in one-half normal saline (pharmacology)

D5½NS
dextrose five percent [5%] in one-half normal saline (pharmacology)

D/NS
dextrose in normal saline (pharmacology)

D5/NS
dextrose five percent [5%] in normal saline (pharmacology)

D$_5$NSS
dextrose five percent [5%] in normal saline solution (pharmacology)

DNT
did not test

DNTP
diethylnitrophenyl thiophosphate (chemistry)

DO
diamine oxidase (chemistry)
Diploma in Ophthalmology (education)

dopamine (cardiovascular and pharmacology) {pronounced "dope-ah"}

dopa
methyldopa [also called *dihydroxyphe-
nylalanine* and *3,4-dihydroxyphenyl-
alanine*] (cardiovascular and pharmacology) {pronounced "dope-ah"}
dopamine (cardiovascular and pharmacology) {pronounced "dope-ah"}

DOPAC
dihydroxyphenylacetic acid [also called
3,4-dihydroxyphenylacetic acid]
(chemistry)

dopase
dopa-oxidase (laboratory)

"dope-ah"
{pronunciation of *DOPA* and *dopa*
[methyldopa (also called *dihydroxy-
phenylalanine* and *3,4-dihydroxyphe-
nylalanine*) (cardiovascular and pharmacology) and dopamine (cardiovascular and pharmacology)]} {not an abbre-
viation}

DOph
Doctor of Ophthalmology (ophthalmology)

DOPS
diffuse obstructive pulmonary syndrome
(respiratory)

DORIDN
Doriden (pharmacology and psychiatry)

DOrth
Diploma in Orthodontics [British] (education)
Diploma in Orthoptics [British] (education)

DORV
double outlet right ventricle (cardiovascular)

DORx
date of treatment

DOS
date of surgery

deoxystreptamine
Doctor of Ocular Science (ophthalmology)
Doctor of Optical Science (ophthalmology)

D.O.S.
Division of Occupational Safety

dos
dosage (pharmacology)
dosis [dose] (pharmacology)

dos.
dosage (pharmacology)
dosis [dose] (pharmacology)

DOSC
Dubois oleic serum complex (bacteriology and laboratory)

DOSS
dioctyl sodium sulfosuccinate [also
called *docusate sodium*] (chemotherapy, gastroenterology, oncology, and
pharmacology) {pronounced "doss"}
distal over-shoulder strap (rehabilitation)

D.O.S.S.
Department of Social Services (social
services)

"doss"
{pronunciation of *DOSS* [dioctyl sodium
sulfosuccinate; also called *docusate
sodium*]} (chemotherapy, gastroenterology, oncology, and pharmacology)
{not an abbreviation}

DOT
died on table [referring to operating
table] (surgery)
Doppler ophthalmic test (ophthalmology)

DOU
definitive observation unit
direct observation unit

DOV
discharged on visit (psychiatry)

DP
deep pulse (cardiovascular)
degradation products (laboratory)
deltopectoral (neurology and orthopedics)
dementia praecox (psychiatry)
dental prosthetics (dentistry)
diastolic pressure (cardiovascular)
diffusion pressure
digestible protein (dietary and laboratory)
diphosgene (chemistry)
diphosphate (chemistry)
dipropionate (pharmacology)
direct puncture
directional preponderance
directione propria [with proper direc-
   tion] (pharmacology)
disability pension
displaced person
distal phalanx (orthopedics and podiatry)
distopulpal (dentistry)
Doctor of Pharmacy (pharmacology)
donor's plasma (laboratory)
dorsalis pedis [pulse] (cardiovascular)

D.P.
directione propria [with proper direc-
   tion] (pharmacology)
Doctor of Pharmacy (pharmacology)
Doctor of Podiatry (podiatry)

D/P
distal interphalangeal [joints] (orthopedics and podiatry)

D-P
Depo-Provera [also called *medroxyprogesterone acetate*] (gynecology and
   pharmacology)

d.p.
directione propria [with proper direc-
   tion] (pharmacology)

DPA
Department of Public Assistance (government)
dextroposition of aorta (cardiovascular)
diphenylamine (chemistry)

dipicolinic acid
dipropylacetate (chemistry)

DPC
delayed primary closure (surgery)
desaturated phosphatidylcholine (laboratory and pharmacology)
direct patient care
discharge planning coordinator
distal palmar crease (neurology and orthopedics)

DPD
Department of Public Dispensary (government)
desoxypyridoxine hydrochloride [also
   called *deoxypyridoxine hydrochloride*] (pharmacology)
diffuse pulmonary disease (respiratory)
diphenamid [also called *diphenyl-di-
   methylacetamide*] (chemistry)
Diploma in Public Dentistry (dentistry
   and education)

DPDA
phosphorodiamidic anhydride (chemistry)

DPDL
diffuse, poorly differentiated lymphoma
   (oncology)

DPDLL
diffuse, poorly differentiated, lymphocytic lymphoma (oncology)

dpdt switch
double-pole double-throw switch

DPF
Dental Practitioners' Formulary (dentistry)

DPG
2,3-diphosphoglycerate [also called *diphosphoglycerate*] (chemistry)
displacement placentogram (radiology)

2,3-DPG
2,3-diphosphoglycerate (chemistry)
2,3-diphosphoglyceric acid (chemistry)

DPGM
diphosphoglycerate mutase (chemistry)

2,3-DPGM
2,3-diphosphoglycerate mutase (chemistry)

DPGP
diphosphoglycerate phosphatase (chemistry)

DPH
Department of Public Health (government)
diphenhydramine (laboratory)
diphenylhydantoin [also called *Dilantin* and *phenytoin*] (neurology and pharmacology)
Diploma in Public Health (education)
Doctor of Public Health (education)
Doctor of Public Hygiene (education)

D.P.H.
Diploma in Public Health (education)

DPh
Doctor of Philosophy (education)

D.Ph.
Doctor of Philosophy (education)

DPhC
Doctor of Pharmaceutical Chemistry (chemistry, education, and pharmacology)

DPhc
Doctor of Pharmacology (education and pharmacology)

DPHEd
Doctor of Public Health Education (education)

DPHEng
Doctor of Public Health Engineering (education)

DPHN
Doctor of Public Health Nursing (education and nursing)

D.P.H.N.
Department of Public Health Nursing

DPhys
Diploma in Physiotherapy (education)

DPhysMed
Diploma in Physical Medicine (education)

DPI
disposable personal income

DPIF
Drug Product Information File (pharmacology)

DPL
dipalmitoyl lecithin (chemistry and laboratory)
distopulpolingual (dentistry)

DPLa
distopulpolabial (dentistry)

DPM
Diploma in Psychological Medicine (education)
discontinue previous medication (pharmacology)
disintegration per minute (physics)
Doctor of Physical Medicine (education)
Doctor of Podiatric Medicine (education and podiatry)
Doctor of Preventive Medicine (education)
Doctor of Psychiatric Medicine (education and psychiatry)

D.P.M.
Diploma in Psychological Medicine (education)
Doctor of Podiatric Medicine (education and podiatry)

dpm
disintegration per minute (physics)

DPN
diphosphopyridine nucleotide [former name for *nicotinamide-adenine dinucleotide (NAD)*] (genetics and laboratory)

DPNase
diphosphopyridine nucleotide [hydrolyzing enzyme] (genetics and laboratory)

DPNH
diphosphopyridine nucleotide [reduced form] (laboratory)

DPP
dimethoxyphenyl penicillin (pharmacology)

DPS
dimethylpolysiloxane (chemistry)

dps
disintegration per second (physics)

DPSS
Department of Public Social Service (government and social services)

dpst switch
double-pole single-throw switch

DPT
Demerol, Phenergan, and Thorazine (pharmacology)
dimethyltryptamine [a hallucinogen] (chemical dependency) {slang}
diphosphothiamine (chemistry)
diphtheria, pertussis, and tetanus [immunization; also called *diphtheria toxoid, pertussis vaccine, and tetanus toxoid*] (pediatrics and pharmacology)
dipropyltryptamine (chemistry)

DPTA
diethylenetriamine penta-acetic acid (chemistry)

DPTI
diastolic pressure time index (cardiovascular)

DPU
delayed pressure urticaria (dermatology)
diphenylhydantoin [also called *phenytoin* and *Dilantin*] (neurology and pharmacology)

DQ
deterioration quotient (physics)
developmental quotient (psychiatry)

DR
daunorubicin [also called *Rubidazone*] (chemotherapy, oncology, and pharmacology)
delivery room (obstetrics)
diabetic retinopathy (endocrinology and ophthalmology)
diagnostic radiology (radiology)
dining room
dorsal root (neurology)
reaction of degeneration (physics)

D.R.
delivery room (obstetrics)
diabetic retinopathy (endocrinology and ophthalmology)

Dr
doctor

Dr.
doctor

dr
dorsal root [of spinal nerves] (neurology and orthopedics)
drachm (pharmacology)
dram (pharmacology)
dressing

dr.
drachm (pharmacology)
dram (pharmacology)
dressing

DRACOG
Diploma of Royal Australian College of Obstetricians and Gynaecologists (education, gynecology, and obstetrics)

DRACR
Diploma of Royal Australasian College of Radiologists (radiology)

dr ap
drachm apothecaries' [weight] (pharmacology)

DSC
disodium cromoglycate (pharmacology and respiratory)
Doctor of Surgical Chiropody (education and podiatry)

D.S.C.
Doctor of Surgical Chiropody (education and podiatry)

DSc
Doctor of Science (education)

DSCG
disodium cromoglycate (pharmacology and respiratory)

DSCS
disodium cromoglycate (pharmacology and respiratory)

DSD
discharge summary dictated (medical records)
dry sterile dressing

dsDNA
double-stranded deoxyribonucleic acid (genetics and laboratory)

DSE
digital subtraction echocardiogram (cardiovascular and radiology)
Doctor of Sanitary Engineering (education)

dsg
dressing(s)

dsg.
dressing(s)

DSI
deep shock insulin (endocrinology)
digital subtraction imaging (cardiovascular and radiology)
Down's Syndrome International (genetics and neurology)

DSIM
Doctor of Science in Industrial Medicine (education)

DSIP
delta sleep-inducing peptide (laboratory and neurology)

dslv
dissolved

DSM
dextrose solution mixture (pharmacology)
Diagnostic and Statistical Manual of Mental Disorders (psychiatry, research, and statistical analysis)
Diploma in Social Medicine [British] (education)
drink skim milk (dietary)

DSM III
Diagnostic and Statistical Manual of Mental Disorders, Third Edition (psychiatry, research, and statistical analysis)

DSMO
dimethyl sulfoxide [topical anti-inflammatory] (dermatology and pharmacology)

D-spine
dorsal spine [the twelve dorsal or thoracic vertebrae] (neurology and orthopedics)

D/spine
dorsal spine [the twelve dorsal or thoracic vertebrae] (neurology and orthopedics)

DSR
dynamic spatial reconstructor (radiology)

dsRNA
double-stranded ribonucleic acid (genetics and laboratory)

DSS
dengue shock syndrome (hematology and infectious diseases)
Developmental Sentence Scoring (speech and language therapy)

dioctyl sodium sulfosuccinate [also called *docusate sodium*] (chemotherapy, gastroenterology, oncology, and pharmacology)

DSSc
Diploma in Sanitary Science (education)

DST
daylight saving time
desensitization test (allergy)
dexamethasone suppression test (laboratory and nephrology)
dihydrostreptomycin (pharmacology)
donor-specific transfusion (hematology and laboratory)

DSUH
direct suggestion under hypnosis (parapsychology and psychiatry)

DSur
Doctor of Surgery (education and surgery)

DSVP
downstream venous pressure (cardiovascular)

DSX
Detrostix (endocrinology, laboratory, and pharmacology)

DT
delirium tremens (chemical dependency, neurology, and psychiatry)
dental technician (dentistry)
diphtheria and tetanus [immunization] (pediatrics and pharmacology)
diphtheria-tetanus [immunization] (pediatrics and pharmacology)
diphtheria toxoid (pharmacology)
discharge tomorrow
dispensing tablet (pharmacology)
distance test
diversional therapy (psychiatry)
duration [of] tetany (cardiovascular)
dye test (laboratory)

D/T
deaths
total ratio (measurement)

dt
diphtheria and tetanus toxoids (pediatrics and pharmacology)

DTBC
D-tubocurarine (pharmacology)
tubocurarine (pharmacology)

DTBN
di-*t*-butyl nitroxide (chemistry)

DTC
day treatment center
D-tubocurarine (pharmacology)

DTCD
Diploma in Tuberculosis and Chest Diseases (education, infectious diseases, and respiratory)

DTCH
Diploma in Tropical Child Health (education and pediatrics)

DTD
Diploma in Tuberculous Diseases [British] (education, infectious diseases, and respiratory)

D.T.D.
datur talis dosis [give of such a dose] (pharmacology)

DTD #30
dispense 30 such doses (pharmacology)

dtd
datur talis dosis [give of such a dose] (pharmacology)

d.t.d.
datur talis dosis [give of such a dose] (pharmacology)

dtdNo iv
dentur tales doses No. iv [let four such doses be given] (pharmacology)

dTDP
thymidine diphosphate (genetics and laboratory)

2-D TEE
two-dimensional transesophageal echocardiography (cardiovascular)

DTF
detector transfer function (chemistry)

D-TGA
dextrotransposition of the great arteries
[right transposition] (cardiovascular,
neonatology, and pediatrics)

d-TGA
dextrotransposition of the great arteries
[right transposition] (cardiovascular,
neonatology, and pediatrics)

DTH
delayed-type hypersensitivity [reaction]
(allergy)
Diploma in Tropical Hygiene (education)

DTIC
5-(3,3-dimethyl-1-triazino)-imidazole-4-
carboxamide [also called *dacarbazine*
and *dimethyl triazene imidazole carboxamide*] (chemotherapy, oncology,
and pharmacology)

D.T.I.C.
5-(3,3-dimethyl-1-triazino)-imidazole-4-
carboxamide [also called *dacarbazine*
and *dimethyl triazene imidazole carboxamide*] (chemotherapy, oncology,
and pharmacology)

D time
dream time (neurology and psychiatry)

DTLA
Detroit Test of Learning Aptitude (psychiatry and rehabilitation)

DTM
dermatophyte test median (laboratory)
Diploma in Tropical Medicine (education)

DTMA
desoxycorticosterone trimethylacetate
(pharmacology)

DTM & H
Diplomate of Tropical Medicine and Hygiene (education)

DTMP
deoxythymidine monophosphate (genetics and laboratory)

dTMP
de novo thymidylate [synthesis] (laboratory)
thymidine-5'-phosphate (laboratory)

DTMV$_{max}$
diastolic transmembrane voltage, maximum (cardiovascular)

DTN
diphtheria toxin, normal (laboratory)

DTNB
dithiobisnitrobenzoic acid (chemistry)
dithionitrobenzene (chemistry)

DTP
diphtheria, tetanus, and pertussis (pediatrics and pharmacology)
distal tingling on percussion [Tinel's
sign] (neurology)

D.T.P.
diphtheria, tetanus, and pertussis (pediatrics and pharmacology)
distal tingling on percussion [Tinel's
sign] (neurology)

DTPA
diethylenetriamine penta-acetic acid
[also called *penetate trisodium calcium, pentetic acid,* and *penthanil
diethylenetriamine penta-acetic
acid*; used for scanning] (chemistry
and radiology)

DTPH
Diploma in Tropical Public Health (education)

DTR
deep tendon reflex (neurology)

D.T.R.
deep tendon reflex (neurology)

DTRs
deep tendon reflexes (neurology)

DTR's
deep tendon reflexes (neurology)

DTS
dense tubular system (anatomy)
donor specific transfusion (hematology)

DTs
delirium tremens (chemical dependency, neurology, and psychiatry)

DT's
delirium tremens (chemical dependency, neurology, and psychiatry)

DTT
diphtheria-tetanus toxoid (pharmacology)
direct transverse traction (orthopedics)
dithiothreitol (chemistry)

dTTP
thymidine triphosphate (laboratory)

DTV
due to void

DT-VAC
diphtheria-tetanus vaccine (infectious diseases and pharmacology)

DTVM
Diploma in Tropical Veterinary Medicine (education and veterinary medicine)

D.T.V.M.
Diploma in Tropical Veterinary Medicine (education and veterinary medicine)

DTX
detoxification (chemical dependency)

DTZ
diatrizoate (chemistry, pharmacology, and radiology)

DU
decubitus ulcer (dermatology)
density [optical] unknown (ophthalmology)
diabetic urine (endocrinology, laboratory, and nephrology)
diagnosis undetermined
dog unit [referring to adrenal cortical hormones] (endocrinology and laboratory)
duodenal ulcer (gastroenterology)
duroxide uptake (radiology)

D$_U$
urea dialysance (laboratory)

DU+
dog unit positive (laboratory)

dU
deoxyuridine (laboratory)

d.u.
dial unit (measurement)

DUB
Dubowitz [score] (obstetrics)
dysfunctional uterine bleeding (gynecology)

DUI
driving under the influence (chemical dependency and law)

dulc
dulcis [sweet] (pharmacology)

dUMP
deoxyuridine monophosphate (laboratory)
deoxyuridine-5'-phosphate (laboratory)
deoxyuridylate (laboratory)

DUNG
dog unit negative (laboratory)

duod
duodenum (gastroenterology)

duod.
duodenum (gastroenterology)

dup
duplicate

DUPL
duplicate

dur
duration
durus [hard] (pharmacology)

dur.
durus [hard] (pharmacology)

dur dol
durante dolore [while the pain lasts]
   (pharmacology)

dur. dolor.
durante dolore [while the pain lasts]
   (pharmacology)

DV
dependent variable
dianhydrogalactitol and VP-16 (chemotherapy, oncology, and pharmacology)
dilute volume [of solutions] (pharmacology)
distemper virus (infectious diseases, laboratory, and veterinary medicine)
divorced
domiciliary visit
double vision (neurology and ophthalmology)

D & V
diarrhea and vomiting (gastroenterology)

D/V
diffusion per unit volume (measurement)

dv
double vibrations [unit for measuring
   frequency of sound waves] (otorhinolaryngology)

d.v.
double vibrations [unit for measuring
   frequency of sound waves] (otorhinolaryngology)

DVA
distance visual acuity (ophthalmology)

duration of voluntary apnea [test] (respiratory)
vindesine (chemotherapy, oncology, and
   pharmacology)

D/V$_A$
diffusion per unit of alveolar volume
   (laboratory and respiratory)

D value
decimal reduction time (measurement)

DVCC
Disease Vector Control Center (government and infectious diseases)

DVD
dissociated vertical divergence (ophthalmology)

DV & D
Diploma in Venereology and Dermatology (dermatology, education, gynecology, infectious diseases, and urology)

DVDALV
double vessel disease with an abnormal
   left ventricle (cardiovascular)

DVE
duck virus enteritis (gastroenterology
   and laboratory)

DVH
Diploma in Veterinary Hygiene (education and veterinary medicine)
Division for the Visually Handicapped
   (ophthalmology and rehabilitation)

DVI
Digital Vascular Imaging [System] (cardiovascular and radiology)

DVIU
direct vision internal urethrotomy (urology)

DVLP
daunomycin, vincristine, L-asparaginase,
   and prednisone (chemotherapy, oncology, and pharmacology)

DVM
digital voltmeter (electricity)
Doctor of Veterinary Medicine (education and veterinary medicine)

D.V.M.
Doctor of Veterinary Medicine (education and veterinary medicine)

DVMS
Doctor of Veterinary Medicine and Surgery (education and veterinary medicine)

D.V.M.S.
Doctor of Veterinary Medicine and Surgery (education and veterinary medicine)

DVO
Divisional Veterinary Office (veterinary medicine)

DVOP
Disabled Veterans Outreach Program (armed forces)

DVORAK
{not an abbreviation} [an alternative design for the typewriter keyboard] (business)

DVPL-ASP
daunorubicin, vincristine, prednisone, and L-asparaginase (chemotherapy, oncology, and pharmacology)

DVR
Department of Vocational Rehabilitation (rehabilitation)
derotational varus osteotomy (orthopedics)
Doctor of Veterinary Radiology (radiology and veterinary medicine)
double valve replacement (cardiovascular)

DVS
Doctor of Veterinary Science (education and veterinary medicine)
Doctor of Veterinary Surgery (education and veterinary medicine)

D.V.S.
Division of Vital Statistics (government and statistics)
Doctor of Veterinary Science (education and veterinary medicine)
Doctor of Veterinary Surgery (education and veterinary medicine)

DVSc
Doctor of Veterinary Science (education and veterinary medicine)

DVSM
Diploma of Veterinary State Medicine (education and veterinary medicine)

DVT
deep vein thrombosis (cardiovascular)
deep venous thrombosis (cardiovascular)

DVXI
direct vision times one (surgery)

DW
deionized water (pharmacology)
dextrose in water (pharmacology)
distilled water (pharmacology)
dry weight (cardiovascular and nephrology)

D/W
dextrose and water (pharmacology)
dextrose in water (pharmacology)

D5W
dextrose five percent [5%] in water (pharmacology)

D_5W
dextrose five percent [5%] in water (pharmacology)

D5/W
dextrose five percent [5%] in water (pharmacology)

D-5-W
dextrose five percent [5%] in water (pharmacology)

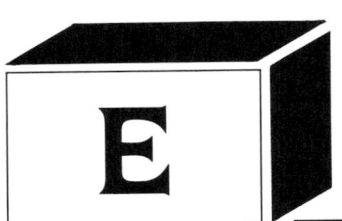

E

ϵ

epsilon [fifth letter of the Greek alphabet]

{not an abbreviation} [symbol for *molar absorptivity*] (chemistry and measurement)

{not an abbreviation} [symbol for the *heavy chain of immunoglobulin E* (IgE)] (laboratory)

{not an abbreviation} [symbol for the ϵ chain of *hemoglobin*] (hematology and laboratory)

η

eta [seventh letter of the Greek alphabet]

{not an abbreviation} [symbol for *viscosity*] (chemistry and laboratory)

E

air dose [also called *air exposure*, referring to radiation exposure] (radiation therapy and radiology)

cortisone [compound E] (pharmacology)

edema (cardiovascular and orthopedics)

elastance [pressure per unit of volume change] (laboratory and respiratory)

electric field vector (physics)

electrode potential (neurology)

electrolyte [panel] (laboratory)

electromotive force (physics)

emmetropia (ophthalmology)

endoplasm (laboratory)

enema (gastroenterology and pharmacology)

energy

Entamoeba (laboratory)

enzyme (laboratory)

epinephrine (pharmacology)

erythrocyte (hematology and laboratory)

Escherichia (laboratory)

esophagus (anatomy and gastroenterology)

esophoria (ophthalmology)

ester (chemistry)

estradiol (endocrinology, gynecology, laboratory, and pharmacology)

ethmoid sinus (allergy and otorhinolaryngology)

ethyl (chemistry)

etiology

exa- [prefix for 10^{18}]

experiment(al)

experimenter

expired (respiratory)

expired gas (chemistry, laboratory, and respiratory)

extraction fraction (chemistry)

extralymphatic

eye (ophthalmology)

internal energy

mathematical expectation (mathematics and statistics)

redox potential (chemistry and laboratory)

{not an abbreviation} [symbol for *elastance* (pressure per unit of volume change)] (laboratory and respiratory)

{not an abbreviation} [symbol for *electromotive force*] (physics)

{not an abbreviation} [symbol for *energy*] (physics)

{not an abbreviation} [symbol for *expectation*] (mathematics and statistics)

ᴇ

expired gas (laboratory and respiratory) [*Note: The abbreviation is subscripted.*]

E.

electromagnetic force (physics)

emmetropia (ophthalmology)

experimenter

eye (ophthalmology)

E′

esophoria (ophthalmology)

E°
standard potential (physics)

γE
gamma-E immunoglobulin (laboratory)
immunoglobulin E (laboratory)

E^+
positron [also called *positive electron*] (physics)

E^-
negative electron (physics)

E_0
electric affinity (physics)

E_1
estrone (endocrinology, gynecology, and laboratory)

E_2
17-beta-estradiol [also called *estradiol*] (endocrinology, gynecology, laboratory, and pharmacology)

E_3
estriol (endocrinology, gynecology, laboratory, and pharmacology)

E_4
estetrol (endocrinology, gynecology, and laboratory)

4E
four plus edema (cardiovascular and orthopedics)

e
base of natural logarithms (mathematics)
electric charge (electricity)
electron (physics)
elementary charge
emergency area (emergency medicine)
erg [unit of energy] (physics)
ex [from]
patient education [on nurse-to-nurse order] (nursing)

EA
early antigen (laboratory)
educational age (pediatrics and psychiatry)
electric affinity (physics)
emergency area (emergency medicine)
endocardiographic amplifier (cardiovascular)
Endometriosis Association (gynecology)
erythrocyte antibody (hematology and laboratory)
estivoautumnal [malaria] (infectious diseases and laboratory)
ethacrynic acid [a diuretic] (cardiovascular, nephrology, and pharmacology)

E-A
E to A changes [saying "E,E,E" comes out as "A,A,A" upon auscultation of lung showing consolidation] (respiratory)

E→A
E to A changes [saying "E,E,E" comes out as "A,A,A" upon auscultation of lung showing consolidation] (respiratory)

ea
each

ea.
each

EAA
electrothermal atomic absorption (physics)
Epilepsy Association of America (neurology)
essential amino acid (laboratory)
extrinsic allergic alveolitis (allergy and respiratory)

EAB
elective abortion (obstetrics)
Ethics Advisory Board [Department of Health and Human Science]

EAC
Ehrlich ascites carcinoma (oncology)
erythrocyte antibody complement (hematology and laboratory)
external auditory canal (otorhinolaryngology)
{not an abbreviation} [used in studies of

complement in which *E* represents erythrocyte, *A* antibody, and *C* complement] (laboratory)

EACA
epsilon-aminocaproic acid [also abbreviated *EACA*] (hematology and pharmacology)

EACD
eczematous allergic contact dermatitis (allergy and dermatology)

EAD.
eadem [the same]

ead
eadem [the same]

ead.
eadem [the same]

EAE
experimental allergic encephalomyelitis (allergy and neurology)
experimental autoimmune encephalitis (immunology and neurology)

EAHF
eczema, allergy, hay fever (allergy and dermatology)
eczema, asthma, hay fever [complex] (allergy and dermatology)

EAHLG
equine antihuman lymphoblast globulin (laboratory)

EAHLS
equine antihuman lymphoblast serum (laboratory)

EAI
Emphysema Anonymous, Incorporated (respiratory)

EAM
external auditory meatus (otorhinolaryngology)

EAMG
experimental autoimmune myasthenia gravis (immunology and neurology)

EAN
experimental allergic neuritis (allergy and neurology)

EAP
electroacupuncture (acupuncture)
employee assistance personnel (psychiatry)
epiallopregnanolone (laboratory and obstetrics)
erythrocyte acid phosphatase (laboratory)

EaR
Entartungs-Reaktion [reaction of degeneration] (physics)

Ea. R.
Entartungs-Reaktion [reaction of degeneration] (physics)

ear ox
ear oximetry (otorhinolaryngology) {pronounced "ear-ox"} [*Note:* Do not confuse with *air ox* (air oximetry).]

"ear-ox"
{pronunciation of *ear ox* [ear oximetry]} (otorhinolaryngology) {not an abbreviation}

EAST
external rotation, abduction, stress test (orthopedics)

EAT
ectopic atrial tachycardia (cardiovascular)
electroaerosol therapy (pharmacology and respiratory)
experimental autoimmune thymitis (immunology and neurology)

EATC
Ehrlich ascites tumor cell (laboratory and oncology)

EB
elementary body [also called *blood platelet* and *inclusion body*] (hema-

tology, infectious diseases, and laboratory)

epidermolysis bullosa (dermatology)

Epstein-Barr [virus] (infectious diseases, laboratory, and oncology)

estradiol benzoate (gynecology and pharmacology)

E.B.

elementary body [also called *blood platelet* and *inclusion body*] (hematology, infectious diseases, and laboratory)

E-B

Epstein-Barr [virus] (infectious diseases, laboratory, and oncology)

E.B.A.A.

Eye Bank Association of America (ophthalmology)

EBAP

vindesine, BCNU [carmustine], Adriamycin, and prednisone (chemotherapy, oncology, and pharmacology)

EBCDIC

extended binary-coded decimal interchange code (computer science)

EBD

epidermolysis bullosa dystrophia (dermatology)

EBDD

epidermolysis bullosa dystrophia dominant (dermatology)

EBDR

epidermolysis bullosa dystrophia recessive (dermatology)

EBF

erythroblastosis fetalis (hematology and neonatology)

EBI

electromagnetic bone stimulator (orthopedics)

emetine and bismuth iodide [an antiemetic] (gastroenterology, infectious diseases, and pharmacology)

EBK

embryonic bovine kidney (laboratory and research)

EBL

estimated blood loss (surgery)

E.B.L.

estimated blood loss (surgery)

EBM

expressed breast milk (obstetrics)

EBNA

Epstein-Barr [virus] nuclear antigen (laboratory)

E/BOD

electrolyte biological oxygen demand (laboratory)

EBP

estradiol-binding protein (laboratory)

EBS

electric brain stimulator (neurology)

emergency bed service (emergency medicine)

epidermolysis bullosa simplex (dermatology)

EBT

early bedtime

EBV

Epstein-Barr virus (infectious diseases, laboratory, and oncology)

EB v

Epstein-Barr virus (infectious diseases, laboratory, and oncology)

EC

ejection click (cardiovascular)

electrochemical (chemistry and laboratory)

electron capture (physics)

enteric-coated [referring to tablets] (pharmacology)

entering complaint

enterochromaffin cells (laboratory)

entrance complaint
Enzyme Commission (laboratory)
epidermal cell (dermatology and laboratory)
Escherichia coli (laboratory)
excitation-contraction (neurology and orthopedics)
excitatory center (neurology)
experimental control (research)
extracellular (laboratory)
eyes closed (neurology and ophthalmology)

E.C.
Enzyme Commission (laboratory)

E/C
endoscopy/cystoscopy (urology)
estrogen to creatinine [ratio] (laboratory)

E-C
ether-chloroform [mixture] (anesthesiology and pharmacology)

ECA
ethacrynic acid [a diuretic] (cardiovascular, nephrology, and pharmacology)
ethylcarboxylate adenosine (laboratory)

ECAT
emission computerized axial tomography

ECBD
exploration of common bile duct (gastroenterology and surgery)

ECBO
enteric cytopathogenic bovine orphan [virus] (laboratory)

ECBO virus
enteric cytopathogenic bovine orphan virus (laboratory)

ECBV
effective circulating blood volume (cardiovascular)

ECC
edema, clubbing, and cyanosis (cardiovascular and orthopedics)
electrocorticogram (neurology)

emergency cardiac care (cardiovascular and emergency medicine)
endocervical cone (gynecology)
endocervical conization (gynecology)
endocervical curettage (gynecology)
endocervical curettings (gynecology)
extracorporeal circulation (cardiovascular)

ECCE
extracapsular cataract extraction (ophthalmology)

E.C.C.L.S.
European Committee for Clinical Laboratory Standards (laboratory)

ECD
electron capture detector (physics)
endocardial cushion defect (cardiovascular)

ECDO
enteric cytopathic dog orphan [virus] (laboratory)

ECDO virus
enteric cytopathogenic dog orphan virus (laboratory)

ECE
early childhood education (education and pediatrics)
endocervical ecchymosis (gynecology)

E.C.E.
early childhood education (education and pediatrics)

ECEMG
evoked compound electromyography (neurology)

ECF
effective capillary flow (cardiovascular)
eosinophilic chemotactic factor (laboratory)
extended care facility
extracellular fluid (endocrinology and laboratory)

ECF-A
eosinophil chemotactic factor of anaphylaxis (laboratory)

ECFMG
Educational Commission for Foreign Medical Graduates (education)

ECFMS
Educational Council for Foreign Medical Students (education)

ECFV
extracellular fluid volume (laboratory)

ECG
echocardiogram (cardiovascular)
electrocardiogram (cardiovascular)

ECGF
endothelial cell growth factor (laboratory)

ECH
extended care hospital

ECHIN
Echinococcus (laboratory)

ECHO
echocardiogram (cardiovascular and radiology) {pronounced "ek-oh"}
echoencephalogram [also called *sonoencephalon*] (neurology and radiology) {pronounced "ek-oh"}
enterocytopathogenic human orphan [virus] (gastroenterology and laboratory) {pronounced "ek-oh"}
etoposide [VP-16], cyclophosphamide, Adriamycin, and vincristine (chemotherapy, oncology, and pharmacology) {pronounced "ek-oh"}

echo
echocardiogram (cardiovascular and radiology) {pronounced "ek-oh"}
echoencephalogram (neurology and radiology) {pronounced "ek-oh"}
echogram (radiology) {pronounced "ek-oh"}

echo EEG
echoencephalogram (neurology and radiology)

ECHO virus
enteric cytopathogenic human orphan virus (laboratory) {pronounced "ek-oh-vi-russ"}

ECI
electrocerebral inactivity (neurology)
extracorporeal irradiation (radiation therapy)

ECIB
extracorporeal irradiation of the blood (radiation therapy)

ECIL
extracorporeal irradiation of lymph (radiation therapy)

ECL
emitter-coupled logic (computer science)
extent of cerebral lesion (neurology)
extracapillary lesions (cardiovascular)

Eclec
eclectic

eclec.
eclectic

ECLT
euglobulin clot lysis time (hematology and laboratory)

ECM
embryo chicken muscle (laboratory and research)
erythema chronicum migrans (dermatology)
extracellular material (laboratory)

E-C mixture
ether-chloroform mixture (anesthesiology, chemistry, and pharmacology)

ECMO
enteric cytopathic monkey orphan [virus] (gastroenterology and laboratory) {pronounced "ek-moe"}
extracorporeal membrane oxygenation

(cardiovascular, neonatology, and respiratory) {pronounced "ek-moe"}

ECMO virus
enteric cytopathogenic monkey orphan
virus (gastroenterology and laboratory) {pronounced "ek-moe-vi-russ"}

ECMP
enterocoated microspheres of pancreli-
pase (gastroenterology and pharmacology)

ECN
extended care nursery (neonatology)

ECOG
Eastern Cooperative Oncology Group
(oncology)

ECoG
electrocorticogram (neurology)
electrocorticography (neurology)

E. coli
Escherichia coli (laboratory) {pro-
nounced "E-co-lie"}

"E-co-lie"
{pronunciation of *E. coli* [*Escherichia
coli*]} (laboratory) {not an abbrevia-
tion}

ECP
erythrocyte coproporphyrin (laboratory)
Escherichia coli polypeptides (laboratory)
estradiol cyclopentaneopropionate
(pharmacology)
free cytoprophyrin in erythrocytes (laboratory)

ECPO
enteric cytopathogenic porcine orphan
[virus] (laboratory)

ECPOG
electrochemical potential gradient
(chemistry)

ECPO virus
enteric cytopathogenic porcine orphan
virus (laboratory)

ECR
emergency chemical restraint

ECRB
extensor carpi radialis brevis [muscle or
tendon] (orthopedics)

ECRL
extensor carpi radialis longus [muscle or
tendon] (orthopedics)

ECS
elective cosmetic surgery (plastic surgery)
electroconvulsive shock (psychiatry)
extracellular-like solution [a cardio-
plegic solution] (pharmacology)

ECSO
enteric cytopathic swine orphan [virus]
(laboratory)

ECSO virus
enteric cytopathogenic swine orphan
virus (laboratory)

ECT
electroconvulsive therapy [also called
electroshock therapy] (psychiatry)
emission computed tomography (radiology)
enhanced computer tomography (radiology)
enteric-coated tablet (pharmacology)
euglobulin clot test (hematology and
laboratory)
European compression technique [bone
screw and internal fixation] (orthopedics)

E.C.T.
electroconvulsive therapy [also called
electroshock therapy] (psychiatry)

ECU
extensor carpi ulnaris [muscle or ten-
don] (orthopedics)

ECV
extracellular volume (laboratory)
extracorporeal volume (cardiovascular)

ECVE
extracellular volume expansion (laboratory)

ECW
extracellular water (laboratory)

ED
Department of Education (education and government)

effective dose (pharmacology and radiation therapy)

Ehlers-Danlos [syndrome] (cardiovascular, dermatology, gastroenterology, genetics, ophthalmology, and orthopedics)

electrodialysis (cardiovascular and nephrology)

emergency department (emergency medicine)

Entner-Doudoroff [metabolic pathway] (chemistry and laboratory)

enzymatic deficiencies (laboratory)

epidural (anesthesiology and neurology)

epileptiform discharge (neurology)

erythema dose (radiation therapy)

ethynodiol (gynecology, obstetrics, and pharmacology)

ethyl dichlorarsine

evidence of disease

exertional dyspnea (respiratory)

extensor digitorum [muscle or tendon] (orthopedics)

external diameter (measurement)

extralow dispersion (laboratory)

E.D.
effective dose (pharmacology and radiation therapy)

emergency department (emergency medicine)

emotionally disturbed (psychiatry)

erythema dose (pharmacology and radiation therapy)

ED$_{50}$
median effective dose [dose that produces desired effect in 50% of the population] (pharmacology and radiation therapy)

E.D.$_{50}$
median effective dose [dose that produces desired effect in 50% of popula-

tion] (pharmacology and radiation therapy)

E$_d$
depth dose (radiation therapy)

Ed
editor (publishing)

ed
edition (publishing)

end-diastolic (cardiovascular)

e.d.
effective dose (pharmacology and radiation therapy)

EDA
end-diastolic area (cardiovascular)

EDB
early dry breakfast (dietary)

ethylene dibromide (chemistry, dietary, laboratory, and oncology)

extensor digitorum brevis [muscle or tendon] (orthopedics)

EDC
emergency decontamination center (emergency medicine)

end-diastolic counts (cardiovascular)

estimated date of conception (obstetrics)

estimated date of confinement (obstetrics)

expected date of confinement (obstetrics)

extensor digitorum communis [muscle or tendon] (orthopedics)

EDD
effective drug duration (pharmacology)

enzyme-digested delta [endotoxin] (laboratory)

expected date of delivery (obstetrics)

edent
edentulous (dentistry and otorhinolaryngology)

E-diol
estradiol (endocrinology, gynecology, laboratory, and pharmacology)

EDL
end-diastolic length (cardiovascular)
extensor digitorum longus [muscle] (orthopedics)

ED/LD
emotionally disturbed/learning disabled (neurology and psychiatry)

EDM
early diastolic murmur (cardiovascular)

EDN
electrodesiccation (surgery)

EDNA
Emergency Department Nurses Association (emergency medicine and nursing)

EDP
electron dense particles (chemistry)
electronic data processing (computer science)
end-diastolic pressure (cardiovascular)
epatite degenerative-proliferative [hepatic virus] (gastroenterology and laboratory)

EDQ
extensor digiti quinti [muscle] (orthopedics)

EDR
effective direct radiation (radiology)
electrodermal response (neurology)
electrodialysis with reversed polarity (cardiovascular and nephrology)

EDS
Ehlers-Danlos syndrome (cardiovascular, dermatology, gastroenterology, genetics, ophthalmology, and orthopedics)

EDTA
ethylenediaminetetra-acetic acid [also called *edathamil* and *edetic acid*] (chemistry)

EDU
eating disorder unit (gastroenterology, dietary, and psychiatry)

EDV
end-diastolic volume (cardiovascular)

EDVI
end-diastolic volume index (cardiovascular)

EDW
estimated dry weight (nephrology)

EDWTH
end-diastolic wall thickness (cardiovascular)

EDX
electrodiagnosis

EDx
electrodiagnosis

EDXA
energy-dispersive X-ray analysis (radiology)

EE
embryo extract (laboratory and pharmacology)
end-to-end [anastomosis] (surgery)
Enterobacteriaceae enrichment [broth] (laboratory)
equine encephalitis (neurology)
eye and ear (ophthalmology and otorhinolaryngology)

E-E
erythematous-edematous [reaction] (radiation therapy)

EEA
electroencephalic audiometry (neurology and otorhinolaryngology)
end-to-end anastomosis (surgery)
{not an abbreviation} [a stapler used for end-to-end anastomosis] (surgery)

EEC
ectrodactyly, ectodermal dysplasia,

clefting [syndrome] (genetics, pediatrics, and plastic surgery)
enteropathogenic *Escherichia coli* (laboratory)

EEC syndrome
ectrodactyly-ectodermal dysplasia-clefting syndrome (dentistry, dermatology, and otorhinolaryngology)

EEE
eastern equine encephalitis (neurology)
eastern equine encephalomyelitis (neurology)
edema, erythema, and exudate (ophthalmology)
equine encephalomyelitis, eastern (neurology)
experimental enterococcal endocarditis (cardiovascular)
external eye examination (ophthalmology)

EEEP
end-expiratory esophageal pressure (gastroenterology and respiratory)

EEE virus
eastern equine encephalomyelitis virus (laboratory and neurology)

EEG
electroencephalogram (neurology)
electroencephalography (neurology)

EEG T
Electroencephalographic Technologist (neurology)

EEME
ethinylestradiol methyl ether (gynecology and pharmacology)

EE3ME
ethinyloestradiol-3-methyl ether [also called *mestranol*] (gynecology and pharmacology)

EENT
eyes, ears, nose, and throat (ophthalmology and otorhinolaryngology)

E.E.N.T.
eyes, ears, nose, and throat (ophthalmology and otorhinolaryngology)

EEPI
extraretinal eye position information (ophthalmology)

EER
electroencephalic response (neurology)

EES
erythromycin ethylsuccinate (pharmacology)
{not an abbreviation} {trade name for erythromycin ethylsuccinate] (pharmacology)

EF
ectopic focus (neurology)
edema factor (cardiovascular and orthopedics)
ejection factor (cardiovascular)
ejection fraction (cardiovascular)
elastic fibril (laboratory)
electric field (chemistry and physics)
elongation factor (laboratory)
embryo-fetal (neonatology and obstetrics)
emergency facilities (emergency medicine)
emotional factor (psychiatry)
encephalitogenic factor (laboratory and neurology)
endurance factor (cardiovascular and rehabilitation)
eosinophilic fasciitis (orthopedics)
equivalent focus
extended field (radiation therapy)
extrafine
extrinsic factor [also called vitamin B_{12}] (pharmacology)

EFA
Epilepsy Foundation of America (neurology)
essential fatty acids (laboratory)
extrafamily adoptees

EFAD
essential fatty acid deficiency (laboratory)

EFC
endogenous fecal calcium (laboratory)

EFE
endocardial fibroelastosis (cardiovascular and pediatrics)

EFF
efficiency

Eff
effacement (obstetrics)

eff
effects
efferent

effect
effective

effer
efferent

EFL
effective focal length (measurement)

EFM
electronic fetal monitoring (obstetrics)
external fetal monitoring (obstetrics)

EFP
effective filtration pressure (laboratory)

EFR
effective filtration rate (laboratory)

E.FRAG
red blood cell fragility [test] (hematology and laboratory)

EFV
extracellular volume (laboratory)

EFVC
expiratory flow-volume curve (respiratory)

EFW
estimated fetal weight (obstetrics)

EG
esophagogastrectomy (gastroenterology)
esophagogastric (gastroenterology)
external genitalia (gynecology, obstetrics, and urology)

eg
exempli gratia [for example]

e.g.
exempli gratia [for example]

EGA
estimated gestational age (neonatology and obstetrics)

EGBPS
equilibrium-grated blood pool study

EGBUS
external genitalia and Bartholin's, urethral, and Skene's [glands] (gynecology)

EGD
esophagogastroduodenoscopy (gastroenterology)

EGDF
embryonic growth and development factor (laboratory)

EGF
epidermal growth factor (laboratory)

EGG
electrogastrogram (gastroenterology)

EGJ
esophagogastric junction (gastroenterology)

EGL
eosinophilic granuloma of the lung (respiratory)

E_3-3GI
estriol-3-glucosiduronate (endocrinology, gynecology, and pharmacology)

E_3-3,16GI
estriol-3,16α-diglucosiduronate (endocrinology, gynecology, and pharmacology)

E_3-16GI
estriol-16α-glucosiduronate (endocrinology, gynecology, and pharmacology)

EGM
electrogram (cardiovascular and neurology)

EGOT
erythrocyte glutamic oxaloacetic transaminase (laboratory)

EGS
electric galvanic stimulation (orthopedics and physical therapy)
ethylene glycol succinate (chemistry)

EGTA
esophagogastric tube airway (respiratory)
ethylene glycol tetra-acetic acid (chemistry)

EH
educationally handicapped (education, neurology, pediatrics, and rehabilitation)
emotionally handicapped (psychiatry)
enlarged heart (cardiovascular)
essential hypertension (cardiovascular)
extramedullary hematopoiesis (hematology)

E & H
environment and heredity (psychiatry)

E_h
redox potential (chemistry and laboratory)

eH
oxidation-reduction potential (chemistry and laboratory)

EHA
Emotional Health Anonymous (psychiatry)
Environmental Health Agency (ecology)

EHAA
epidermic hepatitis-associated antigen (gastroenterology, infectious diseases, and laboratory)

EHB
elevate head of bed

EHBA
extrahepatic biliary atresia (gastroenterology and pediatrics)

EHBF
essential high blood pressure (cardiovascular)
estimated hepatic blood flow (cardiovascular and gastroenterology)
extrahepatic blood flow (cardiovascular and gastroenterology)
exercise hyperemia blood flow (cardiovascular)

EHC
enterohepatic circulation (cardiovascular and gastroenterology)
enterohepatic clearance (gastroenterology and laboratory)
essential hypercholesterolemia (cardiovascular and gastroenterology)
extended health care

EH-CF
Entamoeba histolytica-complement fixation (laboratory)

EHD
epizootic hemorrhagic disease [of poultry] (veterinary medicine)

EHDA
etidronate sodium (orthopedics, pharmacology, and radiology)

EHDP
ethane hydroxydiphosphate (chemistry)

EHF
electrohydraulic fragmentation (nephrology and urology)
epidemic hemorrhagic fever (hematology and infectious diseases)

exophthalmos-hyperthyroid factor (endocrinology, laboratory, and ophthalmology)

EH-IHA
complement histolytica-indirect hemagglutination (hematology and laboratory)

EHL
effective half-life [of radioactive substances] (chemistry, radiation therapy, and radiology)
electrohydraulic lithotriptor (nephrology and urology)
endogenous hyperlipidemia (cardiovascular)
Environmental Health Laboratory (ecology and laboratory)
extensor hallucis longus [muscle] (orthopedics)

EHME
Employee Health Maintenance Examination

EHO
extrahepatic obstruction (gastroenterology)

EHP
di-(2-ethylhexyl) hydrogen phosphate (chemistry)
excessive heat production
extrahigh potency (pharmacology)

EHPAC
Emergency Health Preparedness Advisory Committee (emergency medicine)

EHPH
extrahepatic portal hypertension (cardiovascular and gastroenterology)

EHPT
Eddy hot plate test (laboratory)

EHSDS
Experimental Health Service Delivery System (research)

EHV
electric heat vector (physics)

equine herpes virus (infectious diseases, laboratory, and veterinary medicine)

EI
electrolyte imbalance (cardiovascular, gastroenterology, nephrology, and respiratory)
enzyme inhibitor (laboratory)
eosinophilic index (laboratory)

E/I
expiration-inspiration [ratio] (respiratory)

E & I
endocrine and infertility (endocrinology and obstetrics)

EIA
electroimmunoassay (laboratory)
enzyme immunoassay (laboratory)
exercise-induced anaphylaxis (allergy)
exercise-induced asthma (respiratory)

E.I.A.
Electronics Industries Association

EIAB
extracranial-intracranial arterial bypass (cardiovascular and neurology)

EIB
exercise-induced bronchospasm (respiratory)

EIC
elastase inhibitory capacity (laboratory)

EICT
external isovolumic contraction time (laboratory)

EID
egg-infective dose (pharmacology and radiation therapy)
electroimmunodiffusion (laboratory)
electronic infusion device (pharmacology)

eIF
erythrocyte initiation factor (laboratory)

EIP
extensor indicis proprius [muscle or tendon] (orthopedics)

EIPS
endogenous inhibitor of prostaglandin synthase (endocrinology, gynecology, and laboratory)

EIRnv
extra incidence rate in nonvaccinated groups (research)

EIRv
extra incidence rate in vaccinated groups (research)

EIS
endoscopic injection scleropathy (gastroenterology)
Epidemic Intelligence Service [Centers for Disease Control] (government and research)
Environmental Impact Statement (ecology)

EIT
erythroid iron turnover (laboratory)

EIWA
Escala Inteligencia Wechsler Para Adultes [Wechsler Adult Intelligence Scale] (psychiatry)

EJ
elbow jerk (neurology and orthopedics)
external jugular [pulse or vessel] (cardiovascular)

Ej
elbow jerk (neurology and orthopedics)

EJP
excitatory junction potential (neurology)

ejusd
ejusdem [of the same]

ejusd.
ejusdem [of the same]

EK
erythrokinase (laboratory)

EKC
epidemic keratoconjunctivitis (ophthalmology)

EKG
electrocardiogram (cardiovascular)
epidemic keratoconjunctivitis (ophthalmology)

EKG leads
augmental—aVF, aVL, and aVR
cardiac—I, II, III, IV, VF, VL, VR, and V_1 through V_6

"ek-moe"
{pronunciation of *ECMO* [enteric cytopathic monkey orphan {virus} (gastroenterology and laboratory) and extracorporeal membrane oxygenation (cardiovascular, pediatrics, and respiratory)]} {not an abbreviation}

"ek-moe-vi-russ"
{pronunciation of *ECMO virus* [enteric cytopathogenic monkey orphan virus] (gastroenterology and laboratory) {not an abbreviation}

"ek-oh"
{pronunciation of *ECHO* [echocardiogram (cardiovascular and radiology), echoencephalogram {also called *sonoencephalon*} (neurology and radiology), enterocytopathogenic human orphan {virus} (gastroenterology and laboratory), and etoposide {VP-16}, cyclophosphamide, Adriamycin, and vincristine (chemotherapy, oncology, and pharmacology)] and *echo* [echocardiogram (cardiovascular and radiology), echoencephalogram (neurology and radiology), and echogram (radiology)]} {not an abbreviation}

"ek-oh-vi-russ"
{pronunciation of *ECHO virus* [enteric cytopathogenic human orphan virus]} (laboratory) {not an abbreviation}

EKY
electrokymogram (measurement)

EL
early latent
erythroleukemia (hematology and oncology)
exercise limit (cardiovascular)

E-L
external lids (ophthalmology)

el
elixir (pharmacology)

el.
elixir (pharmacology)

ELAT
enzyme-linked antiglobulin test (laboratory)

ELB
early light breakfast (dietary)

elb.
elbow (orthopedics)

elec
electric(al)
electricity

ELECT
electrolytes (laboratory)

elect
electuarium [electuary] (pharmacology)

elem
elementary

elev
elevate
elevation
elevator

ELF
elective low forceps [delivery] (obstetrics)

ELH
egg-laying hormone (laboratory)
endolymphatic hydrops (neurology and otorhinolaryngology)

ELI
Environmental Language Inventory (speech and language therapy)

EIDP
Early Intervention Developmental Profile (speech and language therapy)

ELIEDA
enzyme-linked immunoelectrodiffusion assay (laboratory)

"E-lie-za"
{pronunciation of *ELISA* [enzyme-linked immunoadsorbent assay; also called *enzyme-linked immunosorbent assay*]} (immunology and laboratory) {not an abbreviation}

ELISA
enzyme-linked immunoadsorbent assay [also called *enzyme-linked immunosorbent assay*] {pronounced "E-lie-za" or "el-sa"} (immunology and laboratory)

Elix.
elixir (pharmacology)

elix
elixir (pharmacology)

elix.
elixir (pharmacology)

ELLP
elliptocytes (laboratory)

ELMT
elements [on urinalysis] (laboratory)

ELMTNO
element numbers [on urinalysis] (laboratory)

ELOP
estimated length of program

ELOS
estimated length of stay
extralymphatic organ site (oncology)

ELP ELP ELP ELP ELP ELP ELP ELP ELP ELP ELP ELP ELP ELP ELP ELP ELP ELP ELP ELP ELP ELP ELP ELP ELP ELP ELP ELP ELP ELP ELP ELP ELP ELP ELP ELP ELP ELP ELP ELP ELP ELP ELP ELP ELP ELP ELP ELP ELP ELP ELP ELP ELP ELP ELP ELP ELP ELP ELP ELP ELP ELP ELP ELP ELP ELP ELP ELP ELP ELP ELP ELP ELP ELP ELP ELP ELP ELP ELP ELP ELP ELP ELP ELP ELP ELP ELP ELP ELP ELP ELP ELP ELP

ELP   **EMCRO**

ELP
electrophoresis (laboratory)
endogenous limbic potential (neurology)

ELP broach
{not an abbreviation} (orthopedics)

"el-sa"
{pronunciation of *ELISA* [enzyme-linked immunoadsorbent assay; also called *enzyme-linked immunosorbent assay*)]} (immunology and laboratory) {not an abbreviation}

EL-SPT
electrolytes on urine spot [test] (laboratory)

ELSS
Emergency Life Support System (emergency medicine)

ELT
euglobulin lysis time (laboratory)

EM
ejection murmur (cardiovascular)
electromechanical
electron microscope (laboratory)
electron microscopy (laboratory)
electrophoretic mobility (laboratory)
emergency medicine
emotionally disturbed (psychiatry)
erythema multiforme (dermatology)
erythrocyte mass (laboratory)
external monitor (obstetrics)

E-M
Embden-Meyerhof [glycolytic pathway] (endocrinology and laboratory)

E & M
endocrine and metabolism (endocrinology)

Em
emmetropia [normal vision] (ophthalmology)

Em.
emmetropia [normal vision] (ophthalmology)

e/m
ratio of charge to mass (physics)

EMA
emergency assistance (emergency medicine)
emergency assistant (emergency medicine)

EMB
embryology
endometrial biopsy (gynecology)
endomyocardial biopsy (cardiovascular)
engineering in medicine and biology
eosin-methylene blue [agar] (laboratory)
ethambutol [also called *Myambutol*] (pharmacology)
explosive mental behavior (psychiatry)

Emb
embryology

EMB agar
eosin-methylene blue agar (laboratory)

EMBASE
Excerpta Medica data base

EMBL
European Molecular Biology Laboratory (laboratory)

embryol
embryology

EMC
electron microscopy (laboratory)
emergency medical care (emergency medicine)
encephalomyocarditis [virus] (laboratory)
endometrial curettage (gynecology)
endometrial curettings (gynecology)

EMC & R
emergency medical care and rescue (emergency medicine)

EMCRO
Experimental Medical Care Review Organization (research)

EMC virus
encephalomyocarditis virus (laboratory)

Emcyt
{not an abbreviation} [brand name for
    estramustine phosphate sodium] (che-
    motherapy, oncology, and pharmacol-
    ogy)

EMD
electromechanical dissociation (cardio-
    vascular)
esophageal motility disorder (gastroen-
    terology)

emend
emendatis [emended]

emer
emergency

emer.
emergency

Emerg
emergency

EMF
electromagnetic flowmeter (physics)
electromotive force (physics)
Emergency Medical Foundation (emer-
    gency medicine)
endomyocardial fibrosis (cardiovascular)
erythrocyte maturation factor (labora-
    tory)
evaporated milk formula (neonatology
    and dietary)

E.M.F.
electromotive force (physics)
erythrocyte maturation factor (labora-
    tory)

EMG
electromyelogram (neurology)
electromyelography (neurology)
electromyogram (neurology)
electromyography (neurology)
essential monoclonal gammopathy (he-
    matology)
exophthalmos, macroglossia, and gigan-
    tism [syndrome] (genetics, ophthal-
    mology, and otorhinolaryngology)

EMGORS
electromyogram sensors (neurology)

EMI
Electric and Musical Industries [develop-
    ers of the first computerized tomo-
    graphic scanner] {pronounced
    "emmy" or "M-E"} (radiology)
Emergency Medical Information (emer-
    gency medicine)

EMIC
emergency maternity and infant care
    (emergency medicine, neonatology,
    and obstetrics)

E-MICR
electron microscopy (laboratory)

EMI scan
Electric and Musical Industries scan [the
    developers of the first computerized
    tomographic scanner] (radiology)
    {pronounced "emmy-scan" or "M-E-
    scan"}

EMIT
enzyme-multiplied immunoassay tech-
    nique (laboratory)

EMJH
Ellinghausen, McCullough, Johnson,
    Harris [medium] (laboratory)

EMMA
eye-movement measuring apparatus
    (ophthalmology)

"emmy"
{pronunciation of *EMI* [Electric and Mu-
    sical Industries, developers of the first
    computerized tomographic scanner]}
    (radiology) {not an abbreviation}

"emmy-scan"
{pronunciation of *EMI* scan [Electric and
    Musical Industries scan by the devel-
    opers of the first computerized tomo-
    graphic scanner]} (radiology) {not an
    abbreviation}

EMO
Epstein and Macintosh, Oxford [ether inhaler and Oxford bellows] (anesthesiology and respiratory)

emot
emotion(al) (psychiatry)

emp
emplastrum [a plaster] (pharmacology)
employee
ex modo prescripto [as directed, after the manner prescribed] (pharmacology)

emp.
emplastrum [a plaster] (pharmacology)
employee
ex modo prescripto [as directed, after the manner prescribed] (pharmacology)

emp vesic
emplastrum vesicatorium [a blistering plaster] (pharmacology)

emp. vesic.
emplastrum vesicatorium [a blistering plaster] (pharmacology)

EMR
educable mentally retarded (education, genetics, neurology, pediatrics, psychiatry, and rehabilitation)
emergency mechanical restraint (emergency medicine)
empty, measure, and record (nursing)

EMRA
Emergency Medicine Residents Association (emergency medicine)

EMS
early morning specimen (laboratory)
electric muscle stimulation (neurology and orthopedics)
electromyostimulation (neurology and orthopedics)
electronic medical service
emergency medical service(s) (emergency medicine)
error mean squares (measurement)
ethyl methane sulfonate (chemistry)

E.M.S.
Emergency Medical Service [British] (emergency medicine)

EMSS
Emergency Medical Service Systems (emergency medicine, government, and law enforcement)

EMT
Emergency Medical Tag (emergency medicine)
Emergency Medical Technician (emergency medicine)
emergency medical treatment (emergency medicine)

E.M.T.
Emergency Medical Technician (emergency medicine)

EMT-P
Emergency Medical Technician-Paramedic (emergency medicine)

EMU
electromagnetic unit (physics)

emu
electromagnetic unit (physics)

emul.
emulsio [emulsion, *emulsum*] (pharmacology)

emuls
emulsio [emulsion, *emulsum*] (pharmacology)

EMV
eye, motor, verbal [grading scale for Glasgow coma scale] (neurology)

EMW
electromagnetic waves (physics)

EN
enema (gastroenterology and pharmacology)
enrolled nurse (nursing)
erythema nodosum (dermatology)

EOR
exclusive operating room (surgery)

EORA
elderly onset rheumatoid arthritis (rheumatology)

EOS
ellipse of skin (surgery)

Eos
eosinophil (laboratory)

eos
eosinophil (laboratory)

eos.
eosinophil (laboratory)

EOSIN
eosinophil (laboratory)

eosin
eosinophil (laboratory)

eosin B
dibromodinitrofluorescein [a dye] (laboratory)

eosin I bluish
dibromodinitrofluorescein [a dye] (laboratory)

eosins
eosinophils (laboratory)

eosin W
water-soluble eosin [a dye] (laboratory)

eosin W-S
water-soluble eosin [a dye] (laboratory)

eosin Y
yellowish eosin [a dye] (laboratory)

EOT
effective oxygen transport (respiratory)

EOU
epidemic observation unit (infectious diseases)

EOWPVT
Expressive One-Word Picture Vocabulary Test (speech and language therapy)

EP
ectopic pregnancy (gynecology and obstetrics)
edible portion [of a food] (dietary)
electrophoresis (laboratory)
electrophysiologic (cardiovascular)
Emergency Procedures (emergency medicine)
endogenous pyrogen (laboratory)
endpoint (laboratory and pharmacology)
enzyme product (laboratory)
epithelial (anatomy)
epithelioid (anatomy)
erythrocyte protoporphyrin (laboratory)
erythrophagocytosis (hematology and laboratory)
erythropoietic porphyria (dermatology, gastroenterology, hematology, and neurology)
erythropoietin (laboratory)
esophageal pressure (gastroenterology)
evoked potential (neurology)
extreme pressure
protroporphyrin [free in lymphocytes] (laboratory)

EPA
eicosapentaenoic acid (chemistry)
erect posterior-anterior [projection] (radiology)
Environmental Protection Agency (ecology and government)

EPB
Environmental Pre-Language Battery (speech and language therapy)
extensor pollicis brevis (neurology and orthopedics)

EPC
electronic pain control [apparatus] (neurology)
epilepsia partialis continua (neurology)
epilepsy partialis continua (neurology)
external pneumatic compression (emergency medicine and surgery)

EPDML
epidemiological (epidemiology)
epidemiologist (epidemiology)
epidemiology

EPE
erythropoietin-producing enzyme (laboratory)

"ep-E"
{pronunciation of *EPI, epi,* and *epi.* [epinephrine]} (pharmacology) {not an abbreviation}

EPEC
enteropathogenic *Escherichia coli* (laboratory)

EPEG
etoposide [also called *VP-16*] (chemotherapy, oncology, and pharmacology)

"ep-E-neff"
{pronunciation of *epineph* [epinephrine]} (pharmacology) {not an abbreviation}

EPF
endothelial proliferating factor (laboratory)
exophthalmos-producing factor (laboratory and ophthalmology)

EPG
eggs per gram (laboratory and parasitology)
electropneumogram (neurology)

EPI
epinephrine (pharmacology) {pronounced "ep-E"}
epithelial (anatomy)
epithelium (anatomy)
evoked potential index (neurology)
Eysenck Personality Inventory (psychiatry)

epi
epidural (anesthesiology, neurology, and obstetrics)
epinephrine (pharmacology) {pronounced "ep-E"}

epi.
epinephrine (pharmacology) {pronounced "ep-E"}

epid
epidemic (infectious diseases)

Epil
epilepsy (neurology)
epileptic (neurology)

epineph
epinephrine (pharmacology) {pronounced "ep-E-neff"}

EPIS
episiotomy (obstetrics)

epis
episiotomy (obstetrics)

epistom
epistomium [a stopper] (pharmacology)

epith
epithelial (anatomy)
epithelium (anatomy)

epith.
epithelial (anatomy)
epithelium (anatomy)

EPK
early prenatal karyotype (genetics, laboratory, and obstetrics)

EPL
extensor pollicis longus (neurology and orthopedics)
{not an abbreviation} [broach, femoral prosthesis, and stem for hip arthroplasty] (orthopedics)

EPLB
Environmental Pre-Language Battery (speech and language therapy)

EPM
electronic pacemaker (cardiovascular)
energy-protein malnutrition (dietary)

EPN
O-ethyl-O-paranitrophenyl benzenethio-
phosphonate [also called *acaracide*;
an insecticide] (chemistry)

EPP
end-plate potential (neurology)
equal pressure point
erythropoietic protoporphyria (dermatology)

EPPS
Edwards Personal Preference Schedule
(psychiatry)

EPR
electron paramagnetic resonance (physics)
electrophrenic respiration (respiratory)
emergency physical restraint (emergency medicine)
estradiol production rate (laboratory)

EPROM
erasable programmable read-only memory (computer science)

EPS
elastosis perforans serpiginosa (dermatology)
electrophysiologic study (cardiovascular)
exophthalmos-producing substance [of
anterior pituitary] (endocrinology,
laboratory, and ophthalmology)
extrapyramidal symptom(s) (neurology
and psychiatry)
extrapyramidal syndrome (neurology
and psychiatry)

ep's
epithelial cells (laboratory) {pronounced
"epz"}

EPSP
excitatory postsynaptic potential (neurology)

EPT
early pregnancy test (laboratory and obstetrics)

e.p.t.
{not an abbreviation} [trade name for an

early pregnancy test product] (laboratory, obstetrics, and pharmacology)

e.p.t. Plus
{not an abbreviation} [trade name for an
early pregnancy test product] (laboratory, obstetrics, and pharmacology)

EPTE
existed prior to enlistment (armed
forces)

EPTS
existed prior to service(s) (armed
forces)

"epz"
{pronunciation of *ep's* [epithelial cells]}
(laboratory) {not an abbreviation}

EQ
educational quotient (education)
encephalization quotient (neurology)

Eq.
equivalent

eq
equation
equivalent

equip
equipment

equiv
equivalent

ER
ejection rate (cardiovascular)
emergency room (emergency medicine)
endoplasmic reticulum (laboratory)
environmental resistance (research)
equivalent roentgen [unit] (radiology)
estrogen receptor (gynecology, laboratory, and oncology)
evoked response (neurology)
extended release (neurology)
external resistance (physics)
external rotation (orthopedics)

E.R.
emergency room (emergency medicine)

E+R
equal and regular (ophthalmology)

E & R
equal and reactive (ophthalmology)
equal and regular (ophthalmology)

Er
erbium (chemistry)
erythrocyte (hematology and laboratory)

49er
Forty-Niner [brace] (orthopedics and sports medicine)

ERA
electrical response activity (neurology)
Electroshock Research Association (psychiatry and research)
Equal Rights Amendment (government)
estrogen receptor assay (gynecology, laboratory, and oncology)
evoked response audiometry (neurology and otorhinolaryngology)

E.R.A.
Electroshock Research Association (psychiatry and research)

ERBF
effective renal blood flow (cardiovascular and nephrology)

ERC
endoscopic retrograde cholangiography (gastroenterology and radiology)
enterocytopathogenic human orphan(ECHO)-rhinocoryza [viruses] (gastroenterology and laboratory)
erythropoietin-responsive cell (laboratory)

ERCP
endoscopic retrograde cannulation of pancreatic duct (gastroenterology and radiology)
endoscopic retrograde cholangiopancreatography (gastroenterology and radiology)

ERD
evoked response detector (neurology)

ERDA
Energy Research and Development Administration (research)

ERE
external rotation in extension (orthopedics)

ERF
Education and Research Foundation (education and research)
external rotation in flexion (orthopedics)
Eye Research Foundation (ophthalmology and research)

E.R.F.
Education and Research Foundation (education and research)

ERFC
erythrocyte rosette forming cells (laboratory)

ERG
electroretinogram (ophthalmology)

ERIA
electroradioimmunoassay (laboratory)

ERL
effective refractory length (ophthalmology)

ERM
electrochemical relaxation methods (psychiatry)

ERP
effective refractory period (ophthalmology)
emergency room physician (emergency medicine)
endoscopic retrograde pancreatography (gastroenterology and radiology)
equine rhinopneumonitis (respiratory)
estrogen receptor protein (gynecology, laboratory, and oncology)

ERPF
effective renal plasma flow (cardiovascular and nephrology)

ERR
error (laboratory)

ERSP
event-related slow-brain potential (neurology)

ERT
estrogen replacement therapy (gynecology and pharmacology)

ERV
expiratory reserve volume (laboratory and respiratory)

ERY
erysipelas (dermatology)

Ery
Erysipelothrix [a bacteria] (laboratory)

Eryc
{not an abbreviation} [a brand name preparation of erythromycin, an antibiotic] (pharmacology)

ERYTHR
erythromycin [an antibiotic] (pharmacology)

erythro
erythrocyte (hematology and laboratory)

erythromycin B
erythromycin berythromycin [an antibiotic] (pharmacology)

ES
Ego Stress [test] (psychiatry)
ejection sound (cardiovascular)
elastic suspensor
electrical stimulation (neurology)
electrical stimulus (neurology)
electroshock (psychiatry)
elopement status (psychiatry)
emergency service (emergency medicine)
emission spectrometry (laboratory)
endoscopic sclerosis (gastroenterology)
endoscopic sphincterotomy (gastroenterology)
end-to-side [anastomosis] (surgery)
enema saponis [soap enema] (gastroenterology and pharmacology)
enzyme substrate (laboratory)
esophageal scintigraphy (gastroenterology and radiology)
esophagus (gastroenterology)
esophoria (ophthalmology)
estimated standard (statistics)
Expectation Score (measurement)
experimental study (research)
exsmoker (respiratory)
exterior surface
extrasystole (cardiovascular)

E.S.
electrical stimulation (neurology and orthopedics)

Es
einsteinium (chemistry)

ESA
Electrolysis Society of America (dermatology)

ESAP
evoked sensory [nerve] action potential (neurology)

ESB
electrical stimulation to brain (neurology)

ESC
electromechanical slope computer (computer science)
end-systolic counts (cardiovascular)
erythropoietin-sensitive stem cells (laboratory)

Esch
Escherichia (laboratory)

Esch.
Escherichia (laboratory)

ESCN
electrolyte-produced and steroid-pro-

duced cardiopathy characterized by necrosis (cardiovascular)

ESD
electronic summation device (computer science)
esophagus, stomach, and duodenum (gastroenterology)

ESE
electrostatische Einheit [electrostatic unit] (physics)

ESF
erythropoietic-stimulating factor (laboratory)

E.S.F.
erythropoietic-stimulating factor (laboratory)

E₃-3S,16Gl
estriol-3-sulfate-16α-glucosiduronate (gynecology, laboratory, and pharmacology)

ESL
end-systolic length (cardiovascular)
English as a second language (education)

ESM
ejection systolic murmur (cardiovascular)

ESN
educationally subnormal (psychiatry)
estrogen-stimulated neurophysin (endocrinology)

ESO
electrospinal orthosis (neurology and orthopedics)
esophagus (gastroenterology)

eso.
esophagoscopy (gastroenterology)
esophagus (gastroenterology)

esoph
esophagus (gastroenterology)

ESP
early systolic paradox (cardiovascular)

effective sensory projection (neurology)
effective systolic pressure (cardiovascular)
electrostatic precipitator (chemistry)
end-systolic pressure (cardiovascular)
eosinophil stimulation promotor (laboratory)
epidermal soluble protein (laboratory and pharmacology)
especially
evoked synaptic potential (neurology)
extrasensory perception (parapsychology)

esp
especial(ly)

"es-pep"
{pronunciation of *SPEP* [serum protein electrophoresis]} (laboratory) {not an abbreviation}

ESR
electric skin resistance (neurology)
electron spin resonance (laboratory)
erythrocyte sedimentation rate (laboratory)

E.S.R.
erythrocyte sedimentation rate (laboratory)

esr
electron spin resonance (laboratory)

ESRD
end-stage renal disease (nephrology)

ESS
erythrocyte-sensitizing substance (laboratory)

ess.
essential

ess. neg.
essentially negative

EST
electroshock therapy [also called *electric shock therapy*] (psychiatry)
esterase (laboratory)

ETOH
alcohol (chemistry)
alcoholic (chemical dependency)
ethanol (chemical dependency and
chemistry)
ethyl alcohol (chemical dependency and
chemistry)

EtOH
ethyl alcohol (chemical dependency and
chemistry)

ETOX
ethylene oxide (chemistry)

ETP
electron transport particle (physics)
entire treatment period
eustachian tube pressure (otorhinolaryngology)

ETR
effective thyroxine ratio (endocrinology,
laboratory, and pharmacology)
epitympanic recess

et seq
et sequentels [and those that follow]

ETT
endotracheal tube (respiratory)
exercise tolerance test (cardiovascular)
exercise treadmill test (cardiovascular)
extrathyroidal thyroxine (endocrinology
and laboratory)

ETU
emergency and trauma unit (emergency
medicine)
emergency treatment unit (emergency
medicine)

ETV
educational television (education)

EU
Ehrlich unit (laboratory)
entropy unit (physics)
enzyme unit (laboratory)
euthyroid (endocrinology)
excretory urogram (radiology)

Eu
europium (chemistry)

EUA
examination under anesthesia (surgery)
examine under anesthesia (surgery)

E.U.A.
examination under anesthesia (surgery)

EUG LY
euglobulin lysis [also called *fibrinolysin*
and *plasmin*] (laboratory)

EUROTOX
European Committee on Chronic Toxicity Hazards (research)

EUS
external urethral sphincter (urology)

EUV
extreme ultraviolet laser (surgery)

EV
emergency vehicle (emergency medicine)
evoked response (neurology)
extravascular (cardiovascular)

eV
electron volt (electricity)

ev
electron volt (electricity)
eversion

EVA
ethylene vinyl acetate (chemistry)
ethyl violet azide [broth] (laboratory)

EVAC
evacuated {pronounced "e-vak"}
evacuation {pronounced "e-vak"}

evac
evacuated {pronounced "e-vak"}
evacuation {pronounced "e-vak"}

"e-vak"
{pronunciation of *EVAC* and *evac* [evac-
uated and evacuation]} {not an abbre-
viation}

eval
evaluation
evaluate

eval.
evaluation
evaluate

evap
evaporated (laboratory)

evap.
evaporated (laboratory)

ever
eversion

evisc.
evisceration (surgery)

EVM
electronic voltmeter (electricity)

EVP
evoked visual potential (neurology)

EVR
evoked response (neurology)

EW
emergency ward (emergency medicine)

ew.
elsewhere

EWB
estrogen withdrawal bleeding (gynecology)

EWL
egg-white lysozyme (laboratory)
evaporative water loss (laboratory)

EWSCLs
extended-wear soft contact lenses (ophthalmology)

Ex
excision (surgery)

ex
exaggerated
examine(d)
example

exercise (rehabilitation)
{not an abbreviation} [Latin for *from*]

ex.
excision (surgery)
exophthalmos (ophthalmology)

ex aff
ex affinis [of affinity]

exag
exaggerated

exam
examination

exam.
examination

EXBF
exercise hyperemia blood flow (cardiovascular)

exc
except(ed)
excision (surgery)

exc.
except(ed)
excision (surgery)

exer
exercise (rehabilitation)

exer.
exercise (rehabilitation)

EXGBUS
external genitalia and Bartholin's, urethral, and Skene's glands (gynecology)

ex gr
ex grupa [of the group of]

exhib
exhibeatur [let it be given] (pharmacology)

exhib.
exhibeatur [let it be given] (pharmacology)

EXP
experienced
expiratory (respiratory)
exploration (surgery)

Exp
expectorant (respiratory)

exp
expect(ed)
expecting
experiment(al) (research)
expiratory (respiratory)
expired (respiratory)

exp.
expired (respiratory)
exploration (surgery)
exponential function (mathematics)
exposure (surgery)

expect
expectorant (pharmacology and respiratory)

exper
experiment(al) (research)

ExPGN
extracapillary proliferative glomerular nephritis (nephrology)

expir
expiration (respiratory)
expiratory (respiratory)

expir.
expiration (respiratory)
expiratory (respiratory)
expired (respiratory)

expl
exploratory (surgery)

exp. lap.
exploratory laparotomy (surgery)

expl. lap.
exploratory laparotomy (surgery)

expt
expect(ed)
experimental (research)

exptl
experimental (research)

EXREM
external radiation dose (radiation therapy and radiology)

EXT
external

Ext
extraction (dentistry)
extremities (orthopedics)

ext
extend [spread]
extension
extensor (orthopedics)
external
extractum [extract] (pharmacology)
extremity (neurology and orthopedics)

ext.
extend [spread]
extensor (orthopedics)
exterior
external
extract (pharmacology)
extractum [extract] (pharmacology)
extremities (orthopedics)

extd
extended
extracted (dentistry)

ext fl
fluid extract (pharmacology)

Extr
extremities (orthopedics)
extremity (orthopedics)

extr.
extremities (orthopedics)
extremity (orthopedics)

EXTREM
external radiation dose (radiation therapy)

ext rot
external rotation (neurology and orthopedics)

ext. rot.
external rotation (neurology and orthopedics)

EX U
excretory urogram (radiology and urology)

exx
examples

EY
egg yolk (laboratory)

EYA
egg yolk-pyruvate-tellurite-glycine agar
(laboratory)

"eye-vak"
{pronunciation of *IVAC* [intravenous accurate control (pharmacology)] and
IVAC {not an abbreviation [manufac-
turer of volumetric infusion pump]}
{not an abbreviation}

Ez
eczema (dermatology)

Ez.
eczema (dermatology)

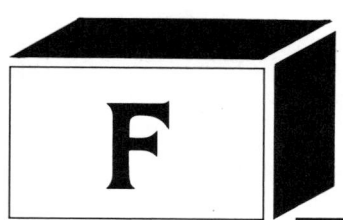

F
facial
facies
factor (laboratory)
Fahrenheit [temperature scale] (measurement)
failure
family
farad (measurement)
Faraday constant (physics)
fasting [test] (laboratory)
fat(s) (dietary)
father
feces (gastroenterology)
Fellow (education)
female
feminine
fertility (gynecology and obstetrics)
fertility factor (laboratory and obstetrics)
fetal (obstetrics)
fibrous [referring to proteins] (laboratory)
field of vision (ophthalmology)
filament
fine
finger (orthopedics)
firm
flow [of blood] (cardiovascular)
fluoride (chemistry)
fluorine (chemistry)
focal length (ophthalmology)
foil (dentistry)
foramen (anatomy)
force
(form of acropectorovertebral dysplasia)
formula
formulary (pharmacology)
fractional [referring to fractional composition of a gas in gas phase] (laboratory and respiratory)
fracture (orthopedics)
fragment of an antibody (laboratory)
free
French [catheter size, language, or nationality]

frontal (neonatology, neurology, and obstetrics)
frontal sinus (otorhinolaryngology)
full [referring to diet] (dietary)
function
Fusarium [a fungus] (laboratory)
Fusiformis [a bacteria] (laboratory)
gilbert [unit of magnetomotive force] (physics)
hydrocortisone (compound F) (pharmacology)
inbreeding coefficient (genetics)
phenylalanine (chemistry and laboratory)
variance ratio

F.
Fahrenheit [temperature scale] (measurement)
fiat [let there be made] (pharmacology)
field of vision (ophthalmology)
Filaria (laboratory)
formula
French [catheter size] (cardiovascular and urology)
Fusiformis (laboratory)
Fusobacterium (laboratory)

μF
microfarad (electricity measurement)

F°
Fahrenheit degree [temperature scale] (measurement)

°F
degree(s) Fahrenheit [temperature scale] (measurement)

F₀
emitted frequency [on Doppler studies] (cardiovascular)

F₁
first filial generation (genetics)

offspring of first generation (genetics)
received frequency [on Doppler studies] (cardiovascular)
{not an abbreviation} [a fluorescent substance found in small amounts in normal urine] (laboratory)

F₂
offspring of second generation (genetics)
second filial generation (genetics)
zinc oxide-eugenol cement (dentistry)
{not an abbreviation} [a substance in urine that develops fluorescence after alkali is added] (laboratory)

f
atomic orbital with angular momentum quantum number 3
breathing frequency (respiratory)
fac [make] (pharmacology)
farad (measurement)
femto- [prefix meaning 10^{-15}] (measurement) {not an abbreviation}
fiat [let it be made] (pharmacology)
fiant [let them be made] (pharmacology)
fluid
focal
forma [form]
frequency
frequently
from
respiratory frequency [breaths per unit of time] (respiratory)

f.
fiat [let it be made] (pharmacology)
fiant [let them be made] (pharmacology)
forma [form]

μf
microfarad (electricity measurement)

FA
false aneurysm (cardiovascular)
Families Anonymous (psychiatry)
far advanced
fatty acid (laboratory)
febrile antigens (laboratory)
femoral artery (cardiovascular)
fetal age (ob)
fibrosing alveolitis (respiratory)
field ambulance (emergency medicine)
filterable agent (laboratory)
first aid (emergency medicine)

fluorescent antibody [technique] (laboratory)
5-fluorouracil and Adriamycin (chemotherapy, oncology, and pharmacology)
folic acid (laboratory and pharmacology)
forearm (anatomy and orthopedics)
fortified aqueous [referring to solutions] (pharmacology)
free acid (chemistry)
Freund's adjuvant (oncology)
functional activities (rehabilitation)

F/A
fetus active (obstetrics)

Fa
Fahrenheit [temperature scale] (measurement)
father

FAAP
family assessment adjustment pass (psychiatry)

FAA sol.
formalin, acetic, and alcohol solution [a fixative] (chemistry)

FAB
antigen-binding fragments (laboratory)
formalin ammonium bromide (chemistry)
French-American-British [classification system for leukemia; classes include L-1, L-2, L-3, M-1, M-2, M-3, M-4, M-5, and M-6] (hematology, oncology, and pathology)
functional arm brace (orthopedics and rehabilitation)

Fab
antigen-binding fragment of an antigen (laboratory)
fragment antigen-binding (laboratory)

FABER
flexion in abduction and external rotation (neurology and orthopedics) {pronounced "fay-burr"}

fabere
flexion, abduction, external rotation, and extension [sign; also called *Patrick's test*] (neurology and orthopedics) {pronounced "fay-burr"}

FAC
factor (laboratory)
5-fluorouracil, Adriamycin [doxorubicin], and cyclophosphamide [Cytoxan] (chemotherapy, oncology, and pharmacology)
fractional area concentration (radiation therapy)
free available chlorine (chemistry)

Fac
factor (laboratory)

FACA
Fellow of the American College of Anesthetists (anesthesiology)
Fellow of the American College of Angiology (cardiovascular)
Fellow of the American College of Apothecaries (pharmacology)

F.A.C.A.
Fellow of the American College of Anesthesiologists (anesthesiology)

FACAG
Fellow of the American College of Angiology (cardiovascular)

FACAL
Fellow of the American College of Allergy (allergy)

FACAI
Fellow of the American College of Allergists (allergy)

FACAN
Fellow of the American College of Anesthesiologists (anesthesiology)

FACAS
Fellow of the American College of Abdominal Surgeons (gastroenterology and surgery)

Facb
fragment antigen and complement binding (laboratory)

FAC-BCG
Ftorafur, Adriamycin, cyclophosphamide, and bacille Calmette-Guérin [BCG] (chemotherapy, oncology, and pharmacology)

FACC
Fellow of the American College of Cardiologists (cardiovascular)
Fellow of the American College of Cardiology (cardiovascular)

F.A.C.C.
Fellow of the American College of Cardiologists (cardiovascular)

FACCP
Fellow of the American College of Chest Physicians (cardiovascular and respiratory)

F.A.C.C.P.
Fellow of the American College of Chest Physicians (cardiovascular and respiratory)

FACCPC
Fellow of the American College of Clinical Pharmacology and Chemotherapy (chemotherapy and pharmacology)

FACD
Fellow of the American College of Dentists (dentistry)

F.A.C.D.
Fellow of the American College of Dentists (dentistry)

FACFP
Fellow of the American College of Family Physicians

FACFS
Fellow of the American College of Foot Surgeons (orthopedics and podiatry)

F.A.C.F.S.
Fellow of the American College of Foot Surgeons (orthopedics and podiatry)

FACG
Fellow of the American College of Gastroenterology (gastroenterology)

FACGE
Fellow of the American College of Gastroenterology (gastroenterology)

FACH
forceps to after-coming head (obstetrics)

FACHA
Fellow of the American College of Health Administrators (administration)

F.A.C.H.A.
Fellow of the American College of Hospital Administrators (administration)

FACLM
Fellow of the American College of Legal Medicine (law)

FACMTA
Federal Advisory Council on Medical Training Aids (education)

FACN
Fellow of the American College of Nutrition (dietary)

FACNHA
Foundation of American Colleges of Nursing Home Administrators (administration)

FACNP
Fellow of the American College of Neuropsychopharmacology (neurology, pharmacology, and psychiatry)

FACO
Fellow of the American College of Otolaryngology (otorhinolaryngology)

FACOG
Fellow of the American College of Obstetricians and Gynecologists (gynecology and obstetrics)

F.A.C.O.G.
Fellow of the American College of Obstetricians and Gynecologists (gynecology and obstetrics)

FACOS
Fellow of the American College of Orthopedic Surgeons (orthopedics)

FACOSH
Federal Advisory Committee on Occupational Safety and Health (government)

FACP
Fellow of the American College of Physicians
Ftorafur, Adriamycin, cyclophosphamide, and cisplatin (chemotherapy, oncology, and pharmacology)

F.A.C.P.
Fellow of the American College of Physicians

FACPM
Fellow of the American College of Preventive Medicine

FACPRM
Fellow of the American College of Preventive Medicine

FACR
Fellow of the American College of Radiology (radiology)

F.A.C.R.
Fellow of the American College of Radiologists (radiology)

FACS
Fellow of the American College of Surgeons (surgery)
fluorescence-activated cell sorter (laboratory)
5-fluorouracil, Adriamycin, cyclophos-

phamide, and streptozocin (chemotherapy, oncology, and pharmacology)

F.A.C.S.
Fellow of the American College of Surgeons (surgery)

FACSM
Fellow of the American College of Sports Medicine (sports medicine)

F.A.C.S.M.
Fellow of the American College of Sports Medicine (sports medicine)

FACT
Flanagan Aptitude Classification Test (psychiatry)

Factor VII
proconvertin (hematology and laboratory) {pronounced "fak-tor-seven"}

FACVP
5-fluorouracil, Adriamycin, cyclophosphamide, and VP-16 (chemotherapy, oncology, and pharmacology)

FAD
familial autonomic dysfunction (genetics and neurology)
Family Assessment Device (psychiatry)
fetal activity-acceleration determination (obstetrics)
flavin adenine dinucleotide (laboratory)

FADF
fluorescent antibody darkfield (laboratory)

FADH₂
flavin adenine dinucleotide (reduced form) (laboratory)

FADIR
flexion in adduction and internal rotation (neurology and orthopedics)

FADN
flavin adenine dinucleotide (laboratory)

FAH
Federation of American Hospitals

Fahr
Fahrenheit [temperature scale] (measurement)

Fahr.
Fahrenheit [temperature scale] (measurement)

FAI
First Aid Instructor (education and emergency medicine)
functional assessment inventory (neurology, psychiatry, and rehabilitation)

"fair-in-go"
{pronunciation of *pharyngo-* [prefix indicating relationship to the pharynx]} (otorhinolaryngology) {not an abbreviation}

FAIT
First Aid Instructor Trainer (education and emergency medicine)

"fak-tor-seven"
{pronunciation of Factor VII [proconvertin]} (hematology and laboratory) {not an abbreviation}

FALG
fowl antimouse lymphocyte globulin (laboratory and research)

FALL
fallopian (gynecology)

"fal-low"
{pronunciation of *phallo-* [prefix indicating relationship to the penis]} (urology) {not an abbreviation}

FAM
family
5-fluorouracil, Adriamycin [doxorubicin], and mitomycin-C (chemotherapy, oncology, and pharmacology)

Fam
family

FAMA
Fellow of the American Medical Association

F.A.M.A.
Fellow of the American Medical Association

FAM-C
5-fluorouracil, Adriamycin, and mitomycin-C (chemotherapy, oncology, and pharmacology)

Fam Doc
family doctor

fam. doc.
family doctor

FAME
fatty acid methyl ester (laboratory)
5-fluorouracil, Adriamycin, and methyl-CCNU [MeCCNU or semustine] (chemotherapy, oncology, and pharmacology)

Fam per par
familial periodic paralysis (neurology)

fam. per. par.
familial periodic paralysis (neurology)

Fam phys
family physician

fam. phys.
family physician

FAN
fuchsin, amido black, and naphthol yellow (chemistry)

FANA
fluorescent antinuclear antibody (laboratory)

"fan-air-oh"
{pronunciation of *phanero-* [prefix meaning *apparent* or *visible*]} {not an abbreviation}

F and R
force and rhythm [of pulse] (cardiovascular)

FANPT
Freeman Anxiety Neurosis and Psychosomatic Test (psychiatry)

FANS
Fellow of the American Neurological Society (neurology)

F.A.N.S.
Fellow of the American Neurological Society (neurology)

FANY
First Aid Nursing Yeomanry [British] (emergency medicine)

FAO
Food and Agricultural Organization [of the United Nations] (government)

FAP
familial amyloid polyneuropathy (neurology)
fibrillating action potentials (neurology)
5-fluorouracil, Adriamycin, and cisplatin (chemotherapy, oncology, and pharmacology)

FAPA
Fellow of the American Psychiatric Association (psychiatry)
Fellow of the American Psychoanalytical Association (psychology)

F.A.P.A.
Fellow of the American Psychiatric Association (psychiatry)
Fellow of the American Psychoanalytical Association (psychology)

FAPHA
Fellow of the American Public Health Association

F.A.P.H.A.
Fellow of the American Public Health Association

FAR
flight aptitude rating (aerospace science)

FC

fast component [of an axon] (laboratory)
fecal coli [broth] (laboratory)
fever and chills
finger clubbing (cardiovascular and orthopedics)
finger counting (neurology and ophthalmology)
Foley catheter (urology)
functional class (rehabilitation)

F + C

flare and cells (ophthalmology)

F & C

foam and condom [birth control methods] (gynecology)

5-FC

5-fluorocytosine [also called *Ancobon* and *flucytosine*] (chemotherapy, oncology, and pharmacology)

Fc

fragment, crystallizable [part of immunoglobulin G molecule] (laboratory)

Fc′

{not an abbreviation} [fragment produced in minute quantities following papain digestion of immunoglobulin molecules] (laboratory)

fc

foot-candle (measurement)

fc.

foot-candle (measurement)

FCA

ferritin-conjugated antibodies (laboratory)
Freund's complete adjuvant (oncology)

FCAP

Fellow of the College of American Pathologists (pathology)

F.C.A.P.

Fellow of the College of American Pathologists (pathology)

F. cath.

Foley catheter (urology)

FCC

familial colonic cancer (gastroenterology and oncology)
family center care
Federal Communications Commission (government)
follicular center cells (laboratory)
fracture, compound and comminuted (orthopedics)

FCCP

Fellow of the American College of Chest Physicians (cardiovascular and respiratory)

FCD

fecal collection device (gastroenterology)

FCDB

fibrocystic disease of the breast (gynecology)

FCG

French catheter gauge (surgery)

F.C.G.P.

Fellow of the College of General Practitioners

FCH

familial combined hyperlipidemia (cardiovascular)

FChS

Fellow of the Society of Chiropodists (podiatry)

fcly

face lying [position]

FCMC

family-centered maternity care (obstetrics)

FCMD

Fukiyama's congenital muscular dystrophy (neurology)

FCMN
family-centered maternity nursing (obstetrics)

FCMS
Fellow of the College of Medicine and Surgery

FCMW
Foundation for Child Mental Welfare (psychiatry)

FCO
Fellow of the College of Osteopathy (osteopathy)

FCP
fasting chemistry profile (laboratory)
final common pathway (neurology)

FCPS
Fellow of the College of Physicians and Surgeons

F.C.P.S.
Fellow of the College of Physicians and Surgeons

FCPSA(SoAf)
Fellow of the College of Physicians and Surgeons, South Africa

FCR
flexor carpi radialis (neurology and orthopedics)
fractional catabolic rate (laboratory)

FCRA
fecal collection receptacle assembly (gastroenterology)
Fellow of the College of Radiologists of Australasia (radiology)

FCRB
flexor carpi radialis brevis (neurology and orthopedics)

FCRC
Frederick Cancer Research Center (oncology and research)

FCS
fecal containment system (gastroenterology)

feedback control system (psychiatry)
Fellow of the Chemical Society (chemistry)
fetal calf serum (laboratory)

FCSNVD
fever, chills, sweating, nausea, vomiting, and diarrhea (gastroenterology)

FCSP
Fellow of the Chartered Society of Physiotherapy (physical therapy and rehabilitation)

FCST
Fellow of the College of Speech Therapists (rehabilitation and speech pathology)

FCT
food composition table (dietary)

FCU
flexor carpi ulnaris (neurology and orthopedics)

FD
familial dysautonomia (neurology)
fan douche (gynecology)
fatal dose (pharmacology, radiation therapy, and radiology)
focal distance (ophthalmology)
foot drape (surgery)
forceps delivery (obstetrics)
freeze-dried (chemistry and laboratory)

F.D.
fatal dose {obsolete} [lethal dose] (pharmacology, radiation therapy, and radiology)
focal distance (ophthalmology)

F & D
fixed and dilated (neurology and ophthalmology)

FD$_{50}$
median fatal dose (pharmacology, radiation therapy, and radiology)

Fd
{not an abbreviation} [heavy chain portion of fragment antigen-binding (Fab) fragment after papain digestion of an immunoglobulin G molecule] (laboratory)

FDA
Food and Drug Administration (dietary, government, and pharmacology)
Frenchay Dysarthria Assessment (speech and language therapy)
frontodextra anterior [right frontoanterior fetal position] (obstetrics)

F.D.A.
Food and Drug Administration (dietary, government, and pharmacology)
frontodextra anterior [right frontoanterior fetal position] (obstetrics)

FDA medium
{not an abbreviation} [also called *extract* agar] (laboratory)

FD & C
Food, Drug, and Cosmetic [Act] (dietary, government, manufacturing, and pharmacology)

FDCPA
Food, Drug, and Consumer Product Agency [Department of Health and Human Science] (dietary, government, manufacturing, and pharmacology)

FDD
Food and Drug Directorate [Canada] (dietary, government, manufacturing, and pharmacology)

FDDC
ferric dimethyl dithiocarbonate (chemistry)

FDE
final drug evaluation (pharmacology)

FDF
fast death factor

FDG
fluorodeoxyglucose (laboratory)

fDG
feeding (dietary)

fdg
feeding (dietary)

FDI
Fédération Dentaire Internationale [International Dental Association] (dentistry)
first dorsal interosseous [muscle or nerve] (neurology and orthopedics)

F.D.I.
Fédération Dentaire Internationale [International Dental Association] (dentistry)

FDIU
fetal death in utero (obstetrics)

FDL
flexor digitorum longus [muscle or nerve] (neurology and orthopedics)

FDLMP
first day of last menstrual period (gynecology and obstetrics)

FDNB
1-fluoro-2,4-dinitrobenzene [also called *fluorodinitrobenzene*] (chemistry)

FDO
Fleet Dental Officer (armed forces and dentistry)

FDP
fibrin degradation product(s) (hematology and laboratory)
fibrinogen degradation product(s) (hematology and laboratory)
flexor digitorum profundus [muscle or nerve] (neurology and orthopedics)
flexor distal phalanx (orthopedics)
frontodextra posterior [right frontoposterior fetal position] (obstetrics)
fructose 1,6-diphosphate [also called *fructose diphosphate*] (chemistry)

F.D.P.
frontodextra posterior [right frontoposterior fetal position] (obstetrics)

FDPase
fructose diphosphatase (chemistry)

fdp/Fdp
fibrin/fibrinogen degradation products (hematology and laboratory)

FDQB
flexor digiti quinti brevis [muscle or nerve] (neurology and orthopedics)

FDS
Fellow in Dental Surgery (dentistry)
flexor digitorum sublimis [muscle or nerve] (neurology and orthopedics)
flexor digitorum superficialis [muscle or nerve] (neurology and orthopedics)
for duration of stay

F.D.S.
Fellow in Dental Surgery (dentistry)

FDSRCSEng
Fellow in Dental Surgery of the Royal College of Surgeons of England (dentistry)

FDT
frontodextra transversa [right fronto-transverse fetal position] (obstetrics)

F.D.T.
frontodextra transversa [right fronto-transverse fetal position] (obstetrics)

FDTVMP
Frostig Developmental Test of Visual-Motor Perception (psychiatry and rehabilitation)

FDTVP
Frostig Developmental Test of Visual Perception (psychiatry and rehabilitation)

FDV
Friend disease virus (laboratory)

FE
fecal emesis (gastroenterology)

fecal energy (gastroenterology)
fetal erythroblastosis (hematology, neonatology, and obstetrics)
fluid extract (pharmacology)

Fe
female
ferrum [iron] (chemistry, laboratory, and pharmacology)

Fe^{59}
radioactive iron (chemistry)

^{59}Fe
radioactive iron (chemistry)

fe
female
ferrum [iron] (chemistry, laboratory, and pharmacology)

feb
febrile
febus [fever]

feb dur
febre durante [while the fever lasts] (pharmacology)

feb. dur.
febre durante [while the fever lasts] (pharmacology)

FEBP
fetoneonatal estrogen-binding protein (laboratory, neonatology, and obstetrics)

FEBRIL
febrile agglutinins (laboratory)

FEBROA
febrile battery-acute (laboratory)

F.E.B.S.
Federation of European Biochemical Societies (biology and chemistry)

FEC
fecal (gastroenterology and laboratory)

forced expiratory capacity (laboratory and respiratory)

free erythrocyte coproporphyrin (hematology and laboratory)

FECG
fetal electrocardiogram (cardiovascular, neonatology, and obstetrics)

FECP
free erythrocyte coproporphyria (hematology and laboratory)

FECT
fibroelastic connective tissue (rheumatology)

FECV
functional extracellular fluid volume (laboratory)

Fed
federal (government)
federation
{not an abbreviation} [slang for *federal government agent*] {pronounced "fed"}

"fed"
{pronunciation of *Fed* [slang for *federal government agent*]} {not an abbreviation}

Fed spec
federal specifications (government and measurement)

FEE
forced equilibrating expiration (laboratory and respiratory)

"fee-oh"
{pronunciation of *phaeo, Pheo,* and *pheo* [phaeochromocytoma, pheochromocytoma (endocrinology and oncology)] and *pheo-* [prefix indicating relationship to brown, dun, or dusky]} {not an abbreviation}

FEF
forced expiratory flow [rate] (laboratory and respiratory)

FEF 0-25
forced expiratory flow zero percent [0%] to twenty-five percent [25%] forced vital capacity (laboratory and respiratory)

FEF 25
forced expiratory flow twenty-five percent [25%] forced vital capacity (laboratory and respiratory)

FEF 25-75
mean forced expiratory flow twenty-five percent [25%] to seventy-five percent [75%] forced vital capacity [mean forced expiratory flow during the middle half of the forced vital capacity; formerly called the *maximum midexpiratory flow rate*] (laboratory and respiratory)

FEF 50
forced expiratory flow fifty percent [50%] forced vital capacity (laboratory and respiratory)

FEF 75
forced expiratory flow seventy-five percent [75%] forced vital capacity [instantaneous forced expiratory flow after 75% of vital capacity has been exhaled] (laboratory and respiratory)

FEF200-1200
mean forced expiratory flow between 200 milliliters and 1200 milliliters of the forced vital capacity [formerly called the *maximum expiratory flow rate*] (laboratory and respiratory)

FEFmax
maximal forced expiratory flow achieved during a forced vital capacity (laboratory and respiratory)

FEF$_x$
forced expiratory flow [related to some portion of the forced vital capacity (FVC) curve, modifiers referring to the amount of FVC already exhaled

when the measurement is made] (laboratory and respiratory)

FEGO
{not an abbreviation} [International Federation of Gynecology and Obstetrics staging of adenocarcinoma] (gynecology, obstetrics, and oncology)

FE INC
iron inclusion bodies (hematology and laboratory)

FEKG
fetal electrocardiogram (cardiovascular, neonatology, and obstetrics)

FEL
familial erythrophagocytic lymphohistiocytosis (hematology)

Fel
Fellow (education)

FEM
femoral (cardiovascular and orthopedics)
femoris [thigh]

Fem
femoral (cardiovascular and orthopedics)
femur (orthopedics)

fem
female
feminine
femoral (cardiovascular and orthopedics)
femoris [thigh]
femur (orthopedics)

FEMED
5-fluorouracil, methotrexate, cyclophosphamide, and prednisone (chemotherapy, oncology, and pharmacology)

Fem intern
femoribus internus [at the inner side of the thighs]

fem. intern.
femoribus internus [at the inner side of the thighs]

fem-pop
femoral-popliteal [also called *femoropopliteal* (bypass)] (cardiovascular) {pronounced "fem-pop"}

"fem-pop"
{pronunciation of *fem-pop* [femoral-popliteal (also called *femoropopliteal* {bypass})]} (cardiovascular) {not an abbreviation}

femto-
{not an abbreviation} [prefix meaning 10^{-15}] (measurement) {pronounced "fem-toe"}

"fem-toe"
{pronunciation of *femto-* [prefix meaning 10^{-15}]} (measurement) {not an abbreviation}

FEN
fluid, electrolytes, and nutrition (dietary and pharmacology)

"fen"
{pronunciation of *phen-* [prefix indicating: (1) a displaying or showing and/or (2) derived from or related to benzene or containing phenyl]} (chemistry) {not an abbreviation}

FE$_{Na}$
excreted fraction of filtered sodium [test] (laboratory)
fractional extraction of sodium (laboratory)

"fen-oh"
{pronunciation of *pheno-* [prefix indicating: (1) a displaying or showing and/or (2) derived from or related to benzene or containing phenyl]} (chemistry) {not an abbreviation}

"fen-ox-E"
{pronunciation of *phenoxy-* [prefix indicating the presence of OC_6H_5]} (chemistry) {not an abbreviation}

FEOM
full extraocular motion (ophthalmology)
full extraocular movement (ophthalmology)

FEP
fluorinated ethylene propylene (chemistry)
free erythrocyte protoporphyrin (hematology and laboratory)

FEPP
free erythrocyte protoporphyrin (hematology and laboratory)

Fer
ferrum [iron] (chemistry, laboratory, and pharmacology)

FERRIT
ferritin (hematology and laboratory)

fertd
fertilized

ferv
fervens [boiling] (pharmacology)

ferv.
fervens [boiling] (pharmacology)

FES
flame emission spectroscopy (laboratory)
forced expiratory spirogram (laboratory and respiratory)

FeSO$_4$
ferrous sulfate (chemistry, laboratory, and pharmacology)

FET
field effect transistor (physics)
fixed erythrocyte turnover (hematology and laboratory)
forced expiratory time (laboratory and respiratory)

FETS
forced expiratory time in seconds (laboratory and respiratory)

FET$_x$
forced expiratory time for a specific period of the forced vital capacity [The symbol "X" refers to the period of the forced vital capacity.] (laboratory and respiratory)

FEUO
for external use only (pharmacology)

FE-UR
iron in urine (laboratory)

FEV
forced expiratory volume (laboratory and respiratory)

FEV 1
forced expiratory volume in one second of expiration (laboratory and respiratory)

FEV$_1$
forced expiratory volume in one second of expiration (laboratory and respiratory)

FEV 1%
forced expiratory volume/forced vital capacity times 100 in one second (laboratory and respiratory)

FEV 2
forced expiratory volume in two seconds of expiration (laboratory and respiratory)

FEV$_2$
forced expiratory volume in two seconds of expiration (laboratory and respiratory)

FEV 2%
forced expiratory volume/forced vital capacity times 100 in two seconds (laboratory and respiratory)

FEV 3
forced expiratory volume in three seconds of expiration (laboratory and respiratory)

FEV₃
forced expiratory volume in three seconds of expiration (laboratory and respiratory)

FEV 3%
forced expiratory volume/forced vital capacity times 100 in three seconds (laboratory and respiratory)

FEVt
forced expiratory volume (timed) (laboratory and respiratory)

FEVt/FVC%
forced expiratory volume (timed) to forced vital capacity ratio [expressed as a percentage] (laboratory and respiratory)

FEV₁/VC
forced expiratory volume [in one second] vital capacity (laboratory and respiratory)

FF
fat-free (dietary)
father factor
fecal frequency (gastroenterology)
fertility factor
filtration factor (laboratory)
filtration fraction (laboratory)
finger-to-finger [test] (neurology)
fixing fluid (laboratory)
flat feet (orthopedics and podiatry)
flip-flop (cardiovascular)
force fluids (dietary)
forearm flow (cardiovascular)
foster father
free fat (laboratory)
fresh frozen (laboratory)
fundus firm (obstetrics)
further flexion (neurology and orthopedics)

F.F.
fat-free (dietary)

F & F
filiform and follower [instruments] (urology)

ff
following

force fluid (dietary)
full field (radiation therapy)
fundus firm (obstetrics)

f/f
fundus firm (obstetrics)

FFA
Fellow of the Faculty of Anaesthetists (anesthesiology and education)
free fatty acids (laboratory)

F.F.A.
free fatty acids (laboratory)

F factor
fertility factor (laboratory)

FFAP
free fatty acid phase (laboratory)

FFARCS
Fellow of the Faculty of Anaesthetists, Royal College of Surgeons (anesthesiology and education)

FFC
fixed flexion contracture (neurology and orthopedics)
free from chlorine (chemistry)

FFCM
Fellow of the Faculty of Community Medicine

FFD
Fellow in the Faculty of Dentistry (dentistry)
focus film distance (radiology)

FFDCA
Federal Food, Drug, and Cosmetic Act (chemistry, dietary, government, manufacturing, and pharmacology)

FFDSRCS
Fellow of the Faculty of Dental Surgery, Royal College of Surgeons (dentistry)

FFDW
fat-free dry weight

FFHom
Fellow of the Faculty of Homeopathy (homeopathic medicine)

FFI
free from infection

FFIT
fluorescent focus inhibition test

FFM
fat-free mass (laboratory)

FFOM
Fellow of the Faculty of Occupational Medicine (occupational medicine and rehabilitation)

FFP
fistful of prisms (ophthalmology)
fresh frozen plasma (hematology)

F.F.P.
fresh frozen plasma (hematology)

FFR
Fellow of the Faculty of Radiologists (radiology)

FFS
fat-free solids (dietary)
fat-free supper (dietary)

FFT
fast-Fourier transforms
flicker fusion threshold (cardiovascular)

F.F.T.
flicker fusion threshold (cardiovascular)

FFU
focus-forming unit

FFWW
fat-free wet weight

FG
fibrinogen (hematology and laboratory)

F-G
Feeley-Gorman [agar] (laboratory)

FGAR
formylglycinamide ribonucleotide (laboratory)

FGD
fatal granulomatous disease (respiratory)

FGF
father's grandfather

FGLU
fasting glucose (endocrinology and laboratory)

FGM
father's grandmother

FGRN
finely granular (laboratory)

FGS
focal glomerulosclerosis (nephrology)

FH
familial hypercholesterolemia (cardiovascular and genetics)
family history
fetal head (obstetrics)
fetal heart (obstetrics)
Frankfort horizontal [plane of skull] (radiology)
fundal height (obstetrics)

F.H.
family history

fh
fiat haustus [let a draught be made] (pharmacology)

f.h.
fiat haustus [let a draught be made] (pharmacology)

FHA
Federal Housing Authority (government)
Fellow of the Institute of Hospital Administrators (administration)

FHF
fulminate hepatic failure (gastroenterology)

FHH
familial hypocalciuric hypercalcemia (nephrology)
fetal heart heard (obstetrics)

FHI
Fuch's heterochromic iridocyclitis (ophthalmology)

FHIP
Family Health Insurance Plan (insurance)

FHNH
fetal heart not heard (obstetrics)

FHR
familial hypophosphatemic rickets (orthopedics)
fetal heart rate (obstetrics)

FHS
fetal heart sounds (obstetrics)
fetal hydantoin syndrome (obstetrics)

FHT
fetal heart (obstetrics)
fetal heart tone(s) (obstetrics)

FHVP
free hepatic vein pressure (cardiovascular)

FHx
family history

F hx
family history

FI
fever caused by infection
fibrinogen (hematology and laboratory)
fixed internal [reinforcement]
forced inspiration (laboratory and respiratory)

FIA
Freund's incomplete adjuvant (oncology)
fluorescent immunoassay (laboratory)

FIAT
Field Information Agency, Technical [of *US Reports*]

FIB
Fellow of the Institute of Biology [British] (biology)
fibrillation {pronounced "fib"} (cardiovascular and neurology)
fibrin (hematology and laboratory)
fibrinogen (hematology and laboratory)
fibrositis (orthopedics)
fibula (orthopedics)

Fib
fibrillation {pronounced "fib"} (cardiovascular and neurology)
fibula (orthopedics)

fib.
fibrillation {pronounced "fib"} (cardiovascular and neurology)
fibrinogen (hematology and laboratory)

"fib"
{pronunciation of *FIB*, *Fib*, and *fib.* [fibrillation]} (cardiovascular and neurology) {not an abbreviation}

FRIBGN
fibrinogen (hematology and laboratory)

fibrill
fibrillation (cardiovascular and neurology)

FIC
fasting intestinal contents (gastroenterology)
Fellow of the Institute of Chemistry (chemistry)

FICA
Federal Insurance Contribution Act [of Social Security] (government) {pronounced "fie-kah"}

FICD
Fellow of the Institute of Canadian Dentists (dentistry)

F.I.C.D.
Fellow of the International College of Dentists (dentistry)

F.I.C.D.
Fellow of the International College of Dentists (dentistry)

FICO$_2$
fraction of inspired carbon dioxide (laboratory and respiratory)

FICS
Fellow of the International College of Surgeons (surgery)

F.I.C.S.
Fellow of the International College of Surgeons (surgery)

FICU
fetal intensive care unit (neonatology)

FID
flame ionization detector (chemistry)
free induction decay or delay (radiology)

"fie-kah"
{pronunciation of *FICA* [Federal Insurance Contribution Act (of Social Security)]} (government) {not an abbreviation}

"fie-ko"
{pronunciation of *phyco-* [prefix indicating relationship to algae or seaweed]} (oceanography) {not an abbreviation}

field H$_1$
fasciculus thalamicus (anatomy and neurology)

field H$_2$
fasciculus lenticularis (anatomy and neurology)

"fie-low"
{pronunciation of *phyllo-* [prefix indicating relationship to leaves]} {not an abbreviation}

"fie-so"
{pronunciation of *physo-* [prefix indicat-

ing relationship to air or gas]} {not an abbreviation}

"fie-toe"
{pronunciation of *phyto-* [prefix indicating relationship to a plant or plants]} {not an abbreviation}

FIF
feedback inhibition factor
fibroblast interferon (hematology, laboratory, and pharmacology)
forced inspiratory flow (laboratory and respiratory)

FIF 25
forced inspiratory flow twenty-five percent [25%] inspiratory vital capacity (laboratory and respiratory)

FIF 50
forced inspiratory flow fifty percent [50%] inspiratory vital capacity (laboratory and respiratory)

FIF 75
forced inspiratory flow seventy-five percent [75%] inspiratory vital capacity (laboratory and respiratory)

FIFR
fasting intestinal flow rate (gastroenterology)

FIFRA
Federal Insecticide, Fungicide, and Rodenticide Act (chemistry and government)

FIF$_X$
forced expiratory flow [The symbol "X" refers to the volume at which flow is being measured.] (laboratory and respiratory)

fig
figuratively
figure

fig.
figuratively
figure

FIGLU
formiminoglutamic acid [an 8-hour histidine loading test] (laboratory)

FIGO
International Federation of Gynecology and Obstetrics (gynecology and obstetrics)

F.I.G.O.
International Federation of Gynecology and Obstetrics (gynecology and obstetrics)
International Federation of Gynecology and Obstetrics Staging Classification (gynecology, obstetrics, and oncology)

FIH
fat-induced hyperglycemia (endocrinology)

fil
filamentous (laboratory)

FILAR
filariasis (infectious diseases)

"fill-E-ah"
{pronunciation of -philia [suffix indicating abnormal or notable attraction or fondness]} {not an abbreviation}

"fill-oh"
{pronunciation of phyllo- [prefix indicating relationship to leaves]} {not an abbreviation}

filt
filtra [filter]

filt.
filtra [filter]

FIM
field ion microscope (laboratory)

FIME
5-fluorouracil, ICRF-159, and methyl-CCNU [MeCCNU or semustine] (chemotherapy, oncology, and pharmacology)

FIMF
International Federation of Physical Medicine (physical medicine and rehabilitation)

FIMLT
Fellow of the Institute of Medical Laboratory Technology (laboratory)

F.I.M.L.T.
Fellow of the Institute of Medical Laboratory Technology (laboratory)

FIN
fine intestinal needle (gastroenterology)

FInstSP
Fellow of the Institute of Sewage Purification (ecology)

F-insulin
fibrous insulin (endocrinology, laboratory, and pharmacology)

FIO$_2$
forced inspiratory oxygen (laboratory and respiratory)
fraction of inspired oxygen (laboratory and respiratory)
fractional concentration of inspired oxygen (laboratory and respiratory)
fractional inspiratory oxygen (laboratory and respiratory)
inspired flow of oxygen (laboratory and respiratory)

FIR
far infrared (laboratory)

FIRDA
frontal intermittent rhythmic delta activity [on an electroencephalogram] (neurology)

fist
fistula (surgery)

fist.
fistula (surgery)

FIT
fluorescein isothiocyanate (chemistry)
fusion inferred threshold [test] (cardiovascular)

FITC
fluorescein isothiocyanate (chemistry)

FITT
frequency, intensity, time, and type [ex-
ercise program] (rehabilitation)

FIUO
for internal use only (pharmacology)

FIVC
forced inspiratory vital capacity (laboratory and respiratory)

"fizz-ed"
{pronunciation of *PhysEd* and *phys ed*
[physical education]} (education) {not
an abbreviation}

"fizz-E-oh"
{pronunciation of *physio* [physio-
therapist, physiotherapy (physical
therapy)] and *physio-* [prefix indicating relationship to nature or indicating physical]} {not an abbreviation}

"fizz-med"
{pronunciation of *PhysMed* [physical
medicine]} {not an abbreviation}

"fizz-ther"
{pronunciation of *PhysTher* [physical
therapy]} {not an abbreviation}

F-J
Fisher-John [melting point method] (laboratory)

FJN
familial juvenile nephrophthisis (nephrology)

FJRM
full joint range of movement (orthopedics)

FL
filtered load
Florida [Postal Service state designation]

fluid (pharmacology)
fluorescence
fluorescent
focal length (laboratory)
frontal lobe [of the brain] (neurology)

Fl
fluid (pharmacology)

fL
foot-lambert (measurement)

fl
flexion (orthopedics)
fluidium [fluid] (pharmacology)

fl.
femtoliter (measurement)
flexion (orthopedics)
fluidus [fluid] (pharmacology)

FLA
frontolaeva anterior [left frontoanterior
fetal position] (obstetrics)

F.L.A.
frontolaeva anterior [left frontoanterior
fetal position] (obstetrics)

fla
fiat lege artis [let it be done according
to rule]

f.l.a.
fiat lege artis [let it be done according
to rule]

flac
flaccid (neurology)

flac.
flaccid (neurology)

Fl Ang
fluorescein angiography (cardiovascular
and radiology)

Fl Ant
fluorescent antibody (laboratory)

flav
flavus [yellow]

flav.
flavus [yellow]

FLC
Friend leukemia cells (hematology, laboratory, and oncology)

fld
field
fluid (pharmacology)

fld.
fluid (pharmacology)

fld ext
fluid extract (pharmacology)

fl dr
fluid dram [also called *fluid drachm*] (measurement)

fl. dr.
fluid dram [also called *fluid drachm*] (measurement)

fld. rest.
fluid restriction (dietary)

fldxt
fluidextractum [fluid extract, fluidextract] (pharmacology)

fldxt.
fluidextractum [fluid extract, fluidextract] (pharmacology)

"fleb"
{pronunciation of *phleb-* [prefix indicating relationship to a vein or veins]} (cardiovascular and hematology) {not an abbreviation}

"flee-bow"
{pronunciation of *phlebo-* [prefix indicating relationship to a vein or veins]} (cardiovascular and hematology) {not an abbreviation}

FLEX
Federal Licensing Examination (government)

flex
flexion (orthopedics)
flexor (orthopedics)

flex.
flexion (orthopedics)

flex sig
flexible sigmoidoscopy (gastroenterology) {pronounced "flex-sig"}

"flex-sig"
{pronunciation of *flex sig* [flexible sigmoidoscopy]} (gastroenterology) {not an abbreviation}

FLK
funny-looking kid [referring to strange facies] (genetics, neonatology, and pediatrics)

flocc
flocculation (laboratory)

flor
flores [flowers]

flor.
flores [flowers]

"flow-go"
{pronunciation of *phlogo-* [prefix indicating relationship to inflammation]} {not an abbreviation}

fl oz
fluid ounce (measurement)

fl. oz.
fluid ounce (measurement)

FLP
few large platelets (hematology and laboratory)
frontolaeva posterior [left frontoposterior fetal position] (obstetrics)

F.L.P.
frontolaeva posterior [left frontoposterior fetal position] (obstetrics)

FLS
Fellow of the Linnean Society (botany)
fibrous long-spacing [collagen] (laboratory)
flashing lights and/or scotoma (neurology and ophthalmology)

FLSA
follicular lymphosarcoma (oncology)

FLSP
fluorescein-labeled serum protein (laboratory)

FLT
frontolaeva transversa [left fronto-transverse fetal position] (obstetrics)

F.L.T.
frontolaeva transversa [left fronto-transverse fetal position] (obstetrics)

FLTA
Fullerton Language Test for Adolescents (psychiatry and speech and language therapy)

FLTAC
Fisher-Logemann Test of Articular Competence (speech and language therapy)

flu
influenza (gastroenterology and infectious diseases)

fluor
fluorescent
fluoroscopy (radiology)

fluor.
fluorometry

fluores
fluorescent

FLUORO
fluoroscopy (radiology) {pronounced "flur-oh"}

fluoro
fluoroscopy (radiology) {pronounced "flur-oh"}

fluoro.
fluoroscopy (radiology) {pronounced "flur-oh"}

fl.-up
flare-up
follow-up

"flur-oh"
{pronunciation of *FLUORO*, *fluoro*, and *fluoro*. [fluoroscopy]} (radiology) {not an abbreviation}

FLV
Friend leukemia virus (hematology, laboratory, and oncology)

FM
face mask (respiratory)
Farnsworth-Munsell [one hundred hue test] (ophthalmology)
feedback mechanism
fetal movements (obstetrics)
fibrin monomer (laboratory)
flavin mononucleotide (laboratory)
flowmeter (electricity)
fluorescent microscopy (laboratory)
forensic medicine (pathology)
formerly married
foster mother
frequency modulation (neurology)
fusobacteria micro-organisms (laboratory)
Fusobacterium micro-organisms (laboratory)

F.M.
fiat mistura [make a mixture] (pharmacology)

F & M
firm and midline [uterus] (gynecology and obstetrics)

Fm
fermium (chemistry)

fm
femtometer (measurement)
fiat mistura [make a mixture] (pharmacology)

fm.
fiat mistura [make a mixture] (pharmacology)

FMB
full maternal behavior (obstetrics)

FMC
fetal movement count (obstetrics)
Flight Medicine Clinic (aerospace medicine)
Foundation for Medical Care

FMCA
Forensic Medicine Consultant-Advisor (pathology)

FMD
family medical doctor
fibromuscular dysplasia (neurology)
foot-and-mouth disease (infectious diseases)

FMDV
foot-and-mouth disease virus (infectious diseases and laboratory)

FME
full-mouth extraction (dentistry)

FMF
familial Mediterranean fever (gastroenterology and genetics)
fetal movement felt (obstetrics)
forced midexpiratory flow (laboratory and respiratory)

FMG
fine mesh gauze (surgery)
foreign medical graduate(s) (education)

FMH
fat-mobilizing hormone (laboratory)
fibromuscular hyperplasia (neurology)

FMIV
forced mandatory intermittent ventilation (respiratory)

FML
{not an abbreviation} [trade name for *fluorometholone*]

f-MLP
formyl-methionyleucylphenylalanine (chemistry)

FMN
flavin mononucleotide (laboratory)

FMNH
flavin mononucleotide, reduced form (laboratory)

FMO
Fleet Medical Officer (armed forces)
Flight Medical Officer (armed forces)

fmol
femtomole (measurement)

FMP
fasting metabolic panel (laboratory)
first menstrual period (gynecology)

FMS
fat-mobilizing substance (laboratory)
Fellow of the Medical Society
full mouth series (dentistry and radiology)

FMX
full mouth radiography (dentistry and radiology)
full mouth x-ray (dentistry and radiology)

FN
false negative (laboratory)
finger-to-nose (neurology)
fluoride number (chemistry)

F-N
finger-to-nose (neurology)

FNA
fine needle aspiration [biopsy] (oncology and surgery)

FNa
filtered sodium (chemistry)

FNAB
fine needle aspiration biopsy (surgery)

FNAC
fine needle aspiration cytology (laboratory)

FNCJ
fine needle catheter jejunostomy (gastroenterology and surgery)

Fneg
false negative (laboratory)

FNF
finger-nose-finger [test] (neurology)

FNH
focal nodular hyperplasia (pathology and surgery)

FNP
Family Nurse Practitioner (nursing)

FNR
false negative rate (laboratory)

FNS
functional neuromuscular stimulation (neurology)

f-number
focal length [of a lens] (laboratory and ophthalmology)

FO
fiberoptic (surgery)
foramen ovale (anatomy)
fronto-occipital (neurology)

fo
fomentation (pharmacology)

FOA
Federation of Orthodontic Associations (dentistry)

"foat"
{pronunciation of *phot-* [prefix indicating relationship to light]} {not an abbreviation}

FOAVF
failure of all vital forces

FOB
father of baby (obstetrics)

fecal occult blood (gastroenterology and laboratory)
feet out of bed
fiberoptic bronchoscopy (respiratory)
foot of bed

F.O.B.
fiberoptic bronchoscopy (respiratory)

FOBT
fecal occult blood test (gastroenterology and laboratory)

FOC
father of child (obstetrics)

FOCAL
formula calculation (pharmacology)

FOD
free of disease

"foe-be-ah"
{pronunciation of *-phobia* [suffix indicating an abnormal dread or fear]} (psychiatry) {not an abbreviation}

"foe-no"
{pronunciation of *phono-* [prefix indicating relationship to sound]} (electronics, otorhinolaryngology, and speech therapy) {not an abbreviation}

"foe-toe"
{pronunciation of *photo* [photograph] and *photo-* [prefix indicating relationship to light]} {not an abbreviation}

FOG
Fluothane, oxygen, and gas [nitrous oxide] (anesthesiology and chemistry)

FOI
flight of ideas (psychiatry)

fol
folium [a leaf]
following

fol.
folia [leaves]

FOM
5-fluorouracil, Oncovin [vincristine], and mitomycin-C (chemotherapy, oncology, and pharmacology)

FOM-1
5-fluorouracil, Oncovin [vincristine], and mitomycin-C (chemotherapy, oncology, and pharmacology)

FOMi
5-fluorouracil, Oncovin [vincristine], and mitomycin-C (chemotherapy, oncology, and pharmacology)

"fon"
{pronunciation of *phon-* [prefix indicating relationship to sound]} (electronics, otorhinolaryngology, and speech therapy) {not an abbreviation}

FOOB
fell out of bed

FOPR
full outpatient rate

FOR
forensic (laboratory and pathology)

for
foreign

"for"
{pronunciation of *-phore* [suffix indicating a carrier of the root word]} {not an abbreviation}

for. body
foreign body (surgery)

"for-E-sis"
{pronunciation of *-phoresis* [suffix indicating transmission]} {not an abbreviation}

form
formation
formula (chemistry and pharmacology)

fort
fortis [strong]

fort.
fortis [strong]

FORTRAN
formula translation [computer language] (computer science) {pronounced "fortran"}

"for-tran"
{pronunciation of *FORTRAN* [formula translation (computer language)]} (computer science) {not an abbreviation}

"foss"
{pronunciation of *phos* [phosphate, phosphorus]} (chemistry and laboratory) {not an abbreviation}

Found
foundation

FOVI
field of vision intact (ophthalmology)

FP
false positive (laboratory)
family planning (gynecology and obstetrics)
family practice
family practitioner
fibrinopeptide (laboratory)
filter paper (laboratory)
flat paper
flat plate (radiology)
flavin phosphate [also called *riboflavine 5'-phosphate*] (laboratory)
flavoprotein (laboratory)
fluid pressure [spinal fluid pressure] (neurology and surgery)
food poisoning (gastroenterology)
freezing point (chemistry)
frontoparietal (neurology)
frozen plasma (hematology)
fundal pressure (gynecology and obstetrics)

F.P.
false positive (laboratory)
family planning (gynecology and obstetrics)

family practice
flat plate (radiology)
frozen plasma (hematology)

F-P
femoral-popliteal (cardiovascular)

Fp
filtered phosphate (laboratory)

F.p.
fiat potio [let a potion be made] (pharmacology)
freezing point (chemistry)

fp
fiat potio [let a potion be made] (pharmacology)
foot-pound (measurement)
forearm pronated (orthopedics)
freezing point (chemistry)

fp.
forearm pronated (orthopedics)
freezing point (chemistry)

f.p.
foot-pound (measurement)

FPA
Family Planning Association (gynecology and obstetrics)
fibrinopeptide A (laboratory)
filter paper activity (laboratory)
fluorophenylalanine (chemistry and laboratory)

F.P.A.
Family Planning Association (gynecology and obstetrics)

fpA
fibrinopeptide A (laboratory)

FPAL
full-term deliveries, premature [preterm] deliveries, abortions, and living children (gynecology and obstetrics)

F.P.A.L.
full-term deliveries, premature [preterm] deliveries, abortions, and living children (gynecology and obstetrics)

FPB
femoral-popliteal bypass [also called *femoropopliteal bypass*] (cardiovascular)
flexor pollicis brevis [muscle] (neurology and orthopedics)

FPC
Family Planning Clinic (gynecology and obstetrics)
Family Practitioner Committee
fish protein concentrate (pharmacology)

FPD
fetopelvic disproportion [also called *fetal-pelvic disproportion*] (obstetrics)
fixed partial denture (dentistry)

FPDVP
Frostig Program for the Development of Visual Perception (psychiatry and rehabilitation)

FPG
fasting plasma glucose (endocrinology and laboratory)
fluorescence plus Giemsa (laboratory)

FPH$_2$
flavin phosphate, reduced (laboratory)

FPHE
formalin-treated pyruvaldehyde-stabilized human erythrocytes (hematology and laboratory)

FPIA
fluorescence-polarization immunoassay (laboratory)

f pil
fiant pilulae [let pills be made] (pharmacology)

f. pil.
fiant pilulae [let pills be made] (pharmacology)

f pil xi
fac pilulas xi [make eleven pills] (pharmacology)

f. pil. xi
fac pilulas xi [make eleven pills] (pharmacology)

FPL
flexor pollicis longus [muscle] (neurology and orthopedics)

F(plasma)
plasma cortisol [also called *plasma F*] (laboratory)

FPM
filter paper microscopic [test] (laboratory)

fpm
feet per minute (measurement)

FPM test
filter paper microscopic test (laboratory)

FPNA
first-pass nuclear angiocardiography (cardiovascular and radiology)

FPO
freezing point osmometer (chemistry)

FPRA
first-pass radionuclide angiogram (cardiovascular and radiology)

F/P ratio
fluid/plasma ratio (laboratory)

FPS
Fellow of the Pathological Society (pathology)
Fellow of the Pharmaceutical Society (pharmacology)

fps
feet per second (measurement)
foot-pound-second (measurement)
frames per second (measurement)

FPSLST
Fluharty Preschool Speech and Language Screening Test (speech and language therapy)

FPT
fixed parenchymal turnover (laboratory and physiology)

FPV
fowl plague virus (infectious diseases, laboratory, and veterinary medicine)

FPVB
femoral-popliteal vein bypass [also called *femoropopliteal vein bypass*] (cardiovascular)

FPZ
fluphenazine (pharmacology)

FPZ-D
fluphenazine decanoate (pharmacology)

FR
failure rate [referring to conception] (gynecology and obstetrics)
fibrinogen-related (hematology and laboratory)
fibron-related (hematology and laboratory)
Fisher-Race [notation]
fixed ratio (laboratory)
flocculation reaction (laboratory)
flow rate (pharmacology)
fractional reabsorption (laboratory)

F.R.
flocculation reaction (laboratory)

F & R
force and rhythm [of pulse] (cardiovascular)

Fr
francium (chemistry)
franklin (measurement and physics)
French [catheter gauge, language, or nationality] (surgery and urology)

Fr.
French [catheter gauge] (surgery and urology)

fr
fracture (orthopedics)
from

FRA
fluorescent rabies antibody (infectious diseases and laboratory)

frac
fracture (orthopedics)

FRACDS
Fellow of the Royal Australasian College of Dental Surgery (dentistry)

FRACGP
Fellow of the Royal Australasian College of General Practitioners

FRACO
Fellow of the Royal Australasian College of Ophthalmologists (ophthalmology)

FRACP
Fellow of the Royal Australasian College of Physicians

FRACR
Fellow of the Royal Australasian College of Radiologists (radiology)

FRACS
Fellow of the Royal Australasian College of Surgeons (surgery)

Fract
fraction (laboratory and mathematics)
fracture (orthopedics)

fract.
fracture (orthopedics)

fract dos
fracta dosi [in divided doses] (pharmacology)

fract. dos.
fracta dosi [in divided doses] (pharmacology)

frag
fragment (laboratory)

frag.
fragility (laboratory)

FRAI
Fellow of the Royal Anthropological Institute (anthropology)

FRANZCP
Fellow of the Royal Australian and New Zealand College of Psychiatrists (psychiatry)

fra(X)
fragile X [chromosome] (genetics and laboratory)

Fr BB
fracture of both bones (orthopedics)

FRC
Federal Radiation Council (radiation therapy and radiology)
functional residual capacity (laboratory and respiratory)
frozen red cells (hematology)
functional reserve capacity (laboratory and respiratory)
functional residual capacity (laboratory and respiratory)

FRCD
Fellow of the Royal College of Dentists (dentistry)

FRCGP
Fellow of the Royal College of General Practitioners

FRCOG
Fellow of the Royal College of Obstetricians and Gynaecologists (gynecology and obstetrics)

FRCP
Fellow of the Royal College of Physicians

F.R.C.P.
Fellow of the Royal College of Physicians

FRCPA
Fellow of the Royal College of Pathologists, Australia (pathology)

FRCPath
Fellow of the Royal College of Pathologists (pathology)

FRCP(C)
Fellow of the Royal College of Physicians of Canada

F.R.C.P.(C.)
Fellow of the Royal College of Physicians of Canada

FRCPE
Fellow of the Royal College of Physicians of Edinburgh

F.R.C.P.E.
Fellow of the Royal College of Physicians of Edinburgh

FRCP(Glasg)
Fellow of the Royal College of Physi-
cians and Surgeons of Glasgow *qua*
Physician

F.R.C.P.(Glasg.)
Fellow of the Royal College of Physi-
cians and Surgeons of Glasgow *qua*
Physician

FRCPI
Fellow of the Royal College of Physicians of Ireland

F.R.C.P.I.
Fellow of the Royal College of Physicians of Ireland

FRCPsych
Fellow of the Royal College of Psychiatrists (psychiatry)

FRCS
Fellow of the Royal College of Surgeons
(surgery)

F.R.C.S.
Fellow of the Royal College of Surgeons
(surgery)

FRCS(C)
Fellow of the Royal College of Surgeons
of Canada (surgery)

F.R.C.S.(C.)
Fellow of the Royal College of Surgeons
of Canada (surgery)

F.R.C.S.E.
Fellow of the Royal College of Surgeons
of Edinburgh (surgery)

FRCSEd
Fellow of the Royal College of Surgeons
of Edinburgh (surgery)

FRCSEng
Fellow of the Royal College of Surgeons
of England (surgery)

FRCS(Glasg)
Fellow of the Royal College of Physi-
cians and Surgeons of Glasgow *qua*
Surgeon (surgery)

F.R.C.S.(Glasg.)
Fellow of the Royal College of Physi-
cians and Surgeons of Glasgow *qua*
Surgeon (surgery)

FRCSI
Fellow of the Royal College of Surgeons
in Ireland (surgery)

F.R.C.S.I.
Fellow of the Royal College of Surgeons
in Ireland (surgery)

FRCVS
Fellow of the Royal College of Veterinary Surgeons (veterinary medicine)

F.R.C.V.S.
Fellow of the Royal College of Veterinary Surgeons (veterinary medicine)

FREIR
Federal Research on Biological and
Health Effects of Ionizing Radiation
(biology, radiation therapy, radiology,
and research)

frem
fremitus vocalis [vocal fremitus] (oto-rhinolaryngology)

frem.
fremitus vocalis [vocal fremitus] (oto-rhinolaryngology)

"fren"
{pronunciation of *phren-* [prefix indicating relationship to the diaphragm or the mind]} (neurology and respiratory) {not an abbreviation}

freq
frequency
frequent

freq.
frequent

FRES
Fellow of the Royal Entomological Society (entomology)

FRF
Fertility Research Foundation (gynecology, obstetrics, and research)
follicle-stimulating hormone releasing factor (endocrinology and laboratory)

F.R.F.P.S.G.
Fellow of the Royal Faculty of Physicians and Surgeons of Glasgow

FRH
follicle-stimulating hormone-releasing hormone (endocrinology and laboratory)

frict
friction (physics)

frict.
friction (physics)

Fried test
Friedman test [for pregnancy] (laboratory and obstetrics)

frig
frigidus [cold]

frig.
frigidus [cold]

FRIPHH
Fellow of the Royal Institute of Public Health and Hygiene (public health)

FRJM
full range of joint movement (orthopedics)
full range of joint motion (orthopedics)
full range of joint movement (orthopedics)

FRM
full range of motion (orthopedics)

FRMedSoc
Fellow of the Royal Medical Society

FRMS
Fellow of the Royal Microscopical Society (laboratory)

FROM
full range of motion (orthopedics)
full range of movement (orthopedics)

FRP
functional refractory period (neurology)

FRS
Fellow of the Royal Society
ferredoxin-reducing substance (laboratory)
furosemide (pharmacology)

F.R.S.
Fellow of the Royal Society

FRSC
Fellow of the Royal Society of Chemistry (chemistry)

FRSE
Fellow of the Royal Society of Edinburgh

FRSH
Fellow of the Royal Society of Health

FRT
Family Relations Test (psychiatry)
full recovery time (rehabilitation)

fru
fructose (chemistry and dietary)

fru.
fructose (chemistry and dietary)

frust
frustillatim [in small pieces] (pharmacology)

frust.
frustillatim [in small pieces] (pharmacology)

FS
factor of safety
flexible sigmoidoscopy (gastroenterology)
forearm supinated (orthopedics)
fracture, simple (orthopedics)
frozen section (pathology and surgery)
full and soft [diet] (dietary and gastroenterology)
full-scale [intelligence quotient] (psychiatry)
function study (laboratory)

F.S.
frozen section (pathology and surgery)

fsa
fiat secundum artem [let it be made skillfully] (pharmacology)

f.s.a.
fiat secundum artem [let it be made skillfully] (pharmacology)

fsar
fiat secundum artem reglas [let it be made according to the rules of the art] (pharmacology)

FSB
fetal scalp blood (laboratory and obstetrics)
Fokes Sentence Builder (speech and language therapy)

FSBM
full-strength breast milk (neonatology)

FSBT
Fowler single breath test (respiratory)

FSC
Food Standards Committee [of the Ministry of Agriculture, Fisheries, and Food of the United Kingdom] (agriculture and dietary)
Forer Sentence Completion Test (psychiatry)
fracture, simple, comminuted (orthopedics)

FSD
focal skin distance (radiology)

FSE
fetal scalp electrode (obstetrics)

FSF
fibrin stabilizing factor [factor XIII] (hematology and laboratory)

FSG
focal and segmental glomerulosclerosis (nephrology)

FSGS
focal segmental glomerulosclerosis (nephrology)

FSH
facioscapulohumeral (neurology)
follicle-stimulating hormone (endocrinology and laboratory)

FSH-LH
follicle-stimulating hormone-luteinizing hormone (endocrinology and laboratory)

FSH/LH-RH
follicle-stimulating hormone and luteinizing hormone releasing hormone (endocrinology and laboratory)

FSHMD
facioscapulohumeral muscular dystrophy (neurology)

FSHRF
follicle-stimulating hormone releasing
factor (endocrinology and laboratory)

FSH-RF
follicle-stimulating hormone releasing
factor (endocrinology and laboratory)

FSHRH
follicle-stimulating hormone releasing
hormone (endocrinology and laboratory)

FSH-RH
follicle-stimulating hormone releasing
hormone (endocrinology and laboratory)

FSI
Food Sanitation Institute (dietary)

FSIA
foot shock-induced analgesia (neurology)

FSMB
Federation of State Medical Boards
(government)

F.S.M.B.
Federation of State Medical Boards
(government)

FSP
fibrin split products (hematology and
laboratory)
fibrinogen split products (hematology
and laboratory)
fibrinolytic split products (hematology
and laboratory)

FSR
Fellow of the Society of Radiographers
(radiology)
fusiform skin revision (plastic surgery)

FSR-3
isoniazid (pharmacology)

FSS
French steel sound [dilator] (surgery)

FST
foam stability test

FSU
family service unit (social services)

FSV
feline fibrosarcoma virus (laboratory,
oncology, research, and veterinary
medicine)

FSW
Field Service Worker (social services)

FT
false transmitter (neurology)
family therapy (psychiatry)
fibrous tissue (pathology)
follow through [after barium meal] (gastroenterology and radiology)
formal toxoid (chemistry)
Fourier transform (radiology)
free thyroxine (endocrinology and laboratory)
full term (obstetrics)
functional test (neurology)

FT₃
free triiodothyronine (endocrinology
and laboratory)

FT₄
free [unbound] thyroxine (endocrinology
and laboratory)

ft
fiant [let them be made] (pharmacology)
fiat [let it be made] (pharmacology)
foot (anatomy, measurement, orthopedics, and podiatry)

ft.
fac [make] (pharmacology)
feet (anatomy, measurement, orthopedics, and podiatry)
fiant [let them be made] (pharmacology)
fiat [let it be made] (pharmacology)

foot (anatomy, measurement, orthopedics, and podiatry)

FTA
fluorescent titer antibody (laboratory)
fluorescent treponemal antibody [test]
(laboratory)

FTA-ABS
fluorescent treponemal antibody-absorp-
tion [test] (laboratory)

FTAT
fluorescent treponemal antibody test
(laboratory)

FTBD
fit to be detained (psychiatry)
full-term born dead (obstetrics)

FTC
Federal Trade Commission (government)
frames to come (ophthalmology)

ft c
foot-candle (measurement)

ft.-c.
foot-candle (measurement)

ft cataplasm
fiat cataplasma [let a poultice be made]
(pharmacology)

ft cerat
fiat ceratum [let a cerate be made]
(pharmacology)

ft chart vi
fiant chartulae vi [let six powders be
made] (pharmacology)

ft collyr
fiat collyrium [let an eyewash be made]
(pharmacology)

ft. collyr.
fiat collyrium [let an eyewash be made]
(pharmacology)

FTD
failure to descend (obstetrics and urology)

femoral total density (orthopedics)

ft emuls
fiat emulsio [let an emulsion be made]
(pharmacology)

ft enem
fiat enema [let an injection (per rectum)
be made] (pharmacology)

FTF
finger-to-finger (neurology)
free thyroxine fraction (endocrinology
and laboratory)

FT₄F
serum free thyroxine fraction (endocrinology and laboratory)

FTG
full thickness graft (dermatology and
plastic surgery)

ft garg
fiat gargarisma [let a gargle be made]
(pharmacology)

ft. garg.
fiat gargarisma [let a gargle be made]
(pharmacology)

FTI
free thyroxine index (endocrinology and
laboratory)

F.T.I.
free thyroxine index (endocrinology and
laboratory)

FT₃ index
free triiodothyronine index (endocrinology and laboratory)

FT₄ index
free thyroxine index (endocrinology and
laboratory)

ft infus
fiat infusum [let an injection be made
(per urethra)] (pharmacology)

ftL
foot-lambert (measurement)

FTLB
full-term living birth (obstetrics)

ft lb
foot-pound (measurement)

ft-lb
foot-pound (measurement)

ft. lb.
foot-pound (measurement)

FTLFC
full-term living female child (obstetrics)

ft linim
fiat linimentum [let a liniment be made]
(pharmacology)

FTLMC
full-term living male child (obstetrics)

FTM
fluid thioglycolate medium (laboratory)
fractional test meal (laboratory and radiology)

ft mas
fiat massa [let a mass be made] (pharmacology)

ft. mas. div. in pil.
fiat massa dividenda in pilulae [let a
mass be made and divided into pills]
(pharmacology)

ft mas div in pil xiv
fiat massa et divide in pilulae xiv [let
fourteen pills be made] (pharmacology)

ft mist
fiat mistura [let a mixture be made]
(pharmacology)

FTN
finger-to-nose (neurology)
full-term nursery (neonatology)

FTND
full-term normal delivery (obstetrics)

F to N
finger-to-nose (neurology)

FTOR-MIM-BCG
Ftorafur, Adriamycin, cyclophosphamide, and bacille Calmette-Guérin
[BCG] (chemotherapy, oncology, and
pharmacology)

FTP
failure to progress [in labor] (obstetrics)

ft pil xxiv
fiat pilulae xxiv [let twenty-four pills be
made] (pharmacology)

ft pulv
fiat pulvis [let a powder be made]
(pharmacology)

ft. pulv.
fiat pulvis [let a powder be made]
(pharmacology)

FTR
for the record

FTSG
full thickness skin graft (dermatology
and plastic surgery)

F.T.S.G.
full thickness skin graft (dermatology
and plastic surgery)

ft solut
fiat solutio [let a solution be made]
(pharmacology)

ft. solut.
fiat solutio [let a solution be made]
(pharmacology)

ft suppos
fiat suppositorium [let a suppository be
made] (pharmacology)

FTT
failure to thrive (neonatology and pediatrics)
Fever Therapy Technician

fixed tissue turnover (laboratory and physiology)

FTU
Florida Technological University (education)
fluorescence thiourea (laboratory)

ft ung
fiat unguentum [let an ointment be made] (pharmacology)

FU
fecal urobilinogen (gastroenterology and laboratory)
fluorouracil (chemotherapy, oncology, and pharmacology)
follow-up
fractional urinalysis (laboratory)

F & U
flanks and upper quadrants (anatomy)

F/U
follow-up
fundus at umbilicus (obstetrics)

F↑U
finger above umbilicus

F↓U
finger below umbilicus

5FU
5-fluorouracil (chemotherapy, oncology, and pharmacology)

5-FU
5-fluorouracil (chemotherapy, oncology, and pharmacology)

Fu
Finsen unit [for ultraviolet rays] (measurement)

FUB
functional uterine bleeding (gynecology)

FU$_{CO}$
functional uptake of carbon monoxide (laboratory and respiratory)

FUDR
floxuridine [also called *fluorode-oxyuridine, 2-fluoro-2'-deoxyuridine* and *5-fluro-2'-deoxy-β-uridine*] (chemotherapy, oncology, and pharmacology) {not an abbreviation} [trade name for *floxuridine*; also called *2-fluoro-2'-deoxyuridine*] (chemotherapy, oncology, and pharmacology)

5-FUDR
5-fluoro-2'-deoxyuridine (chemotherapy, oncology, and pharmacology)

FUdR
floxuridine [also called *fluorode-oxyuridine, 2-fluoro-2'-deoxyuridine* and *5-fluro-2'-deoxy-β-uridine*] (chemotherapy, oncology, and pharmacology)

FUE
fever of undetermined etiology

fulg
fulguration (surgery)

FUM
5-fluorouracil and methotrexate (chemotherapy, oncology, and pharmacology)
fumarate (laboratory)
fumigate
fumigation

FUN
follow-up note (medical records)

func
function

funct
function(al)

FUO
fever of undetermined origin
fever of unknown origin

F.U.O.
fever of undetermined origin
fever of unknown origin

FUR
fluorouracil riboside (chemotherapy, oncology, and pharmacology)

5-FUR
5-fluorouridine (chemotherapy, oncology, and pharmacology)

FURAM
Ftorafur, Adriamycin, and mitomycin-C
(chemotherapy, oncology, and pharmacology)

"fur-ing-go"
{pronunciation of *pharyngo-* [prefix indicating relationship to the pharynx]}
(otorhinolaryngology) {not an abbrevi-
ation}

FV
fluid volume (measurement)
Friend virus (laboratory)

F-V
flow volume (cardiovascular and measurement)

FVC
forced vital capacity (laboratory and
respiratory)

FVC.5
forced vital capacity in one-half second
(laboratory and respiratory)

FVH
focal vascular headache (cardiovascular
and neurology)

FVL
femoral vein ligation (cardiovascular)
flow volume loop

FVR
feline viral rhinotracheitis (laboratory
and veterinary medicine)
forearm vascular resistance (cardiovascular)

F. vs.
fiat venaesectio [let the patient be bled]
(hematology)

f vs
fiat venaesectio [let the patient be bled]
(hematology)

f. vs.
fiat venaesectio [let the patient be bled]
(hematology)

FW
Felix-Weil [reaction or test] (infectious
diseases and laboratory)
Folin and Wu's [method] (laboratory)
forced whisper (otorhinolaryngology)
fragment wound (emergency medicine)

fw
fresh water

FWA
Family Welfare Association (social services)

FWB
full weight bearing (orthopedics and podiatry)

FWHM
full-width half-maximum [tomography]
(radiology)

FWPCA
Federal Water Pollution Control Administration (ecology and government)

FWR
Felix-Weil reaction (infectious diseases
and laboratory)

FWS
Fish and Wildlife Service (government)

FWW
front wheel walker (rehabilitation)

Fx
fractional urine (laboratory)
fracture (orthopedics)

fx
fracture (orthopedics)

fx.
fractional
fracture (orthopedics)
frozen section (pathology and surgery)

Fx-dis
fracture-dislocation (orthopedics)

FXN
function

FXR
fracture (orthopedics)

fx. urine
fractional urine (laboratory)

FY
fiscal year
full year

FYA
Duffy A positive [blood type] (hematology and laboratory)

FYAN
Duffy A negative [blood type] (hematology and laboratory)

FYB
Duffy B positive [blood type] (hematology and laboratory)

FYBN
Duffy B negative [blood type] (hematology and laboratory)

FYI
for your information

F-Y test
fibrinogen qualitative test (hematology and laboratory)

FZ
focal zone

FZRC
frozen red blood cells (hematology and laboratory)

FZS
Fellow of the Zoological Society (zoology)

G

Γ
gamma [third letter of the Greek alphabet]

γ
gamma [third letter of the Greek alphabet]
0.00001 gauss (measurement)
microgram (measurement)
{not an abbreviation} [an immunoglobulin] (laboratory)

G
conductance (neurology and physics)
force [pull of gravity] (physics)
gallop (cardiovascular)
gap [in cell cycle] (laboratory)
gas (anesthesiology and chemistry)
gastrin (laboratory)
gauge (measurement)
gauss (measurement)
Gibbs' free energy theory (physics)
giga- [prefix for 10^9] (measurement) {not an abbreviation}
gingival (dentistry)
globular [referring to proteins] (laboratory)
globulin (laboratory)
glucose (endocrinology, laboratory, and pharmacology)
glycine (dietary, gastroenterology, laboratory, neurology, and pharmacology)
glycogen (gastroenterology and laboratory)
goat (veterinary medicine)
gold inlay (dentistry)
gonidial [colony] (laboratory)
good
Grafenberg spot (gynecology)
gram (measurement)
gravida (gynecology and obstetrics)
gravitational constant [also called *Newtonian constant*] (physics)
Greek [language or nationality]
green
gross [leukemia antigen] (hematology, laboratory, and oncology)

guanidine (chemistry)
guanine (chemistry)
guanosine (chemistry and research)
{not an abbreviation} [an immunoglobulin] (laboratory)
{not an abbreviation} [an unit of force of acceleration] (aviation medicine and physics)
{not an abbreviation} [an unit of force of gravity on earth's surface] (physics)

G.
gingival (dentistry)
glucose (endocrinology, laboratory, and pharmacology)
gonidial [colony] (laboratory)
gram (measurement)

GΩ
gigaohm (measurement)

γG
gamma G immunoglobulin (laboratory)
immunoglobulin G (laboratory)

G1
grade one

G2
grade two

2G%
two grams percent [meaning *two grams per deciliter* or *4+*] (laboratory)

G3
grade three

G4
grade four

g
gender (gynecology, obstetrics, and urology)
giga- [prefix for 10^9] (measurement) {not an abbreviation}
gram(s) (measurement)
gravida (gynecology and obstetrics)
gravity (physics)
gravity [unit of force exerted on body during acceleration] (physics) {pronounced "geez"}
group
{not an abbreviation} [unit of force exerted upon body during acceleration and deceleration] (aeronautics)

g.
gram(s) (measurement)

g%
gram percent [meaning *grams per deciliter*] (laboratory and measurement)

μg
microgram (measurement)

μμg
micromicrogram [picogram] (measurement)

GA
gastric analysis (gastroenterology and laboratory)
general anesthesia (anesthesiology)
general appearance [on physical examination]
Georgia [Postal Service state designation]
gentisic acid (laboratory)
gestational age (obstetrics)
gingivoaxial (dentistry)
glucose/acetone (laboratory)
glucuronic acid (chemistry)
gramicidin A [an antibiotic] (pharmacology)
guessed average
gut-associated (gastroenterology)

G.A.
gastric analysis (gastroenterology and laboratory)

Ga
airway conductance (respiratory)

gallium (chemistry, pharmacology, and radiology)
granulocyte agglutination (laboratory)

ga
gauge [of needles] (measurement)

GABA
gamma-aminobutyric acid (laboratory and neurology)

GABHS
group A beta-hemolytic streptococcus (laboratory)

GAD
glutamic acid decarboxylase (laboratory)

GADH
gastric alcohol dehydrogenase (laboratory)

GADS
gonococcal arthritis/dermatitis syndrome (dermatology, gynecology, infectious diseases, orthopedics, and urology)

GAG
glycosaminoglycan [used in artificial skin] (chemistry and dermatology)

GAL
galactosyl (laboratory)

gal
galactose (laboratory)
gallon (measurement)

gal.
galactose (laboratory)
gallon (measurement)

G-ALB
globulin-albumin (laboratory)

gal-1-P
galactose-1-phosphate (laboratory)

GALT
gut-associated lymphoid tissue (gastroenterology and laboratory) {pro-
nounced "galt"}

"galt"
{pronunciation of *GALT* [gut-associated
lymphoid tissue]} (gastroenterology
and laboratory) {not an abbreviation}

GaLV
gibbon ape lymphosarcoma virus (laboratory)

Galv.
galvanic (electricity)

galv
galvanic (electricity)

galv.
galvanic (electricity)

gamma HCD
gamma heavy chain disease [protein]
(laboratory)

gang
ganglion (neurology and orthopedics)

gangl
ganglion(ic) (neurology and orthopedics)

ganglioside GM$_1$
{not an abbreviation} [a ganglioside with
addition of an *N*-acetyl galactosamine
and a galactose group] (laboratory)

ganglioside GM$_2$
{not an abbreviation} [a ganglioside with
addition of an *N*-acetyl galactosamine
at the terminal] (laboratory)

GAP
Group for the Advancement of Psychiatry (psychiatry)

GAPD
glyceraldehyde-phosphate dehydrogenase (laboratory)

GAPDH
glyceraldehyde-phosphate dehydrogenase (laboratory)

Garg.
gargarismus [gargle] (pharmacology)

garg
gargarismus [gargle] (pharmacology)

garg.
gargarismus [gargle] (pharmacology)

GARP
Global Atmospheric Research Program
(ecology and research)

GAS
gastroenterology
general adaptation syndrome (psychiatry)
generalized arteriosclerosis (cardiovascular)
Global Assessment Score (psychiatry)
{pronounced "gas"}

"gas"
{pronunciation of *GAS* [Global Assessment Score]} (psychiatry) {not an ab-
breviation}

GAST
gastric (gastroenterology)

GASTRN
gastrin (gastroenterology and laboratory)

Gastro
gastroenterology {pronounced "gas-tro"}
gastrointestinal (gastroenterology) {pro-
nounced "gas-tro"}

gastro
gastroenterology {pronounced "gas-tro"}
gastrointestinal (gastroenterology) {pro-
nounced "gas-tro"}

"gas-tro"
{pronunciation of *Gastro* and *gastro*
[gastroenterology and gastrointes-

tinal]} (gastroenterology) {not an abbreviation}

Gastroc
gastrocnemius [muscle] (neurology and orthopedics) {pronounced "gas-trok"}

gastroc
gastrocnemius [muscle] (neurology and orthopedics) {pronounced "gas-trok"}

"gas-trok"
{pronunciation of *Gastroc* and *gastroc* [gastrocnemius (muscle)]} (neurology and orthopedics) {not an abbreviation}

GAT
group adjustment therapy (psychiatry)

GAW
airway conductance [the reciprocal of airway resistance] (laboratory and respiratory)

Gaw
airway conductance [the reciprocal of airway resistance] (laboratory and respiratory)

Gaw/V$_1$
specific conductance [expressed per liter of lung volume at which G is measured] (laboratory and respiratory)

GB
gallbladder (gastroenterology)
goofball [barbiturate pill] (pharmacology) {slang}
Guillain-Barré [syndrome] (neurology)

G.B.
gallbladder (gastroenterology and surgery)

GBA
ganglionic-blocking agent (neurology and pharmacology)
gingivobuccoaxial (dentistry)

GBBHS
group B beta-hemolytic streptococcus (laboratory)

GBD
gallbladder disease (gastroenterology)

GBG
gonadal steroid-binding globulin (endocrinology and laboratory)

GBH
gamma-benzene hydrochloride [also called *lindane*; an insecticide] (chemistry)
graphite-benzalkonium-heparin (chemistry)

GBIA
Guthrie bacterial inhibition assay (laboratory)

GBL
glomerular basal lamina (nephrology and urology)

GBM
glomerular basement membrane (nephrology and urology)

GBP
galactose-binding protein (laboratory)
gastric bypass (gastroenterology and surgery)

GBS
gallbladder series (gastroenterology and radiology)
glycerine-buffered saline (chemistry and pharmacology)
group B beta-hemolytic streptococcus (laboratory)
Guillain-Barré syndrome (neurology)

GBSS
Gey's balanced salt solution (pharmacology)

GC
ganglion cells (laboratory and neurology)
gas chromatography (laboratory)
geriatric care (geriatrics)
geriatric chair [Gerichair] (geriatrics)

glucocorticoid (endocrinology and laboratory)

gonococcal [infection] (laboratory)

gonococcus [Incorrectly used to mean *gonorrhea*.] (gynecology, infectious diseases, laboratory, and urology)

granular cysts (pathology)

granulocyte cytotoxic (laboratory)

guanine cytosine (laboratory)

G-C
gram-negative cocci (laboratory)

G+C
gram-positive cocci (laboratory)

Gc
gonococcus [Incorrectly used to mean *gonorrhea*.] (gynecology, infectious diseases, laboratory, and urology)

group-specific component

GCA
giant cell arteritis (rheumatology)

g-cal
gram-calorie [also called *small calorie*] (dietary)

g-cal.
gram-calorie [also called *small calorie*] (dietary)

GCDFP
gross cystic disease fluid protein (laboratory)

G.C.F.
greatest common factor

GCFT
gonorrhea complement-fixation test (laboratory)

GCIIS
glucose control insulin infusion system (endocrinology and pharmacology)

g-cm.
gram-centimeter (measurement)

GC-MS
gas chromatography–mass spectrometry (laboratory)

GCN
giant cerebral neuron (laboratory and neurology)

GCS
general clinical service
Glasgow Coma Scale (neurology)

Gc/s
gigacycles per second (measurement)

GCT
giant cell tumor (oncology)

GC type
guanine, cytosine type (chemistry)

GCWM
General Conference on Weights and Measures (measurement)

G.C.W.M.
General Conference on Weights and Measures (measurement)

GD
general dispensary (pharmacology)
gonadal dysgenesis (endocrinology and urology)
Graves' disease (endocrinology)

G & D
growth and development (pediatrics)

Gd
gadolinium (chemistry)

GDA
germine diacetate (chemistry)

GDB
Guide Dogs for the Blind (ophthalmology and veterinary medicine)

GDC
General Dental Council [British] (dentistry)

GDD
gay disaster disease [also called *ac-*

quired immunodeficiency syndrome (AIDS)] (immunology)

GDH
glutamic acid dehydrogenase (laboratory)
glycerophosphate dehydrogenase (laboratory)
growth and differential hormone [in insects] (entomology)

GDM
gestational diabetes mellitus (endocrinology and obstetrics)

GDMO
General Duties Medical Officer (armed forces)

GDP
gel diffusion precipitin (laboratory)
guanosine diphosphate (chemistry)

GDS
Gesell Developmental Schedules (psychiatry and speech and language therapy)
gradual dosage schedule (pharmacology)

GE
gastroemotional (gastroenterology)
gastroenteritis (gastroenterology)
gastroenterology
gastroesophageal (gastroenterology)
gastroenterostomy (gastroenterology)
gel electrophoresis (laboratory)
gentamicin [an antibiotic] (pharmacology)
General Electric [corporation] (manufacturing)

G/E
granulocyte-erythroid [ratio] (laboratory)

G-E
gastroenteritis (gastroenterology)

Ge
germanium (chemistry)

g-e
gravity eliminated

GECC
Government Employees' Clinic Centre [British] (government)

GEE
glycine ethyl ester (laboratory)

"gee-for-saz"
{pronunciation of *G-forces* [acceleration forces]} (aviation medicine) {not an abbreviation}

"gee-I-seer-eez"
{pronunciation of *GI series* [gastrointestinal series]} (gastroenterology and radiology) {not an abbreviation}

"geez"
{pronunciation of *g* [gravity; unit of force exerted on body during acceleration]} (physics) {not an abbreviation}

GEF
gonadotropin-enhancing factor (laboratory)

GEJ
gastroesophageal junction (gastroenterology)

gel
gelatin(ous) (laboratory)

gel.
gelatin(ous) (laboratory)

Gel. quav.
gelatina quavis [in any kind of jelly] (pharmacology)

gel quav
gelatina quavis [in any kind of jelly] (pharmacology)

gel. quav.
gelatina quavis [in any kind of jelly] (pharmacology)

GEMS
good emergency mother substitute (pediatrics)

GEN
gender (gynecology, psychiatry, and urology)
generation
genetics
genital (gynecology and urology)

Gen
genealogy
general
generic
genetics

gen.
general
genus

genet
genetics

gen et sp nov
genus et species nova [new genus and species]

gen. et sp. nov.
genus et species nova [new genus and species]

genit
genitalia (gynecology and urology)

gen'l
general

gen nov
genus novum [new genus]

gen. nov.
genus novum [new genus]

GENP
gentamicin peak [level] (laboratory)

gen proc
general procedure

GENT
gentamicin [an antibiotic] (pharmacology) {pronounced "jent"}
gentamicin trough [level] (laboratory)

gentleman {pronounced "jent"}

gent
gentamicin [an antibiotic] (pharmacology) {pronounced "jent"}
gentleman {pronounced "jent"}

GEP
gastroenteropancreatic (gastroenterology)

GER
gastroesophageal reflux (gastroenterology)

Ger
geriatrics
German [language or nationality]

ger.
geriatrics

GERD
gastroesophageal reflux disease (gastroenterology)

geri
geriatrics

Geriat
geriatrics

GERL
Golgi-associated endoplasmic reticulum lysosomes (laboratory)

Gerontol
gerontologist (geriatrics)
gerontology (geriatrics)

GES
glucose electrolyte solution (pharmacology)

GEST
gestation(al) (obstetrics)

GET
gastric emptying time (gastroenterology)

GET½
gastric emptying half-time (gastroenterology)

GETA
general endotracheal anesthesia (anesthesiology)

GeV
giga electron volt [1,000 GeV equal 1 TeV] (electricity and measurement)

GF
gastric fistula (gastroenterology)
gastric fluid (gastroenterology)
germ-free
glass factor [tissue culture] (laboratory)
glomerular filtrate (nephrology)
gluten-free (dietary)
government-funded (government)
grandfather
growth factor (endocrinology and laboratory)
growth fraction

G-F
globular-fibrous [referring to proteins] (laboratory)

gf
gram-force (measurement)

GFAP
glial fibrillary acidic protein (laboratory)

GFD
gluten-free diet (dietary)
Goodenough Figure Drawing (psychiatry)

G-forces
acceleration forces (aviation medicine) {pronounced "gee-for-saz"}

GFR
glomerular filtration rate (laboratory, nephrology, and urology)

G.F.R.
glomerular filtration rate (laboratory, nephrology, and urology)

GFTA
Goldman-Fristoe Test of Articulation (speech and language therapy)

GG
gamma-globulin (laboratory and pharmacology)
glycylglycine (chemistry)
guaifenesin [an expectorant] (otorhinolaryngology, pharmacology, and respiratory)

GGA
general gonadotropic activity (endocrinology and laboratory)

GGE
general gland enlargement (endocrinology)
generalized glandular enlargement (endocrinology)

GGG
gummi guttae gambiae [gamboge] (pharmacology)

G.G.G.
gummi guttae gambiae [gamboge] (pharmacology)

GG or S
glands, goiter, or stiffness (endocrinology)

GGT
gamma-glutamyl transpeptidase [also called *γ-glutamyltransferase*] (laboratory)

GGTP
gamma-glutamyl transpeptidase [also called *γ-glutamyltransferase*] (laboratory)

GH
general hospital
glenohumeral [joint] (orthopedics)
growth [somatotropic] hormone [of anterior pituitary] (endocrinology, laboratory, and pharmacology)

GHA
glucoheptanoic acid (laboratory)

GHAA
Group Health Association of America

G.H.A.A.
Group Health Association of America

GHB
gamma-hydroxybutyrate (laboratory)

GHb
glycosylated hemoglobin (laboratory)

GHD
growth hormone deficiency (endocrinology)

GHDT
Goodenough-Harris Drawing Test (psychiatry)

GH joint
glenohumeral joint (orthopedics)

GHQ
general health questionnaire

GHRF
growth hormone-releasing factor (endocrinology and laboratory)

GH-RF
growth hormone-releasing factor (endocrinology and laboratory)

GHRH
growth hormone releasing hormone (endocrinology and laboratory)

GH-RH
growth hormone releasing hormone (endocrinology and laboratory)

GHRIH
growth hormone release-inhibiting hormone (endocrinology and laboratory)

GH-RIH
growth hormone release-inhibiting hormone (endocrinology and laboratory)

GHz
gigahertz (electricity and measurement)

GI
gastroenterology
gastrointestinal (gastroenterology)
gelatin infusion [medium] (laboratory)
General Infantry [soldier] (armed forces)
globulin insulin (endocrinology and pharmacology)
granuloma inguinale (endocrinology, gynecology, infectious diseases, and urology)
gravida I (gynecology and obstetrics)
growth-inhibiting (endocrinology and laboratory)

G.I.
gastrointestinal (gastroenterology)
globulin insulin (endocrinology and pharmacology)

gi
gill (oceanography)

GIA
gastrointestinal anastomosis (gastroenterology and surgery)
{not an abbreviation} [a stapling device used for gastrointestinal anastomoses] (gastroenterology and surgery)

GIB
gastric ileal bypass [also called *gastroileal bypass*] (gastroenterology and surgery)

GIC
general immunocompetence (immunology)

GIF
growth hormone inhibiting factor (endocrinology and laboratory)

GIFT
gamete intrafallopian transfer (obstetrics) {pronounced "gift"}

"gift"
{pronunciation of *GIFT* [gamete intrafal-

lopian transfer]} (obstetrics) {not an abbreviation}

giga-
{not an abbreviation} [prefix for 10^9] (measurement) {pronounced "gig-ah"}

"gig-ah"
{pronunciation of *giga-* [prefix for 10^9]} (measurement) {not an abbreviation}

GIGO
garbage in, garbage out (computer science)

GIH
gastrointestinal hormone (gastroenterology and laboratory)
growth-inhibiting hormone (endocrinology and laboratory)

GII
gastrointestinal infection (gastroenterology)
gravida two (gynecology and obstetrics)

GIII
gravida three (gynecology and obstetrics)

GIK
glucose, insulin, and potassium [solution] (endocrinology and pharmacology)

GIM
gonadotropin-inhibitory material (laboratory)

ging
gingiva [gum] (dentistry)

ging.
gingiva [gum] (dentistry)

g-ion
gram-ion (measurement and physics)

GIP
gastric inhibitory peptide (gastroenterology and laboratory)
gastric inhibitory polypeptide (gastroenterology and laboratory)

giant cell interstitial pneumonia (respiratory)

GIS
gas in stomach (gastroenterology)
gastrointestinal series (gastroenterology and radiology)
gastrointestinal system (gastroenterology)

GI series
gastrointestinal series (gastroenterology and radiology) {pronounced "gee-I-seer-eez"}

GIT
gastrointestinal tract (gastroenterology)
glutathione-insulin transhydrogenase (laboratory)

GITS
gastrointestinal therapeutic system (gastroenterology)

GITSG
Gastrointestinal Tumor Study Group (gastroenterology and oncology)

GITT
glucose-insulin tolerance test (endocrinology and laboratory)

giv
given

GIVN
given

GIX
{not an abbreviation} [trademark for an insecticidal compound (difluorodiphenyltrichloroethane)] (chemistry)

GJ
gap junctions (cardiovascular and neurology)
gastrojejunostomy (gastroenterology and surgery)

GK
glycerol kinase (laboratory)

Gk
Greek [language or nationality]

GKMDT
Graham-Kendall Memory for Designs
Test (psychiatry and speech and lan-
guage therapy)

GL
glycosphingolipid (laboratory)
greatest length [referring to embryo]
(obstetrics)

Gl
glucinium [also called *beryllium*] (chemistry)

gl
gill (oceanography)
glandula(e) [gland(s)] (endocrinology)

gl.
gill (oceanography)
glandula(e) [gland(s)] (endocrinology)

g/l
grams per liter (measurement)

GLA
gingivolinguoaxial (dentistry)

glac
glacial (chemistry)

gland
glandula [gland] (endocrinology)
glandular (endocrinology)

gland.
glandula [gland] (endocrinology)
glandular (endocrinology)

GLC
gas-liquid chromatography (laboratory)

glc
glaucoma (ophthalmology)

GlcA
gluconic acid (laboratory)

GLI
glicentin [new name for *enteroglucagon*;

also called *intestinal glucagon*] (gastroenterology and laboratory)
glucagon-like immunoreactivity (laboratory)

glio
glioma (neurology)

Gln
glutamine (laboratory)

GLO
glyoxalase I [also called *lactoylgluta-
thione lyase*] (laboratory)

GLOB
globulin (laboratory)

Glob
globular (laboratory)
globulin (laboratory)

glob
globulin (laboratory)

glob.
globulin (laboratory)

globulin X
{not an abbreviation} (laboratory)

GLP
group-living program

GL-PP
postprandial glucose (endocrinology and
laboratory)

Gltn
glomerulotubulonephritis (nephrology)

GLU
glucose (laboratory and pharmacology)

GLU 5
five-hour glucose tolerance test (endocrinology and laboratory)

Glu
glucose (laboratory and pharmacology)
glutamic acid (laboratory)
glutamine (laboratory)

glu
glucose (laboratory and pharmacology)
glutamic acid (laboratory)
glutamine (laboratory)

glu.
glucose (laboratory and pharmacology)

gluc.
glucose (laboratory and pharmacology)

GLUC-S
urine glucose spot [test] (endocrinology and laboratory)

GLUTAM
glutamine (laboratory)

Gly
glycerol (laboratory)
glycine (laboratory)

gly
glycerol (laboratory)
glycine (laboratory)

glyc
glycerin (laboratory)
glyceritum [glycerite] (laboratory)

glyc.
glycerin (laboratory)
glyceritum [glycerite] (laboratory)

GM
gamma [third letter of the Greek alphabet]
gastric mucosa (gastroenterology)
Geiger-Müller [counter] (chemistry)
general medical
general medicine
geometric mean (mathematics)
gram (measurement)
grand mal [seizure] (neurology)
grandmother
grand multiparity (gynecology and obstetrics)
monosialoganglioside [a genetic marker] (genetics and laboratory)

Gm
gamma [third letter of the Greek alphabet]
gram (measurement)

Gm%
gram percent [meaning *grams per deciliter*] (measurement)

gm
gram (measurement)

gm.
gram(s) (measurement)

g-m
gram-meter (measurement)

g/m
gallons per minute (measurement)

GMA
glyceryl methacrylate (chemistry)

GMC
General Medical Council [British]
grivet monkey cell [line] (laboratory)

G.M.C.
General Medical Council [British]
General Motors Corporation (manufacturing)

GM₁ gangliosidosis
{not an abbreviation} [also called *generalized gangliosidosis*] (genetics)

GM₂ gangliosidosis
{not an abbreviation} [also called *Tay-Sachs disease*] (genetics)

GMK
green monkey kidney [cells] (laboratory)
{not an abbreviation} [a preparation used as a virus culture system] (laboratory)
{not an abbreviation} [a green monkey kidney preparation] (laboratory)

gm/l
grams per liter (measurement)

gm-m
gram-meter (measurement)

gm-m.
gram-meter (measurement)

g-mol
gram-molecule (measurement)

g-mol.
gram-molecule (measurement)

GMP
guanosine monophosphate [also called *guanosine-5-phosphate* and *guanylic acid*] (laboratory)

G-MP
G-myeloma proteins (laboratory)

GMS
General Medical Services
Gomori's methenamine silver [stain] (laboratory)

G.M.S.
General Medical Services

GM & S
general medical and surgical
general medicine and surgery

GMSC
General Medical Services Committee [British]

GMT
geometric mean titer (laboratory)
Greenwich Mean Time (time measurement)

GMTs
geometric mean titers (laboratory)

GMV
gram-molecular volume (chemistry)

GMW
gram-molecular weight (chemistry)

GN
glomerulonephritis (nephrology)
Graduate Nurse (nursing)
gram-negative (laboratory)

G.N.
Graduate Nurse (nursing)

G/N
glucose-nitrogen [ratio in urine examinations] (laboratory)

Gn
gonadotropin (endocrinology and laboratory)

Gn.
gonadotropin (endocrinology and laboratory)

GNB
gram-negative bacilli (laboratory)

GNBM
gram-negative bacillary meningitis (laboratory and neurology)

GNC
general nursing care (nursing)
General Nursing Council (nursing)

G.N.C.
General Nursing Council (nursing)

GNID
gram-negative intracellular diplococci (laboratory)

GNP
Gerontological Nurse Practitioner (geriatrics and nursing)

GnRF
gonadotropin-releasing factor (endocrinology and laboratory)

GnRH
gonadotropin-releasing hormone (endocrinology and laboratory)

Gn-RH
gonadotropin-releasing hormone (endocrinology and laboratory)

GNTP
Graduate Nurse Transition Program (nursing)

GO
glucose oxidase (laboratory)

G & O
gas and oxygen (anesthesiology)

g.o.
glucose oxidase (laboratory)

GOE
gas, oxygen, and ether (anesthesiology)

GOG
Gynecologic Oncology Group [of National Cancer Institute] (gynecology and oncology)

GOK
God only knows [slang]

G.O.K.
God only knows [slang]

GOM
God's own medicine [slang]

Gonio
goniometric (physical therapy)

GOO
gastric outlet obstruction (gastroenterology)

GOR
general operating room (surgery)

GORT
Gilmore Oral Reading Test (psychiatry and speech therapy)
Gray Oral Reading Test (psychiatry and speech therapy)

GOT
aspartate aminotransferase (laboratory)
glucose oxidase test (laboratory)
glutamic-oxaloacetic transaminase (laboratory)
glutamine-oxaloacetic transaminase (laboratory)

Gov
government(al)

GP
general paralysis (neurology)
general paresis (neurology)
general practice [a medical specialty]
general practitioner
genetic prediabetes (endocrinology and genetics)
geometric progression (mathematics)
globus pallidus (anatomy and neurology)
glucose phosphate (laboratory)
glutathione peroxidase (laboratory)
glycoprotein (laboratory)
Goodpasture [syndrome] (nephrology and respiratory)
gram-positive (laboratory)
group
guinea pig (research)
gutta-percha (chemistry, dentistry, orthopedics, and surgery)

G.P.
general paresis (neurology)
general practice [a medical specialty]
general practitioner

G/P
gravida/para (gynecology and obstetrics)

G-1-P
glucose-1-phosphate (laboratory)

G3P
glyceraldehyde-3-phosphate (laboratory)

G-3-P
glyceraldehyde-3-phosphate (laboratory)

G_4P_{3104}
four pregnancies [gravid], 3 went to term, one premature, no abortion [or miscarriage], and 4 living children [para] [*This is a sample for format purposes. Other numbers may be used.*] (gynecology and obstetrics)

G-6-P
glucose-6-phosphate (laboratory)

gp
group

gp.
group

GPA
grade point average (education)
gravida, para, and abortus [*When each
letter is followed by a numeral, they
indicate the number of pregnancies,
deliveries, and abortions, respectively.*] (gynecology and obstetrics)
Group Practice Association
guinea pig albumin (research)

g-p-ab
gravida, para, and abortus [*When letters
are followed by numerals, they indicate the number of pregnancies, deliveries, and abortions, respectively.*]
(gynecology and obstetrics)

GPAIS
guinea pig anti-insulin serum (laboratory)

G-6-Pase
glucose-6-phosphatase (laboratory)

GPB
glossopharyngeal breathing (respiratory)

GPBP
guinea pig myelin basic protein (research)

GPC
gastric parietal cell (laboratory)
giant papillary conjunctivitis (ophthalmology)
glycerylphosphorylcholine (chemistry)
gram-positive cocci (laboratory)

GPD
glucose-6-phosphate dehydrogenase
(laboratory)

G3PD
glyceraldehyde-3-phosphate dehydrogenase (laboratory)

G-3-PD
glyceraldehyde-3-phosphate dehydrogenase (laboratory)

G6PD
glucose-6-phosphate dehydrogenase
(laboratory)

G-6-PD
glucose-6-phosphate dehydrogenase
(laboratory)

G-6-PDH
glucose-6-phosphate dehydrogenase
(laboratory)

G-6-PDHA
glucose-6-phosphate dehydrogenase enzyme variant A (laboratory)

GPE
glycerylphosphorylethanolamine (laboratory)

GPF
granulocytosis-promoting factor (hematology and laboratory)

GPGG
guinea pig gamma-globulin (research)

GPh
Graduate in Pharmacy (education and
pharmacology)

GPI
general paralysis of the insane (neurology and psychiatry)
glucose, potassium, and insulin [for-
merly used to reverse myocardial in-
farctions] (cardiovascular and pharmacology) {obsolete}
glucosephosphate isomerase (chemistry)

G.P.I.
general paralysis of the insane (neurology and psychiatry)

GPIMH
guinea pig intestinal mucosal homoge-
nate (laboratory)

GPIPID
guinea pig intraperitoneal infectious
dose (laboratory)

GPK
guinea pig kidney [antigen] (laboratory)

GPKA
guinea pig kidney absorption [test] (laboratory)

Gply
gingivoplasty (dentistry and otorhinolaryngology)

GPM
general preventive medicine

GPMAL
gravida, para, multiple births, abortions,
and live births (gynecology and obstetrics)

GPN
Graduate Practical Nurse (nursing)

GPPQ
General Purpose Psychiatric Questionnaire (psychiatry)

GPRA
General Practice Reform Association

GPS
Goodpasture's syndrome (nephrology
and respiratory)
guinea pig serum (laboratory and research)

GPT
glutamate pyruvate transaminase (laboratory)
glutamic pyruvic transaminase (laboratory)

GpTh
group therapy (psychiatry)

GPU
guinea pig unit (laboratory and research)

GPUT
galactose phosphate uridyl transferase
(laboratory)

GR
gamma ray (radiology)
gastric resection (gastroenterology and
surgery)
general research (research)
glutathione reductase (laboratory)
grain(s) (measurement)

G-R
gram-negative rods (laboratory)

G+R
gram-positive rods (laboratory)

Gr
grain (measurement)
gravida (obstetrics)

gr
gamma roentgen (radiology)
grain(s) (measurement)
gravity (physics)
gray [unit] (radiation therapy and radiology)

gr.
gamma roentgen (radiology)
grain(s) (measurement)
gravity (physics)

gr−
gram-negative [bacteria] (laboratory)

gr+
gram-positive [bacteria] (laboratory)

GRA
gonadotropin-releasing agent (endocrinology and laboratory)

Grad.
gradatim [by degrees, gradually]
gradient
graduate (education)

grad
gradient
graduate(d) (education)

grad.
gradatim [by degrees, gradually]
gradient
graduate (education)

GRAE
generally regarded as effective (pharmacology)

gram-neg
gram-negative (laboratory) {pronounced "gram-neg"}

"gram-neg"
{pronunciation of *gram-neg* [gram-negative]} (laboratory) {not an abbreviation}

"gram-pause"
{pronunciation of *gram-pos* [gram-positive]} (laboratory) {not an abbreviation}

gram-pos
gram-positive (laboratory) {pronounced "gram-pause" or "gram-poz"}

"gram-poz"
{pronunciation of *gram-pos* [gram-positive]} (laboratory) {not an abbreviation}

gran
granulatus [granulated] (pharmacology)

gran.
granulatus [granulated] (pharmacology)

granulo
granulocyte (hematology and laboratory)

GRAS
generally recognized as safe [referring to food additives; United States Food and Drug Administration category] (dietary)

grav
gravid (obstetrics)
gravida (obstetrics)
gravity (physics)
pregnant (obstetrics)

"grav-ah-dah-one"
{pronunciation of *gravida I* [also called *primigravida*, a women who is pregnant for the first time]} (obstetrics) {not an abbreviation}

"grav-ah-dah-two"
{pronunciation of *gravida II* [also called *secundigravida*, a woman who is pregnant for the second time]} (obstetrics) {not an abbreviation}

"grav-ah-dah-three"
{pronunciation of *gravida III* [also called *tertigravida*, a woman who is pregnant for the third time] (obstetrics) {not an abbreviation}

grav I
primigravida [first pregnancy or pregnancy one] (obstetrics)

gravida I
{not an abbreviation} [also called *primigravida*, a woman who is pregnant for the first time] (obstetrics) {pronounced "grav-ah-dah-one"}

gravida II
{not an abbreviation} [also called *secundigravida*, a woman who is pregnant for the second time] (obstetrics) {pronounced "grav-ah-dah-two"}

gravida III
{not an abbreviation} [also called *tertigravida*, a woman who is pregnant for the third time] (obstetrics) {pronounced "grav-ah-dah-three"}

grav II
secundigravida [second pregnancy or pregnancy two] (obstetrics)

GRD
gastroesophageal reflux disease (gastroenterology)

grd
ground

GRF
gonadotropin-releasing factor (endocrinology and laboratory)
growth hormone-releasing factor (endocrinology and laboratory)

GRH
growth hormone-releasing hormone (endocrinology and laboratory)

G Rh
{not an abbreviation} [trademark for preparation of $Rh_0(D)$ immune serum globulin] (hematology, immunology, and pharmacology)

GRID
gay-related immunodeficiency [former name for *acquired immunodeficiency syndrome* (AIDS)] (immunology)

GRIF
growth hormone release-inhibiting factor (endocrinology and laboratory)

Gris-PEG
{not an abbreviation} [trademark for preparation of griseofulvin] (pharmacology)

GRN
granules
green

gros
grossus [coarse]

gros.
grossus [coarse]

GrP
gram-positive [bacilli] (laboratory)

grp
group

Gr₁P₀AB₁
gravida one, para none, and abortus one [*This is included as a sample for format purposes. The numbers may vary.*] (gynecology and obstetrics)

one pregnancy, no births, and one abortion [*This is included as a sample for format purposes. The numbers may vary.*] (gynecology and obstetrics)

GRPS
glucose-Ringer-phosphate solution (pharmacology)

GRS
beta-glucuronidase (chemistry)

GS
gastric shield (gastroenterology)
general surgery (surgery)
Gilbert's syndrome (gastroenterology and genetics)
glomerular sclerosis (nephrology)

G/S
glucose and saline (pharmacology)

g/s
gallons per second (measurement)

GSA
general somatic afferent [nerve] (neurology)
Girl Scouts of America
Gross [sarcoma] virus antigen (laboratory)
guanidinosuccinic acid (laboratory)

GSBG
gonadal steroid-binding globulin (endocrinology and laboratory)

GSC
gas-solid chromatography (laboratory)
Glasgow [coma] scale (neurology)
gravity-settling culture [plate] (laboratory)

GSCN
giant serotonin-containing neuron (neurology)

GSD
genetically significant dose [of roentgen rays] (radiation therapy and radiology)

guid
guidance

GUS
genitourinary sphincter (urology)
genitourinary system (gynecology and
   urology)

Gus
conductance of upstream segment
   (physics)

gutt
gutturi [to the throat] (pharmacology)

Guttat.
guttatim [drop by drop] (pharmacology)

guttat
guttatim [drop by drop] (pharmacology)

guttat.
guttatim [drop by drop] (pharmacology)

Gutt. quibusd.
guttis quibusdam [with a few drops]
   (pharmacology)

gutt quibusd
guttis quibusdam [with a few drops]
   (pharmacology)

gutt. quibusd.
guttis quibusdam [with a few drops]
   (pharmacology)

"guy-knee"
{pronunciation of *gyne* [gynecology]}
   (gynecology) {not an abbreviation}

GV
gentian violet (laboratory and pharmacology)
gingivectomy (dentistry and otorhinolaryngology)
gross virus [nodules] (laboratory)

GVA
general visceral afferent [nerve] (neurology)

GFBD
germinal vesicle breakdown (laboratory)

GVE
general visceral efferent [nerve] (neurology)

GVF
good visual fields (ophthalmology)

GVG
gamma-vinyl-gamma-aminobutyric acid
   [GABA] (laboratory)

GVH
graft versus host [disease or reaction]
   (transplantation)

GvH
graft versus host [disease or reaction]
   (transplantation)

GVHD
graft versus host disease (transplantation)

GVHR
graft versus host reaction (transplantation)

Gvty
gingivectomy (dentistry and otorhinolaryngology)

GW
germ warfare (armed forces)
glycerine in water (pharmacology)
group work

G/W
glucose and water (pharmacology)

GWA
gunshot wound of the abdomen (emergency medicine)

GWT
gunshot wound of the throat (emergency
   medicine)

GXD
graded

GXD EKG
graded exercise electrocardiogram (cardiovascular)

GXT
graded exercise test (cardiovascular)

Gy
gray (radiation therapy and radiology)

Gy.
gray (radiation therapy and radiology)

gym
gymnasium (rehabilitation and sports medicine)

GYN
gynecologist (gynecology)
gynecology (gynecology)

gyn
gynecology (gynecology)

gyn.
gynecology (gynecology)

gyne
gynecology {pronounced "guy-knee"} (gynecology)

gyro
gyroscope {pronounced "ji-row"}

gyro-
{not an abbreviation} [prefix meaning round or indicating relationship to a gyrus]

GZ
Guilford-Zimmerman [personality test] (psychiatry)

²H
deuterium [also called *heavy hydrogen*]
(chemistry)

H₂
{not an abbreviation} [H₂ receptor blockers, H₂ referring to the histamine receptor site] (gastroenterology and
pharmacology)

H³
tritium [isotope of hydrogen mass 3]
(chemistry)

3H
high, hot, and a helluva lot (slang)

μH
microhenry (measurement)

h
haustus [a draught] (pharmacology)
hecto- [prefix for 10²] (measurement)
{not an abbreviation}
height (measurement)
henry [unit of electrical inductance]
(electricity)
hora [hour] (measurement)
horizontal
hour (measurement)
Planck's constant [also called *quantum
constant*] (physics)

HA
hallux abductus (orthopedics and podiatry)
headache (neurology)
hearing aid (otorhinolaryngology)
height age (measurement and pediatrics)
hemadsorbent (laboratory)
hemadsorption [test] (laboratory)
hemagglutinating activity (laboratory)
hemagglutinating antibody (laboratory)
hemagglutinating antigen (laboratory)
hemagglutination (laboratory)
hemolytic anemia (hematology)
hepatic artery (cardiovascular and gastroenterology)
hepatitis A (gastroenterology and infectious diseases)
hepatitis-associated [virus] (gastroenterology, infectious diseases, and laboratory)

Heyden antibiotic (pharmacology)
high anxiety (psychiatry)
hospital admission
Hospital Apprentice
Hounsfield [unit; on computerized to-
mography] (radiology)
hyaluronic acid (laboratory)
hydroxyapatite (laboratory)
hyperalimentation (gastroenterology and
pharmacology)
hypothalmic amenorrhea (gynecology
and endocrinology)
{not an abbreviation} [general symbol for
acid] (chemistry)

H/A
headache (neurology)

HA1
hemadsorption [virus], type 1 (laboratory)

Ha
absolute hypermetropia (ophthalmology)
hahnium (chemistry)

HAA
hearing aid amplifier (otorhinolaryngology)
hemolytic anemia antigen (hematology
and laboratory)
hepatitis-associated antigen [also called
Australia antigen] (gastroenterology,
infectious diseases, and laboratory)
hospital activity analysis (statistics)

HAB
hepatitis B [virus] (gastroenterology, infectious diseases, and laboratory)

HABA
hydroxybenzeneazobenzoic acid (laboratory)

HABF
hepatic artery blood flow (cardiovascular and gastroenterology)

HAC
hexamethylmelamine, Adriamycin, and

cyclophosphamide (chemotherapy, oncology, and pharmacology)

HAChT
high-affinity choline transport (laboratory)

HACS
hyperactive child syndrome (neurology, pediatrics, and psychiatry)

HAD
hearing aid dispenser (otorhinolaryngology)
hemadsorption (laboratory)
hexamethylmelamine, Adriamycin, and cisplatin (chemotherapy, oncology, and pharmacology)
hospital administration (administration)
hospital administrator (administration)

HADD
hydroxyapatite deposition disease (laboratory)

HAE
hearing aid evaluation (otorhinolaryngology)
hepatic artery embolization (cardiovascular and gastroenterology)
hereditary angioedema (cardiovascular and genetics)

HAAg
hepatitis A antigen (gastroenterology, infectious diseases, and laboratory)

HAGG
hyperimmune antivariola gamma globulin (laboratory)

HAHTG
horse antihuman thymus globulin (laboratory)

HAI
hemagglutinating-inhibiting [antibody] (hematology and laboratory)
hemagglutination inhibition (hematology and laboratory)
hemagglutinin inhibition (hematology and laboratory)
hepatic arterial infusion (chemotherapy, oncology, and pharmacology)

H & A Ins
health and accident insurance (insurance)

HAL
hyperalimentation (gastroenterology and pharmacology)

hal.
halothane (anesthesiology and chemistry)

HaLV
hamster leukemia virus (laboratory)

halluc
hallucination (psychiatry)

HAM
hearing aid microphone (otorhinolaryngology)
hexamethylmelamine, Adriamycin, and L-phenylalanine mustard (chemotherapy, oncology, and pharmacology)

HAM-A
Hamilton Anxiety [scale] (psychiatry)

HAM-D
Hamilton Depression [scale] (psychiatry)

HAM-II
hexamethylmelamine, Adriamycin, and methotrexate (chemotherapy, oncology, and pharmacology)

HAMP
hexamethylmelamine, Adriamycin, methotrexate, and cisplatin (chemotherapy, oncology, and pharmacology)

HAN
heroin-associated nephropathy (chemical dependency and nephrology)
hyperplastic alveolar nodules (respiratory)

H and A staining
hematoxylin and eosin staining (laboratory)

HANDICP
handicapped (rehabilitation)

H and P
history and physical (medical records)

H and V
hemigastrectomy and vagotomy (gastroenterology and surgery)

HANE
hereditary angioneurotic edema (cardiovascular and genetics)

HANES
Health and Nutritional Examination Survey (statistics)

H antigens
{not an abbreviation} [antigens localized in flagella of motile bacteria] (laboratory)

HAO
hearing aid follow-up and orientation (otorhinolaryngology)
hospitals, administrators, and organizations (administration)

HAP
Handicapped Aid Program (rehabilitation)
Health Alliance Plan
heredopathia atactica polyneuritiformis [also called *Refsum's disease*] (cardiovascular, genetics, neurology, ophthalmology, and otorhinolaryngology)
histamine phosphate acid (laboratory)
hydrolysed animal protein (laboratory)

HAPA
hemagglutination antipenicillin antibody (laboratory)

HAPC
hospital-acquired penetration contact

HAPE
high-altitude pulmonary edema (respiratory and sports medicine)

HAPS
hepatic arterial perfusion scintigraphy (cardiovascular and radiology)

HAPT
haptoglobin (hematology and laboratory)

HAQ
Headache Assessment Questionnaire (neurology)

HAS
highest asymptomatic [dose] (pharmacology and radiation therapy)
hyperalimentation solution (pharmacology)
hypertensive arteriosclerosis (cardiovascular)
hypertensive arteriosclerotic (cardiovascular)

HASCVD
hypertensive arteriosclerotic cardiovascular disease (cardiovascular)

hash
{not an abbreviation} [slang for *hashish*] (chemical dependency and pharmacology) {pronounced "hash"}

"hash"
{pronunciation of *hash* [slang for *hashish*]} (chemical dependency and pharmacology) {not an abbreviation}

HASHD
hypertensive arteriosclerotic heart disease (cardiovascular)

H & ASHD
hypertensive and arteriosclerotic heart disease (cardiovascular)

HASP
Hospital Admission and Surveillance Program (statistics)

HAsP
Health Aspects of Pesticides (chemistry)

HAT
harmonic attenuation table [also called *harmonic attenuation test*] (otorhinolaryngology)
head, arms, and trunk (anatomy)

HATH
Heterosexual Attitudes Towards Homo-
sexuality [scale] (psychiatry)

haust.
haustus [a draft, a draught] (pharmacology)

HAV
hallux abducto valgus (orthopedics and
podiatry)
hepatitis A virus (gastroenterology and
laboratory)

HB
bundle of His (cardiovascular)
Health Board
heart block (cardiovascular)
hemoglobin (hematology and laboratory)
hepatitis B (gastroenterology, infectious
diseases, and laboratory)
His bundle (cardiovascular)
hold breakfast (dietary)
hospital bed
house-bound (rehabilitation)

H.B.
hospital bed

HB 1°
first-degree heart block (cardiovascular)

HB 2°
second-degree heart block (cardiovascular)

HB 3°
third-degree heart block (cardiovascular)

Hb
hemoglobin (hematology and laboratory)

H^b
deuterium [also called *heavy hydrogen*]
(chemistry)

h.b.
heart block (cardiovascular)

HbA
hemoglobin A [the normal adult hemo-
globin] (hematology and laboratory)

Hb A
hemoglobin A [the normal adult hemo-
globin] (hematology and laboratory)

Hb A$_1$
hemoglobin A$_1$ [the normal adult hemo-
globin] (hematology and laboratory)

Hb A$_2$
hemoglobin A$_2$ [the minor fraction of
adult hemoglobin] (hematology and
laboratory)

Hb A$_{1a}$
hemoglobin A$_{1a}$ [a glycosylated he-
moglobin] (hematology and laboratory)

HB Ab
hepatitis B antibody (gastroenterology,
infectious diseases, and laboratory)

Hb A$_{1b}$
hemoglobin A$_{1b}$ [a glycosylated he-
moglobin] (hematology and laboratory)

HBABA
hydroxybenzeneazobenzoic acid (chemistry)

Hb A$_{1c}$
hemoglobin A$_{1c}$ [a glycosylated he-
moglobin] (hematology and laboratory)

HB Ag
hepatitis B antigen (gastroenterology,
infectious diseases, and laboratory)
{pronounced "H-bag"}

HbAg
hepatitis B antigen (gastroenterology,
infectious diseases, and laboratory)
{pronounced "H-bag"}

"H-bag"
{pronunciation of *HB Ag* and *HbAg* [hepatitis B antigen]} (gastroenterology, infectious diseases, and laboratory) {not an abbreviation}

HBB
hospital blood bank (hematology)
hydroxybenzyl benzimidazole (chemistry)

HB Barts
Bart's hemoglobin (laboratory)

HBBW
hold breakfast blood work (laboratory)

HB$_c$
hepatitis B core [antibody or antigen] (gastroenterology, infectious diseases, and laboratory)

Hb C
hemoglobin C [an abnormal hemoglobin] (hematology and laboratory)

HB$_c$Ab
hepatitis B core antibody (gastroenterology, infectious diseases, and laboratory)

HB$_c$Ag
hepatitis B core antigen (gastroenterology, infectious diseases, and laboratory)

Hb CO
carboxyhemoglobin (hematology and laboratory)

Hb CS
hemoglobin Constant Spring [an abnormal hemoglobin] (hematology and laboratory)

HBD
has been drinking (chemical dependency and emergency medicine)
hydroxybutyrate dehydrogenase (laboratory)
hydroxybutyric acid dehydrogenase (laboratory)

Hb D
hemoglobin D [an abnormal hemoglobin] (hematology and laboratory)

HBDH
hydroxybutyrate dehydrogenase (laboratory)

HBE
His bundle electrogram (cardiovascular)

HBe
hepatitis B e [antibody or antigen; also called *hepatitis B early antibody* or *antigen*] (gastroenterology, infectious diseases, and laboratory)

Hb E
hemoglobin E [an abnormal hemoglobin] (hematology and laboratory)

HB$_e$Ab
hepatitis B e antibody [also called *hepatitis B early antibody*] (gastroenterology, infectious diseases, and laboratory)

HB$_e$Ag
hepatitis B e antigen [also called *hepatitis B early antigen*] (gastroenterology, infectious diseases, and laboratory)

HBF
hand blood flow (cardiovascular and orthopedics)
hepatic blood flow (cardiovascular and gastroenterology)

HbF
hemoglobin F [also called *fetal hemoglobin*] (hematology and laboratory)

Hb F
hemoglobin F [also called *fetal hemoglobin*] (hematology and laboratory)

HBGM
home blood glucose monitoring (endo-

crinology, laboratory, and pharmacology)

Hb H
hemoglobin H [an abnormal hemoglobin] (hematology and laboratory)

HBHC
home-based hospital care (hospice and rehabilitation)

HBI
hemibody irradiation (oncology and radiation therapy)
high serum-bound iron (laboratory)

HBIG
hepatitis B immunoglobulin (gastroenterology, infectious diseases, and laboratory) {pronounced "H-big"}

HBIg
hepatitis B immunoglobulin (gastroenterology, infectious diseases, and laboratory) {pronounced "H-big"}

"H-big"
{pronunciation of *HBIG* and *HBIg* [hepatitis B immunoglobulin]} (gastroenterology, infectious diseases, and laboratory) {not an abbreviation}

Hb Kansas
hemoglobin Kansas [a mutant hemoglobin with a low affinity for oxygen] (hematology and laboratory)

Hb Lepore
hemoglobin Lepore [an abnormal hemoglobin] (hematology and laboratory)

HBLLSB
heard best at left lower sternal border (cardiovascular)

H$_2$ blocker
{not an abbreviation} [H$_2$ receptor blockers, H$_2$ referring to the histamine receptor site] (gastroenterology and pharmacology)

HBLUSB
heard best at left upper sternal border (cardiovascular)

HBLV
human B-lymphotropic virus (immunology and laboratory)

Hb M
hemoglobin M [an abnormal hemoglobin] (hematology and laboratory)

HBO
Home Box Office (cable television)
hyperbaric oxygen [therapy or unit] (neurology, respiratory, and sports medicine)

H$_3$BO$_3$
boric acid (chemistry and pharmacology)

HbO$_2$
oxyhemoglobin (laboratory)

HBOT
hyperbaric oxygen therapy [experimental use in many specialties] (neurology, respiratory, and sports medicine)

HBP
high blood pressure (cardiovascular)

HbP
primitive hemoglobin [also called *fetal hemoglobin*] (laboratory)

HBr
hydrobromic acid (chemistry)

HBS
Health Behavior Scale (psychiatry)
hemoglobin S [an abnormal hemoglobin associated with sickle cell disease] (hematology and laboratory)

HB$_s$
hepatitis B surface [antibody or antigen] (gastroenterology, infectious diseases, and laboratory)

Hb S
hemoglobin S [an abnormal hemoglobin

associated with sickle cell disease]
(hematology and laboratory)

HB$_s$Ab
hepatitis B surface antibody (gastroenterology, infectious diseases, and laboratory)

HB$_s$Ag
hepatitis B surface antigen (gastroenterology, infectious diseases, and laboratory)

HBSS
Hank's balanced salt solution (pharmacology)

HBT
human breast tumor (endocrinology, gynecology, oncology, and pathology)

HBV
hepatitis B vaccine (gastroenterology, infectious diseases, and pharmacology)
hepatitis B virus (gastroenterology, infectious diseases, and laboratory)
honey bee venom (laboratory)

HBW
high birth weight (neonatology)

HC
hair cell (laboratory)
handicapped (rehabilitation)
head circumference (neonatology and pediatrics)
head compression
heart cycle (cardiovascular)
hepatic catalase (laboratory)
Hickman catheter (surgery)
hippocampus (anatomy and neurology)
home care
Hospital Corps (armed forces)
hospital course
house call
Huntington's chorea (neurology)
hyaline casts (laboratory)
hydrocarbon (chemistry)
hydrocortisone (pharmacology)
hydroxycorticoid (pharmacology)

HCA
health care aide (rehabilitation)

heart cell aggregate (laboratory)
hepatocellular adenoma (gastroenterology and oncology)
Hospital Corporation of America (administration)
hydrocortisone acetate (pharmacology)

HCAP
handicapped (rehabilitation)
hexamethylmelamine, Adriamycin, cyclophosphamide, and cisplatin (chemotherapy, oncology, and pharmacology)

HCC
hepatitis contagiosa canis [virus] (laboratory)
hepatocellular carcinoma (gastroenterology and oncology)
hydroxycholecalciferol (gastroenterology and laboratory)

HCD
heavy chain disease [protein] (laboratory)
homologous canine distemper [antiserum] (pharmacology)

γHCD
gamma-heavy chain disease [protein] (laboratory)

HCF
high carbohydrate, high fiber [diet] (dietary)
highest common factor (statistics)

HCFA
Health Care Financing Administration (administration)

HCG
human chorionic gonadotropin (endocrinology, laboratory, oncology, and urology)

hCG
human chorionic gonadotropin (endocrinology, laboratory, oncology, and urology)

HCGN
hypocomplementemic glomerulonephritis (nephrology)

hCG-α subunit
human chorionic gonadotropin-alpha subunit (endocrinology, laboratory, oncology, and urology)

hCG-β subunit
human chorionic gonadotropin-beta subunit (endocrinology, laboratory, oncology, and urology)

HCH
hexachlorocyclohexane [also called *benzene hexachloride* and *1,2,3,4,5,6-hexachlorocyclohexane*] (chemistry)

H chains
heavy chains (laboratory)

HCHO
formaldehyde (chemistry and laboratory)

HcImp
hydrocolloid impression (dentistry)

HCL
hair cell leukemia (hematology and oncology)
hairy cell leukemia (hematology and oncology)
hard contact lens (ophthalmology)
human cultured lymphoblastoid [cells] (laboratory)

HCl
hydrochloric acid (chemistry)
hydrochloride (chemistry and pharmacology)
hydrogen chloride (chemistry)

HCLF
high carbohydrate, low fiber [diet] (dietary)

HCLs
hard contact lenses (ophthalmology)

HCM
health care maintenance (administration)

hypertrophic cardiomyopathy (cardiovascular)

HCO₃
bicarbonate (laboratory and pharmacology)

HCP
handicapped (rehabilitation)
hepatocatalase peroxidase (laboratory)
hereditary coproporphyria (rheumatology)

H & CP
Hospital and Community Psychiatry (psychiatry)

HCR
heme-controlled repressor (genetics)
human-controlled repressor (genetics)
hydrochloric acid (chemistry and laboratory)
hysterical conversion reaction (psychiatry)

HCRE
Homeopathic Council for Research and Education (education and research)

H'crit
hematocrit (hematology and laboratory)

HCS
hospital car service
hourglass contraction of stomach (gastroenterology)
human chorionic somatomammotropin [also called *human placental lactogen*] (endocrinology and laboratory)
human cord serum (hematology, laboratory, and pharmacology)

H.C.S.
Harvey Cushing Society (endocrinology)

17-HCS
17-hydroxycorticosteroids (laboratory and pharmacology)

hCS
human chorionic somatomammotropin (endocrinology and laboratory)

HCSD
Health Care Studies Division (administration and statistics)

HCSM
human chorionic somatomammotropin [also called *human placental lactogen*] (endocrinology and laboratory)

hCSM
human chorionic somatomammotropin [also called *human placental lactogen*] (endocrinology and laboratory)

HCT
heart-circulation training (cardiovascular and rehabilitation)
hematocrit (hematology and laboratory)
histamine challenge test (laboratory)
homocytotropic (laboratory)
human chorionic placental thyrotropin (endocrinology and laboratory)
hydrochlorothiazide (cardiovascular and pharmacology)
hydrocortisone (pharmacology)

Hct
hematocrit (hematology and laboratory)

hct
hematocrit (hematology and laboratory)
hydrochlorothiazide (cardiovascular and pharmacology)

HCTU
home cervical traction unit (chiropractic medicine, orthopedics, and physical therapy)

HCTZ
hydrochlorothiazide (cardiovascular and pharmacology)

HCU
homocystinuria (laboratory and urology)

HCVD
hypertensive cardiovascular disease (cardiovascular)

HD
Hajna-Damon [broth] (laboratory)
Hansen's disease [leprosy] (infectious diseases)
hearing distance (otorhinolaryngology)
heart disease (cardiovascular)
heloma durum [a hard corn] (orthopedics and podiatry)
hemodialysis (nephrology)
hemolysing dose (laboratory)
herniated disc (neurology and orthopedics)
high density
high dosage (pharmacology and radiation therapy)
high dose (pharmacology and radiation therapy)
hip disarticulation (orthopedics)
Hodgkin's disease (oncology)
hospital day
Huntington's disease (neurology)
hydatid disease (gastroenterology and infectious diseases)

H-2D
{not an abbreviation} [a gene cluster] (genetics and laboratory)

HD 2
{not an abbreviation} [a hip prosthesis] (orthopedics)

HD$_{50}$
hemolyzing dose of complement that lyses 50 percent of a suspension of sensitized red blood cells (laboratory)

Hd
heart disease (cardiovascular)
Hodgkin's disease (oncology)

hd
hora decubitus [at bedtime, at hour of lying down] (pharmacology)

h.d.
hora decubitus [at bedtime, at hour of lying down] (pharmacology)

HDA
Huntington's Disease Association (neurology)
hydroxydopamine (cardiovascular and pharmacology)

HDARAC
high-dose cytarabine [Ara C] (chemotherapy, oncology, and pharmacology)

HDBD
hydroxybutyric dehydrogenase (laboratory)

HDC
histidine decarboxylase (laboratory)
human diploid cell (laboratory)

HDCCAMS
high-dose cyclophosphamide and Adriamycin (chemotherapy, oncology, and pharmacology)

HDCS
human diploid cell strain (laboratory)

HDCV
human diploid cell rabies vaccine (pharmacology)

HDD
Higher Dental Diploma (dentistry and education)

HDF
human diploid fibroblast (laboratory)

HDFP
Hypertension Detection and Follow-Up Program (cardiovascular)

HDH
heart disease history (cardiovascular)

HD II
{not an abbreviation} [a hip prosthesis] (orthopedics)

HDL
high-density lipoprotein [one of the cholesterol levels] (cardiovascular and laboratory)

HDL-c
high density lipoprotein-cell surface [receptor] (laboratory)
high density lipoprotein [fraction] (laboratory)

HDLW
distance at which a watch is heard by the left ear (otorhinolaryngology)

HDMTX
high-dose methotrexate (chemotherapy, oncology, and pharmacology)

HDN
hemolytic disease of the newborn (hematology and neonatology)
high-density nebulizer (pharmacology and respiratory)

hDNA
deoxyribonucleic acid, histone (laboratory)

HDP
hexose diphosphate (laboratory)
hydroxydimethylpyrimidine (laboratory)

HDPAA
heparin-dependent platelet-associated antibody (laboratory)

HDRF
Heart Disease Research Foundation (cardiovascular and research)

HDRS
Hamilton Depression Rate Scale (psychiatry)

HDRV
human diploid cell strain rabies vaccine (pharmacology)

HDRW
distance at which a watch is heard by the right ear (otorhinolaryngology)

HDS
herniated disc syndrome (neurology and orthopedics)
Hospital Discharge Survey (statistics)

HDU
hemodialysis unit (nephrology)

HdU
hemodialysis unit (nephrology)

HE
hard exudate (ophthalmology)
Hearing Examiner
hemagglutinating encephalomyelitis
 (neurology)
hemoglobin electrophoresis (hematology
 and laboratory)
hepatic encephalopathy (gastroenterology and neurology)
hereditary elliptocytosis (hematology)
high explosive (chemistry)
hollow enzyme (laboratory)
human enteric [virus] (gastroenterology
 and laboratory)
hypogonadotropic eunuchoidism (endocrinology)
hypophysectomy (endocrinology, neurology, and neurosurgery)

H & E
hematoxylin and eosin [stain] (laboratory)
hemorrhage and exudate (ophthalmology)
heredity and environment

H-E
heat exchanger [for cardiopulmonary
 bypass and extracorporeal membrane
 oxygenation] (cardiology, neonatology, and surgery)

He
Hedstrom number (chemistry)
helium (chemistry)

³He
helium-3 (chemistry)

⁴He
helium-4 (chemistry)

he.
head (anatomy)

HEA
hexone-extracted acetone (chemistry)

human erythrocyte antigen (hematology
 and laboratory)

He antigen
MNS blood group antigen (hematology
 and laboratory)

HEART
Health Evaluation and Risk Tabulation
 (cardiovascular and statistics)

HEAT
human erythrocyte agglutination test
 (laboratory)

HEB
hematoencephalic barrier [also called
 blood brain barrier] (anatomy, cardiovascular, and neurology)

HEBDOM
hebdomada [a week; referring to the
 first week of life] (neonatology)

hebdom.
hebdomada [a week; referring to the
 first week of life] (neonatology)

HEC
hamster embryo cell (laboratory and research)
Health Education Council [British]
health evaluation center
human endothelial cell (laboratory)
hydroxyergocalciferol (laboratory)

"heck-toe"
{pronunciation of *hecto-* [prefix for 10^2]}
 (measurement) {not an abbreviation}

hecto-
{not an abbreviation} [prefix for 10^2]
 (measurement) {pronounced "heck-
 toe" or "hek-toe"}

HED
Haut-Einheits-Dosis [unit skin dose of
 roentgen rays] (radiation therapy)

Haut-Erythem-Dosis [skin erythema
dose] (radiation therapy)
hydrotropic electron donor (physics)

HEDSPA
^{99m}Tc Etidronate [also called *ethane-1-hy-droxyl-1,1-diphosphonate*] (radiology)

HEENT
head, ears, eyes, nose, and throat
head, eyes, ears, nose, and throat

H'EENT
head, ears, eyes, nose, and throat
head, eyes, ears, nose, and throat

HEE syndrome
hemiconvulsion, hemiplegia, and epilepsy syndrome (neurology)

HEF
hamster embryo fibroblast (laboratory and research)

HEG
hemorrhagic erosive gastritis (gastroenterology)

HEHR
highest equivalent heart rate (cardiovascular)

HEI
high-energy intermediate
homogeneous enzyme immunoassay (laboratory)

HE inj.
hyperextension injury (neurology and orthopedics)

HEIR
health effects of ionizing radiation (dermatology, oncology, radiation therapy, and radiology)
high-energy ionizing radiation (radiation therapy and radiology)

HEIS
high-energy ion scattering (radiation therapy, radiology, and physics)

HEK
human embryo kidney [cell culture] (laboratory)
human embryonic kidney [cells] (laboratory)

"hek-toe"
{pronunciation of *hecto-* [prefix for 10^2] (measurement) {not an abbreviation}

HEL
hen's egg-white lysozyme (laboratory)
human embryonic lung [cell culture] (laboratory)
human embryonic lung [cells] (laboratory)
human erythroleukemia (hematology and oncology)

HeLa
Helen Lake [tumor cells] (laboratory)
{not an abbreviation} [a carcinoma cell line for tissue cultures; name from patient, Henrietta Lacks] (laboratory and oncology)

HELF
human embryonic lung fibroblasts (laboratory)

HELLP
hemolysis, elevated liver enzymes, and low platelet [count] (laboratory)

HELM
helmet cells (laboratory)

HELP
Hawaii Early Learning Profile (education, pediatrics, and speech and language therapy)
Health Education Library Program (education and library science)
Health Emergency Loan Program [Planned Parenthood] (gynecology and obstetrics)
Health Evaluation and Learning Program (education)
Health Evaluation through Logical Processing (computer science)
heat escape lessening posture

Henry's Emergency Lessons for People
Heroin Emergency Life Project (chemical dependency and emergency medicine)
Hospital Equipment Loan Project

HEM
hematology

Hem
hematology
hemolysis (hematology and laboratory)
hemolytic (hematology and laboratory)

hem
hemolysis (hematology and laboratory)
hemolytic (hematology and laboratory)

hem.
hematuria (urology)
hemolysis (hematology and laboratory)
hemolytic (hematology and laboratory)
hemorrhage (hematology)
hemorrhoid (gastroenterology)

HEMA
Health Education Media Association
hematology profile (hematology and laboratory)

HEMAT
hematology

hemat
hematocrit (laboratory)
hematology

hematem.
hematemesis (gastroenterology)

hematol.
hematologist (hematology)
hematology

"hem-E"
{pronunciation of *hemi* [hemiparalysis, hemiplegia]} (neurology) {not an abbreviation}

Hemi
hemisphere (neurology)

hemi
hemiparalysis (neurology) {pronounced "hem-E"}
hemiplegia (neurology) {pronounced "hem-E"}

HEMO
hemolyzed (laboratory)

hemo
hemoglobin (hematology and laboratory)
hemophilia (hematology)

hemocyt.
hemocytometer (hematology and laboratory)

hemorr.
hemorrhage (hematology)

HEMPAS
hereditary erythroblastic multinuclearity with a positive acidified serum [test] (hematology and laboratory)
hereditary erythrocytic multinuclearity with a positive acidified serum [test] (hematology and laboratory)

HEMSID
hemosiderin (laboratory)

HEN
hemorrhages, exudates, and/or nicking (ophthalmology)

He-Ne
helium-neon [laser surgery] (surgery)

HEP
hepatic (gastroenterology)
hepatology (gastroenterology)
high egg passage [strain of virus] (laboratory)
high-energy phosphate (laboratory)
histamine equivalent prick (allergy)
human epithelial cells (laboratory)

hep
hepatitis (gastroenterology)

HEPA
high-efficiency particulate air [filter]
(respiratory)

HEP-AC
hepatitis battery-acute (gastroenterology and laboratory)

HEPES
hydroxyethylpiperazine ethanesulphonic
acid (chemistry)

HEPM
human embryonic palatal mesenchymal
[cells] (laboratory)

herb recent
herbarium recentium [fresh herbs]
(pharmacology)

herb. recent.
herbarium recentium [fresh herbs]
(pharmacology)

hered
heredity (genetics)

hern
hernia (gastroenterology and surgery)
herniated

HERS
Health Evaluation and Referral Service
National Heart Education Research Society (cardiovascular, education, and
research)

HES
hypereosinophilic syndrome (hematology)
hydroxyethyl starch (chemistry)

HESCA
Health Sciences Communications Association

HESO
Hospital Educational Services Officer
(education)

HET
Health Education Telecommunications
(education)

helium equilibration time (laboratory
and respiratory)
heterozygous (genetics)

HET-BE
heterophile beef (laboratory)

HET-GP
heterophile guinea pig (laboratory)

HETP
height equivalent to a theoretical plate
hexaethyltetraphosphate (laboratory)

HET-PR
heterophile presumptive (laboratory)

HEV
health and environment

HEW
Department of Health, Education, and
Welfare [now *Department of Health
and Human Services*] (government)

H.E.W.
Department of Health, Education, and
Welfare [now *Department of Health
and Human Services*] (government)

Hex
hexamethylmelamine (chemotherapy,
oncology, and pharmacology)

HEXA-CAF
hexamethylmelamine, cyclophosphamide, 5-fluorouracil, and methotrexate (chemotherapy, oncology, and
pharmacology)

HEXL
methohexital [a barbiturate] (pharmacology)

HF
Hageman factor [coagulation factor XII]
(hematology and laboratory)
hard-filled [capsules] (pharmacology)
hay fever (allergy, otorhinolaryngology,
and respiratory)
heart failure (cardiovascular)

hemorrhagic factor (hematology and
    laboratory)
hemorrhagic fever (hematology and in-
    fectious diseases)
high fat [diet] (dietary)
high flow (respiratory)
high frequency (electricity, neurology,
    and otorhinolaryngology)
hollow fiber [dialyzer] (nephrology)
house formula [an in-house formula
    found in a particular hospital or clinic]
    (pharmacology)
human fibroblasts (laboratory)

H/F
HeLa/fibroblast [hybrid] (laboratory)

Hf
hafnium (chemistry)

hf
half (measurement)

HFC
hand-filled capsules (pharmacology)
hard-filled capsules (pharmacology)
high-frequency current (electricity)

HFD
high forceps delivery (obstetrics)

HFDK
human fetal diploid kidney [cells] (labo-
    ratory)

HFHL
high-frequency hearing loss (otorhi-
    nolaryngology)

HFI
hereditary fructose intolerance (gastro-
    enterology)

H field
{not an abbreviation} (anatomy)

HFIF
human fibroblast interferon (laboratory)

HFJV
high-frequency jet ventilation (respi-
    ratory)

"H-flew"
{pronunciation of *H flu* [*Hemophilus in-
    fluenzae*] (bacteriology and labora-
    tory)} {not an abbreviation}

H flu
Hemophilus influenzae (bacteriology
    and laboratory) {pronounced "H-
    flew"}

HFMA
Healthcare Financial Management Asso-
    ciation

HFO
high-frequency oscillation (respiratory)

HFOV
high-frequency oscillatory ventilation
    (respiratory)

HFP
hexafluoropropylene (chemistry)
hypofibrinogenic plasma (laboratory)

HFPPV
high-frequency positive pressure ventila-
    tion (respiratory)

HFR
high frequency of recombination (chem-
    istry and laboratory)

Hfr
high frequency (electricity, neurology,
    and otorhinolaryngology)
high frequency of recombination (chem-
    istry and laboratory)

HFRS
hemorrhagic fever with renal syndrome
    (hematology, infectious diseases, and
    nephrology)

HFSH
human follicle-stimulating hormone (en-
    docrinology and laboratory)

hFSH
human follicle-stimulating hormone (en-
    docrinology and laboratory)

HFST
hearing-for-speech test [British] (otorhinolaryngology)

HFT
high-frequency transduction (electricity)

HG
hemoglobin (hematology and laboratory)
herpes genitalis (gynecology, infectious
diseases, and urology)
herpes gestationis (infectious diseases
and obstetrics)
human gonadotropin (endocrinology and
laboratory)
human growth [factor] (endocrinology
and laboratory)

Hg
hemoglobin (hematology and laboratory)
hydrargyrum [mercury] (chemistry)

hg
hectogram (measurement)

hg.
hectogram (measurement)

HGA
homogentisic acid (laboratory)

HGB
hemoglobin (hematology and laboratory)

Hgb
hemoglobin (hematology and laboratory)

Hgb.
hemoglobin (hematology and laboratory)

hgb
hemoglobin (hematology and laboratory)

HGB EL
hemoglobin electrophoresis (hematology
and laboratory)

HGB Elect
hemoglobin electrophoresis (hematology
and laboratory)

Hgb F
hemoglobin F [also called *fetal hemoglobin*] (hematology and laboratory)

Hgb & Hct
hemoglobin and hematocrit (hematology
and laboratory)

HGB-PL
hemoglobin plasma (hematology and
laboratory)

HGBS
methemoglobin-sulfhemoglobin (hematology and laboratory)

HGF
hyperglycemic-glycogenolytic factor
[glucagon] (endocrinology and laboratory)

Hg F
hemoglobin F [also called *fetal hemoglobin*] (hematology and laboratory)

Hg-F
hemoglobin F [also called *fetal hemoglobin*] (hematology and laboratory)

HGG
human gamma globulin (infectious diseases, laboratory, and pharmacology)

hGG
human gamma globulin (infectious diseases, laboratory, and pharmacology)

HGH
human [pituitary] growth hormone (endocrinology and laboratory)

hGH
human [pituitary] growth hormone (endocrinology and laboratory)

hgm
hectogram (measurement)

HGMCR
human genetic mutant cell repository
(genetics and laboratory)

HGO
hepatic glucose output (endocrinology,
gastroenterology, and laboratory)

HGPRT
hypoxanthine-guanine phosphoribosyltransferase (laboratory)

HG-PRTase
hypoxanthine-guanine phosphoribosyltransferase (laboratory)

HGRM
hemogram (hematology and laboratory)

hgt.
height (measurement)

HH
hard of hearing (otorhinolaryngology)
Henderson and Haggard [inhaler] (respiratory)
hiatal hernia (gastroenterology and surgery)
holistic health (holistic medicine)
home health (rehabilitation)
home help (rehabilitation)
hydroxyhexamide (chemistry)
hypogonadism (endocrinology)
hypogonadotrophic (endocrinology)

H & H
hemoglobin and hematocrit (hematology
and laboratory)

H/H
hemoglobin and hematocrit (hematology
and laboratory)

HHA
hereditary hemolytic anemia (hematology)
home health agency (rehabilitation)
hypothalamic-hypophyseal-adrenal (endocrinology)

H.H.A.
home health agency (rehabilitation)
home health aid (rehabilitation)

HHb
reduced hemoglobin (hematology and
laboratory)
un-ionized hemoglobin (hematology and
laboratory)

HHC
home health care (rehabilitation)

HHD
hypertensive heart disease (cardiovascular)

HHFM
high-humidity face mask (respiratory)

HHHO
hypotonia-hypomentia-hypogonadism-
obesity (endocrinology and neurology)

H. H. inhaler
{not an abbreviation} [named for the in-
ventors] (respiratory)

H. + Hm.
compound hypermetropic astigmatism
(ophthalmology)

HHN
hand-held nebulizer (pharmacology and
respiratory)

HHNK
hyperglycemic, hyperosmolar, nonketotic [coma] (endocrinology and neurology)

HHS
Department of Health and Human Services (government)

HHSSA
Home Health Services and Staffing Association (rehabilitation)

HHT
hereditary hemorrhagic telangiectasia (dermatology, gastroenterology, genetics, hematology, and otorhinolaryngology)
12-L-hydroxy-5,8,10-heptadecatrienoic acid (chemistry)

HI
Hawaii [Postal Service state designation]
head injury (neurology)
health insurance (insurance)
hemagglutination inhibition [titer] (hematology and laboratory)
hepatobiliary imaging (gastroenterology and radiology)
high impulsiveness (psychiatry)
homicidal ideation (psychiatry)
hospital insurance (insurance)
hydriodic acid (chemistry)
hydroxyindole (laboratory)

Hi
histidine (chemistry and laboratory)

HIA
heat infusion agar (laboratory)
hemagglutination-inhibition antibody (laboratory)

HIAA
Health Insurance Association of America (insurance)

5-HIAA
5-hydroxyindoleacetic acid (laboratory)

HIB
Hemophilus influenzae, type B (bacteriology and laboratory)
Hemophilus influenzae, type B [vaccine] (pharmacology)

HIBAC
Health Insurance Benefits Advisory Council (insurance)

HIC
Heart Information Center (cardiovascular)

hi-cal
high caloric (dietary) {pronounced "hi-kal"}

high calorie (dietary) {pronounced "hi-kal"}

HiCN
cyanmethemoglobin (laboratory)

HID
headache, insomnia, depression [syndrome] (neurology and psychiatry)

HIDA
hepatoiminodiacetic acid [scan; also called *lidofenin scan* and *technetium scan*] (radiology)

"hi-drow"
{pronunciation of *Hydro* [hydrotherapy]} (physical therapy) {not an abbreviation}

HIE
hypoxic-ischemic encephalopathy (neurology)

HIF
higher integrative functions (neurology)

HIFBS
heat-inactivated fetal bovine serum (laboratory)

HIFC
hog intrinsic factor concentrate (laboratory)

HIg
human immunoglobulin (laboratory)

HIHA
high impulsiveness, high anxiety (psychiatry)

HII
Health Industries Institute
Health Insurance Institute (insurance)
hemagglutination-inhibition immunoassay (laboratory)

"hi-kal"
{pronunciation of *hi-cal* [high caloric,

HKS
heel-knee-shin [test] (neurology)

HL
hairline
half-life (chemistry and physics)
hallux limitus (podiatry)
haloperidol (pharmacology)
harelip (genetics and surgery)
hearing level (otorhinolaryngology)
hearing loss (otorhinolaryngology)
heparin lock (pharmacology)
Hickman line (cardiovascular)
histiocytic lymphoma (oncology)
histocompatibility locus (laboratory)
Hodgkin's lymphoma (oncology)
Hygienic Laboratory (laboratory)
hypertrichosis lanuginosa (endocrinology)

H/L
hydrophile/lipophile [number] (chemistry and laboratory)

H & L
heart and lungs (cardiovascular and respiratory)

Hl
latent hypermetropia (ophthalmology)
latent hyperopia (ophthalmology)

hl
hectoliter (measurement)

h.l.
hearing loss (otorhinolaryngology)

HLA
histocompatibility locus A [system] (laboratory)
histocompatibility locus antigen (laboratory)
homologous leukocytic antibody (laboratory)
human leukocyte antigen [system] (laboratory)
Human Life Amendment (law)
human lymphocyte antigen (laboratory)
hypoplastic left atrium (cardiovascular)

HLA-A
{not an abbreviation} [subdetermination of human leukocyte antigen] (laboratory)

HLA-B
{not an abbreviation} [subdetermination of human leukocyte antigen] (laboratory)

HLA-B8
{not an abbreviation} [subdetermination of human leukocyte antigen] (laboratory)

HLA-B27
{not an abbreviation} [subdetermination of human leukocyte antigen] (laboratory)

HLA-C
{not an abbreviation} [subdetermination of human leukocyte antigen] (laboratory)

HLA-C8
{not an abbreviation} [subdetermination of human leukocyte antigen] (laboratory)

HLA-D
{not an abbreviation} [subdetermination of human leukocyte antigen] (laboratory)

HLA-DR
{not an abbreviation} [subdetermination of human leukocyte antigen] (laboratory)

HLA-DR2
{not an abbreviation} [subdetermination of human leukocyte antigen] (laboratory)

HL-A factor
{not an abbreviation} (laboratory)

HLALD
horse liver alcohol dehydrogenase (laboratory)

HL-A-LD
human lymphocyte-antigen—lymphocyte defined (laboratory)

HL-A-SD
human lymphocyte-antigen—serologically defined (laboratory)

HLB
hydrophile-lipophile balance [with reference to surfactants] (laboratory)
hypotonic lysis buffer (laboratory)

HLC
Human Lactation Center (obstetrics)

HLD
herniated lumbar disc (neurology and orthopedics)
hypersensitivity lung disease (respiratory)

HL-D
haloperidol decanoate (pharmacology)

HLDH
heat-stable lactic dehydrogenase (laboratory)

HLF
heat-labile factor (laboratory)

HLH
human luteinizing hormone (endocrinology and laboratory)
hypoplastic left heart [syndrome] (cardiovascular and neonatology)

hLH
human luteinizing hormone (endocrinology and laboratory)

HLHS
hypoplastic left heart syndrome (cardiovascular)

HLK
heart, liver, and kidneys [on physical examination] (anatomy)

HLN
hyperplastic liver nodules (gastroenterology)

H-2 locus
{not an abbreviation} (genetics and laboratory)

HLP
hyperlipoproteinemia (cardiovascular and laboratory)

HLR
heart-lung resuscitation (cardiovascular and respiratory)
heart-lung resuscitator (cardiovascular and respiratory)

HLS
Health Learning Systems (education)

hLT
human lymphocyte transformation (laboratory)

hlth.
health

HLV
herpes-like virus (laboratory)
hypoplastic left ventricle (cardiovascular)

HM
hand motion [vision] (neurology and ophthalmology)
hand movement(s) (neurology and ophthalmology)
heart murmur (cardiovascular)
heloma molle [a soft corn] (orthopedics and podiatry)
human milk (neonatology)
human semisynthetic insulin (pharmacology)
hydatidiform mole (gynecology and obstetrics)
hyperimmune mice (laboratory)

Hm
home
manifest hypermetropia (ophthalmology)
manifest hyperopia (ophthalmology)

Hm.
manifest hypermetropia (ophthalmology)
manifest hyperopia (ophthalmology)

hm
hectometer (measurement)

HMAC
Health Manpower Advisory Council

HMAS
hyperimmune mice ascitic [fluid] (laboratory)

HMB
homatropine methobromide [an anticholinergic] (ophthalmology and pharmacology)
homatropine methylbromide [an anticholinergic] (gastroenterology and pharmacology)

HMC
heroin, morphine, cocaine (chemical dependency and pharmacology)
hydroxymethyl cytosine (genetics and laboratory)

HMD
hyaline membrane disease (neonatology and respiratory)

HMD type I
hyaline membrane disease type I [also called *classical hyaline membrane disease*] (neonatology and respiratory)

HMD type II
hyaline membrane disease type II [also called *drowning syndrome* and *neonatal wet lung*] (neonatology and respiratory)

HMDP
hydroxymethylene diphosphonate

HME
Health Media Education (education)
heat and moisture exchanger
heat, massage, and exercise (physical therapy)

HMF
hydroxymethylfurfural (chemistry)

HMG
human menopausal gonadotropin (endocrinology and laboratory)
hydroxymethylglutaryl (endocrinology, genetics, and laboratory)

hMG
human menopausal gonadotropin (endocrinology and laboratory)

HMG CoA
hepatic hydroxymethylglutaryl coenzyme A (endocrinology, genetics, and laboratory)

HMI
healed myocardial infarction (cardiovascular)

HML
human milk lysozyme (laboratory)

hML
human milk lysozyme (laboratory)

HM & LP
hand motion and light perception (neurology and ophthalmology)

HMM
heavy meromyosin (chemistry)
hexamethylmelamine (chemotherapy, oncology, and pharmacology)

HMMA
4-hydroxy-3-methoxymandelic acid (chemistry)

HMO
health maintenance organization [a type of health care system and insurance] (insurance)
heart minute output (cardiovascular)

HMP
hexose monophosphate [also called *hexosephosphate*] (laboratory)

hexose monophosphate pathway (laboratory)
hot moist packs (physical therapy)

HMPA
hexamethylphosphoramide (chemistry)

HMPG
4-hydroxy-3-methoxyphenylethylene glycol (chemistry)

HMPS
hexose monophosphate shunt

HMR
histocytic medullary reticulosis (hematology)

H-mRNA
H-chain messenger ribonucleic acid (genetics and laboratory)

HMS
Health Mobilization Series

HMS
Hospital Marketing Services (manufacturing)

HMSAS
hypertrophic muscular subaortic stenosis (cardiovascular)

HMT
human molar thyrotropin (endocrinology and laboratory)

hMT
hydroxymethyl uracil (chemistry)

HMW
high molecular weight (chemistry)

HMX
heat-massage-exercise (physical therapy)

HN
head nurse (nursing)
hereditary nephritis (genetics and nephrology)
high nitrogen (chemistry and laboratory)
hilar node (respiratory)

Home Nursing (nursing)
Hospitalman [Navy] (armed forces)
human nutrition (dietary)

H.N.
head nurse (nursing)

H & N
head and neck (anatomy)

HN$_2$
nitrogen mustard [also called *methyl bis (β-chloroethyl)-amine*] (chemistry, chemotherapy, oncology, and pharmacology)

hn
hoc nocte [tonight] (pharmacology)

h.n.
hoc nocte [tonight] (pharmacology)

HNA
heparin neutralizing activity (cardiovascular, hematology, laboratory, and pharmacology)

HNB
2-hydroxy-5-nitrobenzyl bromide (chemistry)

HNC
hypothalamic-neurohypophyseal complex (endocrinology and neurology)

HNO$_3$
nitric acid (chemistry)

HNP
herniated nucleus pulposus (neurology and orthopedics)

H.N.P.
herniated nucleus pulposus (neurology and orthopedics)

HNRNA
heterogeneous nuclear ribonucleic acid (genetics and laboratory)

hnRNA
heterogeneous nuclear ribonucleic acid
(genetics and laboratory)

HNS
head, neck, and shaft [of a bone] (orthopedics)
Home Nursing Supervisor (nursing)

HNSHA
hereditary nonspherocytic hemolytic leukemia (hematology and oncology)

HNV
has not voided (urology)

HO
heterotopic ossification (radiology, orthopedics)
high oxygen (respiratory)
House Officer
hyperbaric oxygen (neurology, respiratory, and sports medicine)

H/O
hematology and oncology
history of

H₂O
water [also called *hydrogen monoxide*] (chemistry)

H₂O₂
hydrogen peroxide (laboratory and pharmacology)

Ho
holmium (chemistry)

H₀
null hypothesis

HOAP
Adriamycin, cytosine arabinoside, vincristine, and prednisone (chemotherapy, oncology, and pharmacology)

HoaRhLG
horse antirhesus lymphocyte globulin (immunology and laboratory)

HoaTTG
horse antitetanus toxoid globulin (immunology and laboratory)

HOB
head of bed

HOBUPSOB
head of bed up for shortness of breath (respiratory)

HOC
Health Officer Certificate
human ovarian cancer (gynecology and oncology)
hydroxycorticoid (laboratory)

HOCM
hypertrophic obstructive cardiomyopathy (cardiovascular) {pronounced "hoe-come"}

hoc vesp
hoc vespere [this evening, tonight] (pharmacology)

hoc vesp.
hoc vespere [this evening, tonight] (pharmacology)

HOD
hyperbaric oxygen drenching (neurology, respiratory, and sports medicine)

HoD
Hodgkin's disease (oncology)

"hoe-come"
{pronunciation of *HOCM* [hypertrophic obstructive cardiomyopathy]} (cardiovascular) {not an abbreviation}

"hoe-moe"
{pronunciation of *homo* and *homo.* [homosexual]} (psychiatry) {not an abbreviation}

HofF
height of fundus (obstetrics)

Hoff
Hoffmann [reflex] (neurology and orthopedics)

HOG
halothane, oxygen, and gas [nitrous oxide] (anesthesiology)

HOH
hard of hearing (otorhinolaryngology)

HoIg
horse immunoglobulin (immunology and laboratory)

HOLD
hemostatic occlusive leverage device (cardiovascular)

HOM
hexamethylmelamine, Oncovin [vincristine], and methotrexate (chemotherapy, oncology, and pharmacology)

Homeo.
homeopathy (homeopathic medicine)

Homeop
homeopathy (homeopathic medicine)

homo
homosexual (psychiatry) {pronounced "hoe-moe"}

homo.
homosexual (psychiatry) {pronounced "hoe-moe"}

homolat.
homolateral

HOOD
hereditary osteo-onychodysplasia (orthopedics)

HOP
Adriamycin, vincristine, and prednisone (chemotherapy, oncology, and pharmacology)
high oxygen pressure (respiratory)
high-pressure oxygen (respiratory)

HOPE
health-oriented physical education (physical education)

HOPI
history of present illness

hor
horizontal

hor decu
hora decubitus [at bedtime] (pharmacology)

hor. decu.
hora decubitus [at bedtime] (pharmacology)

hor decub
hora decubitus [at bedtime] (pharmacology)

hor. decub.
hora decubitus [at bedtime] (pharmacology)

hor interm
horis intermediis [at the intermediate hours] (pharmacology)

hor. interm.
horis intermediis [at the intermediate hours] (pharmacology)

hor som
hora somni [at bedtime] (pharmacology)

hor. som.
hora somni [at bedtime] (pharmacology)

hor un spatio
horae unius spatio [at the end of one hour] (pharmacology)

hor. un. spatio
horae unius spatio [at the end of one hour] (pharmacology)

HOS
human osteosarcoma (oncology and orthopedics)

HoS
horse serum (immunology and laboratory)

HPS
hematoxylin-phloxine-saffron (chemistry
and laboratory)
high protein supplement (dietary and
pharmacology)
hypertrophic pyloric stenosis (gastroenterology)

HPT
human placental thyrotropin (endocrinology and laboratory)
hyperparathyroidism (endocrinology)

hPT
human placental thyrotropin (endocrinology and laboratory)

HPV
Hemophilus pertussis vaccine (pharmacology and respiratory)
human papillomavirus (laboratory)
hypoxic pulmonary vasoconstriction
(cardiovascular and respiratory)

HPVD
hypertensive pulmonary vascular disease (cardiovascular and respiratory)

HPV–DE
high-passage virus—duck embryo (laboratory)

HPV–DK
high-passage virus—dog kidney (laboratory)

HPVG
hepatic portal venous gas (laboratory)

HPZ
high-pressure zone

HQC
hydroquinone cream (pharmacology)

HR
hallux rigidus (orthopedics and podiatry)
Halstead-Reitan [neuropsychological
battery] (psychiatry)
Harrington rod (orthopedics)
heart rate (cardiovascular)
hemorrhagic retinopathy (ophthalmology)

heterosexual relations [scale] (psychiatry)
higher rate
hospital record (medical records)
Hospital Recruit
hospital report (medical records)
hour (measurement)

H-R
Holland-Rantos [company] (pharmacology)

H & R
hysterectomy and radiation (gynecology
and radiation therapy)

2HR
two-hour pregnancy test (laboratory and
obstetrics)

hr
hour (measurement)

hr.
hour (measurement)

HRA
Health Resources Administration
heart rate audiometry (cardiovascular)
histamine releasing activity (laboratory)

HRBC
horse red blood cells (laboratory)

HRC
horse red cells (laboratory)
Human Rights Committee

HRE
high-resolution electrocardiogram (cardiovascular)
high-resolution electrocardiography
(cardiovascular)

HRG
Health Research Group (research)

HRI
Harrington rod instrumentation (orthopedics)

HRIG
human rabies immune globulin (immunology and laboratory)

HRIg
human rabies immune globulin (immunology and laboratory)

HRL
head rotated left (neurology)

HRLA
human reovirus-like agent (laboratory)

hRNA
heterogeneous ribonucleic acid (genetics and laboratory)

HRP
horseradish peroxidase (chemistry)

hr pp
hours postprandial [usually preceded by a numeral] (laboratory and pharmacology)

HRR
head rotated right (neurology)
heart rate range (cardiovascular)

HRRC
Walt Disney Hearing Rehabilitation Research Center (otorhinolaryngology and research)

HRS
Hamilton Rating Scale
hepatorenal syndrome (gastroenterology and nephrology)
hormone receptor site (endocrinology and laboratory)

HRT
heart rate (cardiovascular)

HRV
human rotavirus (laboratory)

HS
half-strength
Hartman's solution (pharmacology)
head sling
heart sounds (cardiovascular)
heat stable (chemistry and laboratory)

heel spur (orthopedics)
heel stick [for blood samples] (laboratory)
heme synthetase (laboratory)
Henoch-Schönlein [syndrome; also called *allergic purpura*] (cardiovascular, dermatology, gastroenterology, nephrology, and rheumatology)
hereditary spherocytosis (hematology)
herpes simplex (infectious diseases and laboratory)
homologous serum (laboratory)
hora somni [at bedtime] (pharmacology)
horse serum (laboratory)
Hospital Ship
Hospital Staff
hour of sleep (pharmacology)
House Supervisor
House Surgeon
Hurler's syndrome (genetics)

H & S
hysterotomy and sterilization (gynecology)

H-S
heel-to-shin [test] (neurology)

H→S
heel-to-shin [test] (neurology)

hs
hora somni [at bedtime] (pharmacology)

h.s.
hora somni [at bedtime] (pharmacology)

HSA
Health Services Administration
Health Systems Agency (psychiatry)
horse serum albumin (pharmacology)
Hospital Savings Association
human serum albumin (gastroenterology, hematology, nephrology, and pharmacology)
hypersomnia-sleep apnea syndrome (neurology and respiratory)

HSAA
Health Sciences Advancement Award

HSAG
HEPES-saline-albumin-gelatin [*HEPES* is *hydroxyethylpiperazine ethanesulphonic acid.*] (chemistry)

HSAS
hypertrophic subaortic stenosis (cardiovascular)

HSBG
heel stick blood gas (cardiovascular, laboratory, and respiratory)

HSC
Health and Safety Commission [British]
hematopoietic stem cell (hematology and laboratory)

HSCA
Health Sciences Communications Association

HS-CoA
coenzyme A, reduced (laboratory)
reduced coenzyme A (laboratory)

HS-Co A
coenzyme A, reduced (laboratory)
reduced coenzyme A (laboratory)

HSD
hydroxysteroid dehydrogenase (laboratory)

HSE
Health and Safety Executive (administration)
herpes simplex encephalitis (neurology)

HSG
herpes simplex genitalis (gynecology, infectious diseases, and urology)
hysterosalpingogram (gynecology and radiology)

HSGB
hysterosalpingography (gynecology and radiology)

hSGF
human skeletal growth factor (endocrinology and laboratory)

HSHP
High School for Health Professions (education)

HSI
herpes simplex I [titer and virus] (dermatology and laboratory)

HS I
herpes simplex I [titer and virus] (dermatology and laboratory)

HSJ
Hôpital St Joseph [Paris, France]

HSL
herpes simplex labialis (gynecology and infectious diseases)

HSM
hepatosplenomegaly (gastroenterology)
holosystolic murmur (cardiovascular)

HSMHA
Health Services and Mental Health Administration (administration)

HSN
hereditary sensory neuropathy (neurology)

H₂SO₄
sulfuric acid (chemistry)

HSP
Health Systems Plan
Henoch-Schönlein purpura [also called *allergic purpura*] (cardiovascular, dermatology, gastroenterology, nephrology, and rheumatology)
Hospital Service Plan [British]
human serum prealbumin (laboratory)

HSQB
Health Standards and Quality Bureau

HSR
Harleco synthetic resin (chemistry)
heated serum reagin (laboratory)
homogeneous staining region (laboratory)

HSRA
Health Services and Resources Administration (administration)

HSRC
Human-Subjects Review Committee (research)

HSRD
hypertension secondary to renal disease (cardiovascular and nephrology)

HSRI
Health Systems Research Institute (research)

HSS
high-speed supernatant (laboratory)
Hospital and Specialist Service
hypertrophic subaortic stenosis (cardiovascular)

HSSE
high soap suds enema (gastroenterology)

HST
health screening tests (laboratory)

HSTF
human serum thymus factor (laboratory)

HSV
herpes simplex virus (infectious diseases and laboratory)

HSVE
herpes simplex virus encephalitis (infectious diseases and neurology)

HSV I
herpes simplex virus I (infectious diseases and laboratory)

HSV II
herpes simplex virus II (infectious diseases and laboratory)

HT
hammer toe (orthopedics and podiatry)
haustus [a draft, a draught] (pharmacology)
heart (cardiovascular)
heart transplant (cardiovascular)
height (measurement)
hemagglutination titer (laboratory)
high temperature (chemistry)
Histologic Technician (laboratory)
Histologic Technologist (laboratory)
home treatment (rehabilitation)
hospital train (transportation)
Hubbard tank (physical therapy)
Huhner test (laboratory)
human thrombin (hematology, laboratory, and pharmacology)
hydrotherapy (physical therapy)
hydroxytryptamine [serotonin] (pharmacology)
hypermetropia, total (ophthalmology)
hyperopia (ophthalmology)
hypertension (cardiovascular)
hyperthyroidism (endocrinology)
hypodermic tablet (pharmacology)
hypothalamus (neurology)

H.T.
hypodermic tablet (pharmacology)

H & T
hospitalization and treatment

3-HT
dopamine [also called *3-hydroxytyramine*] (pharmacology)

³HT
tritiated thymidine (genetics and laboratory)

5-HT
serotonin [also called *5-hydroxytryptamine*] (pharmacology)

Ht
total hypermetropia (ophthalmology)

Ht.
heart (cardiovascular)
height (measurement)
total hyperopia (ophthalmology)

ht
heart tones (cardiovascular)
heat
height (measurement)
high tension

HTA
hypophysiotropic area [of the hypothalamus] (neurology)
5-hydroxytryptamine [also called *serotonin*] (pharmacology)

5-HTA
5-hydroxytryptamine [also called *serotonin*] (pharmacology)

HTACS
human thyroid adenyl-cyclase stimulator (laboratory)

ht. aer.
heated aerosol (pharmacology)

HT(ASCP)
Histologic Technician (American Society of Clinical Pathologists) (laboratory)
Histologic Technologist (American Society of Clinical Pathologists) (laboratory)

HTAT
human tetanus antitoxin (pharmacology)

HTB
hot tub bath (physical therapy)

HTC
hepatoma cells (laboratory)
homozygous typing cells (laboratory)
hypertensive crisis (cardiovascular)

HTD
human therapeutic dose (pharmacology and radiation therapy)

HTF
heterothyrotropic factor (laboratory)
house feeding tube (dietary and gastroenterology)

HTH
homeostatic thymus hormone (endocrinology and laboratory)

HTHD
hypertensive heart disease (cardiovascular)

HTL
hearing threshold level (otorhinolaryngology)
human thymic leukemia (hematology and oncology)
hypermetropia, left (ophthalmology)

HTLA
high titer, low acidity (laboratory)

HTLV
human T-cell leukemia virus (hematology and laboratory)
human T-cell lymphotropic virus (immunology and laboratory)

HTLV-I
human T-cell lymphotropic virus type I (immunology and laboratory)

HTLV-II
human T-cell lymphotropic virus type II (immunology and laboratory)

HTLV-III
human T-cell lymphotropic virus type III (immunology and laboratory)

HTLV-III/LAV
human T-cell lymphotropic virus type III/lymphadenopathy-associated virus (immunology and laboratory)

HTN
hypertension (cardiovascular)
hypertensive (cardiovascular)

htn.
hypertension (cardiovascular)
hypertensive (cardiovascular)

HTO
heterotopic ossification (orthopedics)

high tibial osteotomy (orthopedics)
hospital transfer order
tritiated water (chemistry)

HTOH
hydroxytryptophol (laboratory)

HTP
House-Tree-Person [test] (psychiatry)
hydroxytryptophan (laboratory and
pharmacology)

5-HTP
5-hydroxytryptophan (laboratory and
pharmacology)

HTR
hypermetropia, right (ophthalmology)

HTS
heel-to-shin [test] (neurology)
human thyroid stimulator (endocrinology and laboratory)

H-TSH
human thyroid-stimulating hormone (endocrinology and laboratory)

hTSH
human thyroid-stimulating hormone (endocrinology and laboratory)

HTST
high temperature–short time [pasteur-
ization] (laboratory)

HTV
herpes-type virus (laboratory)

HTVD
hypertensive vascular disease (cardiovascular)

HU
Harvard University (education)
heat unit (physics)
hemagglutinating unit (laboratory)
hemolytic unit (laboratory)
hydroxyurea (chemotherapy, oncology,
and pharmacology)
hyperemia unit

HUC
hypouricemia (laboratory and nephrology)

HUIFM
human leukocyte interferon milieu (laboratory)

HUR
hydroxyurea (chemotherapy, oncology,
and pharmacology)

HUS
hemolytic-uremic syndrome (nephrology)
hyaluronidase unit for semen (laboratory)

HUTHAS
human thymus antiserum (laboratory)

HV
hallux valgus (orthopedics and podiatry)
has voided (urology)
hepatic vein (cardiovascular and gastroenterology)
hepatic venous (cardiovascular and gastroenterology)
herpes virus (laboratory)
home visit
hospital visit
hyperventilation (respiratory)

H & V
hemigastrectomy and vagotomy (gastroenterology and surgery)

HVA
homovanillic acid (laboratory)
3-methoxy-4-hydroxyphenylacetic acid
(laboratory)

H vag
Hemophilus vaginalis (gynecology and
laboratory)

HVC
Health Visitor's Certificate [British]

HVc
hyperstriatum ventrale, pars caudale (neurology)

HVD
hypertensive vascular disease (cardiovascular)

HVE
high-voltage electrophoresis (laboratory)

HVEM
high voltage electron microscope (laboratory)

HVG
host versus graft [response] (transplantation surgery)

HVH
herpes virus hominis (laboratory)

HVJ
hemagglutinating virus of Japan (laboratory)

HVL
half-value layer [also called *half-value thickness*] (radiation therapy and radiology)

HVM
high-velocity missile (armed forces)

HVR
hypoxic ventilatory response (respiratory)

HVS
herpes virus of Saimiri (laboratory)

HVSD
hydrogen-detected ventricular septal defect (cardiovascular)

HW
heparin well (pharmacology)
housewife

h wave
{not an abbreviation} [an occasional late filling wave on phlebograms] (cardiovascular)

HWB
hot water bottle (physical therapy)

hwb
hot water bottle (physical therapy)

HWC
Health and Welfare, Canada (government)

HWD
Hynson, Westcott, and Dunning [company] (pharmacology)

HW & D
Hynson, Westcott, and Dunning [company] (pharmacology)

HWS
hot water-soluble (pharmacology)

HWY
hundred woman years [of exposure]

Hx
history
hospitalization
hypoxanthine (laboratory)

Hx.
history
hospitalization

HXM
hexamethylmelamine (pharmacology)

HXV
herpes simplex virus (dermatology, infectious diseases, and laboratory)

Hy
hypermetropia (ophthalmology)
hypothenar (neurology and orthopedics)

Hy.
hypermetropia (ophthalmology)
hyperopia (ophthalmology)

hy.
hysteria (psychiatry)

HYD
hydrated
hydroxyurea (chemotherapy, oncology,
and pharmacology)

HYD'PR
hydroxyproline (laboratory)

hydra
hydraulic

hydrarg
hydrargyrum [mercury] (chemistry)

HYDRAT
chloral hydrate (neurology, pharmacology, and psychiatry)

Hydro
hydrotherapy (physical therapy) {pronounced "hi-drow"}

Hyg
hygiene

Hygst
Hygienist

HYL
hydroxylysine (laboratory)

HYLO
hyaline

HYP
hypnosis (psychiatry)

Hyp
hydroxyproline (laboratory)
hyperresonance
hypertrophy

hyperal.
hyperalimentation (gastroenterology)
{pronounced "hi-purr-al"}

hyper-al
hyperalimentation (gastroenterology)
{pronounced "hi-purr-al"}

hyperpara
hyperparathyroidism (endocrinology)
{pronounced "hi-per-par-ah"}

hyper. T & A
hypertrophy of tonsils and adenoids
(otorhinolaryngology)

Hypn
hypertension (cardiovascular)

hypno
hypnosis (psychiatry) {pronounced "hip-know"}
hypnotism (psychiatry) {pronounced "hip-know"}

hypo
hypochromasia (hematology and laboratory) {pronounced "hi-poe"}
hypochromia (laboratory) {pronounced "hi-poe"}
hypodermic [injection] (pharmacology) {pronounced "hi-poe"}

hypo-
{not an abbreviation} [prefix meaning *under*] {pronounced "hi-poe"}

HYPOC
hypochromasia (hematology and laboratory)

Hypox
hypophysectomized (endocrinology and neurosurgery)

HYPP
hypersegmented neutrophil (hematology and laboratory)

HypRho-D
{not an abbreviation} [trademark for a preparation of $Rh_o(D)$ immune serum globulin] (pharmacology)

Hypro
hydroxyproline (laboratory)

hys
hysteria (psychiatry)
hysterical (psychiatry)

hys.
hysteria (psychiatry)

HYST
hysterectomy (gynecology)

hyst
hysterectomy (gynecology)

hyster.
hysterectomy (gynecology)

HZ
herpes zoster (dermatology and neurology)

Hz
hertz (electricity and neurology)

Hz.
hertz (electricity and neurology)

HZO
herpes zoster ophthalmicus (ophthalmology)

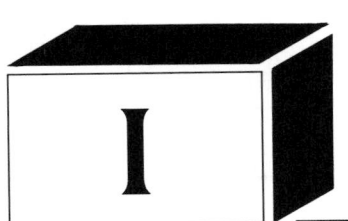

I

ι
iota [ninth letter of the Greek alphabet]

I
electric current (electricity)
impression
incisal (dentistry)
incisor [permanent] (dentistry)
independent
index
indicated
induction (anesthesiology)
inhibitor
inosine (laboratory)
inspired (respiratory)
intact
intensity of magnetism (physics)
internist
iodine (chemistry, laboratory, and pharmacology)
ionic strength (physics)
iota [ninth letter of the Greek alphabet]
moment of inertia (physics)
one [Roman numeral]
permanent incisor (dentistry)

I°
primary

I₂
iodine (chemistry, laboratory, and pharmacology)

I-123
radioactive iodine (radiology)

I¹²⁵
radioactive iodine (radiology)

¹²⁵I
radioactive iodine (radiology)

¹³⁰I
radioactive iodine (radiology)

I-131
radioactive iodine (radiology)

I¹³¹
radioactive iodine (radiology)

¹³¹I
radioactive iodine (radiology) {obsolete}

I-132
radioactive iodine (radiology)

I¹³²
radioactive iodine (radiology) {obsolete}

¹³²I
radioactive iodine (radiology)

i
deciduous incisor (dentistry)
incisor [deciduous] (dentistry)
insoluble
isochromosome (genetics)
optically inactive (chemistry)

i.
deciduous incisor (dentistry)
insoluble
optically inactive (chemistry)

IA
image amplification (radiology and surgery)
immune adherence (laboratory)
impedance angle (electricity)
incurred accidentally
indolaminergic-accumulating [cells] (laboratory)
indulin agar (laboratory)
infected area
inferior angle
internal auditory (otorhinolaryngology)
intra-amniotic (obstetrics)
intra-aortic (cardiovascular)
intra-arterial (cardiovascular)

intra-articular (orthopedics)
intra-atrial (cardiovascular)
intra-auricular (cardiovascular)
Iowa [Postal Service designation]

I.A.
impedance angle

I & A
irrigation and aspiration (ophthalmology)

I/A
irrigation and aspiration (ophthalmology)

Ia
immune region associated antigen (laboratory)
immune response gene-associated antigen (laboratory)

IAA
indole-3-acetic acid (laboratory)
International Antituberculosis Association (infectious diseases and respiratory)
interrupted aortic arch (cardiovascular)

IAB
identa-band [for patient identification]
Industrial Accident Board
intra-abdominal (surgery)
intra-aortic balloon [catheter and pump] (cardiovascular)

IABC
intra-aortic balloon catheter (cardiovascular)
intra-aortic balloon counterpulsation (cardiovascular)

IABP
intra-aortic balloon pump (cardiovascular)

IAC
internal auditory canal (otorhinolaryngology)
intra-arterial chemotherapy (chemotherapy, oncology, and pharmacology)
isolated adrenal cell (endocrinology and laboratory)

IACB
intraaortic counterpulsation balloon

IAC-CPR
interposed abdominal compressions—cardiopulmonary resuscitation (cardiovascular and respiratory)

IACP
intra-aortic counterpulsation (cardiovascular)

IACPA
Inter-American Council of Psychiatric Associations (psychiatry)

IACS
International Academy of Cosmetic Surgery (plastic surgery)

IACVF
International Association of Cancer Victims and Friends (oncology)

IAD
internal absorbed dose (radiation therapy)

IADH
inappropriate antidiuretic hormone (laboratory)

IADHS
inappropriate antidiuretic hormone syndrome (endocrinology)

IADR
International Association for Dental Research (dentistry and research)

IA DSA
intra-arterial digital subtraction arteriography (cardiovascular and radiology)

IAE
intra-atrial electrocardiogram (cardiovascular)

IAEA
International Atomic Energy Agency (chemistry and physics)

IAFI
infantile amaurotic familial idiocy (genetics and neurology)

IAG
International Association of Gerontology (geriatrics)

IAGP
International Association of Geographic Pathology (pathology)

IAGUS
International Association of Genito-Urinary Surgeons (urology)

IAH
implantable artificial heart (cardiovascular)

IAHA
immune adherence hemagglutination (laboratory)

IAHD
idiopathic acquired hemolytic disease (hematology)

IAHP
International Association of Heart Patients (cardiovascular)

IAHS
International Association for Hospital Security

IAI
intra-abdominal infection (gastroenterology and surgery)

IAL
International Association of Laryngectomees (otorhinolaryngology)

IAM
Institute of Aviation Medicine (aerospace medicine)
internal acoustic meatus (otorhinolaryngology)
internal auditory meatus (otorhinolaryngology)

IAMM
International Association of Medical Museums

IAN
interim admission note (medical records)
intern admission note (medical records)

I and O
intake and output (nursing)

IAO
immediately after onset
intermittent aortic occlusion (cardiovascular)

IAP
Institute of Animal Physiology [British] (veterinary medicine)
intermittent acute porphyria (nephrology)
International Academy of Pathology (pathology)
International Academy of Proctology (gastroenterology)

IAPB
International Association for Prevention of Blindness (ophthalmology)

IAPM
International Academy of Preventive Medicine

IAPP
International Association for Preventive Pediatrics (pediatrics)

IARC
International Agency for Research on Cancer (oncology and research)

IAS
interatrial septum (cardiovascular)
intra-amniotic saline [infusion] (obstetrics)

IASD
interatrial septal defect (cardiovascular)

IASHS
Institute for Advanced Study in Human
Sexuality (psychiatry)

IASL
International Association for Study of
the Liver (gastroenterology)

IASP
International Association for the Study
of Pain (neurology)

IAT
indirect antiglobulin test (laboratory)
invasive activity test (laboratory)
iodine azide test (laboratory)
Iowa Achievement Test (psychiatry)

IAV
intra-arterial vasopressin (cardiovascular and pharmacology)

IB
immune body (laboratory)
inclusion body (laboratory)
index of body build (measurement)
infectious bronchitis (respiratory)
Institute of Biology [British] (biology)
isolation bed (infectious diseases)

ib
ibidem [in the same place]

IBA
Industrial Biotechnology Association

IBB
intestinal brush border (gastroenterology)

IBC
Institutional Biosafety Committee
iodine-binding capacity (laboratory)
iron-binding capacity (laboratory)

IBD
inflammatory bowel disease (gastroenterology)
ischemic bowel disease (gastroenterology)

IBE
International Bureau for Epilepsy (neurology)

IBED
InterAfrican Bureau for Epizootic Diseases (veterinary medicine)

iB-EP
immunoreactive beta-endomorphin (laboratory)

IBF
immature brown fat [cells] (laboratory)
immunoglobulin-binding factor (immunology and laboratory)

I/B/F
{not an abbreviation} [a total knee instrumentation designed by John In-
stall, M.D., Albert Berstein, Ph.D., and
M.A.R. Freeman, M.D.] (orthopedics)

IBI
intermittent bladder irrigation (urology)

ibid
ibidem [in the same place]

IBK
infectious bovine keratoconjunctivitis
(infectious diseases and ophthalmology)

IBM
International Business Machines Corporation [manufacturer] (business)

IBMP
International Board of Medicine and
Psychology (psychology)

IBNR
incurred but not reported

IBP
International Biological Program (biology)
iron-binding protein (laboratory)

IBPMS
indirect blood pressure measuring system (cardiovascular)

IBR
infectious bovine rhinotracheitis (infectious diseases and otorhinolaryngology)

IBRO
International Brain Research Organization (neurology and research)

IBRV
infective bovine rhinotracheitis virus (laboratory)

IBS
irritable bowel syndrome (gastroenterology)

IBT
Industrial Bio-Test Laboratories (laboratory)
ink blot test [Rorschach test] (psychiatry)
isatin-beta-thiosemicarbosone (laboratory)

IBU
international benzoate unit (chemistry)

IBV
infectious bronchitis vaccine (pharmacology and respiratory)

IBW
ideal body weight (measurement)

IC
icteric (dermatology, gastroenterology, and ophthalmology)
ileocecal (gastroenterology)
iliococcygeal [muscle] (orthopedics)
iliocostal [muscle] (orthopedics)
immune complex (laboratory)
immune cytotoxicity (laboratory)
immunocytochemistry (laboratory)
incomplete
indirect calorimetry (physiology)
individual counseling (psychiatry)
inferior colliculus (neurology and otorhinolaryngology)
inhibiting concentration
inorganic carbon (chemistry)
inspiratory capacity [also called *respiratory capacity*] (laboratory and respiratory)

inspiratory center (respiratory)
Institutional Care [British]
instruction counter (computer science)
integrated circuit (electronics)
intensive care
intercostal [space] (respiratory)
intermediate care
intermittent catheterization (urology)
intermittent claudication (cardiovascular)
internal capsule (neurology)
internal carotid [artery] (cardiovascular)
internal cerebral (neurology)
internal cholecystectomy (gastroenterology and surgery)
internal conjugate [diameter] (gynecology)
International Classification
interstitial cells (laboratory)
intracardiac (cardiovascular)
intracarotid (cardiovascular)
intracavitary
intracellular (laboratory)
intracellular concentration (laboratory)
intracerebral (neurology)
intracisternal (neurology)
intracranial (neurology)
intracutaneous [injection] (pharmacology)
intrapleural catheter (respiratory)
irritable colon (gastroenterology)
islet cells [of the pancreas] (endocrinology and laboratory)
isovolumic contraction

Ic
intermittent catheterization (urology)

ic
inter cibos [between meals] (pharmacology)

i.c.
inter cibos [between meals] (pharmacology)

ICA
Institute of Clinical Analysis
internal carotid artery (cardiovascular and neurology)

intracranial aneurysm (cardiovascular and neurology)
islet cell antibodies (laboratory)

ICAA
International Council on Alcohol and Addictions (chemical dependency)
Invalid Children's Aid Association (pediatrics)

ICAMI
International Committee Against Mental Illness (psychiatry)

ICAO
internal carotid artery occlusion (cardiovascular and neurology)

ICAV
intracavitary

ICBP
intracellular binding protein (laboratory)

ICBT
intercostobronchial trunk (respiratory)

ICC
immunocompetent cell (laboratory)
immunocytochemistry (chemistry and laboratory)
Indian childhood cirrhosis (gastroenterology and pediatrics)
Information Center Complex
intensive coronary care (cardiovascular)
Internal Conversion Coefficient (radiology)

ICCE
intracapsular cataract extraction (ophthalmology)

ICCM
idiopathic congestive cardiomyopathy (cardiovascular)

ICCR
International Committee for Contraceptive Research (gynecology, obstetrics, and research)

ICCU
intensive coronary care unit (cardiovascular)
intermediate coronary care unit (cardiovascular)

ICD
immune complex disease (immunology)
instantaneous cardiac death (cardiovascular)
Institute for Crippled and Disabled (rehabilitation)
International Center for the Disabled (rehabilitation)
International Classification of Diseases [of the World Health Organization]
International College of Dentists (dentistry)
intrauterine contraceptive device (gynecology)
isocitrate dehydrogenase (laboratory)

I.C.D.
International Classification of Diseases [of the World Health Organization]

ICDA
International Classification of Diseases, Adapted

ICD 9 CM
International Classification of Diseases, Ninth Revision, Clinical Modification

ICDH
isocitric dehydrogenase (laboratory)

ICEA
International Childbirth Education Association (education and obstetrics)

ICF
indirect centrifugal flotation (laboratory)
Intensive Care Facility
Intermediate Care Facility
International Cardiology Foundation (cardiovascular)
intracellular fluid (laboratory)
intravascular coagulation and fibrinolysis [syndrome] (hematology)

ICF(M)A
International Cystic Fibrosis (Mucovisci-dosis) Association (respiratory)

ICFMR
Intermediate Care Facility for the Mentally Retarded (psychiatry)

ICG
indocyanine green (laboratory)

ICH
infectious canine hepatitis (gastroenterology and infectious diseases)
intracranial hemorrhage (cardiovascular and neurology)

ICJ
ileocecal junction (gastroenterology)

ICLA
International Committee on Laboratory Animals (laboratory, research, and veterinary medicine)

ICLE
intracapsular lens extraction (ophthalmology)

ICLH
Imperial College, London Hospital [orthopedic device] (orthopedics)

ICM
infracostal margin (anatomy)
inner cell mass (laboratory)
intercostal margin (anatomy)
International Confederation of Midwives (obstetrics)

ICN
Intensive Care Nursery (neonatology)
International Council of Nurses (nursing)

I.C.N.N.D.
Interdepartmental Committee on Nutrition in National Defense (armed forces and dietary)

ICON
{not an abbreviation} [a serum pregnancy test] (laboratory and obstetrics)

ICP
Infection-control Practitioner (infectious diseases)
intracranial pressure (neurology)

ICPA
International Committee for the Prevention of Alcoholism (chemical dependency)

ICPC
intracranial pressure catheter (neurology)

ICPI
Intersociety Committee on Pathology Information (pathology)

I, C, PM, M
incisors, canines, premolars, molars
[*When each portion is followed by a fraction, the complete expression is the formula of permanent dentition.*] (dentistry)

ICPP
intubated continuous positive pressure (respiratory)
Isochromic Color Perception Plates (ophthalmology)

ICR
distance between iliac crests (orthopedics and surgery)
Institute for Cancer Research (oncology and research)
intensive care room
International Congress of Radiology (radiology)
intracranial reinforcement (maxillofacial surgery and neurology)

ICRC
International Committee of the Red Cross (emergency medicine)

ICRD
Index of Codes for Research Drugs (pharmacology and research)

ICRETT
International Cancer Research Technology Transfer (oncology and research)

ICREW
International Cancer Research Workshop (oncology and research)

ICRF
Imperial Cancer Research Fund [British] (oncology and research)

ICRF-159
razoxane (chemotherapy, oncology, and pharmacology)

ICRFSDD
Independent Citizens Research Foundation for the Study of Degenerative Diseases (research)

ICRP
International Commission on Radiological Protection (radiology)

ICRU
International Commission on Radiological Units and Measurements (radiology)

ICS
Imperial College of Science [British]
impulse-conducting system (electricity)
Intensive Care, Surgical (surgery)
intercostal space (anatomy)
International Cardiovascular Study (cardiovascular and research)
International College of Surgeons (surgery)
International Craniopathic Society (neurology)
intracellular-like solution [cardioplegic solution] (cardiovascular and pharmacology)
intracranial stimulation (neurology)

ICSH
International Committee for Standardization in Haematology [Hematology] (hematology)
interstitial cell-stimulating hormone [luteinizing hormone] (endocrinology and laboratory)

I.C.S.P.
International Council of Societies of Pathology (pathology)

ICSS
intracranial self-stimulation (neurology)

ICSU
International Council of Scientific Unions

ICT
icterus (dermatology, gastroenterology, and ophthalmology)
indirect Coombs' test (laboratory)
inflammation of connective tissue (rheumatology)
insulin coma therapy (endocrinology and neurology)
intensive conventional therapy
intermittent cervical traction (orthopedics)
isometric contraction time
isovolumic contraction time

I.C.T.
intermittent cervical traction (orthopedics)

iCT
immunoreactive calcitonin (laboratory)

ICTH
International Committee on Thrombosis and Homeostasis (cardiovascular and hematology)

ict. ind.
icterus index (dermatology, gastroenterology, and ophthalmology)

Ict Index
icterus index (dermatology, gastroenterology, and ophthalmology)

ICTMM
International Congress on Tropical Medicine and Malaria (infectious diseases)

ICTV
International Committee on Taxonomy
   of Viruses (virology)

ICU
intensive care unit
intermediate care unit

ICV
intracerebroventricular (neurology)

ICVH
ischemic cerebrovascular headache
   (cardiovascular and neurology)

ICVS
International Cardiovascular Society
   (cardiovascular)

ICW
intracellular water (laboratory)

ID
Idaho [Postal Service designation]
idem [the same]
identification
identify
iditol dehydrogenase (laboratory)
immunodeficiency (immunology)
immunodiffusion (laboratory)
inclusion disease
index of discrimination
infant deaths (neonatology)
infectious disease(s)
infective dose
inferior division
inhibitory dose
initial dose
injected dose
inside diameter
internal diameter
intradermal (dermatology)
intraduodenal (gastroenterology)

I.D.
infective dose

I & D
incision and drainage (surgery)
irrigation and debridement (surgery)
irrigation and drainage (surgery)

ID$_{50}$
median infectious dose

median infective dose

Id
idem [the same]
intradermal (dermatology)

id
idem [the same]

id.
idem [the same]

IDA
image display and analysis
iron deficiency anemia (hematology)
iminodiacetic acid

id. ac
idem ac [the same as]

IDAMIS
Integrated Dose Abuse Management Informational Systems (chemical dependency and pharmacology)

IDARP
Integrated Drug Abuse Reporting Process (chemical dependency, pharmacology, and statistics)

IDB
incomplete data base (statistics)

IDBR
indirect bilirubin (laboratory)

IDCF
immunodiffusion complement fix (immunology and laboratory)

IDD
insulin-dependent diabetes [mellitus]
   (endocrinology)

IDDM
insulin-dependent diabetes mellitus (endocrinology)

IDDS
implantable drug delivery system (pharmacology)

IDE
Investigational Device Exemption (research)

ID/ED
internal diameter to external diameter
[ratio for cardiac valve replacement]
(cardiovascular)

IDFC
immature dead female child (neonatology and obstetrics)

IDH
isocitric dehydrogenase (laboratory)

IDI
induction-delivery interval (obstetrics)
Instant Drug Index [publication] (pharmacology)

IDIC
Internal Dose Information Center (radiology)

IDK
internal derangement of knee [joint] (orthopedics)

IDL
intermediate-density lipoprotein (laboratory)

IDM
idiopathic disease of the myocardium
(cardiovascular)
indirect method
infant of diabetic mother (neonatology)

IDMC
immature dead male child (neonatology
and obstetrics)

ID-MS
isotope dilution-mass spectrometry (laboratory)

idon vehic
idoneo vehiculo [in a suitable vehicle]
(pharmacology)

IDP
immunodiffusion procedures
initial dose period

inosine diphosphate (laboratory)
instantaneous diastolic pressure (cardiovascular)

IDPH
idiopathic pulmonary hemosiderosis
(hematology and respiratory)

IDPN
beta-iminodipropionitrile [*β-iminodipro-
pionitrile* or *iminodipropionitrile*]
(laboratory)

IDR
intradermal reaction (dermatology)

IDS
immunity deficiency state (immunology)
Infectious Disease Service (infectious
diseases)
incremented dynamic scanning
Investigative Dermatological Society
(dermatology and research)

IDSA
Infectious Disease Society of America
(infectious diseases)
Intraoperative digital subtraction angiography

IDT
International Diagnostic Technology
(laboratory)

IDU
idoxuridine (ophthalmology and pharmacology)
iododeoxyuridine (pharmacology)

IdUA
iduronic acid (laboratory)

IDV
intermittent demand ventilation (respiratory)

IDVC
indwelling venous catheter (cardiovascular)

IE
immunitäts Einheit [immunizing unit]
(laboratory)
immunoelectrophoresis (laboratory)
intake energy [unit of food] (dietary)

I/E
inspiratory-expiratory [ratio] (respiratory)

I:E
inspiratory-expiratory [ratio] (respiratory)

I.E.
immunitäts Einheit [immunizing unit]
(laboratory)

ie
id est [that is]

i.e.
id est [that is]

IEA
immunoelectroadsorption (laboratory)
immunoenzyme assay (laboratory)
International Epidemiological Association (epidemiology)
intravascular erythrocyte aggregation
(hematology and laboratory)

IEC
injection electrode catheter (cardiovascular)
inpatient exercise center (rehabilitation)
intraepithelial carcinoma (dermatology
and oncology)
ion exchange chromatography (physics)

IEE
inner enamel epithelium (dentistry)

IEF
International Eye Foundation (ophthalmology)
isoelectric focusing (laboratory)

IEL
intraepithelial lymphocytes (laboratory)

IEM
immune electron microscopy (laboratory)
inborn error of metabolism (laboratory)

IEMG
integrated electromyogram (neurology)

IEOP
immunoelectro-osmophoresis (laboratory)

IEP
immunoelectrophoresis (laboratory)
individual(ized) education(al) program
(education)
isoelectric point (laboratory)

IF
immunofluorescence [test] (laboratory
and ophthalmology)
infrared (chemistry)
inhibiting factor (laboratory)
interferon (laboratory and pharmacology)
intermediate frequency
internal fixation (orthopedics)
interstitial fluid (respiratory)
intrinsic factor (laboratory)
involved field (radiation therapy)

IFA
immunofluorescence assay (laboratory)
indirect fluorescent antibody [test] (laboratory)
International Fertility Association (gynecology, obstetrics, and urology)
International Filariasis Association (infectious diseases)

IFC
intrinsic factor concentrate (laboratory)

IFCC
International Federation of Clinical
Chemistry (chemistry)

IFCR
International Foundation for Cancer Research (oncology and research)

IFCS
inactivated fetal calf serum (laboratory)

IFFH
International Foundation for Family Health

IFGO
International Federation of Gynecology and Obstetrics (gynecology and obstetrics)

IFHP
International Federation of Health Professionals

IFHPMSM
International Foundation for Hygiene, Preventive Medicine, and Social Medicine

IFLrA
recombinant human leukocyte interferon A (laboratory and pharmacology)

IFM
intrafusal muscle (orthopedics)

IFMBE
International Federation for Medical and Biological Engineering (engineering)

IFME
International Federation for Medical Electronics (electronics)

IFMP
International Federation for Medical Psychotherapy (psychiatry)

IFMSA
International Federation of Medical Student Associations (education)

IFMSS
International Federation of Multiple Sclerosis Societies (neurology)

IFN
interferon (laboratory and pharmacology)

If nec
if necessary

IFPM
International Federation of Physical Medicine (rehabilitation)

IFR
infrared (chemistry)
inspiratory flow rate (respiratory)

IFRA
indirect fluorescent rabies antibody [test] (laboratory)

IFRP
International Fertility Research Program (gynecology, obstetrics, and research)

IFSM
International Federation of Sports Medicine (sports medicine)

IFT
International Frequency Tables

IFV
intracellular fluid volume (laboratory)

IG
immunoglobulin (immunology and laboratory)
intragastric (gastroenterology)

Ig
gamma immunoglobulin [*immunoglobulin* or *γ-immunoglobulin*] (immunology and laboratory)

IgA
gamma A immunoglobulin [*immunoglobulin A*] (immunology and laboratory)

IgA1
{not an abbreviation} [an immunoglobulin A subclass] (immunology and laboratory)

IgA2
{not an abbreviation} [an immunoglobu-

lin A subclass] (immunology and laboratory)

IgD
gamma D immunoglobulin [*immunoglobulin D*] (immunology and laboratory)

IGDM
infant of gestational diabetic mother (neonatology)

IgE
gamma E immunoglobulin [*immunoglobulin E*] (immunology and laboratory)

IGF
insulin-like growth factor (endocrinology and laboratory)

IGFET
insulated gate field effect transistor (electronics)

IgG
gamma G immunoglobulin [*immunoglobulin G*] (immunology and laboratory)

IgG1
{not an abbreviation} [an immunoglobulin G subclass] (immunology and laboratory)

IgG2
{not an abbreviation} [an immunoglobulin G subclass] (immunology and laboratory)

IgG3
{not an abbreviation} [an immunoglobulin G subclass] (immunology and laboratory)

IgG4
{not an abbreviation} [an immunoglobulin G subclass] (immunology and laboratory)

IGH
idiopathic growth hormone (endocrinology and laboratory)

immunoreactive growth hormone (endocrinology and laboratory)

IGIV
immune globulin intravenous (immunology and pharmacology)

IgM
gamma M immunoglobulin [*immunoglobulin M*] (immunology and laboratory)

IGP
intestinal glycoprotein (laboratory)

IGR
intrauterine growth retardation (neonatology and obstetrics)

IGS
inappropriate gonadotropin secretion (endocrinology)

IGT
impaired glucose tolerance (endocrinology)

IgT
{not an abbreviation} [a hypothetical antigen receptor on T cell surfaces] (laboratory)

IGV
intrathoracic gas volume (laboratory and respiratory)

IH
immediate hypersensitivity (allergy)
indirect hemagglutination (laboratory)
Industrial Hygienist
infectious hepatitis (gastroenterology and infectious diseases)
inguinal hernia (gastroenterology and surgery)
inhibiting hormone (laboratory)
inner half
in-patient hospital
iron hematoxylin (laboratory)

I.H.
infectious hepatitis (gastroenterology and infectious diseases)

IHA
indirect hemagglutination [test] (laboratory)
infusion hepatic arteriography (radiology)

IHAC
Industrial Health and Advisory Committee [British]

IHAS
idiopathic hypertrophic aortic stenosis (cardiovascular)

IHB
incomplete heart block (cardiovascular)

IHBTD
incompatible hemolytic blood transfusion disease (hematology)

IHC
idiopathic hemochromatosis (hematology)
idiopathic hypercalciuria (nephrology)
immobilization hypercalcemia
inner hair cell [of the cochlea] (otorhinolaryngology)

IHCP
Institute of Hospital and Community Psychiatry (psychiatry)

IHD
intrahepatic duct (gastroenterology and surgery)
intrahepatic ductulus (gastroenterology and surgery)
ischemic heart disease (cardiovascular)

IHF
Industrial Health Foundation
International Hospital Federation

IHH
idiopathic hypogonadotropic hypogonadism (endocrinology)

IHL
International Homeopathic League (homeopathic medicine)

IHO
idiopathic hypertrophic osteoarthropathy (orthopedics)

IHOP
Adriamycin, isophosphamide, vincristine, and prednisone (chemotherapy, oncology, and pharmacology)

IHP
idiopathic hypoparathyroidism (endocrinology)
inverted hand position (neurology and orthopedics)

IHPH
intrahepatic portal hypertension (cardiovascular and nephrology)

IHPP
Intergovernmental Health Project Policy (government)

IHR
intrahepatic resistance (gastroenterology)
intrinsic heart rate (cardiovascular)

IHRB
Industrial Health Research Board [British] (research)

IHS
Idiopathic Headache Score (neurology)
inactivated horse serum (laboratory)
Indian Health Service
International Health Society

IHs
iris hamartoma (oncology and ophthalmology)

IHSA
iodinated human serum albumin (laboratory)

IHSS
idiopathic hypertrophic subaortic stenosis (cardiovascular) {pronounced "ash"}

IHT
insulin hypoglycemia test (endocrinology and laboratory)
intravenous histamine test (allergy)

IHW
inner heel wedge (orthopedics and podiatry)

II
image intensification (radiology and surgery)
two [Roman numeral]

ii
{not an abbreviation} [symbol for *bid in die* (twice a day)] (pharmacology)

IICP
increased intracranial pressure (neurology)

IICU
infant intensive care unit (neonatology)

IID
insulin-dependent diabetes [mellitus] (endocrinology)

I-IDDM
type I insulin-dependent diabetes mellitus (endocrinology)

IIF
immune interferon (laboratory and pharmacology)
indirect immunofluorescence (laboratory)
indirect immunofluorescent (laboratory)

III
three [Roman numeral]

iii
{not an abbreviation} [symbol for *ter in die* (three times a day)] (pharmacology)

III-para
tertipara (obstetrics)

IIME
Institute of International Medical Education (education)

II-NIDD
type II noninsulin-dependent diabetes [mellitus] (endocrinology)

II-para
secundipara (obstetrics)

IIS
International Institute of Stress (psychiatry)

IJ
ileojejunal (gastroenterology and surgery)
internal jugular (cardiovascular)

I-J
internal jugular (cardiovascular)

IJP
inhibitory junction potential (neurology)
internal jugular pressure (cardiovascular)

IK
immunekörper [immune body] (laboratory)
immunoconglutinin (laboratory)
infusoria killing [unit] (laboratory)

I.K.
immunekörper [immune body] (laboratory)

IL
Illinois [Postal Service designation]
incisolingual (dentistry)
interleukin [1, 2, and 3] (chemotherapy, oncology, and pharmacology)
Intralipid (pharmacology)
intraocular lens (ophthalmology)

IL 1
interleukin 1 (chemotherapy, oncology, and pharmacology)

IL 2
interleukin 2 (chemotherapy, oncology, and pharmacology)

IL 3
interleukin 3 (chemotherapy, oncology, and pharmacology)

Il
illinium [previous name for *promethium*] (chemistry)
illustration

ILA
insulin-like activity (endocrinology and laboratory)
International Leprosy Association (infectious diseases)

ILa
incisolabial (dentistry)

ILB
infant low birth [weight] (neonatology and obstetrics)

ILBW
infant low birth weight (neonatology and obstetrics)

ILC
incipient lethal concentration (radiation therapy)

ILD
interstitial lung disease (respiratory)
ischemic leg disease (cardiovascular and orthopedics)
ischemic limb disease (cardiovascular and orthopedics)

Ile
isoleucine (laboratory)

Ileu
isoleucine (laboratory)

ILFC
immature living female child (neonatology and obstetrics)

ILL
intermediate lymphocytic lymphoma (oncology)

ill
illusion (psychiatry)

illus
illustrated
illustration

ILM
insulin-like material (endocrinology and laboratory)
internal limiting membrane (neurology)

ILMC
immature living male child (neonatology and obstetrics)

ILMI
inferolateral myocardial infarct(ion) (cardiovascular)

ILMN
incomplete lower motor neuron [lesion] (neurology)

ILo
iodine lotion (pharmacology)

ILS
infrared live scanner (radiology)

ILSI
International Life Sciences Institute

ILSS
Integrated Life Support Systems (emergency medicine)

IM
immunosuppression method
Index Medicus (publishing)
Industrial Medicine
infectious mononucleosis (infectious diseases)
intermetatarsal (orthopedics and podiatry)
intermuscular (orthopedics and surgery)
Internal Medicine

internal monitor (obstetrics)
intramedullary (hematology and orthopedics)
intramuscular [injection] (pharmacology)
Institute of Medicine
invasive mole (dermatology)

I.M.
intramuscular [injection] (pharmacology)
intramuscularly

IMA
Industrial Medical Association
inferior mesenteric artery (cardiovascular)
Interchurch Medical Assistance (religion)
internal mammary artery (cardiovascular)
Irish Medical Association

IMAA
iodinated macroaggregated albumin
(gastroenterology, laboratory, nephrology, and pharmacology)

^{131}IMAA
radioiodinated macroaggregated albumin (radiology)

IMAG
internal mammary artery graft (cardiovascular)

IMB
Institute of Microbiology (microbiology)
intermenstrual bleeding (gynecology)

IMBC
indirect maximum breathing capacity
(respiratory)

IMBI
Institute of Medical and Biological Illustrators (publishing)

IMC
internal mammary chain

IMD
immunologically mediated diseases (immunology)

ImD$_{50}$
the immunizing dose of vaccine or antigen sufficient to protect 50 percent of
the animals in a particular test group
(immunology, pharmacology, and research)

IME
independent medical examination
independent medical examiner

IMEM
improved minimum essential medium
(laboratory)

IMF
intermaxillary fixation (dentistry and
oral surgery)

IMG
inferior mesenteric ganglion (neurology)
internal medicine group [group prac-
tices]

IMH
idiopathic myocardial hypertrophy (cardiovascular)
indirect microhemagglutination [test]
(laboratory)

IMHP
1-iodomercuri-2-hydroxypropane (chemistry)

IMI
imipramine (pharmacology)
inferior myocardial infarction (cardiovascular)
intramuscular injection (pharmacology)

IMIG
intramuscular immunoglobulin (immunology and pharmacology)

IMIC
International Medical Information Center (statistics)

IMM
inhibitor-containing minimal medium
(laboratory)

immat
immature (laboratory)

immed
immediately

immobil
immobilize (orthopedics and rehabilitation)

Immu-G
{not an abbreviation} [trademark for a preparation of immune globulin] (pharmacology)

immun
immunity (immunology)
immunization (immunology, pediatrics, and pharmacology)

IMMUNO
immunoglobulin (immunology and laboratory)

Immunol
immunology

IMN
internal mammary [lymph] node

IMNS
Imperial Military Nursing Service (armed forces and nursing)

IMP
impacted (dentistry, gastroenterology, and orthopedics)
impaction (dentistry, gastroenterology, and orthopedics)
impression
inosine monophosphate (laboratory)
inosine-5'-monophosphate (laboratory)
inosinic acid (laboratory)
intramembranous particle

imp
impacted (dentistry, gastroenterology, and orthopedics)
imperfect
important
impression
improved

IMPA
incisal mandibular plane angle (dentistry and otorhinolaryngology)

IMPAC
Immediate Psychiatric Aid and Referral Center (psychiatry)

IMPC
International Myopia Prevention Centre (ophthalmology)

IMPL
impulse

IMPRV
improvement

IMPS
Inpatient Multidimensional Psychiatric Scale (psychiatry)

Impx
impaction (dentistry, gastroenterology, and orthopedics)

IMR
Individual Medical Record (medical records)
infant mortality rate (neonatology and statistics)
Institute for Medical Research (research)
International Medical Research (research)

IMRAD
introduction, methods, results, and discussion

IMS
incurred in military service (armed forces)
Indian Medical Service
Integrated Medical Services
International Medication Systems (pharmacology)
International Metric System (measurements)

IMSS
In-flight Medical Support System (emergency medicine)

IMT
induced muscular tension (neurology)

IMTLYM
immature lymphocytes (hematology and laboratory)

IMV
inferior mesenteric vein
intermittent mandatory ventilation (respiratory)
intermittent mechanical ventilation (respiratory)
isophosphamide, vincristine, and methotrexate (chemotherapy, oncology, and pharmacology)

IMViC
indole, methyl red, Voges-Proskauer, citrate [reaction and test] (laboratory)

imvic
indole, methyl red, Voges-Proskauer, citrate [reaction and test] (laboratory)

IMVP-16
isophosphamide, methotrexate, and VP-16 (chemotherapy, oncology, and pharmacology)

IMVS
Institute of Medical and Veterinary Sciences [Australia] (veterinary medicine)

IN
icterus neonatorum (dermatology, gastroenterology, neonatology, and ophthalmology)
Indiana [Postal Service designation]
initial [dose] (pharmacology and radiation therapy)
insulin (pharmacology)
interneuron (neurology)
intranasal (otorhinolaryngology)

In
indium (chemistry)
inulin (chemistry)

in
inch (measurement)

in.
inch (measurement)

5 in 1
five in one [procedure done for ligamentous repair of knee rotary instability] (orthopedics)

INA
International Neurological Association (neurology)
Jena Nomina Anatomica [with reference to anatomical terminology] (anatomy)

INAD
infantile neuroaxonal dystrophy (neonatology, neurology, and pediatrics)

INAH
isonicotinic acid hydrazide [also called *isoniazid* and *INH*] (infectious diseases, pharmacology, and respiratory)

INC
including
incomplete
inconclusive
incontinent (gastroenterology and urology)
increase(d)
increasing
inside-the-needle catheter (cardiovascular, radiology, and surgery)

Inc
including
incorporated
increase

inc
including
increase
incurred

Inc Ab
incomplete abortion (obstetrics)

IncB
inclusion body (laboratory)

incl.
including

incomp
incomplete

incompl
incomplete

incont
incontinent (gastroenterology and urology)

inc (R)
increase (relative)

incr
increase(d)
increasing
increment

INCS
incomplete resolution, scan to follow (radiology)

incur
incurable

IND
industrial
Investigational New Drug (pharmacology)

ind
independent
induction (anesthesiology)

in d
in dies [daily] (pharmacology)

in d.
in dies [daily] (pharmacology)

INDEP
independent (occupational therapy)

INDIA
India ink [cerebrospinal fluid test] (laboratory)

indic
indicated
indication

INDIR
indirect Coombs test (hematology and laboratory)

INDIV
individual

INDM
infant of nondiabetic mother (neonatology)

IndMed
Index Medicus (publishing)

Ind. Med.
Index Medicus (publishing)

indust
industrial

INE
infantile necrotizing encephalomyelopathy (neurology)

INEX
inexperienced

INF
infant(ile) (neonatology)
infected
infection
inferior
infirmary
infunde [pour in] (pharmacology)
infusum [infusion] (chemotherapy and pharmacology)

inf
infant (neonatology, obstetrics, and pediatrics)
infected
inferior
infunde [pour in] (pharmacology)
infusum [infusion] (chemotherapy and pharmacology)

infect
infection
infectious

INFH
ischemic necrosis of femoral head (orthopedics)

infil
infiltrate (respiratory and radiology)
infiltrated

inflam
inflammation
inflammatory

INFM
infectious mononucleosis (infectious diseases)

inf. mono.
infectious mononucleosis (infectious diseases)

info
information {pronounced "in-foe"}

"in-foe"
{pronunciation of *info* [information]} {not an abbreviation}

INFORM
International Reference Organization in Forensic Medicine and Sciences (forensic medicine)

ING
inguinal (gastroenterology and surgery)

ing
inguinal (gastroenterology and surgery)

InGP
indolglycerophosphate

INH
inhalation (respiratory)
isonicotine hydrazine [also called *isoniazid, isonicotinic acid hydrazide,* and *isonicotinoylhydrazine*] (infectious diseases, pharmacology, and respiratory) {not an abbreviation} [brand name for *isoniazid* (isonicotinic acid hydra-

zide)] (infectious diseases, pharmacology, and respiratory)

inhal
inhalatio [inhalation] (respiratory)

inhib
inhibition
inhibitory

INI
intranuclear inclusion [agent] (laboratory)

inj
inject (pharmacology)
injectable (pharmacology)
injection (pharmacology)
injurious
injury

inject
injection (pharmacology)

inj enem
injiciatur enema [let an enema be injected] (pharmacology)

inj. enem.
injiciatur enema [let an enema be injected] (pharmacology)

inl.
inlay (dentistry)

in litt
in litteris [in correspondence]

INN
International Nonproprietary Name

I.N.N.
International Nonproprietary Name

innerv
innervated (neurology)
innervation (neurology)

INO
intranuclear ophthalmoplegia (ophthalmology) [*Note:* Do not confuse with

I and O or *I & O* (in and out or intake and output)]

ino
inosine (genetics and laboratory)

inoc
inoculate(d) (immunology and pharmacology)
inoculation (immunology and pharmacology)

inop
inoperable (oncology)
inoperative (oncology)

inorg
inorganic (chemistry and laboratory)

inor phos
inorganic phosphorus (chemistry and laboratory)

INPH
iproniazid phosphate (pharmacology)

INPRONS
information processing in the central nervous system (neurology)

IN-PT
inpatient

in pulm
in pulmento [in gruel] (pharmacology)

INPV
intermittent negative-pressure assisted ventilation (respiratory)

INREM
internal radiation dose (radiation therapy)

INS
idiopathic nephrotic syndrome (nephrology)
insurance

Ins.
insulin (endocrinology and pharmacology)

ins
insurance

INS AB
insulin antibody (endocrinology and laboratory)

INSDEN
Inspector of Dental Activities (dentistry)

"in-sigh-too"
{pronunciation of *in situ* [in natural or normal position]} {not an abbreviation}

in situ
{not an abbreviation} [in natural or normal position] {pronounced "in-sigh-too"}

insol
insoluble (chemistry)

INSP
inspiration (respiratory)
inspiratory (respiratory)

Insp
inspection
inspiration (respiratory)
inspiratory (respiratory)

INSPEC
inspection
inspector

inspir
inspiration (respiratory)
inspiratory (respiratory)

INST
instrumental delivery (obstetrics)

Inst
institute

Instn
institution

Instr
instruction
instructor

INSU
intensive neurosurgery unit (neurosurgery)

insuf
insufficient
insufflatio [an insufflation]

insuff
insufflation

INT
intermittent
intern (education)
internal
internist
internship (education)
internal

int
intermediate
intermittent
internal

int cib
inter cibos [between meals] (pharmacology)

int. cib.
inter cibos [between meals] (pharmacology)

INTEG
integument (dermatology)

intell
intelligence (psychiatry)

intern
internal {pronounced "in-turn"}

internat
international

INTEST
intestinal (gastroenterology)

INTH
intrathecal (anesthesiology and neurology)

INTL
internal

INTMD
intermediate

IntMed
internal medicine

int. med.
internal medicine

int noct
inter noctem [during the night] (pharmacology)

int. noct.
inter noctem [during the night] (pharmacology)

int. obst.
intestinal obstruction (gastroenterology)

INTOX
intoxicate(d) (chemical dependency)
intoxication (chemical dependency)

INTR
intermittent

int rot
internal rotation (orthopedics)

int-rot
internal rotation (orthopedics)

"in-turn"
{pronunciation of *intern* [internal]} {not an abbreviation}

in utero
{not an abbreviation} [within the uterus] (obstetrics)

InV
{not an abbreviation} [an allotypic antigenic site and part of human immunoglobulins] (laboratory)

inv
inversion
involuntary

inver
inversion

invest
investigation

in vitro
{not an abbreviation} [within glass,
    within a test tube] (laboratory and ob-
    stetrics)

in vivo
{not an abbreviation} [within a living
    body]

invol
involuntary

IO
incisal opening (dentistry)
inferior oblique [muscle] (anatomy)
initial opening [pressure] (measurement)
internal os (gynecology, obstetrics, and
    urology)
intestinal obstruction (gastroenterology)
intraocular (ophthalmology)

I/O
input/output

I & O
in and out
intake and output

Io
ionium (chemistry)

IOA
International Osteopathic Association
    (osteopathy)

IOC
in our culture
intern on call
intraoperative cholangiogram (gastroen-
    terology, radiology, and surgery)

IOCG
intraoperative cholecystogram (gastro-
    enterology, radiology, and surgery)

IOD
injured on duty (armed forces)
interorbital distance (ophthalmology)

IODA
Iron Overload Diseases Association (he-
    matology)

IODM
infant of diabetic mother (endocrinology
    and neonatology)

IOEBT
intraoperative electron beam therapy

IOF
intraocular fluid (ophthalmology)

IOFB
intraocular foreign body (ophthalmol-
    ogy)

I of L
Institute of Living

IOH
idiopathic orthostatic hypotension (car-
    diovascular and neurology)

IOL
intraocular lens (ophthalmology)

IOM
Institute of Medicine [of National Acad-
    emy of Sciences]

IOML
infraorbitomeatal line

IOMP
International Organization for Medical
    Physics (physics)

ION
ischemic optic neuropathy (neurology
    and ophthalmology)

IOP
intraocular pressure (ophthalmology)

IORT
intraoperative radiation therapy (radia-
    tion therapy)

IOS
intraoperative sonography (radiology)

IOT
intraocular tension (ophthalmology)
intraocular transfer (ophthalmology)
ipsilateral optic tectum (ophthalmology)

IOTA
information overload testing aid

IOU
intensive therapy observation unit

IOV
initial office visit

IP
icterus praecox (dermatology, gastroenterology, neonatology, and ophthalmology)
iliopsoas [muscle] (orthopedics and surgery)
immune precipitate (laboratory)
incisoproximal (dentistry)
incisopulpal (dentistry)
incubation period (infectious diseases and laboratory)
induced protein (laboratory)
induction period (anesthesiology)
infection prevention (infectious diseases)
infundibulopelvic [ligament] (gynecology, obstetrics, and surgery)
initial pressure [on lumbar puncture] (neurosurgery)
inosine phosphorylase (genetics and laboratory)
inpatient
in plaster
instantaneous pressure
International Pharmacopoeia (pharmacology)
interphalangeal (orthopedics and podiatry)
intraperitoneal (surgery)
ionization potential (physics)
isoelectric point (cardiovascular, electricity, and neurology)

I.P.
intraperitoneal (gastroenterology and surgery)

isoelectric point (cardiovascular, electricity, and neurology)

IPA
Individual Practice Association
International Pediatric Association (pediatrics)
International Psychoanalytical Association (psychiatry)
invasive pulmonary aspergillosis (respiratory)
isopropyl alcohol (chemistry and pharmacology)

I.P.A.A.
International Psychoanalytical Association (psychiatry)

I-para
primipara (obstetrics)

IPC
interpenduncular cistern (neuro, radiology)
International Poliomyelitis Congress (infectious diseases and neurology)
isopropyl chlorophenyl (chemistry)

IPCD
infantile polycystic disease (neonatology, nephrology, and pediatrics)

IPCS
intrauterine progesterone contraceptive system [an intrauterine device] (gynecology and pharmacology)

IPD
immediate pigment darkening (laboratory)
inflammatory pelvic disease (gynecology)
intermittent peritoneal dialysis (nephrology)
Inventory of Psychosocial Development (psychiatry)

IPE
initial psychiatric evaluation (psychiatry)

IPEH
intravascular papillary endothelial hyperplasia (cardiovascular)

IPF
idiopathic pulmonary fibrosis (respiratory)

IPFD
intrapartum fetal distress (obstetrics)

IPG
impedance plethysmography (neurology)
individually polymerized grass
inspiratory gas phase (respiratory)

iPGE
immunoreactive prostaglandin E (gynecology and pharmacology)

IPH
idiopathic pulmonary hemosiderosis (hematology and respiratory)
interphalangeal (orthopedics and podiatry)

IPJ
interphalangeal joint (orthopedics and podiatry)

IPK
interphalangeal keratosis (orthopedics and podiatry)
intractable plantar keratosis (orthopedics and podiatry)

IPL
intrapleural (respiratory)

IPM
impulses per minute (measurement)
inches per minute (measurement)

IPMI
inferoposterior myocardial infarct(ion) (cardiovascular)

IPMicro–ELISA
{not an abbreviation} [a trademark name for one *ELISA* (enzyme-linked immunoadsorbent assay) test] (immunology and laboratory)

IPN
infantile periarteritis nodosa (cardiovascular, neonatology, pediatrics, and rheumatology)

intern's progress note (medical records)
interpeduncular nucleus (neurology)
interpenetrating polymer network

IPO
initial planning option

IPP
inferior point [of the] pubic [bone] (orthopedic, radiology)
inflatable penile prosthesis (urology)
intermittent positive pressure (respiratory)
intrapleural pressure (respiratory)
L'Institut Pasteur Productions

IPPA
inspection, palpation, percussion, and auscultation (respiratory)

IPPB
intermittent positive pressure breathing (respiratory)

I.P.P.B.
intermittent positive pressure breathing (respiratory)

IPPB/I
intermittent positive pressure breathing/inspiratory (respiratory)

IPPF
International Planned Parenthood Federation (gynecology, obstetrics, and urology)

IPPI
interruption of pregnancy for psychiatric indication (obstetrics and psychiatry)

IPPNW
International Physicians for the Prevention of Nuclear War

IPPO
intermittent positive pressure inflation with oxygen (respiratory)

IPPR
intermittent positive pressure respiration (respiratory)

IPPV
intermittent positive pressure ventilation (respiratory)

IPQ
intimacy potential quotient (psychiatry)

IPRT
interpersonal reaction test (psychiatry)

IPS
infundibular pulmonic stenosis (cardiovascular and respiratory)
initial prognostic score
intermittent photic stimulation (neurology)
intraperitoneal shock

ips
inches per second (measurement)

IPSID
immunoproliferative small intestinal disease (gastroenterology)

IPSP
inhibitory postsynaptic potential (neurology)

I.P.T.
intermittent pelvic traction (neurology, orthopedics, and rehabilitation)

IPTG
isopropyl thiogalactoside (chemistry)

IPTH
immunoreactive parathyroid hormone (endocrinology, immunology, and laboratory)

iPTH
immunoreactive parathyroid hormone (endocrinology, immunology, and laboratory)

IPU
inpatient unit

IPV
inactivated poliomyelitis vaccine (infectious diseases, neurology, and pharmacology)
inactivated poliovaccine (infectious diseases, neurology, and pharmacology)
infectious pustular vaginitis (gynecology)
infectious pustular vulvovaginitis [of cattle] (veterinary medicine)

IQ
intelligence quotient (psychiatry)

I.Q.
intelligence quotient (psychiatry)

i.q.
idem quod [the same as]

IQ & S
iron, quinine, and strychnine [elixir] (pharmacology)

I.Q. & S.
iron, quinine, and strychnine [elixir] (pharmacology)

IR
immune response (immunology and laboratory)
immunization rate (immunology and laboratory)
immunoreactive (immunology and laboratory)
index of response
inferior rectus [muscle] (ophthalmology)
infrared (laboratory, orthopedics, and physical therapy)
insoluble residue (laboratory)
intelligence ratio (psychiatry)
internal resistance
internal rotation (orthopedics)

I.R.
infrared (laboratory, orthopedics, and physical therapy)

I-R
Ito-Reenstierna [reaction and test] (dermatology)

Ir
iridium (chemistry)
{not an abbreviation} [immune response gene] (genetics and laboratory)

IRA
immunoregulatory alpha-globulin (immunology and laboratory)
Individual Retirement Account (banking)
Irish Republican Army (armed forces)

IRB
institutional review board

IRBBB
incomplete right bundle-branch block (cardiovascular)

IRC
infrared coagulator (hematology and laboratory)
inspiratory reserve capacity (respiratory)
International Red Cross (emergency medicine)

IRCC
International Red Cross Committee (emergency medicine)

IRDS
idiopathic respiratory distress syndrome (respiratory)
infant respiratory distress syndrome (neonatology and respiratory)

IRE
internal rotation in extension (orthopedics)

IRF
internal rotation in flexion (orthopedics)

IRG
immunoreactive glucagon (immunology and laboratory)

Ir gene
{not an abbreviation} [immune response gene] (genetics and immunology)

IRGH
immunoreactive growth hormone (endocrinology and laboratory)

IRGI
immunoreactive glucagon (immunology and laboratory)

IRH
Institute for Research in Hypnosis (parapsychology)
Institute of Religion and Health (religion)

IRHCS
immunoradioassayable human chorionic somatomammotropin (endocrinology and laboratory)

IRhGH
immunoreactive human grown hormone (endocrinology and laboratory)

IRI
immunoreactive insulin (endocrinology and laboratory)

IRICU
Intermountain Respiratory Intensive Care Unit (respiratory)

irid
iridescent (laboratory)

IRIg
insulin-reactive immunoglobulin (endocrinology and laboratory)

IRIS
International Research Information Service (research)

IRM
innate releasing mechanism
Institute of Rehabilitation Medicine (rehabilitation)

IRMA
immunoradiometric assay (immunology and laboratory)

intraretinal microangiopathy (ophthalmology)
intraretinal microvascular abnormalities
  (ophthalmology)

IRMP
Intermountain Regional Medical Program

IRN
iron (chemistry, hematology, laboratory,
  and pharmacology)

iRNA
immune ribonucleic acid (genetics and
  laboratory)

IRO
International Refugee Organization
  (emergency medicine and social services)

IRONS
iron and total iron binding capacity (hematology and laboratory)

IROS
ipsilateral routing of signal (neurology)

IRP
immunoreactive proinsulin (laboratory)
International Reference Preparation

IRR
intrarenal reflux (nephrology)
irritant
irritation

irr
irrigate(d)

irr.
irradiation (radiation therapy and radiology)

IRRD
Institute for Research in Rheumatic Diseases (research and rheumatology)

IRRG
irrigate(d)
irrigation

irrig.
irrigate
irrigation

IRS
infrared spectrophotometry (laboratory)
instrument retrieval system [containers]
  (surgery)
Internal Revenue Service (government)
International Rhinologic Society (otorhinolaryngology)

IRSA
idiopathic refractory sideroblastic anemia (hematology)

IRT
isometric relaxation time (neurology
  and orthopedics)
instrument retrieval containers (surgery)

IRU
Industrial Rehabilitation Unit (rehabilitation)
interferon reference unit (laboratory)

IRV
inspiratory reserve volume (laboratory
  and respiratory)

IS
immune serum (laboratory)
immunosuppressive (laboratory)
incentive spirometry (respiratory)
induced sputum (otorhinolaryngology
  and respiratory)
intercostal space (anatomy)
interspace (anatomy, neurology, and orthopedics)
intraspinal (neurology and orthopedics)
invalided from service (armed forces)
inventory of systems

I.S.
incentive spirometer (respiratory)
intercostal space (anatomy)

I-10-S
invert sugar (10%) in saline (pharmacology)

Is
{not an abbreviation} [gene that governs
formation of suppressor T-lympho-
cytes] (genetics and laboratory)

is
island

ISA
Instrument Society of America
iodinated serum albumin (pharmacology)

ISA$_S$
internal surface area of lung at volume
of five liters (respiratory)

ISADH
inappropriate secretion of antidiuretic
hormone (endocrinology)

IS and R
information storage and retrieval

ISB
incentive spirometry breathing (respiratory)

ISBI
International Society for Burn Injuries
(dermatology and emergency medicine)

ISBP
International Society for Biochemical
Pharmacology (pharmacology)

ISBT
International Society for Blood Transfusion (hematology)

ISC
insoluble collagen (laboratory)
International Society of Cardiology (cardiovascular)
International Society of Chemotherapy
(chemotherapy)
International Statistical Classification
(statistics)
interstitial cell (laboratory)
irreversibly sickled cell (hematology and
laboratory)

I.S.C.L.T.
International Society for Clinical Laboratory Technology (laboratory)

ISCM
International Society of Cybernetic
Medicine (cybernetics)

ISCP
International Society of Clinical Pathology (pathology)

I.S.C.P.
International Society of Comparative
Pathology (pathology)

ISCS
International Society for Cardiovascular
Surgery (cardiovascular and surgery)

ISCs
irreversible sickle cells (hematology and
laboratory)

ISCV
International Society for Cardiovascular
Surgery (cardiovascular and surgery)

ISD
Information Services Division [Scottish
Health Service]
inhibited sexual desire (gynecology, psychiatry, and urology)
isosorbide dinitrate (pharmacology)

ISDN
isosorbide dinitrate (pharmacology)

ISE
inhibited sexual excitement (gynecology, psychiatry, and urology)
International Society of Endocrinology
(endocrinology)
International Society of Endoscopy (gastroenterology, respiratory, and urology)
ion-selective electrode (laboratory)

ISEK
International Society of Electromyo-

graphic Kinesiology (neurology and orthopedics)

ISF
interstitial fluid (respiratory)

ISG
immune serum globulin (laboratory and pharmacology)

ISGE
International Society of Gastroenterology (gastroenterology)

Is gene
{not an abbreviation} [gene that governs formation of suppressor T-lymphocytes] (genetics and laboratory)

ISH
icteric serum hepatitis (gastroenterology)
inner self helper [in multiple personality disorder] (psychiatry)
International Society of Hematology (hematology)
isolated systolic hypertension (cardiovascular)

ISI
infarct size index (cardiovascular and neurology)
injury severity index (emergency medicine)
Institute for Scientific Information
International Sensitivity Index
interstimulus interval (neurology)

ISKDC
International Society of Kidney Diseases in Children (nephrology and pediatrics)

ISM
International Society of Microbiologists (laboratory and microbiology)
intersegmental muscles (neurology and orthopedics)

ISMA
infantile spinal muscular atrophy (neonatology, neurology, and pediatrics)

ISMED
International Society on Metabolic Eye Disorders (ophthalmology)

ISMH
International Society of Medical Hydrology

ISMHC
International Society of Medical Hydrology and Climatology

ISN
International Society of Nephrology (nephrology)
International Society of Neurochemistry (chemistry and neurology)

ISO
International Standards Organization (measurement)
isoproterenol (pharmacology)

iso.
isoproterenol (pharmacology)

Is of Lang
islands of Langerhans (laboratory)

isol
isolate(d)
isolation

isom
isometric (neurology, orthopedics, and rehabilitation)

ISP
distance between iliac spines (measurement)
interspace (anatomy, neurology, and orthopedics)
interspinal (neurology and orthopedics)
intraspinal (neurology and orthopedics)

ISPO
International Society for Prosthetics and Orthotics (orthopedics and rehabilitation)

ISPT
interspecies ovum penetration test (laboratory)

isq
in status quo [unchanged]

i.s.q.
in status quo [unchanged]

ISR
information storage and retrieval
Institute for Sex Research (endocrinology, gynecology, obstetrics, psychiatry, research, and urology)
Institute of Surgical Research [Army] (armed forces, research, and surgery)
integrated secretory response (laboratory)

ISRM
International Society of Reproductive Medicine (gynecology, obstetrics, and urology)

ISS
Injury Severity Score (emergency medicine)
International Society of Surgery (surgery)

ISSVD
International Society for the Study of Vulvar Disease (gynecology)

IST
insulin sensitivity test (laboratory)
insulin shock therapy (endocrinology)
International Society on Toxicology (laboratory and toxicology)

ISTD
International Society of Tropical Dermatology (dermatology)

ISU
International Society of Urology (urology)

I-sub
inhibitor substance (laboratory)

ISW
interstitial water (respiratory)

ISY
intrasynovial (orthopedics)

IT
iliotibial (orthopedics)
immunity test (laboratory)
implantation test
inferior turbinate (otorhinolaryngology)
inhalation test (respiratory)
Inhalation Therapist (respiratory)
inhalation therapy (respiratory)
inspiratory time (respiratory)
intact
intensive therapy (rehabilitation)
intertrochanteric (orthopedics)
intertuberous
intradermal test (allergy and dermatology)
intrathecal (anesthesiology and neurology)
intrathoracic (anatomy)
intratracheal (otorhinolaryngology)
intratracheal tube (anesthesiology, otorhinolaryngology, and respiratory)
intratumoral
ischial tuberosity (orthopedics)
isomeric transition (chemistry)

I.T.
Inhalation Therapist (respiratory)
inhalation therapy (respiratory)

I/T
intensity/duration [of contractions] (obstetrics)

ITA
International Tuberculosis Association (infectious diseases and respiratory)

ITC
imidazolyl-thioguanine chemotherapy (chemotherapy, oncology, and pharmacology)
Interagency Testing Committee

ITc
International Table calorie (dietary)

intraventricular catheter (cardiovascular)
isovolumic contraction [period]

IVCC
intravascular consumption coagulopathy
  (hematology)

IVCD
interventricular conduction delay (cardiovascular)
intraventricular conduction defect (cardiovascular)

IVCh
intravenous cholangiogram (gastroenterology and radiology)
intravenous cholangiography (gastroenterology and radiology)

IVCP
inferior vena cava pressure (cardiovascular)

IVCU
isotope-voiding cystourethrogram (urology, radiology)

IVCV
inferior venacavography (cardiovascular
  and radiology)

IVD
intervertebral disk (neurology and orthopedics)
intravenous drip (pharmacology)

IVDA
intravenous drug abuse(r) (chemical dependency)

IVF
intravascular fluid (pharmacology)
intravenous fluid(s) (pharmacology)
in vitro fertilization (obstetrics)

IVFE
intravenous fat emulsion

IVG
isotopic ventriculogram (cardiovascular
  and radiology)

IVGTT
intravenous glucose tolerance test (endocrinology and laboratory)

IVH
intravenous hyperalimentation (dietary
  and gastroenterology)
intraventricular hemorrhage (cardiovascular and neurology)

IVIG
intravenous immunoglobulin (pharmacology)

IVJC
intervertebral joint complex (orthopedics)

IVLBW
infant of very low birth weight (neonatology)

IVM
intravascular mass (cardiovascular)

IVN
intravenous nutrition (dietary and gastroenterology)

IVP
intravenous Pitocin (obstetrics and
  pharmacology)
intravenous push (pharmacology)
intravenous pyelogram (radiology and
  urology)
intravenous pyelography (radiology and
  urology)

IVp
intravenous push (pharmacology)

IVPB
intravenous piggyback [method of drug
  administration] (pharmacology)

IVPD
in vitro protein digestibility (laboratory)

IVPF
isovolume pressure flow [curve]

IVR
idioventricular rhythm (cardiovascular)
internal visual reference
isolated volume responders (laboratory)
isovolumic relaxation [time]

IVRD
in vitro rumen digestibility (laboratory)

IVS
interventricular septum (cardiovascular)

IVSA
International Veterinary Students Association (education and veterinary medicine)

IVSD
interventricular septal defect (cardiovascular)

IVSS
intravenous Soluset

IVT
intravenous transfusion (hematology)
intraventricular (cardiovascular)

I.V.T.
intravenous transfusion (hematology)

IVTTT
intravenous tolbutamide tolerance test (laboratory)

IVU
intravenous urogram (radiology and urology)
intravenous urography (radiology and urology)

IVV
intravenous vasopressin (pharmacology)

IV vol
intravenous volume (laboratory)

I-5-W
invert sugar (5%) in water (pharmacology)

IWL
insensible water loss

IWMI
inferior wall myocardial infarction (cardiovascular)

IYDP
International Year of Disabled Persons (rehabilitation)

IYS
inverted Y-suspensor (laboratory)

IZS
insulin zinc suspension (endocrinology and pharmacology)

J

chain [not an abbreviation] (laboratory)
Jewish [ethnic origin or religion]
joint (orthopedics)
joule (measurement and physics)
Joule's equivalent (measurement and physics)
journal
juice (dietary)
Jurassic [geological time division] (geology)
juvenile
juvenile (amaurotic idiocy) (genetics, neurology, pediatrics, and psychiatry)

J

flux density (physics)
joule (measurement and physics)
mechanical equivalent (physics)

J.

Jewish [ethnic origin or religion]
joint (orthopedics)
journal
juice (dietary)

J1

Jaeger test type number 1 (ophthalmology)

J-1

Jaeger test type number 1 (ophthalmology)

J2

Jaeger test type number 2 (ophthalmology)

J-2

Jaeger test type number 2 (ophthalmology)

J3

Jaeger test type number 3 (ophthalmology)

J-3

Jaeger test type number 3 (ophthalmology)

j

juice (dietary)
yellow
{not an abbreviation} [Used as the lower case Roman numeral *i* [*one*] or at the end of a number (e.g. j, ij, iij, vij) in writing prescriptions.] (pharmacology)

JA

juvenile atrophy (neurology, orthopedics, and pediatrics)
juxta-articular (orthopedics)

JAI

juvenile amaurotic idiocy (neurology and pediatrics)

JAMA

Journal of the American Medical Association (publishing)

JAMG

juvenile autoimmune myasthenia gravis (neurology and pediatrics)

JAR

Junior admitting resident (education)

JAS

Jenkins Activity Survey (psychiatry)
Job Attitude Scale (psychiatry)

jaund

jaundice (dermatology, gastroenterology, and ophthalmology)

jaund.

jaundice (dermatology, gastroenterology, and ophthalmology)

JBC
Jesness Behavior Checklist (psychiatry)

JBE
Japanese B encephalitis (neurology)

JC
Jakob-Creutzfeldt [disease or syndrome]
   (neurology)
junior clinicians [medical students] (education)

J/C
joule per coulomb (measurement)

jc
juice (dietary)

JCA
juvenile chronic arthritis (orthopedics
   and pediatrics)

JCAE
Joint Committee on Atomic Energy
   [United States of America] (govern-
   ment and physics)

J.C.A.E.
Joint Committee on Atomic Energy
   [United States of America] (govern-
   ment and physics)

JACH
Joint Commission on Accreditation of
   Hospitals [of the American Medical
   Association] (administration)

J.C.A.H.
Joint Commission on Accreditation of
   Hospitals [of the American Medical
   Association] (administration)

JCAHO
Joint Commission on Accreditation of
   Healthcare Organizations

JCAHPO
Joint Commission on Allied Health Personnel in Ophthalmology (ophthalmology)

JCAST
Joint Commission on Archives of Science and Technology

JCC
Joint Commission on Contraception (gynecology and obstetrics)

JCF
juvenile calcaneal fracture (orthopedics
   and pediatrics)

J chain
{not an abbreviation} [a part of the immunoglobulin molecular structure]
   (immunology and laboratory)

JCL
job control language (computer science)

JCM
juvenile chronic myelocytic [leukemia]
   (hematology, oncology, and pediatrics)
juvenile chronic myelogenous [leuke-
   mia] (hematology, oncology, and pediatrics)

JCMHC
Joint Commission on Mental Health of
   Children (pediatrics and psychiatry)

JCMIH
Joint Commission on Mental Illness and
   Health (psychiatry)

JCML
juvenile chronic myelocytic leukemia
   (hematology, oncology, and pediatrics)

JCPA
Joint Commission on Public Affairs (psychiatry)

jct
junction

JCV
Jamestown Canyon virus (laboratory
   and virology)

JC virus
{not an abbreviation} [initials of patient

from whom it was first isolated] (laboratory)

JD
jejunal diverticulitis (gastroenterology)
jugulodigastric [node] (gastroenterology and surgery)
juvenile delinquent (law enforcement and psychiatry)
juvenile diabetes (endocrinology and pediatrics)

JDC
Joslin Diabetes Center (endocrinology)

JDF
Juvenile Diabetes Foundation (endocrinology and pediatrics)

JDM
juvenile-onset diabetes mellitus (endocrinology and pediatrics)

JDMS
juvenile dermatomyositis (dermatology, pediatrics, and rheumatology)

JE
Japanese encephalitis (neurology)
junctional escape (cardiovascular)

JEE
Japanese equine encephalitis (neurology)

JEJ
jejunum (gastroenterology)

jej
jejunum (gastroenterology)

jej.
jejunum (gastroenterology)

JEMBEC
{not an abbreviation} [agar plates] (laboratory)

JEN
Journal of Emergency Nursing (emergency medicine, nursing, and publishing)

"jent"
{pronunciation of *GENT* and *gent* [gentamicin (pharmacology) and gentleman]} {not an abbreviation}

jentac
jentaculum [breakfast]

JEPI
Junior Eysenck Personality Inventory (psychiatry)

JER
Japanese erection ring (urology)

JEV
Japanese encephalitis virus (laboratory and virology)

JF
joint fluid (orthopedics)
jugular foramen (anatomy, cardiovascular, and orthopedics)
junctional fold

JFET
junction field effect transistor (electronics)

JFS
jugular foramen syndrome [also called *Vernet's syndrome*] (neurology and otorhinolaryngology)

J.F.S.
Jewish Family Service (social services)

JG
June grass [test] (allergy)
juxtaglomerular (nephrology)

JGA
juxtaglomerular apparatus (laboratory)

JGC
juxtaglomerular cell (laboratory)

j-g complex
juxtaglomerular complex (laboratory)

JGCT
juxtaglomerular cell tumor (nephrology)

JGI
jejunogastric intussusception (gastroenterology)
juxtaglomerular granulation index (laboratory)
juxtaglomerular index (laboratory)

JGP
juvenile general paralysis (neurology and pediatrics)

JH
echovirus 28 (laboratory and virology)
juvenile hormone [of insects] (chemistry)

j_H
heat transfer factor (physics)

JHA
juvenile hormone analogue (endocrinology and pediatrics)

JHM
J Howard Mueller [virus] (laboratory)

JHMO
Junior Hospital Medical Officer (administration)

JHR
Jarisch-Herxheimer reaction (immunology)

JHU
John Hopkins University (education)

JI
jejunoileal (gastroenterology)
jejunoileitis (gastroenterology)
jejunoileostomy (gastroenterology and surgery)

JIB
jejunoileal bypass (gastroenterology and surgery)

JIH
joint interval histogram (laboratory)

"ji-row"
{pronunciation of *gyro* [gyroscope]} {not an abbreviation}

JJ
jaw jerk (neurology)
jejunojejunostomy (gastroenterology and surgery)

J & J
{not an abbreviation} [Johnson and Johnson] (pharmacology)

Jk
Kidd system blood group [used in alleles Jk^a, Jk^b, anti-Jk^a, and anti-Jk^b] (hematology and laboratory)

Jk^a
Kidd A [blood group] (hematology and laboratory)

Jk^b
Kidd B [blood group] (hematology and laboratory)

JKST
Johnson-Kenney Screening Test (psychiatry)

JL
Jadassohn-Lewandowsky [syndrome; also called *pachyonychia congenita* (thickening of nails)] (dermatology and genetics)
Jaffe-Lichtenstein [syndrome; also called *fibrous dysplasia*] (orthopedics)

JLP
juvenile laryngeal papilloma (otorhinolaryngology and pediatrics)

JM
jugomaxillary (dentistry and maxillofacial surgery)

j_M
mass transfer factor (physics)

JMH
John Milton Hagen [antibody] (laboratory)

JMS
junior medical student (education)

JMSB
John Milton Society for the Blind (ophthalmology)

JNA
Jena Nomina Anatomica [also abbreviated *INA*] (anatomy)

JND
just noticeable difference

jnt
joint (orthopedics)

JOD
juvenile-onset diabetes (endocrinology and pediatrics)

JODM
juvenile-onset diabetes mellitus (endocrinology and pediatrics)

JOMAC
judgment, orientation, memory, abstraction, and calculation (neurology and psychiatry)

JOMACI
judgment, orientation, memory, abstraction, and calculation intact (neurology and psychiatry)

Jour
journal

jour.
journal

JP
Jackson-Pratt [drain] (surgery)
Jobst pump (surgery)
juvenile periodontitis (dentistry and pediatrics)

JPB
junctional premature beat (cardiovascular)

JPC
junctional premature contraction (cardiovascular)

JPD
juvenile plantar dermatosis (orthopedics, pediatrics, and podiatry)

JPI
Jackson Personality Inventory (psychiatry)

JPS
joint position sense (neurology)

JPSA
Joint Program for the Study of Abortions (obstetrics)

J.P.S.A.
Joint Program for the Study of Abortions (obstetrics)

JR
Jolly's reaction (neurology)
junctional rhythm (cardiovascular)
juvenile rheumatoid arthritis (orthopedics, pediatrics, and rheumatology)

Jr.
junior

jr.
junior

JRA
juvenile rheumatoid arthritis (orthopedics, pediatrics, and rheumatology)

JRC
Junior Red Cross (emergency medicine)

JRC-CVT
Joint Review Committee on Education in Cardiovascular Technology (cardiovascular and education)

JRC-DMS
Joint Review Committee on Education in Diagnostic Medical Sonography

(cardiovascular, obstetrics, and radiology)

JRC-EEG
Joint Review Committee on Education in Electroencephalographic Technology (education and neurology)

JRC-EMT-P
Joint Review Committee on Educational Programs for the Emergency Medical Technician-Paramedic (education and emergency medicine)

JRCERT
Joint Review Committee on Education in Radiologic Technology (education and radiology)

JRC-NMT
Joint Review Committee on Educational Programs in Nuclear Medicine Technology (education and radiology)

JRC-OMA
Joint Review Committee on Educational Programs for the Ophthalmic Medical Assistant (education and ophthalmology)

JRC-PA
Joint Review Committee on Educational Programs for Physician Assistants (education)

JRCPE
Joint Review Committee for Perfusion Education (cardiovascular and education)

JRCRTE
Joint Review Committee for Respiratory Therapy Education (education and respiratory)

JRC-ST
Joint Review Committee on Education for the Surgical Technologist (education and surgery)

J receptor
juxtapulmonary-capillary receptor (laboratory)

jrl.
journal

JRN
Junior resident note (medical records)

JrNAD
Junior National Association for the Deaf (otorhinolaryngology)

jrnl.
journal

JS
jejunal segment (gastroenterology)
junctional slowing (cardiovascular)
Junkman-Schoeller [unit of thyrotropin] (endocrinology and laboratory)

Js^a
Sutter antigen [of Kell system blood group] (hematology and laboratory)

Js^b
{not an abbreviation} [an antigen of Kell system blood group] (hematology and laboratory)

JSI
Jansky Screening Index (psychiatry)

JS unit
Junkman-Schoeller unit [of thyrotropin] (endocrinology and laboratory)

JT
joint (orthopedics)

jt
joint (orthopedics)

jt.
joint (orthopedics)

jt. asp.
joint aspiration (orthopedics)

jucund
jucunde [pleasantly]

jug
jugular (cardiovascular)

jug. comp.
jugular compression [test] (neurology)

junct.
junction

juscul.
jusculum [broth, soup]

juv
juvenile (pediatrics)

juve
juvenile (pediatrics)

JUXT
juxta [near]

JV
jugular vein (cardiovascular)
jugular venous [pressure and pulse] (cardiovascular)

JVD
jugular venous distention (cardiovascular)

JVIS
Jackson Vocational Interest Survey (psychiatry)

JVP
jugular vein pulse (cardiovascular)
jugular venous pulse (cardiovascular)
jugular venous pressure (cardiovascular)

JVPT
jugular venous pulse tracing (cardiovascular)

JW
jump walker (rehabilitation)

j.w.
jump walker (rehabilitation)

JXG
juvenile xanthogranuloma (dermatology and pediatrics)

K₄
vitamin K₄ [also called *menadiol sodium diphosphate*] (hematology and pharmacology)

K-10
{not an abbreviation} [a gastric tube] (gastroenterology)

17K
17-ketosteroid excretion (endocrinology and laboratory)

17-K
17-ketosteroids (endocrinology and laboratory)

37K
{not an abbreviation} [a protein with a molecular weight of 37,000 daltons] (chemistry and laboratory)

⁴⁰K
potassium-40 [a radionuclide] (radiology)
total body potassium (laboratory)

⁴²K
potassium-42 [a radionuclide] (radiology)

⁴³K
potassium-43 [a radionuclide] (radiology)

KΩ
kilohm (measurement)

k
Boltzmann constant (chemistry)
constant
kilo- [prefix for 10^3 or thousand] (measurement)
kilogram (measurement)
thousand [as in "white blood count 3K" for *3,000*]
reaction rate constant (chemistry and laboratory)

k
constant
magnetic susceptibility (physics)
rate

velocity (electricity, neurology, and physics)

KA
alkaline phosphatase (laboratory)
kathodal [obsolete for cathodal] (laboratory and radiology)
kathode [obsolete for cathode] (laboratory and radiology)
keratoacanthoma (dermatology)
ketoacidosis (endocrinology)
King-Armstrong [unit] (chemistry and laboratory)

K-A
King-Armstrong [unit] (chemistry and laboratory)

K/A
ketogenic to antiketogenic ratio (laboratory)

Ka
kathodal [obsolete for cathodal] (laboratory and radiology)
kathode [obsolete for cathode] (laboratory and radiology)

Kₐ
acid ionization constant (physics)

ka
kathodal [obsolete for cathodal] (laboratory and radiology)
kathode [obsolete for cathode] (laboratory and radiology)

KAAD mixture
kerosene, alcohol, acetic acid, dioxane mixture (chemistry)

KAB
knowledge, attitude, behavior (psychiatry)

KABC
Kaufman Assessment Battery for Children (psychiatry and speech and language therapy)

KAF
killer-assisting factor (laboratory)
kinase-activating factor (laboratory)

KAFO
knee-ankle-foot orthosis (orthopedics)

KAFO's
knee-ankle-foot orthoses (orthopedics)

KaI
kalium [potassium] (chemistry, dietary,
  laboratory, and pharmacology)

KaI.
kalium [potassium] (chemistry, dietary,
  laboratory, and pharmacology)

KAO
knee-ankle orthosis (orthopedics)

KAP
knowledge, attitudes, and practice [with
  reference to fertility] (obstetrics)

K/A ratio
ratio of ketogenic to antiketogenic substances (laboratory)

KAS
Katz Adjustment Scale (psychiatry)

KAST
Kindergarten Auditory Screening Test
  (otorhinolaryngology)

kat
katal [enzyme unit] (laboratory)

kat.
katal [enzyme unit] (laboratory)

KAU
King-Armstrong unit (chemistry and laboratory)

"kay-ode"
{pronunciation of *KO'd* [knocked out]}
  (neurology and sports medicine) {not
  an abbreviation}

KB
Kashin-Beck [disease] (orthopedics)
ketone bodies (laboratory)

kilobyte (computer science)
knee brace (orthopedics)

K/B
knee bearing [prosthesis] (orthopedics)

Kb
kilobase (genetics and laboratory)

K$_b$
base ionization constant (physics)
dissociation constant of a base (physics)

kb
kilobase (genetics and laboratory)

kbp
kilobase pair (genetics and laboratory)

kb pair
kilobase pair (genetics and laboratory)

KBr
potassium bromide [an anticonvulsant
  and sedative] (chemistry, neurology,
  pharmacology, and psychiatry)

KBS
Klüver-Bucy syndrome (neurology and
  psychiatry)

KB splint
knuckle-bender splint (orthopedics)

KC
kathodal [obsolete for cathodal] closing
  (laboratory and radiology)
keratoconus (ophthalmology)
keratoma climacterium (dermatology)
kilo characters [per second] (computer
  science)
knees to chest [position]
knuckle cracking (orthopedics)
Kupffer cells [also called *stellate cells of
  liver and von Kupffer cells*] (gastroenterology and laboratory)

kc
kilocycle (measurement)

kc.
kilocycle (measurement)

K Cal
kilocalorie [1,000 calories or 1 Calorie] (dietary and measurement)

Kcal
kilocalorie [1,000 calories or 1 Calorie] (dietary and measurement)

kcal
kilocalorie [1,000 calories or 1 Calorie] (dietary and measurement)

kcal.
kilocalorie [1,000 calories or 1 Calorie] (dietary and measurement)

KCC
kathodal [obsolete for cathodal] closing contraction (laboratory and radiology)

KCCT
kaolin-cephalin clotting time (hematology and laboratory)

K cell
killer cell (laboratory)

KCG
kinetocardiogram (cardiovascular)

kCi
kilocurie (measurement and radiology)

KCL
potassium chloride [used as an electrolyte replenisher] (pharmacology) [*Note:* Do not confuse with the brand name drug *Kayciel.*]

KCl
potassium chloride [used as an electrolyte replenisher] (pharmacology) [*Note:* Do not confuse with the brand name drug *Kayciel.*]

K complex
{not an abbreviation} [found on electroencephalograms] (neurology)

kcps
kilocycles per second (measurement)

kc.p.s.
kilocycles per second (measurement)

kc/s
kilocycles per second (measurement)

KCS
keratoconjunctivitis sicca (ophthalmology)

KCT
kathodal [obsolete for cathodal] closing tetanus (laboratory and radiology)

KCTe
kathodal [obsolete for cathodal] closing tetanus (laboratory and radiology)

KD
kathodal [obsolete for cathodal] duration (laboratory and radiology)
Kawasaki's disease [also called *mucocutaneous lymph node syndrome*] (dermatology, ophthalmology, otorhinolaryngology, and pediatrics)
Keto-Diastix (endocrinology and pharmacology)
killed
knee disarticulation (orthopedics)

K_d
dissociation constant (physics)
distribution coefficient [also called *partition coefficient*] (physics)

kd
kilodalton (measurement and physics)

KDA
known drug allergies
{not an abbreviation} [a panel of laboratory tests] (laboratory)

KDC
kathodal [obsolete for cathodal] duration contraction (laboratory and radiology)

KDO
2-keto-3-deoxy-octonate (laboratory)

KDS
Kaufman Developmental Scale (psychiatry)

kd/sec
kilocycles per second (measurement)

KDSM
keratizing desquamative squamous metaplasia (dermatology and pathology)

KDT
kathodal [obsolete for cathodal] duration tetanus (laboratory and radiology)

KDTe
kathodal [obsolete for cathodal] duration tetanus (laboratory and radiology)

KE
Kendall's "Compound E" [cortisone] (pharmacology)
kinetic energy (physics)

K$_e$
exchangeable body potassium (laboratory)

KEC
Klebsiella, Enterobacter, Citrobacter [bacteriae] (laboratory)

Ke/Kg
exchangeable potassium per kilogram of body weight (laboratory)

KELN
Kell negative (hematology and laboratory)

"kem"
{pronunciation of *CHEM, chem,* and *chem.* [chemistry]} (chemistry) {not an abbreviation}

Kemo Tx
chemical therapy [also called *chemotherapy*] (chemotherapy, oncology, and pharmacology)

Kera
keratitis (ophthalmology)

KERV
Kentucky equine respiratory virus (laboratory, respiratory, and virology)

17-KET
17-ketosteroids (endocrinology and laboratory)

KET BD
ketone bodies (endocrinology and laboratory)

keto
17-ketosteroid test (endocrinology and laboratory) {pronounced "key-tow"}

KETONE
ketones—qualitative (endocrinology and laboratory)

keV
kiloelectron-volt (electricity and measurement)

kev
kiloelectron-volt (electricity and measurement)

kev.
kiloelectron-volt (electricity and measurement)

"key-low"
{pronunciation of *KILO* and *kilo.* [kilogram and kilometer (measurement)], *kilo.* [thousand (as in "10 kilos." meaning *10,000*) {slang}], and *kilo-* [prefix for 10^3] {not an abbreviation}

"key-tow"
{pronunciation of *keto* [17-ketosteroid test]} (endocrinology and laboratory) {not an abbreviation}

KF
Kenner-fecal medium (laboratory)
kidney function (nephrology)

Klippel-Feil [syndrome] (neurology and orthopedics)
{not an abbreviation} [KF streptococcal medium] (laboratory)

kf.
{not an abbreviation} [symbol for flocculation speed in antigen-antibody reactions] (laboratory)

KFAB
kidney-fixing antibody (laboratory)

K factor
gamma-ray dose (radiation therapy)

KFAO
knee-foot-ankle orthosis (orthopedics)

KFD
Kinetic Family Drawing [Test] (psychiatry)
Kyasanur Forest disease [of South India] (veterinary medicine)

KFDT
Kinetic Family Drawing Test (psychiatry)

KFS
Klippel-Feil syndrome (neurology and orthopedics)

αKG
alpha-ketoglutarate (chemistry and laboratory)

KG-1
Koeffler Golde-1 [cell line] (laboratory)

kG
kilogauss (measurement)

kg
kilogram (measurement)

kg.
kilogram (measurement)

KGB
Komitet Gosudarstvennoi Bezopasnosti [Soviet State Security Committee] (government and psychiatry)

KGC
Keflin, gentamicin, and carbenicillin [antibiotics] (pharmacology)

Kg-cal
kilogram-calorie [large calorie] (dietary and measurement)

kg-cal
kilogram-calorie [large calorie] (dietary and measurement)

kg.-cal.
kilogram-calorie [large calorie] (dietary and measurement)

kg/cal
kilogram-calorie [large calorie] (dietary and measurement)

KGHT
kidney Goldblatt hypertension (cardiovascular and nephrology)

kgm
kilogram (measurement)

kg-m
kilogram-meter (measurement)

kg.-m.
kilogram-meter (measurement)

kgps
kilogram per second (measurement)

kg.p.s.
kilogram per second (measurement)

KGS
ketogenic steroid (endocrinology and laboratory)

17-KGS
17-ketogenic steroid (endocrinology and laboratory)

KH
Krebs-Henseleit [cycle; also called *ornithine cycle*] (laboratory)

K24H
potassium, urine 24 hour (laboratory)

KHB
Krebs-Henseleit bicarbonate buffer (laboratory)

KHb
potassium hemoglobinate (laboratory)

KHC
kinetic hemolysis curve (laboratory)

KHD
kinky hair disease [also called *Menkes' syndrome* and *steely-hair syndrome*] (cardiovascular, genetics, and neurology)

"khem-o"
{pronunciation of *chemo* [chemotherapy]} (chemotherapy) {not an abbreviation}

KHF
Korean hemorrhagic fever [also called *epidemic hemorrhagic fever*] (infectious diseases, laboratory, and virology)

K hgb.
potassium hemoglobinate (laboratory)

KHN
Knoop hardness number (chemistry and laboratory)

KHP
Honorary Physician to the King [British]

KHS
Honorary Surgeon to the King [British]

KHZ
kilohertz (measurement)

kHz
kilohertz (measurement)

kHz.
kilohertz (measurement)

KI
karyopyknotic index (laboratory)

Krönig's isthmus [also called *Krönig's fields*] (respiratory)
potassium iodide [used as an antifungal and used as an iodine source for various thyroid conditions] (endocrinology and pharmacology)

K$_I$
dissociation of enzyme-inhibitor complex (laboratory)
inhibition constant (laboratory)

KIA
killed in action (armed forces)
Kliger iron agar [medium] (laboratory)

KIC
ketoisocaproate [also called *ketoisocaproic acid*] (chemistry)

KICB
killed intracellular bacteria (laboratory)

KID
keratitis, ichthyosis, and deafness [syndrome] (dermatology, ophthalmology, and otorhinolaryngology)
kidney (nephrology)

KIDS
Kent Infant Development Scale (neonatology)

KILO
kilogram (measurement) {pronounced "key-low"}
kilometer (measurement) {pronounced "key-low"}

kilo.
kilogram (measurement) {pronounced "key-low"}
kilometer (measurement) {pronounced "key-low"}
thousand [as in "10 kilos." meaning *10,000*] {slang}

kilo-
{not an abbreviation} [prefix for 10^3] (measurement) {pronounced "key-low"}

KIMSA
Kirsten murine sarcoma [virus] (laboratory and oncology)

KIMSV
Kirsten murine sarcoma virus (laboratory and oncology)

Ki-MSV
Kirsten murine sarcoma virus (laboratory and oncology)

KIP
key intermediary proteins (laboratory)

KIS
Krankenhaus Information System

KISS
key integrative social system (psychiatry)
saturated solution of potassium iodide (pharmacology)

KIU
kallikrein inactivation unit (laboratory)
kallikrein-inhibiting unit (laboratory)

KJ
knee jerk (neurology and orthopedics)

kJ
kilojoule (measurement)

kj
knee jerk (neurology and orthopedics)

k.j.
knee jerk (neurology and orthopedics)

KJV
King James Version [of Bible] (religion)

KK
knee kick [same as *knee jerk*] (neurology and orthopedics)

kk
knee kick [same as *knee jerk*] (neurology and orthopedics)

k.k.
knee kick [same as *knee jerk*] (neurology and orthopedics)

KKK
Kolmer, Kline, Kahn [test for syphilis] (gynecology, infectious diseases, laboratory, obstetrics, and urology)
Ku Klux Klan [a secret society] (sociology and religion)

KL
kidney lobe (nephrology)
kiloliter (measurement)
Kleine-Levin [syndrome] (neurology and psychiatry)

kl
kiloliter (measurement)

kl.
kiloliter (measurement)
Klang [musical overtone] (otorhinolaryngology)

KL bac.
Klebs-Löeffler bacillus [diphtheria bacillus] (infectious diseases, laboratory, and respiratory)

K.L. bac.
Klebs-Löeffler bacillus [diphtheria bacillus] (infectious diseases, laboratory, and respiratory)

Kleb.
Klebsiella [a bacteria] (laboratory)

Klebs
Klebsiella [a bacteria] (laboratory)

KLH
keyhole limpet hemocyanin (chemistry)

K level
lowest level (radiology)

K lines
Kerley's lines [meaning *Kerley's A lines* and *Kerley's B lines*] (radiology and respiratory)

KLS
kidney(s), liver, and spleen [on physical

examination] (anatomy, gastroenterology, and nephrology)

KLST
Kindergarten Language Screening Test (education and speech and language therapy)

KM
kanamycin [an antibiotic] (pharmacology)
K-immunoglobulin light chains (immunology and laboratory)
Kraepelin-Morel [disease] (psychiatry)

Km
Michaelis-Menten dissociation constant (laboratory)

K$_m$
Michaelis constant (laboratory)
Michaelis-Menten dissociation constant (laboratory)

km
kilometer (measurement)

km.
kilometer (measurement)

kMc
kilomegacycle (measurement)

kMc.
kilomegacycle (measurement)

K-MCM
potassium-containing minimal capacitation medium (laboratory)

kMcps
kilomegacycles per second (measurement)

kMc.p.s.
kilomegacycles per second (measurement)

KMDAT
Key Math Diagnostic Arithmetic Test (psychiatry)

KMEF
keratin, myosin, epidermin, fibrin [class of proteins] (laboratory)

KMnO
potassium permanganate [astringent, bactericide, fungicide, oxidizer, and topical anti-infective] (pharmacology)

KMnO$_4$
potassium permanganate [astringent, bactericide, fungicide, oxidizer, and topical anti-infective] (pharmacology)

kmps
kilometers per second (measurement)

km.p.s.
kilometers per second (measurement)

km/s
kilometers per second (measurement)

KMV
killed measles virus vaccine (infectious diseases, pediatrics, and pharmacology)

KN
knee (orthopedics)

Kn
knee (orthopedics)
Knudsen number [referring to gas flow] (chemistry)

kn.
knee (orthopedics)

K nail
Kuntscher nail (orthopedics)

KNL
Darrow's solution [for antidiarrhea potassium therapy] (gastroenterology and pharmacology)

KNO
keep needle open [referring to intravenous fluid lines] (pharmacology)

knork
knife and fork (psychiatry)

KNRK
normal rat kidney cells transformed by Kirsten sarcoma virus (laboratory, oncology, and research)

KO
keep on [continue]
keep open [referring to intravenous fluid lines] (pharmacology)
knee orthosis (orthopedics)
knocked out (neurology)

K/O
keep open [referring to intravenous fluid lines] (pharmacology)
knocked out (neurology)

K/o
keep on [continue]

KOC
kathodal [obsolete for cathodal] opening contraction (laboratory and radiology)

KO'd
knocked out (neurology and sports medicine) {pronounced "kay-ode"}

KOH
potassium hydroxide [also called *caustic potash, potassa,* and *potassa caustica,* used as an alkalizer in pharmaceutic preparations] (chemistry and pharmacology)

KOIS
Kuder Occupational Interest Survey (psychiatry)

"kok-see"
{pronunciation of *cocci* [coccidioidomycosis]} (laboratory) {not an abbreviation}

KOM
Kentucky, Ohio, Michigan [Medical Library Network] (library sciences)

"koo-sah"
{pronunciation of *CUSA* [Cavitron Ultrasonic Surgical Aspirator]} (neurosur-gery and ophthalmology) {not an abbreviation}

KOT
Knowledge of Occupations Test (psychiatry)

KP
Kaufmann-Peterson base
keratitic precipitates (laboratory, ophthalmology, and pathology)
keratitis punctata (ophthalmology)
keratoprecipitate (laboratory, ophthalmology, and pathology)
kidney protein (laboratory and nephrology)
kidney punch [in boxing] (sports medicine)
kidney punch [test in physical examination; also called *Murphy's test*] (nephrology)
killed parenteral [vaccine] (immunology, infectious diseases, and pharmacology)
kitchen patrol (armed forces)
Klebsiella pneumoniae [a bacteria] (laboratory)

K.P.
keratitic precipitates (laboratory, ophthalmology, and pathology)
keratitis punctata (ophthalmology)

K-P
Kaiser-Permanente [diet] (dietary)

kPa.
kilopascal (measurement and physics)

K-pad
Aqua-K module with pad (rehabilitation)

KPB
kalium (potassium) phosphate buffer (laboratory)
ketophenylbutazone [an antirheumatic; also called *kebuzone*] (orthopedics, pharmacology, and rheumatology)

KPE
Kelman phakoemulsification (ophthalmology)

KPI
karyopyknotic index (laboratory)

K-PL
potassium–plasma (laboratory)

K.P.M.
kilo/pound/meters (cardiovascular and rehabilitation)

KPR
key pulse rate (cardiovascular)
Kuder Preference Record (psychiatry)

KPR-V
Kuder Preference Record-Vocational (psychiatry)

KP's
keratitic precipitates (laboratory, ophthalmology, and pathology)
keratoprecipitates (laboratory, ophthalmology, and pathology)

KPs
keratic precipitates [also called *keratitic precipitates*] (laboratory, ophthalmology, and pathology)

KPT
kidney punch test [on physical examination; also called *Murphy's test*] (nephrology)
Kuder Performance Test (psychiatry)

KPTI
Kunitz pancreatic trypsin inhibitor (laboratory)

KPTT
kaolin partial thromboplastin time (hematology and laboratory)

KPV
killed parenteral vaccine (immunology, infectious diseases, and pharmacology)

KR
knowledge of results

Kopper Reppart [medium] (laboratory)

Kr
krypton (chemistry)

^{79}Kr
radioactive isotope of krypton (chemistry)

^{85}Kr
radioactive isotope of krypton (chemistry)

KRA
Klinefelter-Reifenstein-Albright [syndrome] (dermatology, endocrinology, and genetics)

KRB
Krebs-Ringer bicarbonate buffer (laboratory)

KRBB
Krebs-Ringer bicarbonate buffer (laboratory)

KRBG
Krebs-Ringer bicarbonate buffer (containing) glucose (laboratory)

KRBS
Krebs-Ringer bicarbonate solution (laboratory)

"krit"
{pronunciation of *Crit* and *crit* [hematocrit]} (laboratory) {not an abbreviation}

KRP
Kolmer test with Reiter protein (laboratory)
Krebs-Ringer phosphate (laboratory)

KRPS
Krebs-Ringer phosphate buffer solution (laboratory)

KRRS
kinetic resonance Raman spectroscopy (laboratory)

KS
Kansas [Postal Service state designation]
Kaposi's sarcoma (dermatology, immunology, and oncology)
Kartagener's syndrome (cardiovascular, genetics, otorhinolaryngology, and respiratory)
ketosteroid (laboratory)
Klinefelter's syndrome (endocrinology and genetics)
Kugel-Stoloff [syndrome]
Kveim-Siltzbach [test] (laboratory)

17-KS
17-ketosteroids (endocrinology and laboratory)

KSA
knowledge, skills, and abilities (psychiatry)

KSC
kathodal [obsolete for cathodal] closing contraction (laboratory and radiology)

KSCN
potassium thiocyanate [broth; also called *potassium sulfocyanate;* used as a reagent and previously as an antihypertensive] (cardiovascular, chemistry, laboratory, and pharmacology)

KSK
Kathodenschließungs-Kontaktion [kathodal (obsolete for cathodal) closing contraction] (laboratory and radiology)

KS/OI
Kaposi's sarcoma and opportunistic infections (immunology, infectious diseases, and oncology)

KSP
kidney-specific protein (laboratory and nephrology)

K$_{sp}$
potassium solubility product (laboratory)

K-SPT
potassium−urine [spot] (laboratory)

KSR
keyboard send-receive [set] (computer science)

KST
Kathodenschließungs-Tetanus [kathodal (obsolete for cathodal) closing tetanus] (laboratory and radiology)

KStJ
Knight Commander, Order of Saint John of Jerusalem

K stoff
chloromethyl chloroformate (chemistry)

K.S.U.
Kent State University (education)
Kent State University [Speech Discrimination Test] (speech and language therapy)

KT
kidney transplant (nephrology and transplantation surgery)
Klippel-Trenaunay [syndrome] (dermatology and orthopedics)
Kuder Test (psychiatry)

kt
kiloton (measurement)

KTS
kethoxal thiosemicarbazone [an antiviral] (pharmacology)
Kiersley Temperament Sorter (psychiatry)

KTSA
Kahn Test of Symbol Arrangement (psychiatry)

KTU
kidney transplant unit (nephrology and transplantation surgery)

KU
Karmen units

K-U
Kremers-Urban [company] (pharmacology)

KUB
kidney and upper bladder (nephrology and urology)
kidney(s), ureter(s), and bladder [x-ray] (radiology)

K.U.B.
kidney and upper bladder (nephrology and urology)
kidney(s), ureter(s), and bladder [x-ray] (radiology)

KUF
kidney ultrafiltration rate (laboratory and nephrology)

KUS
kidney(s), ureter(s), and spleen (gastroenterology, nephrology, and urology)

KV
kanamycin-vancomycin [antibiotics] (pharmacology)
killed virus (laboratory and pharmacology)
kilovolt (electricity and measurement)

kV
kilovolt (electricity and measurement)

kV.
kilovolt (electricity and measurement)

kv
kilovolt (electricity and measurement)

kv.
kilovolt (electricity and measurement)

kVA
kilovolt-ampere (electricity and measurement)

kVa
kilovolt-ampere (electricity and measurement)

kva
kilovolt-ampere (electricity and measurement)

K value
{not an abbreviation} [proportion of affected relatives divided by frequency of birth of same sex in general population] (genetics)

KVBA
kanamycin-vancomycin blood agar (laboratory)

KVCP
kilovolt constant potential (physics)

kVcp
kilovolt constant potential (physics)

kV.c.p.
kilovolt constant potential (physics)

kvcp
kilovolt constant potential (physics)

KVE
Kaposi's varicelliform eruption (dermatology, immunology, infectious diseases, and oncology)

KVLBA
kanamycin-vancomycin laked blood agar (laboratory)

KVO
keep vein open [referring to intravenous fluid lines] (pharmacology)

KVO C D5W
keep vein open cum [with] dextrose five percent (5%) in water (pharmacology)

KVP
kilovolt peak [also called *peak kilovoltage*] (electricity measurement)

kVP
kilovolt peak [also called *peak kilovoltage*] (electricity measurement)

kVp
kilovolt peak [also called *peak kilovoltage*] (electricity measurement)

kVp.
kilovolt peak [also called *peak kilovoltage*] (electricity measurement)

kvp
kilovolt peak [also called *peak kilovoltage*] (electricity measurement)

kvp.
kilovolt peak [also called *peak kilovoltage*] (electricity measurement)

KW
Keith-Wagener [test and classification for hypertensive retinopathy, graded I to IV] (ophthalmology)
Kimmelstiel-Wilson [syndrome] (nephrology)
Kugelberg-Welander [disease] (genetics, neurology, orthopedics, and pediatrics)

K-W
Keith-Wagener [test and classification for hypertensive retinopathy, graded I to IV] (ophthalmology)

K.W.
killer weed [slang for *phencyclidine*; also called *PCP* and *Sernyl*] (chemical dependency and law enforcement) {slang}

K_w
dissociation constant of water (physics)

kW
kilohm [unit of electrical resistance; previously *k*] (measurement)
kilowatt (electricity and measurement)

kW.
kilowatt (electricity and measurement)

kw
kilowatt (electricity and measurement)

kw.
kilowatt (electricity and measurement)

KWB
Keith, Wagener, Barker [classification of hypertension] (cardiovascular and ophthalmology)

KWE
Keith-Welti-Ernst [method] (radiology)

kWh
kilowatt-hour (electricity and measurement)

kW-hr
kilowatt-hour (electricity and measurement)

kW.-hr.
kilowatt-hour (electricity and measurement)

kw hr
kilowatt-hour (electricity and measurement)

kw-hr
kilowatt-hour (electricity and measurement)

kw.-hr.
kilowatt-hour (electricity and measurement)

KWIC
keyword in context (computer science)

"kwint"
{pronunciation of *quint* [quintuplet]} (neonatology and obstetrics) {not an abbreviation}

K wire
Kirschner wire (orthopedics)

K-wire
Kirschner wire (orthopedics)

KWOC
keyword out of context (computer science)

"kwod"
{pronunciation of *quad* [quadriceps (muscle) (neurology, orthopedics, and physical therapy) and quadriplegic (neurology)]} {not an abbreviation}

"kwort"
{pronunciation of *QUART* [quandrantectomy, axillary dissection, and radiotherapy (treatment for breast cancer)]} (oncology and surgery) {not an abbreviation}

KY
Kentucky [Postal Service state designation]

KYB
know your body

kyph.
kyphosis (orthopedics)

KZ
Kaplan-Zuelzer [syndrome]

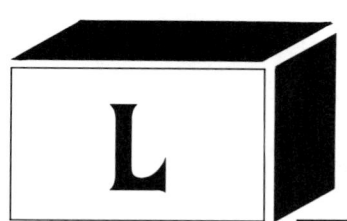

L

λ
decay constant (physics, radiation therapy, and radiology)
lambda [eleventh letter of the Greek alphabet]

L
angular momentum (physics)
Avogadro's constant [also called *Avogadro's number*] (measurement and physics)
coefficient of induction (physics)
fifty [Roman numeral]
inductance (electricity and physics)
Lactobacillus [a bacteria] (laboratory)
lambert [unit of luminance] (physics)
lambda [eleventh letter of the Greek alphabet]
Latin [language or ethnic origin]
left
left eye (ophthalmology)
Legionella [a bacteria] (laboratory)
Leishmania [a protozoan parasite] (laboratory)
length (measurement)
Lente insulin (endocrinology and pharmacology)
Leptospira [a bacteria] (laboratory)
Leptotrichia [a bacteria] (laboratory)
lesser
lethal (pharmacology, radiation therapy, radiology, and research)
leucine (laboratory)
Leuconostoc [an algae] (laboratory)
lewisite [a lethal gas] (armed forces and chemistry)
liber [book] (library sciences)
libra [pound] (measurement)
licensed to practice
lidocaine (anesthesiology, pharmacology, and surgery)
ligament (orthopedics)
light
light [chain of protein molecules] (laboratory)
light sense (ophthalmology)
lilac [a color]

limen [threshold] (anatomy)
limes [boundary] (pharmacology and research)
lingual (dentistry and otorhinolaryngology)
liquor (chemical dependency)
Listeria [a bacteria] (laboratory)
liter (measurement)
liver (anatomy and gastroenterology)
living
longitudinal [referring to sections] (laboratory)
low [when used with another abbreviation, e.g. *LBW* (low birth weight)]
lower
lowest
lues [also called *syphilis*] (gynecology, infectious diseases, and urology)
lumbar (neurology and orthopedics)
lumen (anatomy)
lung (respiratory)
lymph [a fluid] (laboratory)
lymphocyte (laboratory)
lymphogranuloma (pathology)
lysosome (laboratory)
{not an abbreviation} [heat labile component of protein antigen of vaccinia and variola viruses] (laboratory)

L.
coefficient of induction (physics)
Lactobacillus (laboratory)
Latin [language or ethnic origin]
left
length (measurement)
libra [balance, pound]
light sense (neurology and ophthalmology)
limes [boundary] (pharmacology and research)
liter (measurement)
lumbar (neurology and orthopedics)
{not an abbreviation} [Ehrlich's symbol for lethal; also called *Ehrlich's symbol for fatal*] (research)

(L)
left

L_+
limes death [*limes tod*, fatal dose toxin-
antitoxin mixture] (pharmacology and
research)

L-
{not an abbreviation} [a chemical prefix]
(chemistry and pharmacology)

L_0
limes zero [*limes nul*, neutralized toxin-
antitoxin mixture] (pharmacology and
research)

L1
first lumbar nerve (neurology and orthopedics)
first lumbar vertebra (neurology and orthopedics)

L_1
first lumbar nerve (neurology and orthopedics)
first lumbar vertebra (neurology and orthopedics)

L-1
first lumbar nerve (neurology and orthopedics)
first lumbar vertebra (neurology and orthopedics)

L2
second lumbar nerve (neurology and orthopedics)
second lumbar vertebra (neurology and
orthopedics)

L_2
second lumbar nerve (neurology and orthopedics)
second lumbar vertebra (neurology and
orthopedics)

L-2
second lumbar nerve (neurology and orthopedics)
second lumbar vertebra (neurology and
orthopedics)

L3
third lumbar nerve (neurology and orthopedics)
third lumbar vertebra (neurology and
orthopedics)

L_3
third lumbar nerve (neurology and orthopedics)
third lumbar vertebra (neurology and
orthopedics)

L-3
third lumbar nerve (neurology and orthopedics)
third lumbar vertebra (neurology and
orthopedics)

L/3
lower third [referring to long bones] (orthopedics)

L4
fourth lumbar nerve (neurology and orthopedics)
fourth lumbar vertebra (neurology and
orthopedics)

L_4
fourth lumbar nerve (neurology and orthopedics)
fourth lumbar vertebra (neurology and
orthopedics)

L-4
fourth lumbar nerve (neurology and orthopedics)
fourth lumbar vertebra (neurology and
orthopedics)

L5
fifth lumbar nerve (neurology and orthopedics)
fifth lumbar vertebra (neurology and orthopedics)

L_5
fifth lumbar nerve (neurology and orthopedics)
fifth lumbar vertebra (neurology and orthopedics)

L-5
fifth lumbar nerve (neurology and orthopedics)
fifth lumbar vertebra (neurology and orthopedics)

l
left
left eye (ophthalmology)
length (measurement)
lethal (pharmacology, radiation therapy,
radiology, and research)
levo [left or counterclockwise; a chemical prefix] (chemistry and pharmacology)
levorotatory (physics)
line
liter (measurement)
long
longitudinal [referring to sections] (laboratory)
lumen (anatomy)

l.
levo [left or counterclockwise; a chemical prefix] (chemistry and pharmacology)
line
liter (measurement)
long

l-
levo [left or counterclockwise; a chemical prefix] (chemistry and pharmacology)

μl
microliter (measurement)

LA
lactic acid (laboratory)
language age (speech and language therapy)
large amount
late antigen (laboratory)
latex agglutination (laboratory)
Latin America (geography)
Latin American [ethnic origin]
left angle (orthopedics)
left angulation (orthopedics)
left arm (anatomy and orthopedics)
left atrial (cardiovascular)
left atrium [image on transesophageal
echocardiography] (cardiovascular)

left auricle (cardiovascular and otorhinolaryngology)
left auricular (cardiovascular and otorhinolaryngology)
leucine aminopeptidase (laboratory)
leucoagglutinating (laboratory)
leukemia antigen (hematology, laboratory, and oncology)
levator ani [muscle] (gastroenterology
and surgery)
lichen amyloidosis (dermatology)
Lightwood-Albright [syndrome] (nephrology)
linguoaxial (dentistry)
linoleic acid (dietary)
lobuloalveolar (respiratory)
local anesthesia (anesthesiology and surgery)
long acting [referring to drugs] (pharmacology)
long-arm [cast] (orthopedics)
Louisiana [Postal Service state des-
ignation]
low anxiety (psychiatry)
Ludwig's angina (otorhinolaryngology
and respiratory)

L + A
light and accommodation (neurology
and ophthalmology)
living and active

L & A
light and accommodation (neurology
and ophthalmology)
living and active

La
labial (dentistry)
lanthanum (chemistry)

la
lege artis [according to the art]

l.a.
lege artis [according to the art]

l & a
light and accommodation (neurology
and ophthalmology)

LAA
left atrial abnormalities (cardiovascular)
left atrial appendage (cardiovascular)
left auricular appendage (cardiovascular)
leukemia-associated antigen (hematology, laboratory, and oncology)
leukocyte ascorbic acid (laboratory)

LAAM
l-acetyl-α-methadol [also called *levomethadyl acetate*] (pharmacology)

LAAO
l-amino acid oxidase (laboratory)

LAB
Leisure Activities Blank (psychiatry)

Lab
laboratory {pronounced "lab"}

lab
laboratory {pronounced "lab"}
{not an abbreviation} [rennet (German)] (laboratory)

"lab"
{pronunciation of *Lab* and *lab* [laboratory]} {not an abbreviation}

lab proc
laboratory procedure (laboratory)

LABS
Laboratory Admission Baseline Studies (laboratory)

LABVT
left atrial ball-valve thrombus (cardiovascular)

LAC
laceration (dermatology)
La Crosse subtype encephalitis (neurology)
lactose (dietary, laboratory, and pharmacology)
left atrial contraction (cardiovascular)
lingoaxiocervical (dentistry)
long-arm cast (orthopedics)
Los Angeles County (government)
low amplitude contraction (neurology)

LaC
labiocervical (dentistry)

lac
laceration(s) (dermatology)
{not an abbreviation} [milk]

lac.
laceration(s) (dermatology)
lactate (obstetrics)
lactation (obstetrics)

lac. & cont.
lacerations and contusions (dermatology and emergency medicine)

lacr.
lacrimal (ophthalmology)

LACT
lactic acid (laboratory)
Lindamood Auditory Conceptualization Test (psychiatry)

LAC T
lactose tolerance (gastroenterology)

lact.
lactate (obstetrics)
lactating (obstetrics)

LAC/USC
Los Angeles County/University of Southern California Medical Center

LAD
lactic acid dehydrogenase (laboratory)
language acquisition device (otorhinolaryngology and speech and language therapy)
left anterior descending [coronary artery] (cardiovascular)
left axis deviation (cardiovascular)
linoleic acid depression (laboratory)
lipoamide dehydrogenase (laboratory)
lymphocyte-activating determinant (laboratory)

LADA
laboratory animal dander allergy (allergy)

left acromiodorsoanterior [position] (obstetrics)
left anterior descending artery (cardiovascular)

LADCA
left anterior descending coronary artery (cardiovascular)

LADD
left anterior descending diagonal [branch of coronary artery] (cardiovascular)

LADH
lactic acid dehydrogenase (laboratory)
liver alcohol dehydrogenase (laboratory)

LADME
liberation, absorption, distribution, metabolism, excretion (dietary, gastroenterology, laboratory, and urology)

LADP
left acromiodorsoposterior [position] (obstetrics)

LAD-MIN
left axis deviation minimal (cardiovascular)

LADu
lobuloalveolar-ductal (respiratory)

LAE
left atrial enlargement (cardiovascular)
long above-elbow [cast] (orthopedics)

laev
laevus [left]

LAF
laminar airflow
Latin American female [ethnic origin and sex]
leukocyte-activating factor (laboratory)
lymphocyte-activating factor (laboratory)
lymphocyte-activation factor (laboratory)

LAFB
left anterior fascicular block (cardiovascular)

LAFR
laminar airflow room

LAFU
laminar airflow unit

LAG
labiogingival (dentistry)
linguoaxiogingival (dentistry)
lymphangiogram (radiology)
lymphangiography (radiology)

LaG
labiogingival (dentistry)

Lag.
lagena [flask] (pharmacology)

lag
lagena [bottle, flask] (pharmacology)

lag.
lagena [bottle, flask] (pharmacology)

LAH
lactalbumin hydrolysate (laboratory)
left anterior hemiblock (cardiovascular)
left atrial hypertrophy (cardiovascular)
Licentiate of Apothecaries Hall, Dublin [Ireland] (pharmacology)
lithium-aluminum hydride [also called *aluminum lithium hydride*] (laboratory)

L.A.H.
left atrial hypertrophy (cardiovascular)

LAHV
leukocyte-associated herpes virus (laboratory)

LAI
latex (particle) agglutination inhibition (laboratory)
leukocyte adherence inhibition [assay] (laboratory)

LaI
labioincisal (dentistry)

LAIF
leukocyte adherence inhibition factor (laboratory)

LAIT
latex agglutination inhibition test [for pregnancy] (laboratory)

LAK
leukocyte-activated killer [cells] (oncology and laboratory)

LAL
left axillary line (anatomy)
limulus amebocyte lysate (bacteriology and laboratory)

LaL
labiolingual (dentistry)

L-Ala
L-alanine (laboratory)

LALI
lymphocyte antibody lymphocytolytic interaction (laboratory)

LAM
lamina(e) (neurology and orthopedics)
L-asparaginase and methotrexate (chemotherapy, oncology, and pharmacology)
late ambulatory monitoring (rehabilitation)
Latin American male (ethnic origin and sex)
left anterior measurement (measurement)
left atrial myxoma (cardiovascular)
lymphangioleiomyomatosis (pathology and surgery)

Lam
laminectomy (neurology and orthopedics)
laminogram (radiology)

lam
laminectomy (neurology and orthopedics) {pronounced "lam"}
laminogram (radiology)

"lam"
{pronunciation of *lam* [laminectomy]}
(neurology and orthopedics) {not an abbreviation}

LA-MAX
maximal left atrial [dimension] (cardiovascular)

"lam-e"
{pronunciation of *lami* [laminotomy]} (neurology and orthopedics) {not an abbreviation}

lam & fus
laminectomy and fusion (neurology and orthopedics)

lami
laminotomy (neurology and orthopedics) {pronounced "lam-e"}

LAMMA
laser microprobe mass analyzer (laboratory)

LAN
long-acting neuroleptic (neurology and pharmacology)
lymphadenopathy (multiple specialties)

LANC
long-arm navicular cast (orthopedics)

Lang
language (grammar and speech and language therapy)

LANV
left atrial neovascularization (cardiovascular)

LAO
left anterior oblique (radiology)
left anterior occipital [position] (obstetrics)
left atrial overloading (cardiovascular)
Licentiate in Obstetric Science (obstetrics)
Licentiate of the Art of Obstetrics (obstetrics)

LAP
laparoscopy (gynecology) {pronounced
    "lap"}
laparotomy (surgery) {pronounced
    "lap"}
laparotomy [sponges] (surgery) {pro-
    nounced "lap"}
left arterial pressure (cardiovascular)
left atrial pressure (cardiovascular)
leucine aminopeptidase (laboratory)
leukocyte alkaline phosphatase [stain]
    (laboratory)
low atmospheric pressure (weather)
lyophilized anterior pituitary [tissue]
    (endocrinology and laboratory)

lap
laparoscopy (gynecology) {pronounced
    "lap"}
laparotomy (surgery) {pronounced
    "lap"}

"lap"
{pronunciation of *LAP* and *lap* [laparos-
    copy, laparotomy, and laparotomy
    (sponges)]} (gynecology and surgery)
    {not an abbreviation}

lapid
lapideum [stony]

LAPMS
long arm posterior molded splint (ortho-
    pedics)

LAPOCA
L-asparaginase, prednisone, vincristine
    [Oncovin], cytosine arabinoside, and
    Adriamycin [doxorubicin] (chemo-
    therapy, oncology, and pharmacology)

LAPSE
long-term ambulatory physiological sur-
    veillance [a vital sign monitor] (car-
    diovascular and respiratory)

LAPW
left atrial posterior wall (cardiovascular)

LAR
laryngology (otorhinolaryngology)
late asthmatic response (respiratory)
left arm recumbent [blood pressure and
    pulse measurement] (cardiovascular)

lar
larynx (otorhinolaryngology and respira-
    tory)
left arm reclining [blood pressure and
    pulse measurement] (cardiovascular)
left arm recumbent [blood pressure and
    pulse measurement] (cardiovascular)

LARC
leukocyte automatic recognition com-
    puter (laboratory)

LARS
Language-Structured Auditory Reten-
    tion Span [Test] (psychiatry)
leucyl-transfer ribonucleic acid [tRNA]
    synthetase (genetics and laboratory)

laryn.
laryngeal (otorhinolaryngology)
laryngitis (otorhinolaryngology)
laryngoscopy (otorhinolaryngology)

Laryng
laryngology (otorhinolaryngology)

Laryngol
laryngologist (otorhinolaryngology)
laryngology (otorhinolaryngology)

LAS
Laboratory Automation System (labora-
    tory)
Lapidus Airfloat System
laxative abuse syndrome (gastroenterol-
    ogy)
left anterior-superior (anatomy)
left arm sitting [blood pressure and
    pulse measurement] (cardiovascular)
leucine acetylsalicylate (laboratory)
linear alkyl sulfonate (laboratory)
local adaptation syndrome
long-arm splint (orthopedics)
lower abdominal surgery (gastroenterol-
    ogy, gynecology, surgery, and urol-
    ogy)
lymphadenopathy syndrome [former
    name for *acquired immunodeficiency
    syndrome* (AIDS)] (immunology, in-
    fectious diseases, and oncology)

LBWR
lung-body weight ratio (measurement)

LC
Laennec's cirrhosis (gastroenterology)
Langerhan's cells (laboratory)
lethal concentration (radiation therapy)
life care
linguocervical (dentistry)
lipid cytosomes (laboratory)
living children (gynecology and obstetrics)
long-chain [triglycerides] (laboratory)
low calorie [diet] (dietary)

L.C.
low calorie [diet] (dietary)

LCA
Leber's congenital amaurosis (genetics and ophthalmology)
left carotid artery (cardiovascular)
left coronary artery (cardiovascular)

LCAR
late cutaneous anaphylactic reaction (allergy)

LCAT
lecithin cholesterol acetyltransferase (laboratory)

LCC
lactose coliform count (laboratory)

LCCA
left circumflex coronary artery (cardiovascular)
left common carotid artery (cardiovascular and neurology)
leukocytoclastic angiitis (cardiovascular)

LCCS
low cervical cesarean section (obstetrics)

LCD
liquid crystal display (electronics)
liquor carbonis detergens [also called *coal tar solution*] (dermatology and pharmacology)
localized collagen dystrophy (dermatology and orthopedics)

LCF
left common femoral [artery] (cardiovascular)

LCFA
long-chain fatty acid (laboratory)

LCGU
local cerebral glucose utilization (laboratory)

LCH
local city hospital

LCh
Licentiate in Surgery (surgery)

L.Ch.
Licentiate in Surgery (surgery)

L chain
light chain (laboratory)

LCL
lateral collateral ligament (orthopedics)
Levinthal-Coles-Lillie [cytoplasmic inclusion bodies] (laboratory and respiratory)
lymphocytic leukemia (hematology and oncology)
lymphocytic lymphosarcoma (oncology)

LCLC
large cell lung carcinoma (oncology and respiratory)

LCM
left costal margin (anatomy)
lowest common multiple (mathematics)
lymphatic choriomeningitis (neurology)
lymphocyte choriomeningitis (neurology)

LCME
Liaison Committee on Medical Education (education)

LCMG
long-chain monoglyceride (laboratory)

LCMV
lymphocytic choriomeningitis virus (laboratory)

LCP
Legge-Calvé-Perthes [disease] (orthopedics)
long-chain polysaturated [fatty acids] (laboratory)

LCPS
Licentiate of the College of Physicians and Surgeons

LCR
late cutaneous reaction (allergy)
leurocristine [also called *vincristine*] (chemotherapy, oncology, and pharmacology)

LCS
lichen chronicus simplex (dermatology)
Life Care Services (emergency medicine)
low constant suction (surgery)
low continuous suction (surgery)

LCSW
Licensed Clinical Social Worker (social services)

LCT
long-chain triglycerides (laboratory)
Luscher Color Test (psychiatry)
lymphocytotoxicity test (laboratory)

L.C.T.
long chain triglyceride (laboratory)
low cervical transverse [position] (obstetrics)
lymphocytotoxicity (laboratory)

LCV
low cervical vertical [incision] (obstetrics)

LCX
left circumflex coronary artery (cardiovascular)

LCx
left circumflex coronary artery (cardiovascular)

LD
labor and delivery (obstetrics)
laboratory data (laboratory)
labyrinthine defect (otorhinolaryngology)
lactate dehydrogenase [formerly *LDH*] (cardiovascular and laboratory)
lactic dehydrogenase [formerly *LDH*] (cardiovascular and laboratory)
left deltoid (neurology and orthopedics)
legionnaire's disease (respiratory)
lethal dose (laboratory, pharmacology, radiation therapy, and research)
levodopa (obstetrics)
light-dark
light difference [on perception] (ophthalmology)
light difference, perception of (ophthalmology)
linguodistal (dentistry)
liver disease (gastroenterology)
living donor (transplant surgery)
loading dose (pharmacology)
Lombard-Dowell [broth medium] (laboratory)
long day [in plant growth] (agriculture)
low density (radiology)
low dosage (pharmacology)
lymphocyte-defined (laboratory)
lymphocytically determined (laboratory)

L.D.
learning disability (education, psychiatry, and speech and language therapy)
left deltoid (neurology and orthopedics)
light difference (neurology and ophthalmology)

L-D
Leishman-Donovan [bodies; also called *amastigote*] (laboratory and parasitology)

L & D
labor and delivery (obstetrics and neonatology)

L/D
light-dark [ratio] (ophthalmology)

LD$_1$
{not an abbreviation} [a fraction of lactate dehydrogenase; also called LDH_1] (cardiovascular and laboratory)

LD$_2$
{not an abbreviation} [a fraction of lactate dehydrogenase; also called LDH_2] (cardiovascular and laboratory)

LD$_3$
{not an abbreviation} [a fraction of lactate dehydrogenase; also called LDH_3] (cardiovascular and laboratory)

LD$_4$
{not an abbreviation} [a fraction of lactate dehydrogenase; also called LDH_4] (cardiovascular and laboratory)

LD$_5$
{not an abbreviation} [a fraction of lactate dehydrogenase; also called LDH_5] (cardiovascular and laboratory)

LD$_{50}$
median lethal dose (pharmacology and radiation therapy)

LDA
left dorsoanterior [position] (obstetrics)
linear displacement analysis

LDB
legionnaire's disease bacterium (laboratory)

LDD
light-dark discrimination (ophthalmology)

LDDS
local dentist (dentistry)

LDE
lauric diethamide (laboratory)

LD-EYA
Lombard-Dowell egg yolk agar (laboratory)

LDH
lactate dehydrogenase [obsolete, now *LD*; also called *lactic dehydrogenase*

and *serum lactic dehydrogenase*] (cardiovascular and laboratory)

LDH$_1$
{not an abbreviation} [a fraction of lactate dehydrogenase; also called LD_1] (cardiovascular and laboratory)

LDH$_2$
{not an abbreviation} [a fraction of lactate dehydrogenase; also called LD_2] (cardiovascular and laboratory)

LDH$_3$
{not an abbreviation} [a fraction of lactate dehydrogenase; also called LD_3] (cardiovascular and laboratory)

LDH$_4$
{not an abbreviation} [a fraction of lactate dehydrogenase; also called LD_4] (cardiovascular and laboratory)

LDH$_5$
{not an abbreviation} [a fraction of lactate dehydrogenase; also called LD_5] (cardiovascular and laboratory)

LDHI
lactic dehydrogenase isoenzymes (cardiovascular and laboratory)

LDISO
lactic dehydrogenase isoenzymes (cardiovascular and laboratory)

LDL
loudness discomfort level (otorhinolaryngology)
low-density lipoprotein [cholesterol level and fraction] (cardiovascular, endocrinology, and laboratory)

LDLP
low-density lipoprotein [cholesterol level and fraction] (cardiovascular, endocrinology, and laboratory)

LD-NEYA
Lombard-Dowell neomycin egg yolk agar (laboratory)

L-DOPA
levodopa [also called *3-hydroxy-L-ty-rosine*] (neurology and pharmacology)

L-dopa
levodopa [also called *3-hydroxy-L-ty-rosine*] (neurology and pharmacology)

LDP
left dorsoposterior [position] (obstetrics)

L/D ratio
light/dark ratio

LDS
Latter Day Saints [Mormon religion]
Licentiate in Dental Surgery (dentistry)
ligating and dividing stapler (surgery)

L.D.S.
Licentiate in Dental Surgery (dentistry)

LDSc
Licentiate in Dental Science (dentistry)

LDUB
long double upright brace (orthopedics)

LDV
lactic dehydrogenase virus (laboratory)
laser Doppler velocimetry (cardiovascular)

LE
left eye (ophthalmology)
leukoerythrogenetic (laboratory)
lower extremity (orthopedics)
lupus erythematosus (rheumatology)

Le
Leonard [unit for cathode rays] (radiology)

LEA
Lewis A (laboratory)

L.E.A.
local education agency (education and government)

LEAB
Lewis (A+B) (laboratory)

lead I
{not an abbreviation} [an electrocardiographic lead; difference of potential between left arm and right arm] (cardiovascular)

lead II
{not an abbreviation} [an electrocardiographic lead; difference of potential between left leg and right arm] (cardiovascular)

lead III
{not an abbreviation} [an electrocardiographic lead; difference of potential between left arm and right arm] (cardiovascular)

LEAN
Lewis A negative (laboratory)

LEB
Lewis B (laboratory)

LEBN
Lewis B negative (laboratory)

LE cell
lupus erythematosus cell (laboratory)

Lect
lecturer (education)

LED
light-emitting diode (electronics)
lupus erythematosus disseminatus (rheumatology)

"lee-mah"
{pronunciation of *LIMA* [left internal mammary artery]} (cardiovascular) {not an abbreviation}

LEE W
Lee White tritium [clotting time] (hematology and laboratory)

LE factor
{not an abbreviation} (laboratory)

leg
legal
legally

leg com
legally committed (psychiatry)

LEHPZ
lower esophageal high pressure zone
(gastroenterology)

leio
leiomyoma (gynecology and obstetrics)
{pronounced "lie-oh"}

LEL
lowest effect level [of toxicity] (chemotherapy, oncology, pharmacology, and
radiation therapy)

LEM
lateral eye movements (ophthalmology)
Leibovitz-Emory medium (laboratory)
leukocyte endogenous mediator (laboratory)

lenit
leniter [gently]

lenit.
leniter [gently]

LEOD
lens extraction, oculus dexter [right eye]
(ophthalmology)

LEOS
lens extraction, oculus sinister [left eye]
(ophthalmology)

LEP
low egg passage [strain of virus] (laboratory)
lipoprotein electrophoresis (laboratory)
lupus erythematosus preparation (laboratory and rheumatology)

LE prep
lupus erythematosus preparation (laboratory and rheumatology)

LE process
{not an abbreviation} [the process by
which the lupus erythematosus cell

(LE) is formed] (laboratory and rheumatology)

LEPT
leptocytes (laboratory)

Lept
Leptospira (laboratory)

LEPTOS
leptospirosis agglutinins (laboratory)

L-ERX
leukoerythroblastic reaction (laboratory)

LES
lateral epithelial space (anatomy)
Lawrence Experimental Station [agar]
(laboratory)
local excitatory state (neurology)
Locke egg serum [medium] (laboratory)
lower esophageal sphincter (gastroenterology)
systemic lupus erythematosus (rheumatology)

LE's
lower extremities (orthopedics)

les
lesbian (psychiatry) {pronounced "lez"}

l.e.s.
local excitatory state (neurology)

LESS
lateral electrical spine stimulation (orthopedics)

LESP
lower esophageal sphincter pressure
(gastroenterology)

lessy
lesbian (psychiatry) {pronounced
"leze"}

LET
linear energy transfer (physics)

leth
lethal (pharmacology and radiation therapy)

Leu
leucine (laboratory)

leu.
leucine (laboratory)

LEUK
leukocyte (laboratory) {pronounced "luke"}

leuk.
leukemia (hematology and oncology)

LEUKAP
leukocyte alkaline phosphatase (laboratory)

LEV
Leibovitz-Emory medium [for viral cultures] (laboratory)

lev
levis [light]

lev.
levis [light]

levo-
{not an abbreviation} [chemical prefix and prefix denoting left]

LEVT
left extremity venous tracing (cardiovascular and radiology)
lower extremity venous tracing (cardiovascular and radiology)

"lewdz"
{pronunciation of *ludes* [Quaaludes (methaqualone)]} (chemical dependency, pharmacology, and psychiatry) {slang} {not an abbreviation}

LEX
Lewis X (laboratory)

l/ext
lower extremity (orthopedics)

"lez"
{pronunciation of *les* [lesbian]} (psychiatry) {not an abbreviation}

"lez-e"
{pronunciation of *lessy* [lesbian]} (psychiatry) {not an abbreviation}

LF
laryngofissure (otorhinolaryngology)
left foot (orthopedics and podiatry)
limit of flocculation (laboratory)
low forceps (obstetrics)
low frequency (otorhinolaryngology)

Lf
limit flocculation (laboratory)
limit of flocculation (laboratory)

lf
low frequency (otorhinolaryngology)

LFA
left femoral artery (cardiovascular)
left frontoanterior [position] (obstetrics)
low friction arthroplasty (orthopedics)

L.F.A.
left frontoanterior [position] (obstetrics)

LFC
living female child (obstetrics)

LFD
lactose-free diet (dietary)
least fatal dose [of a toxin] (pharmacology)
low-fat diet (dietary)
low forceps delivery (obstetrics)

L.F.D.
least fatal dose [of a toxin] (pharmacology)

LFH
left femoral hernia (gastroenterology and surgery)

LFN
lactoferrin (laboratory)

LIB
left in bottle (emergency medicine and pharmacology)

Lib.
libra [pound] (measurement)

lib
liberation [as in *women's liberation*] {slang} {pronounced "lib"}
libra [pound] (measurement)

lib.
libra [pound] (measurement)

"lib"
{pronunciation of *liberation* [as in women's liberation]} {slang} {not an abbreviation}

LIBC
latent iron-binding capacity (laboratory)

LIBR
Librium (pharmacology and psychiatry)

LIC
least incompatible (laboratory)
left iliac crest (orthopedics)
left internal carotid [artery] (cardiovascular)
limiting isorrheic concentration

Lic
Licentiate

LICA
left internal carotid artery (cardiovascular)

LICM
left intercostal margin (anatomy)

LicMed
Licentiate in Medicine

Lic.Med.
Licentiate in Medicine

LiCO₃
lithium carbonate (pharmacology and psychiatry)

LICS
left intercostal space (anatomy)

"lie-oh"
{pronunciation of *leio* [leiomyoma]} (gynecology and obstetrics) {not an abbreviation}

LIF
left iliac fossa (orthopedics)
leukocyte inhibitory factor (laboratory)
leukocytosis-inducing factor (laboratory)
liver (migration) inhibitory factor (laboratory)

LIG
ligament (orthopedics)

lig
ligament (orthopedics)
ligamentum (orthopedics)
ligation (surgery)
ligature (surgery)

ligg.
ligamenta (orthopedics)
ligaments (orthopedics)
ligature (surgery)

LIH
left inguinal hernia (gastroenterology and surgery)

LIHA
low impulsiveness, high anxiety (psychiatry)

LII
lues II [also called *secondary syphilis*] (gynecology, infectious diseases, and urology)

LIII
lues III [also called *tertiary syphilis*] (gynecology, infectious diseases, and urology)

LILA
low impulsiveness, low anxiety (psychiatry)

lim
limit

LIMA
left internal mammary artery [graft] (cardiovascular) {pronounced "lee-mah"}

"lim-fah"
{pronunciation of *lymph* [lymphocyte]} (laboratory) {not an abbreviation}

"lim-foes"
{pronunciation of *lymphos* [lymphocytes]} (laboratory) {not an abbreviation}

"limps"
{pronunciation of *lymphs* [lymphocytes]} (laboratory) {not an abbreviation}

lin
linear

LINAC
linear accelerator (physics)

LINE
{not an abbreviation} [refers to a specimen obtained from an intravenous line] (laboratory)

LINES
long interspersed repeated segments [of deoxyribonucleic acid (DNA)] (genetics and laboratory)

linim
liniment (pharmacology)

LINK
Literature in Nursing Kardex [Cardex] (nursing and publishing)

Linn
Linnaeus (biology)
Linnaean (biology)

LIO
left inferior oblique (radiology)

L.I.P.
lymphocytic interstitial pneumonia (respiratory)

Lip
lipoate [also called *lipoic acid*] (laboratory)

lip
lipemic (cardiovascular and laboratory)

LIP P
lipid profile (cardiovascular and laboratory)

LIPT
Leiter International Performance Test (psychiatry)

LIQ
liquid (pharmacology)
lower inner quadrant (anatomy)

Liq.
liquor (chemical dependency and pharmacology)

liq
liquor [a liquor, liquid] (chemical dependency and pharmacology)

LIR
left iliac region (orthopedics)
left inferior rectus [muscle] (ophthalmology and surgery)

LIRBM
liver, iron, red bone marrow (hematology and laboratory)

LIS
left intercostal space (anatomy)
lobular in situ [carcinoma] (oncology)
low intermittent suction (surgery)

LISP
List Processing Language

LISS
low ionic strength saline [medium test] (laboratory)

lit
literal
literally

"lites"
{pronunciation of *LYTES* and *lytes* [electrolytes]} (laboratory) {not an abbreviation}

LITH
lithium (pharmacology and psychiatry)

litho
lithotripsy (gastroenterology, nephrology, and urology) {pronounced "lith-oh"}

"lith-oh"
{pronunciation of *litho* [lithotripsy]} (gastroenterology, nephrology, and urology) {not an abbreviation}

LIV
law of initial value
left innominate vein (cardiovascular)
liver battery test (gastroenterology)
living

LIVER S RB
liver scan rose bengal (gastroenterology and radiology)

LIVER S TECHN
liver scan technetium (gastroenterology and radiology)

LIVER S W FLOW
liver scan with flow (gastroenterology and radiology)

LJL
lateral joint line (orthopedics)

LJM
Löwenstein-Jensen medium (laboratory)

LK
left kidney (anatomy and nephrology)

LKID
left kidney (anatomy and nephrology)

LKKS
liver, kidneys, and spleen (anatomy)

LKQCPI
Licentiate of the King and Queen's College of Physicians in Ireland

L.K.Q.C.P.I.
Licentiate of the King and Queen's College of Physicians in Ireland

LKS
liver, kidneys, and spleen (anatomy)

LKS NP
liver, kidneys, and spleen not palpable [on physical examination] (anatomy)

LKV
laked kanamycin vancomycin [agar] (laboratory)
Lengyel-Kerman-Vargar [rating] (psychiatry)

LL
large lymphocyte (laboratory)
left lateral
left leg (orthopedics)
left lower
left lung (respiratory)
lower leg (orthopedics)
lower lid (ophthalmology and plastic surgery)
lower lip (otorhinolaryngology)
lower lobe (respiratory)
lumbar length (orthopedics)
lymphoblastic lymphoma
lysolecithin (hematology and laboratory)

L.L.
left lateral (anatomy)

L lam
lumbar laminectomy (neurology and orthopedics)

LLAT
left lateral (radiology)

LLB
long leg brace (orthopedics)

LLBCD
left lower border of cardiac dullness (cardiovascular)

LLC
long-leg cast (orthopedics)
lymphocytic leukemia, chronic (hematology and oncology)

LLD
cyanocobalamin factor [vitamin B$_{12}$] (laboratory)
Lactobacillus lactis Dorner factor [vitamin B$_{12}$] (laboratory)
leg length discrepancy (neurology, orthopedics, physical therapy, and rehabilitation)

LLDH
liver lactate dehydrogenase (laboratory)

LLE
left lower extremity (orthopedics)

LLF
factor XIII (hematology and laboratory)
fibrin-stabilizing factor (hematology and laboratory)
Laki-Lorand factor [fibrinase] (hematology and laboratory)
left lateral femoral [site of injection] (pharmacology)

LL-GXT
low-level graded exercise test (cardiovascular)

L lines
{not an abbreviation} (radiology)

LLL
left lower lid (ophthalmology and plastic surgery)
left lower limb (neurology and orthopedics)
left lower lobe [lung] (respiratory)
left lower lung (respiratory)

L.L.L.
left lower lobe [of lung] (respiratory)

LLM
localized leukocyte mobilization (laboratory)

LLO
Legionella-like organism (laboratory)

LLQ
left lower quadrant [of abdomen] (anatomy and gastroenterology)

LLR
left lateral rectus [eye muscle] (ophthalmology)
left lumbar region (neurology and orthopedics)

LLS
lazy leukocyte syndrome (hematology)
long leg splint (orthopedics)

LLSB
left lower sternal border (anatomy)

LLT
left lateral (anatomy)
left lateral thigh (orthopedics)

LLVAH
Loma Linda Veterans Administration Hospital (administration, armed forces, and government)

LLUMC
Loma Linda University Medical Center (administration)

LLWC
long-leg walking cast (orthopedics)

LM
labiomental [lip and chin] (dentistry, otorhinolaryngology, and surgery)
laryngeal muscle (otorhinolaryngology)
lateral malleolus (orthopedics)
legal medicine (law)
Licentiate in Medicine
Licentiate in Midwifery (obstetrics)
light microscopy (laboratory)
light minimum (neurology and ophthalmology)
linguomesial (dentistry)
lipid mobilizing [hormone] (cardiovascular and laboratory)

longitudinal muscle (neurology and orthopedics)
lower motor [neuron] (neurology)

L.M.
Licentiate in Midwifery (obstetrics)
light minimum (neurology and ophthalmology)
linguomesial (dentistry)

lm
lumen (measurement)

LMA
left mentoanterior [position] (obstetrics)
liver membrane autoantibody (gastroenterology and laboratory)

L.M.A.
left mentoanterior [position] (obstetrics)

LMB
Laurence-Moon-Biedl [syndrome] (genetics)
leiomyblastoma (gastroenterology and pathology)

LMBBS
Laurence-Moon-Biedl-Bardet syndrome (genetics)

LMC
living male child (obstetrics)
lymphomyeloid complex (laboratory)

LMCA
left main coronary artery (cardiovascular)
left middle cerebral artery (cardiovascular and neurology)

LMCAD
left main coronary artery disease (cardiovascular)

LMCC
Licentiate of the Medical Council of Canada

LMD
local medical doctor
low molecular weight dextran (pharmacology)

LMDX
low molecular weight dextran (pharmacology)

LME
left mediolateral episiotomy (obstetrics)

LMed & Ch
Licentiate in Medicine and Surgery

LMEE
left middle ear exploration (otorhinolaryngology)

LMF
chlorambucil, methotrexate, and 5-fluorouracil (chemotherapy, oncology, and pharmacology)
leukocyte mitogenic factor (laboratory)

L/min
liters per minute (measurement)

LML
large and medium lymphocytes (laboratory)
left mediolateral [episiotomy] (obstetrics)
left middle lobe [of lung] (respiratory)

LMM
Lactobacillus maintenance medium (laboratory)
lentigo maligna melanoma (dermatology)
light meromyosin (laboratory)

LMN
lower motor neuron (neurology)

LMNL
lower motor neuron lesion (neurology)

LMP
last menstrual period (gynecology and obstetrics)
left mentoposterior [position] (obstetrics)
lumbar puncture (neurology)

L.M.P.
left mentoposterior [position] (obstetrics)

LMR
left medial rectus [eye muscle] (ophthalmology)
localized magnetic resonance

LMRCP
Licentiate in Midwifery of the Royal College of Physicians (obstetrics)

L.M.R.C.P.
Licentiate in Midwifery of the Royal College of Physicians (obstetrics)

LMS
leiomyosarcoma (oncology)
Licentiate in Medicine and Surgery

L.M.S.
Licentiate in Medicine and Surgery

LMSSA
Licentiate in Medicine and Surgery of the Society of Apothecaries, London (pharmacology)

L.M.S.S.A.
Licentiate in Medicine and Surgery of the Society of Apothecaries (pharmacology)

LMT
left mentotransverse [position] (obstetrics)

L.M.T.
left mentotransverse [position] (obstetrics)

Lmt.
limited

LMW
low molecular weight (chemistry)

LMWD
low molecular weight dextran (pharmacology)

LN
labionasal [lip and nose] (otorhinolaryngology)
lipoid nephrosis (nephrology)
lupus nephritis (nephrology)
lymph node

L/N
letter-numerical [system]

ln
logarithm, natural (mathematics)

LNB
lymph node biopsy (surgery)

LND
lymph node dissection (surgery)

LNI
logarithm neutralization index (mathematics)

LNMP
last normal menstrual period (gynecology and obstetrics)

LNNB
Luria-Nebraska Neuropsychological Battery (psychiatry)

LNPF
lymph node permeability factor (laboratory)

LNR
lymph node region (oncology and surgery)

LO
lateral oblique [x-ray view] (radiology)
lenticular opacity (ophthalmology)
linguo-occlusal (dentistry)
love object (psychiatry)
low

LOA
leave of absence
left anterior oblique [view] (radiology)
left occipitoanterior [position; also

(chemotherapy, oncology, and pharmacology)

L-phenylalanine, procarbazine, Adriamycin, and methotrexate (chemotherapy, oncology, and pharmacology)

LPC
laser photocoagulation (ophthalmology)
late positive component
lysophosphatidylcholine (laboratory)

LPD
luteal phase defect (gynecology)

LPE
lipoprotein electrophoresis (cardiovascular and laboratory)

LPF
leukocytosis-promoting factor (hematology and laboratory)
localized plaque formation (cardiovascular)
low-power field (laboratory)
low-powered field (laboratory)
lymphocytosis-promoting factor (hematology and laboratory)

L.P.F.
leukocytosis-promoting factor (hematology and laboratory)

lpf
low-power field (laboratory)
low-powered field (laboratory)

LPH
left posterior hemiblock (cardiovascular)
lipotropic pituitary hormone [also called *lipotropin*] (laboratory)

LPL
lamina propria lymphocytes (laboratory)
lipoprotein lipase (laboratory)

LPLIS
lipoprotein lipase inactivation system (laboratory)

LPM
liters per minute (measurement)

lpm
liters per minute (measurement)

LPN
Licensed Practical Nurse (nursing)

L.P.N.
Licensed Practical Nurse (nursing)

LPO
hypothalamic-pituitary-ovarian (endocrinology, gynecology, and obstetrics)
left posterior oblique (radiology)
left posterior occipital [position] (obstetrics)
light perception only (neurology and ophthalmology)
lobus parolfactorius (neurology and otorhinolaryngology)

LpOH
lysopine dehydrogenase (laboratory)

LPP
lipoprotein lipase (laboratory)

LPR
lactate-pyruvate ratio (laboratory)

L/P ratio
liver to plasma concentration ratio (laboratory)
lymph plasma ratio (laboratory)

LPR ratio
lactate-pyruvate ratio (laboratory)

LPS
Lanterman-Petris-Short Act (psychiatry)
last Papanicolaou smear (gynecology)
lipase (laboratory)
lipopolysaccharide (laboratory)

lps
liters per second (measurement)

LP shunt
lumbar-peritoneal shunt [also called *lumboperitoneal shunt*] (neurosurgery)

LPV
left pulmonary vein (cardiovascular and
    respiratory)
lymphopathia venereum (gynecology,
    infectious diseases, and urology)

lpw
lumens per watt (electricity)

Lp.-X
lipoprotein-X (laboratory)

LQ
longevity quotient (statistics)
lordosis quotient (orthopedics)
lowest quadrant (anatomy)

lq
liquid (pharmacology)

LR
labor room (obstetrics)
laboratory references (laboratory)
laboratory report (laboratory)
lactated Ringer's [solution] (pharmacol-
    ogy)
latency relaxation (neurology)
lateral rectus [muscle] (ophthalmology)
left-right
light reaction (neurology and ophthal-
    mology)
light reflex (neurology and ophthalmol-
    ogy)

L/R
left to right [ratio]

L & R
left and right

L→R
left to right

Lr
lawrencium (chemistry)

LRA
left renal artery (nephrology, radiology)

LRC
lower rib cage (anatomy)

LRCP
Licentiate of the Royal College of Physi-
    cians

L.R.C.P.
Licentiate of the Royal College of Physi-
    cians

LRCP & SI
Licentiate of the Royal College of Physi-
    cians and Surgeons, Ireland

L.R.C.P. & S.I.
Licentiate of the Royal College of Physi-
    cians and Surgeons, Ireland

LRCS
Licentiate of the Royal College of Sur-
    geons

L.R.C.S.
Licentiate of the Royal College of Sur-
    geons

LRCSE
Licentiate of the Royal College of Sur-
    geons, Edinburgh

L.R.C.S.E.
Licentiate of the Royal College of Sur-
    geons, Edinburgh

LRCSI
Licentiate of the Royal College of Sur-
    geons, Ireland

LRD
living related donor (transplant surgery)
living renal donor (nephrology and
    transplant surgery)

L.R.E.
least restrictive environment (psychia-
    try)

LRF
latex and resorcinol formaldehyde (labo-
    ratory)
liver residue factor (laboratory)
luteinizing hormone-releasing factor (en-
    docrinology and laboratory)

LRH
luteinizing hormone-releasing hormone
(endocrinology and laboratory)

LRL
Lunar Research Laboratory (aerospace
science and research)

LRM
left radical mastectomy (surgery)

LRND
left radical neck dissection (surgery)

LRQ
lower right quadrant (anatomy)

LRR
labyrinthine righting reflex (neurology
and otorhinolaryngology)

LRS
lactated Ringer's solution (pharmacology)
Lights Retention Scale (psychiatry)

LRSF
lactating rat serum factor (laboratory)

LRT
lower respiratory tract (respiratory)

LRTI
lower respiratory tract illness (respiratory)
lower respiratory tract infection (respiratory)

LRV
left renal vein (nephrology, radiology)

LS
lateral suspensor [ligament] (anatomy)
left sacrum (orthopedics)
left side
legally separated
leiomyosarcoma (oncology)
Licentiate in Surgery
Life Science
liminal sensation (neurology and psychiatry)
liminal sensitivity (neurology and psychiatry)
liver and spleen (anatomy)

lumbosacral (neurology and orthopedics)
lymphosarcoma (oncology)

L/S
lactase/sucrase [ratio] (laboratory)
lecithin/sphingomyelin [ratio] (laboratory and obstetrics)

L-S
lumbosacral (neurology and orthopedics)

L → S
lumen-to-serosa (anatomy)

L$_s$-
{not an abbreviation} [chemical prefix]
(chemistry and pharmacology)

LSA
Language Sampling Analysis [by Tyack
and Gottsleben] (speech and language
therapy)
left sacroanterior [position] (obstetrics)
lichen sclerosis et atrophicus (dermatology)
lipid-bound sialic acid (laboratory)
lymphosarcoma (oncology)

L.S.A.
left sacroanterior [position] (obstetrics)
Licentiate of Society of Apothecaries
(pharmacology)

LSA 1
cyclophosphamide plus radiotherapy
plus consolidation (chemotherapy, oncology, pharmacology, and radiation
therapy)

LSA 212
cyclophosphamide plus radiotherapy
plus consolidation (chemotherapy, oncology, pharmacology, and radiation
therapy)

LSAR
lymphosarcoma cell(s) (laboratory)

LSA/RCS
lymphosarcoma-reticulum cell sarcoma (oncology)

LSB
left sternal border (cardiovascular and respiratory)

LS BPS
laparoscopic bilateral partial salpingectomies (gynecology)

LSC
late systolic click (cardiovascular)
left-side colon [cancer] (gastroenterology and oncology)
lid(s), sclera(e), and conjunctiva(e) (ophthalmology)
liquid scintillation counting (laboratory)

LSCA
left subclavian artery (surgery, radiology)

LScA
left scapuloanterior [position] (obstetrics)

L.Sc.A.
left scapuloanterior [position] (obstetrics)

LScP
left scapuloposterior [position] (obstetrics)

L.Sc.P.
left scapuloposterior [position] (obstetrics)

LSCS
lower segment cesarean section (obstetrics)

LSCV
left subclavian vein (surgery, radiology)

LSD
least significant difference
least significant digit (mathematics)
lysergic acid diethylamide [also called *lysergide*] {This is the drug used in psychiatric treatment and as a street drug in the 1960's and early 1970's and re-emerging as a street drug in the 1980's.} (pharmacology and psychiatry)
low-salt diet (cardiovascular and dietary)

LSD 25
D-lysergic acid diethylamine tartrate 25 (pharmacology)

LSE
left sternal edge (anatomy)
local side effects (pharmacology)

l/sec
liters per second (measurement and respiratory)

LSF
low saturated fat [diet] (cardiovascular and dietary)
lymphocyte-stimulating factor (laboratory)

LSH
lutein stimulating hormone (endocrinology and laboratory)
lymphocyte-stimulating hormone [factor] (endocrinology and laboratory)

LSHTM
London School of Hygiene and Tropical Medicine (education)

LSI
large scale integrated [circuits] (electronics)
large scale integration (electronics)

LSK
liver, spleen, and kidney(s) (anatomy)

LSKM
{slang} liver-spleen-kidney-megaly (gastroenterology and nephrology)

LSL
left sacrolateral [position] (obstetrics)

LSM
late systolic murmur (cardiovascular)

lymphocyte separation medium (laboratory)

lysergic acid morpholide (pharmacology)

LSO
lateral superior olive [of the brain] (neurology)
left salpingo-oophorectomy (gynecology)

LSP
left sacroposterior [position] (obstetrics)
liver-specific [membrane] lipoprotein (laboratory)

L.S.P.
left sacroposterior [position] (obstetrics)

LSp
left span (measurement)
life span (measurement)

L-sp
lumbar spine (neurology and orthopedics)

L-Spar
Elspar [asparaginase] (pharmacology)

L-spine
lumbar spine (neurology and orthopedics)

L/S ratio
lecithin/sphingomyelin ratio (laboratory and obstetrics)

LSS
liver-spleen scan (gastroenterology and radiology)
lumbosacral spine (neurology, orthopedics, and radiology)

LSSA
lipid-soluble secondary antioxidant (laboratory)

LST
left sacrotransverse [position] (obstetrics)

L.S.T.
left sacrotransverse [position] (obstetrics)

LSTL
laparoscopic tubal ligation (gynecology)

LST tract
lateral spinothalamic tract (neurology)

LSU
lactose-saccharose-urea [agar] (laboratory)
Louisiana State University (education)

L.S.U.
lactose-saccharose-urea [medium] (laboratory)

LSV
left subclavian vein (cardiovascular)

LSWA
large-amplitude, slow wave activity (neurology)

LSX
Labstix (endocrinology and laboratory)

LT
heat-labile enterotoxin (laboratory)
left
left thigh (anatomy and orthopedics)
left triceps (anatomy, neurology, and orthopedics)
leukotriene (allergy, laboratory, otorhinolaryngology, and respiratory)
Levin tube (gastroenterology)
levothyroxine (endocrinology and pharmacology)
light
long term
low temperature
low transverse [incision] (obstetrics)
lumbar traction (neurology and orthopedics)
lymphotoxin (laboratory)

Lt.
left

lt
left
light
low tension

LTA
leukotriene A (allergy, laboratory, oto-rhinolaryngology, and respiratory)
lipoate transacetylase (laboratory)
lipoteichoic acid (laboratory)

LTAS
lead tetra-acetate Schiff (laboratory)

LTB
laparoscopic tubal banding [ligation] (gynecology)
laryngotracheobronchitis (otorhinolar-yngology)
leukotriene B (allergy, laboratory, oto-rhinolaryngology, and respiratory)

LTC
left to count
leukotriene C (allergy, laboratory, oto-rhinolaryngology, and respiratory)
long-term care (nursing and rehabilita-tion)

LTCF
long-term care facility (nursing and re-habilitation)

LTCS
low transverse cesarean section (obstet-rics)

LTD
leukotriene D (allergy, laboratory, oto-rhinolaryngology, and respiratory)

ltd
limited

LTDQ
limited quantity [refers to a test per-formed on a scanty specimen] (labora-tory)

LTE
leukotriene E (allergy, laboratory, oto-rhinolaryngology, and respiratory)

LTF
lipotropic factor [or hormone] (labora-tory)
lymphocyte transforming factor (labora-tory)

LTG
long-term goals (occupational and physi-cal therapy)

LTGA
left transposition of the great arteries [also called *corrected transposition*] (cardiovascular)

L-TGA
levo-transposition of the great vessels [also called *corrected transposition*] (cardiovascular)

l-TGA
levotransposition of the great arteries [also called *corrected transposition*] (cardiovascular)

LTH
low-temperature holding [pasteurization] (laboratory)
luteotropic hormone [also called *lacto-genic hormone* and *prolactin*] (endo-crinology and laboratory)

LtH
luteotropic hormone [also called *lacto-genic hormone* and *prolactin*] (endo-crinology and laboratory)
left-handed (neurology and orthopedics)

LTL
laparoscopic tubal ligation (gynecology)

lt lat
left lateral

LTP
long-term potentiation

LTPP
lipothiamide-pyrophosphate (labora-tory)

LVFP
left ventricular filling pressure (cardiovascular)

L.V.G.
left ventrogluteal (anatomy)

LVH
large vessel hematocrit (hematology and
laboratory)
left ventricular hypertrophy (cardiovascular)

L.V.H.
left ventricular hypertrophy (cardiovascular)

LVI
left ventricular insufficiency (cardiovascular)

LVID
left ventricular internal dimension (cardiovascular)

LVL
left vastus lateralis (anatomy)

L.V.L.
left vastus lateralis (anatomy)

LVLG
left ventrolateral gluteal [injection site]
(anatomy and pharmacology)

LVMM
left ventricular muscle mass (cardiovascular)

LVN
Licensed Visiting Nurse (nursing)
Licensed Vocational Nurse (nursing)

L.V.N.
Licensed Visiting Nurse (nursing)

LVO
left ventricular overactivity (cardiovascular)

LVOA
left ventricular overactivity (cardiovascular)
Licensed Vocational Nurse (nursing)

LVP
large volume parenteral (pharmacology)
left ventricular pressure (cardiovascular)
8-lysine-vasopressin (cardiovascular and
pharmacology)

L.V.P.
lysine-vasopressin (cardiovascular and
pharmacology)

LVPW
left ventricular posterior wall (cardiovascular)

LVPWT
left ventricular posterior wall thickness
(cardiovascular)

LVS
left ventricular strain (cardiovascular)

LV$_S$
mean left ventricular systolic pressure
(cardiovascular)

LVs
mean left ventricular systolic pressure
(cardiovascular)

LVSP
left ventricular systolic pressure (cardiovascular)

LVSV
left ventricular stroke volume (cardiovascular)

LVSW
left ventricular septal wall (cardiovascular)
left ventricular stroke work (cardiovascular)

LVSWI
left ventricular stroke work index (cardiovascular)

LVT
left ventricular tension (cardiovascular)
lysine vasotonin (pharmacology)

LVV
left ventricular volume (cardiovascular)

LVVP
chlorambucil, vinblastine, vincristine, and prednisone (chemotherapy, oncology, and pharmacology)

LVW
left ventricular work (cardiovascular)

LVWI
left ventricular work index (cardiovascular)

LW
lacerating wound (dermatology and emergency medicine)

LW
lateral wall [image on transesophageal echocardiography] (cardiovascular)
Lee-White [method, clotting test] (hematology and laboratory)

L.W.
Lee-White [method, clotting test] (hematology and laboratory)

L & W
living and well

L/W
living and well

L-10-W
Levulose (10%) in water (pharmacology)

Lw
lawrencium (physics)

l & w
living and well

LWCT
Lachar-Wrobel Critical Items (psychiatry)
Lee-White clotting time (laboratory)

LX
local irradiation (radiation therapy)

lx
lux [the metric unit of illumination] (chemistry)

LXT
left exotropia (ophthalmology)

LY
lactoalbumin-yeastolate [media] (laboratory)

Ly
{not an abbreviation} [various T-cell antigens] (laboratory)

ly
langley [unit of sun's heat] (physics)

LYG
lymphomatoid granulomatosis (infectious diseases and oncology)

lym
lymphocyte (laboratory)

LYMPH%
percent of lymphocytes [in differential count] (laboratory)

lymph
lymphocyte (laboratory) {pronounced "lim-fa"}

lymphos
lymphocytes (laboratory) {pronounced "lim-foes"}

lymphs
lymphocytes (laboratory) {pronounced "limps"}

LYP
lactose, yeast, peptone [agar] (laboratory)

Lys
lysine [an amino acid] (laboratory)

LYTES
electrolytes (laboratory) {pronounced "lites"}

lytes
electrolytes (laboratory) {pronounced
  "lites"}

LZM
lysozyme (laboratory)

lzm
lysozyme (laboratory)

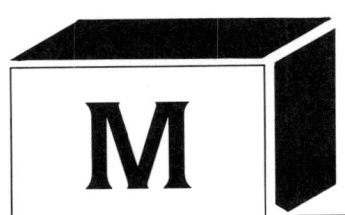

M

μ
micro- [a prefix meaning *small*] {not an abbreviation}
micrometer (measurement)
micron (measurement)
mu [twelfth letter of the Greek alphabet]

M
internal medicine [specialty]
macerare [macerate]
male
malignant [referring to tumors] (oncology)
married
masculine (endocrinology)
mass
massage (physical therapy)
maternally contributing (genetics)
matrix
mature
maximal
maximum
mean (laboratory and mathematics)
medial
median
mediator [chemical released in tissues] (laboratory)
medical
medicine (pharmacology)
medium (laboratory)
mega- [prefix for 10^6 (measurement) or big or huge as a word prefix] {not an abbreviation}
memory [associative] (neurology and psychiatry)
mentum [chin] (anatomy)
meridies [noon]
mesial
metabolite (laboratory)
meter (measurement)
methionine [an amino acid] (chemistry, dietary, and laboratory)
methotrexate (chemotherapy, oncology, and pharmacology)
Micrococcus [a bacterium] (laboratory)
Microsporum [a fungus] (dermatology and laboratory)

mild
mille [thousand]
minim (measurement)
minimum
minute (measurement)
misce [mix] (pharmacology)
mistura [mixture] (pharmacology)
mitte [send]
mixture (pharmacology)
mol [also called mole] (measurement)
molar [solution] (chemistry)
molar [tooth, permanent] (dentistry)
molecular weight (chemistry)
Monday
monkey (research and veterinary medicine)
monocyte (laboratory)
month
morphine (chemical dependency and pharmacology)
mortis [death]
mother
motile [referring to bacteria] (laboratory)
mu [twelfth letter of the Greek alphabet]
mucoid [referring to bacterial colonies] (laboratory)
mucoid colony (laboratory)
multipara (gynecology and obstetrics)
murmur [heart] (cardiovascular)
muscle (neurology and orthopedics)
mutitas [dullness]
Mycobacterium [a bacterium] (laboratory)
Mycoplasma [a bacterium] (laboratory)
myopia (ophthalmology)
permanent molar [tooth] (dentistry)
strength of pole (chemistry)

M.
macerare [macerate]
maximal
maximum
meter (measurement)
mil [mille, thousand]

486

minim (measurement)
misce [mix] (pharmacology)
mistura [mixture] (pharmacology)
mucoid [colony] (bacteriology)
muscle (neurology and orthopedics)
myopia (ophthalmology)

MΩ

megaohm [also called *megohm*] (measurement)

γM

gamma M immunoglobulin [also called *immunoglobulin M*] (immunology and laboratory)

μM

micromolar (measurement)

M₁

mitral first heart sound (cardiovascular)
slight dullness [on auscultation] (respiratory)
sphenoidal segment of middle cerebral artery (cardiovascular and neurology)

M₂

insular segment of middle cerebral artery (cardiovascular and neurology)
marked dullness [on auscultation] (respiratory)
mitral second heart sound (cardiovascular)
square meter (measurement)
square meter [of body surface] (radiation therapy)

M²

square meter (measurement)

M-2

M-2 protocol [vincristine (Oncovin), carmustine (BCNU), cyclophosphamide (Cytoxan), melphalan, and prednisone] (chemotherapy, oncology, and pharmacology)

α₂M

alpha₂-macroglobulin (laboratory)

M₃

absolute dullness [on auscultation] (respiratory)

opercular segment of middle cerebral artery (cardiovascular and neurology)

M/3

middle third [of long bones] (orthopedics)

M₄

cortical segment of middle cerebral artery (cardiovascular and neurology)

M/10

tenth molar (chemistry)

M/100

hundredth molar (chemistry)

M-300

{not an abbreviation} [a panel of tests] (laboratory)

m

deciduous molar [tooth] (dentistry)
macerare [macerate]
magnetic moment (physics)
manipulus [handful] (pharmacology)
mass
mean
median
medium (laboratory)
melts at [when followed by a number indicating temperature] (chemistry)
mentum [chin] (anatomy)
mesial
meter (measurement)
mil [thousand]
milli- [prefix for 10^{-3}] (measurement)
minim (measurement)
minute (measurement)
misce [mix] (pharmacology)
mistura [mixture] (pharmacology)
mitte [send]
molar [tooth, deciduous] (dentistry)
motile (laboratory)
murmur [heart] (cardiovascular)
sample mean (laboratory)

m.

meter (measurement)

Multilingual Aphasia Examination (speech and language therapy)

MAEEW
moves all extremities equally well (neurology and rehabilitation)

MAF
macrophage activating factor (laboratory)
macrophage activation factor (laboratory)
macrophage agglutinating factor (laboratory)
minimum audible field (otorhinolaryngology)
movement aftereffect

MAFAs
movement-associated fetal [heart rate] accelerations (obstetrics)

MAFH
macroaggregated ferrous hydroxide (laboratory)

Mag
magnesium (chemistry, laboratory, and pharmacology)

mag
magnification (laboratory, ophthalmology, and surgery)
magnus [large]

mag cit
magnesium citrate (pharmacology)

MAggF
macrophage agglutination factor (laboratory)

Magic
microprobe analysis generalized intensity corrections (laboratory)

magn
magnus [large]

mag sulf
magnesium sulfate (pharmacology)

mag sulfate
magnesium sulfate (pharmacology)

MAHA
macroangiopathic hemolytic anemia (hematology)

"mah-tab"
{pronunciation of *metab* [metabolic and metabolism]} {not an abbreviation}

MAI
Mycobacterium avium intracellulare (bacteriology and laboratory)

MAILED
mailed out (laboratory)

MAIT
methotrexate and cytosine arabinoside [intrathecal] (chemotherapy, oncology, and pharmacology)

MAKA
major karyotypic abnormality (genetics and laboratory)

MAL
midaxillary line (anatomy)
malfunction

Mal
malate (laboratory and pharmacology)
Malayan [nationality]

mal
malum [ill]

MALA
malarial parasites (infectious diseases, laboratory, and respiratory)

MALAR
malaria (infectious diseases, laboratory, and respiratory)

Mal-BSA
maleated bovine serum albumin (laboratory)

malig
malignant (oncology and pathology)

MALIMET
Master List of Medical Indexing Terms
  [EMBASE thesaurus] (publishing and
  reference)

MALT
mucosa-associated lymphoid tissue (pathology)

MAM
methylazomethanol (gastroenterology
  and laboratory)

M+Am
compound myopic astigmatism (ophthalmology)
myopic astigmatism (ophthalmology)

mam
milliampere-minute (measurement)

MAMA
monoclonal antimalignin antibody (laboratory and neurology)

MAMC
midarm muscle circumference (neurology and orthopedics)

ma-min
milliampere-minute (electricity)

mammo
mammography (gynecology and radiology) {pronounced "mam-oh"}

"mam-oh"
{pronunciation of *mammo* [mammogra-
  phy]} (gynecology and radiology) {not
  an abbreviation}

m-AMSA
acridinyl anisidide (chemotherapy, hematology, pharmacology, and oncology)

MAN
magnocellular nucleus [of anterior neo-
  striatum] (neurology)

Man.
manipulus [handful] (pharmacology)

man
mane [morning]
manipulate (orthopedics, physical therapy, and rehabilitation)
manipulus [handful] (pharmacology)

mand
mandible (dentistry and otorhinolaryngology)
mandibar (dentistry and otorhinolaryngology)

manifest
manifestation

Manip.
manipulus [handful] (pharmacology)

manip
manipulation (orthopedics, physical
  therapy, and rehabilitation)
manipulus [handful] (pharmacology)

MANOVA
multivariate analysis of variance (physics)

MAN-6-P
mannose-6-phosphate (chemistry)

Man-6-P
mannose-6-phosphate (chemistry)

Man. pr.
mane primo [early in the morning]

man pr
mane primo [early in the morning]

man. pr.
mane primo [early in the morning]

manu
manufacture (manufacturing)

MAO
Master of the Art of Obstetrics (education and obstetrics)
maximal acid output (laboratory)
medial ankle orthosis (orthopedics and
  rehabilitation)

Marsh-Bender factor (laboratory)
Medicinae Baccalaureus [Bachelor of Medicine] (education)
mesiobuccal (dentistry)
methyl bromide [a toxic insect fumigant] (chemistry)
methylene blue [dye] (laboratory and surgery)
microbiological assay (laboratory)
{not an abbreviation} [measurement of creatine phosphokinase isoenzyme MB bands of cardiac muscle] (cardiovascular and laboratory)

M.B.
Medicinae Baccalaureus [Bachelor of Medicine] (education)

Mb
myoglobin tritium (hematology and laboratory)

mb
millibar (measurement)
misce bene [mix well] (pharmacology)

m.b.
misce bene [mix well] (pharmacology)

MBA
methylbovine albumin (laboratory)

MBAC
Member of the British Association of Chemists

M-BACOD
methotrexate, citrovorum factor, bleomycin, Adriamycin, cyclophosphamide, vincristine, and dexamethasone (chemotherapy, oncology, and pharmacology)

mbar.
millibar (measurement)

MBAS
methylene blue active substance (laboratory)

MB bands
{not an abbreviation} [measurement of creatine phosphokinase isoenzyme MB bands of cardiac muscle] (cardiovascular and laboratory)

MBC
maximum breathing capacity (respiratory)
methylthymol blue complex (laboratory)
minimal bactericidal concentration (laboratory)

MB-CK
{not an abbreviation} [a creatinine kinase isoenzyme] (laboratory)

MBD
methotrexate, bleomycin, and cis-platinum (chemotherapy, oncology, and pharmacology)
methylene blue dye (laboratory and surgery)
minimal brain damage (neurology)
minimal brain dysfunction (neurology)
Morquio-Brailsford disease [also called *Morquio-Brailsford syndrome, Morquio's syndrome,* and *mucopolysaccharidosis IV* (MPS IV)] (cardiovascular, genetics, neurology, ophthalmology, and orthopedics)

MBE
may be elevated

MBF
myocardial blood flow (cardiovascular)

MB factor
Marsh-Bender factor (laboratory)

MBFLB
monaural bifrequency loudness balance (otorhinolaryngology)

MBH
medial basal hypothalamus (neurology)

MBH₂
methylene blue reduced (laboratory)

MBI
methylene blue installation (radiology and surgery)

MBK
methyl butyl ketone (laboratory)

MBL
Marine Biological Laboratory [Woods Hole, Massachusetts] (biology, laboratory, oceanography, and research)
medium brown loose [stool] (gastroenterology)
menstrual blood loss (gynecology)
minimal bactericidal level (laboratory)

MBLA
methylbenzyl linoleic acid (chemistry)

MBM
mineral basal medium (laboratory)
mother's breast milk (neonatology and obstetrics)

MBNOA
Member British Naturopathic and Osteopathic Association (naturopathy and osteopathy)

MBO
mesiobucco-occlusal (dentistry)

MBP
MB band present (cardiovascular and laboratory)
mean blood pressure (cardiovascular)
melitensis bovine, porcine [antigen from *Brucella melitensis, Brucella bovis,* and *Brucella suis*] (laboratory)
mesiobuccopulpul (dentistry)
myelin basic protein (laboratory)

MBR
methylene blue reduced (laboratory)

MBRT
methylene blue reduction time (laboratory)

MBSA
methylated bovine serum albumin (immunology and laboratory)

MC
Magister Chirurgiae [Master of Surgery] (education and surgery)
mast cell (laboratory)
maximum concentration (laboratory)

Medical Corps (armed forces)
medium-chain [triglycerides] (laboratory)
Merkel cell (laboratory)
mesenteric collateral (cardiovascular and gastroenterology)
mesiocervical (dentistry)
metacarpal (orthopedics)
metatarsocuneiform (orthopedics and podiatry)
mineralocorticoid [referring to adrenal cortical hormones] (endocrinology and laboratory)
miscarriage (obstetrics)
mitomycin (chemotherapy, oncology, and pharmacology)
mitomycin-C (chemotherapy, oncology, and pharmacology)
mitochondrial complementation (laboratory)
mitotic cycle (laboratory)
mixed cellularity (laboratory)
mixed cryoglobulinemia (cardiovascular, dermatology, gastroenterology, hematology, nephrology, neurology, and orthopedics)
monkey cells (laboratory and research)
myocarditis (cardiovascular)
monocomponent highly purified pork insulin (endocrinology and pharmacology)

M.C.
Magister Chirurgiae [Master of Surgery] (education and surgery)
Medical Corps (armed forces)

M-C
medico-chirurgical [referring to medicine and surgery]
mineralocorticoid [referring to adrenal cortical hormones] (endocrinology and laboratory)

M & C
morphine and cocaine (chemical dependency and pharmacology)

Mc
megacurie (measurement, radiation therapy, and radiology)
megacycle (measurement)

mC
millicoulomb (electricity)

mc
millicurie (measurement, radiation therapy, and radiology)

mμc
millimicrocurie [also called nanocurie] (measurement, radiation therapy, and radiology)

MCA
main coronary artery (cardiovascular)
major coronary arteries (cardiovascular)
Manufacturing Chemists Association (chemistry and manufacturing)
Maternity Center Association (obstetrics)
methylcholanthrene [a procarcinogen] (chemistry, laboratory, oncology, and research)
middle cerebral aneurysm (cardiovascular and neurology)
middle cerebral artery (cardiovascular and neurology)
monoclonal antibodies (laboratory)
motorcycle accident (emergency medicine)
multichannel analyzer (laboratory)

M.C.A.
middle cerebral artery (cardiovascular and neurology)

MCAT
Medical College Admission Test (education)

m caute
misce caute [mix cautiously] (pharmacology)

m. caute
misce caute [mix cautiously] (pharmacology)

MCB
membranous cytoplasmic body (laboratory)

McB
McBurney's [point] (anatomy, gastroenterology, and surgery)

MCBM
muscle capillary basement membrane (laboratory)

MCBP
melphalan, cyclophosphamide, carmustine [BCNU], and prednisone (chemotherapy, oncology, and pharmacology)

MCB pt
McBurney's point (anatomy, gastroenterology, and surgery)

MCBR
minimum concentration of bilirubin (laboratory)

MCC
marked cocontraction (neurology and orthopedics)
mean corpuscular hemoglobin concentration (laboratory)
midstream clean-catch [urine] (laboratory)
minimum complete-killing concentration (laboratory)

McC
McCarthy [panendoscope] (urology)
McCoy [antibodies] (laboratory)

MCCNU
methyl-1-(-2-chloroethyl)-3-cyclohexyl-1-nitrosourea [also called *methyl-CCNU* and *semustine*] (chemotherapy, oncology, and pharmacology)

MCCU
Mobile Coronary Care Unit (cardiovascular and emergency medicine)

MCD
mean cell diameter (laboratory)
mean corpuscular diameter (laboratory)
mean of consecutive differences
medium corpuscular density (cardiovascular)

medullary cystic disease [also called *familial juvenile nephronophthisis*] (nephrology)

metacarpal cortical density (orthopedics)

millicuries destroyed (radiation therapy)

minimal changes disease

multiple carboxylase deficiency [also called *holocarboxylase synthetase deficiency*] (dermatology, endocrinology, genetics, and psychiatry)

mcd
millicuries destroyed (radiation therapy)

MCDT
mast cell degranulation test (allergy and laboratory)

MCF
macrophage chemotactic factor (laboratory)

medium corpuscular fragility (hematology)

myocardial contractile force (cardiovascular)

MCFA
medium-chain fatty acid (laboratory)

mcg
microgram (measurement)

MCGN
minimal-change glomerular nephritis [also called *minimal-change glomerulonephritis*] (nephrology)

mixed cryoglobulinemia associated with glomerulonephritis (cardiovascular, dermatology, gastroenterology, hematology, nephrology, neurology, and orthopedics)

MCH
Maternal and Child Health (gynecology, neonatology, obstetrics, and pediatrics)

mean cell hemoglobin (hematology and laboratory)

mean corpuscular hemoglobin (hematology and laboratory)

mean corpuscular hemoglobin and red cell indices (hematology and laboratory)

muscle contraction headache (neurology)

MCh
Magister Chirurgiae [Master of Surgery] (education and surgery)

mc h
millicurie-hour (measurement, radiation therapy, and radiology)

mc.h.
millicurie-hour (measurement, radiation therapy, and radiology)

mc-h
millicurie-hour (measurement, radiation therapy, and radiology)

MCHb
mean corpuscular hemoglobin (hematology and laboratory)

MCHbC
mean corpuscular hemoglobin concentration (hematology and laboratory)

mean corpuscular hemoglobin count (hematology and laboratory)

MCHC
mean corpuscular hemoglobin concentration (hematology and laboratory)

mean corpuscular hemoglobin concentration and red cell indices (hematology and laboratory)

mean corpuscular hemoglobin count (hematology and laboratory)

MChD
Master of Dental Surgery (dentistry and education)

MCHg
mean corpuscular hemoglobin (hematology and laboratory)

MCHgb
mean corpuscular hemoglobin (hematology and laboratory)

MChir
Magister Chirurgiae [Master of Surgery]
(education and surgery)

MCHL
mean corpuscular hemoglobin [count]
(hematology and laboratory)

MChOrth
Master of Orthopedic Surgery (education and orthopedics)

MChOtol
Master of Otology (education and otorhinolaryngology)

MCHR
Medical Committee for Human Rights
(ethics)

mc.hr.
millicurie-hour (measurement, radiation
therapy, and radiology)

mc-hr
millicurie-hour (measurement, radiation
therapy, and radiology)

MCHS
Maternal and Child Health Service (gynecology, neonatology, obstetrics, and
pediatrics)

MChS
Member of the Society of Chiropodists
(podiatry)

MCI
mean cardiac index (cardiovascular)

MCi
megacurie (measurement, radiation
therapy, and radiology)

Mci
millicurie (measurement, radiation therapy, and radiology)

mCi
millicurie (measurement, radiation therapy, and radiology)

mCi-hr
millicurie-hour (measurement, radiation
therapy, and radiology)

MCKD
multicystic kidney disease (nephrology)

MCL
medial collateral ligament (neurology
and orthopedics)
midclavicular line (anatomy)
midcostal line (anatomy)
modified chest lead [on electrocardio-
gram] (cardiovascular)
most comfortable level [referring to
sound level] (otorhinolaryngology)
most comfortable loudness [level on au-
diometry] (otorhinolaryngology)

MCLL
most comfortable loudness level [on au-
diometry] (otorhinolaryngology)

MCLNS
mucocutaneous lymph node syndrome
[also called *Kawasaki's disease*] (dermatology, ophthalmology, otorhinolaryngology, and pediatrics)

MClSci
Master of Clinical Science (education)

MCMAI
Millon Clinical Multi-Axial Inventory
(psychiatry)

M colony
mucoid colony (laboratory)

MCommH
Master of Community Health (education)

mcoul
millicoulomb (electricity and measurement)

MCP
Medical College of Pennsylvania (education)

Medical Continuation Pay (armed forces)

melphalan, cyclophosphamide, and prednisone (chemotherapy, oncology, and pharmacology)

metacarpophalangeal [joint] (orthopedics)

mitotic-control protein (laboratory)

MCPA
Member of the College of Pathologists, Australasia (pathology)

MCPH
metacarpophalangeal (orthopedics)

MCPS
Member of the College of Physicians and Surgeons

Mcps
megacycles per second (measurement)

Mc.p.s.
megacycles per second (measurement)

mc. p. s.
megacycles per second (measurement)

MCQ
multiple choice question [on testing] (education and psychiatry)

MCR
Medical Corps Reserve (armed forces)
message competition ratio
metabolic clearance rate (laboratory)

MCRA
Member of the College of Radiologists, Australasia (radiology)

MCS
microculture and sensitivity (laboratory)
myocardial contractile state (cardiovascular)

MCSA
minimal cross-sectional area (laboratory and radiology)

MCSP
Member of the Chartered Society of

Physiotherapists [British] (physical therapy and rehabilitation)

M.C.S.P.
Member of the Chartered Society of Physiotherapists [British] (physical therapy and rehabilitation)

MCT
mean cell thickness (laboratory)
mean cell threshold (laboratory)
mean circulation time (pharmacology)
mean corpuscular thickness (hematology and laboratory)
medium-chain triglyceride (laboratory)
medullary cancer of the thyroid (endocrinology and oncology)
multiple compressed tablet (pharmacology)

MCTC
metrizamide computerized tomographic cisternography (neurosurgery and radiology)

MCTD
mixed connective tissue disease (rheumatology)

MCT Oil
{not an abbreviation} [a dietary supplement] (pharmacology)

MCU
Malaria Control Unit [Army] (armed forces, infectious diseases, and respiratory)
maximum care unit
millicurie (measurement, radiation therapy, and radiology)
Mobile Care Unit (emergency medicine)

mcU
micro unit (measurement)

MCV
mean cell volume (laboratory)
mean clinical value (clinical research)
mean corpuscular volume (hematology and laboratory)

mcv

mean corpuscular volume and red cell indices (hematology and laboratory)

mcv

microvolt (measurement)

MCZ

Museum of Comparative Zoology [Harvard University] (zoology)

MD

main duct (anatomy)

malic dehydrogenase (laboratory)

manic-depression (psychiatry)

manic-depressive (psychiatry)

Mantoux diameter [result of Mantoux test (a tuberculin test)] (immunology, infectious diseases, and laboratory)

March of Dimes (genetics, neurology, orthopedics, and research)

Marek's disease [a herpesvirus-caused lymphoproliferative disease of chickens] (veterinary medicine)

Maryland [Postal Service state designation]

maternal deprivation (neonatology and obstetrics)

mean deviation (statistics)

medical department (administration)

medical doctor

Medicinae Doctor [Doctor of Medicine] (education)

medium dosage (pharmacology and radiation therapy)

mental deficiency (neurology and psychiatry)

mentally deficient (neurology and psychiatry)

mesiodistal (dentistry)

mitral disease (cardiovascular)

monocular deprivation (ophthalmology)

movement disorder (neurology)

muscular dystrophy (neurology)

myocardial damage (cardiovascular)

myocardial disease (cardiovascular)

M.D.

Medicinae Doctor [Doctor of Medicine] (education)

Md

mendelevium [a radioactive chemical element] (chemistry)

md

mean diastolic (cardiovascular)

median

MDA

malondialdehyde (laboratory)

manual dilation of the anus (gastroenterology)

mentodextra anterior [right mentoanterior position] (obstetrics)

3-4-methylenedioxyamphetamine [also called *methylenedioxyamphetamine*; an illegal amphetamine] (chemical dependency, pharmacology, and psychiatry)

monodehydroascorbate (laboratory)

motor discriminative acuity (neurology)

multivariant discriminant analysis

Muscular Dystrophy Association (neurology and research)

M.D.A.

mentodextra anterior [right mentoanterior position] (obstetrics)

motor discriminative acuity (neurology)

MDAC

multiplying digital-to-analog converter (radiology)

MDAP

Machover Draw-A-Person Test (psychiatry)

MDBDF

March of Dimes Birth Defect Foundation (genetics, neurology, orthopedics, and research)

MDBK

Madin-Darby bovine kidney [cells] (laboratory)

MDC

medial dorsal cutaneous [nerve] (neurology)

minimum detectable concentration (laboratory)

MDCK
Madin-Darby canine kidney [cell line] (laboratory)

MDD
Doctor of Dental Medicine (dentistry and education)
major depressive disorder (psychiatry)
manic depressive disorder (psychiatry)
mean daily dose

MDentSc
Master of Dental Science (dentistry and education)

MDF
mean dominant frequency (neurology)
myocardial depressant factor (cardiovascular and laboratory)

MDH
malic dehydrogenase (laboratory)
medullary dorsal horn (neurology)

MDHR
maximum determined heart rate (cardiovascular)

MDI
diphenylmethane diisocyanate [a gas] (chemistry)
manic-depressive illness (psychiatry)
metered dose inhaler (pharmacology and respiratory)
multiple daily injection (pharmacology)

m dict
more dicto [in the manner directed] (pharmacology)

m. dict.
more dicto [in the manner directed] (pharmacology)

MDII
multiple daily insulin injection (endocrinology and pharmacology)

MDL
Master Drug List (pharmacology)

MDM
mid-diastolic murmur (cardiovascular)

minor determinant mix [of penicillin] (laboratory)
minor determinant mixture (laboratory)

MDMA
3,4-methylene dioxymethamphetamine (pharmacology and psychiatry)

mdn
median

MDNB
metadinitrobenzene [a poisonous substance] (chemistry)

MDOPA
alpha-methyl-dopa (pharmacology)

MDP
mandibular dysostosis and peromelia (dentistry, genetics, oral surgery, and orthopedics)
manic-depressive psychosis (psychiatry)
maximum deliverable pressure
mentodextra posterior [right mentoposterior position] (obstetrics)
^{99m}Tc medronate methylene diphosphonate (chemistry and radiology)
muramyldipeptide (laboratory)

M.D.P.
mentodextra posterior [right mentoposterior position] (obstetrics)

MDQ
minimum detectable quantity (laboratory)

MDR
mammalian diving response (emergency medicine, respiratory, and trauma)
minimum daily requirement (dietary and pharmacology)

M.D.R.
minimum daily requirement (dietary and pharmacology)

MDS
Master of Dental Surgery (dentistry and education)

maternal deprivation syndrome (neonatology and obstetrics)
microsurgery drill system (surgery)
myocardial depressant substance (cardiovascular)

MDSO
mentally disordered sex offender (psychiatry)

MDT
median detection threshold
mentodextra transversa [right mentotransverse position] (obstetrics)

M.D.T.
mentodextra transversa [right mentotransverse position] (obstetrics)

MDTA
McDonald Deep Test of Articulation (speech and language therapy)

MDTP
multidisciplinary treatment plan (rehabilitation)

MDTR
mean diameter-thickness ratio (laboratory)

MDU
Medical Defence Unit [British]

MDUO
myocardial disease of unknown origin (cardiovascular)

MDV
Marek's disease virus [of chickens] (laboratory and veterinary medicine)

MDY
month, date, year

ME
macular edema (ophthalmology)
Maine [Postal Service state designation]
maximum effort
medial episiotomy (obstetrics)
median eminence [of hypothalamus] (neurology)
medical education (education)

Medical Examiner (government and pathology)
mercaptoethanol (chemistry and laboratory)
metabolizable energy
middle ear (otorhinolaryngology)
mouse epithelial [cells] (hematology and laboratory)

M/E
myeloid/erythrocyte [ratio] (hematology and laboratory)

"M-E"
{pronunciation of *EMI* [Electric and Musical Industries, developers of the first computerized tomographic scanner; *EMI* is the trade name of the scanner.]} (radiology) {not an abbreviation}

2ME
2-mercaptoethanol (chemistry and laboratory)

Me
methyl [CH$_3$] (chemistry)

MEA
Medical Exhibition Association
mercaptoethylamine (chemistry)
multiple endocrine abnormalities (endocrinology)
multiple endocrine adenomata [adenomas] (endocrinology)
multiple endocrine adenomatosis (endocrinology)
multiple endocrine adenopathy (endocrinology)

Mead-J
Mead Johnson [manufacturer] (pharmacology)

MEA-I
multiple endocrine adenomatosis type I (endocrinology)

meas
measure
measurement

MEB
Medical Evaluation Board (armed
    forces)

MeB
Medical Board
methylene blue (chemistry, laboratory,
    and surgery)

MEC
middle ear cells (otorhinolaryngology)
minimum effective concentration (labo-
    ratory, pharmacology, and radiation
    therapy)

mec
meconium (laboratory, neonatology, and
    obstetrics)

Mecano
mechanotherapy (physical therapy)

Me-CCNU
methyl-CCNU [also called *methyl-1-(-2-
chloroethyl)-3-cyclohexyl-1-nitroso-
urea, nitrosourea,* and *semustine*]
(chemotherapy, oncology, and pharmacology)

MECG
maternal electrocardiogram (cardiovas-
    cular and obstetrics)

mech
mechanical

MED
medial
median erythrocyte diameter (hematol-
    ogy and laboratory)
medical {pronounced "med"}
medication (pharmacology) {pro-
    nounced "med"}
medicine (pharmacology) {pronounced
    "med"}
medium (bacteriology and laboratory)
minimal effective dose (laboratory,
    pharmacology, and radiation therapy)
minimal erythema dose (radiation ther-
    apy)

M.E.D.
minimal effective dose (laboratory,
    pharmacology, and radiation therapy)

minimal erythema dose (radiation ther-
    apy)

med
medial
median
medical {pronounced "med"}
medication (pharmacology) {pro-
    nounced "med"}
medicine (pharmacology) {pronounced
    "med"}
medium (bacteriology and laboratory)

med.
medial
medication (pharmacology) {pro-
    nounced "med"}

"med"
{pronunciation of *MED, med,* and *med*
    [medical, medication (pharmacology),
    and medicine (pharmacology)]} {not
    an abbreviation}

MEDAC
multiple endocrine deficiency–Addison's
    disease–candidiasis [syndrome] (endo-
    crinology, immunology, and infectious
    diseases)
multiple endocrine deficiency–autoim-
    mune–candidiasis (endocrinology, im-
    munology, and infectious diseases)

MEDEX
médecin extension [extension of the
    physician—referring to recruitment
    program]

MEDF
midexpiratory dynamic flow rate (respi-
    ratory)

MEDICO
Medical Information Cooperation
Medical International Cooperation

MEDICS
Medical Information and Career Service
    [British]

MEP
mean effective pressure
motor end-plate (neurology and orthopedics)
multimodality evoked potential (neurology)

mep
meperidine [an analgesic] (pharmacology)

MEPH
mephobarbital [a sedative and anticonvulsant] (pharmacology)

MEPP
miniature end-plate potential (neurology)

MEPROB
meprobamate [an anticonvulsant, muscle relaxant, and tranquilizer] (neurology, orthopedics, pharmacology, and psychiatry)

MEq
milliequivalent (measurement)

mEq
milliequivalent (measurement)

meq
milliequivalent (measurement)

MEq/L
milliequivalent per liter (measurement)

mEq/L
milliequivalent per liter (measurement)

MER
ethamoxytriphetol [an antiestrogen] (pharmacology)
mean ejection rate (cardiovascular)
methanol-extracted residue of bacille Calmette-Guérin [BCG] (chemotherapy, laboratory, oncology, and pharmacology)
methanol-extruded residue of bacille Calmette-Guérin [BCG] (chemotherapy, laboratory, oncology, and pharmacology)
myeloid-erythrocyte ratio (hematology and laboratory)

myeloid-erythroid ratio (hematology and laboratory)

MER-29
triparanol (pharmacology) [*Note: A cholesterol biosynthesis inhibitor removed from market due to side effects.*]

M/E ratio
myeloid/erythroid ratio (hematology and laboratory)

M:E ratio
myeloid:erythroid ratio (hematology and laboratory)

MERB
Medical Examination and Review Board [Department of Defense] (armed forces and education)

MERCRY
mercury (chemistry)

MES
maintenance electrolyte solution (pharmacology)
maximum electroshock seizure (psychiatry)
morpholino-ethanesulphonic acid (laboratory)

Mesc
mescaline [A psychedelic and poisonous plant used as a hallucinogenic drug in the 1960's.] (chemical dependency, chemistry, and pharmacology) {slang}

"M-E-scan"
{pronunciation of *EMI scan* [Electric and Musical Industries scan by the developers of the first computerized tomographic scanner. *EMI* is the trade name of the scanner.]} (radiology) {not an abbreviation}

MeSH
Medical Subject Heading [a part of *MEDLARS*] (computer sciences and library science)

MET
metabolic equivalent of the task (cardiovascular)
metastasis (oncology)
midexpiratory time (respiratory)

Met
methionine (chemistry and laboratory)

met
metallic [referring to breath sounds]
(respiratory)
metastasis (laboratory, oncology, and
pathology)
{not an abbreviation} [unit of measurement of heat production by the body]

META
metamyelocyte (hematology and laboratory) {pronounced "met-ah"}

META 1
Metabolic Profile 1 [also called *SMA-6*; a
panel of tests] (laboratory)

meta
metacarpal (orthopedics)
metatarsal (orthopedics and podiatry)

meta-
{not an abbreviation} [prefix referring to
change, exchange, or transformation]

metab
metabolic {pronounced "mah-tab"}
metabolism {pronounced "mah-tab"}

"met-ah"
{pronunciation of *META* [metamyelo-
cyte]} (hematology and laboratory)
{not an abbreviation}

metaph
metaphysics (parapsychology)

metas
metastasis (oncology)
metastasize (oncology)

METH
methicillin [an antibiotic] (pharmacology) {pronounced "meth"}

Meth
methedrine [also called *methylamphetamine hydrochloride*] (chemical
dependency and pharmacology) {pro-
nounced "meth"}

meth
methyl (chemistry and laboratory) {pro-
nounced "meth"}

"meth"
{pronunciation of *METH* [methicillin
(pharmacology)], *Meth* [methedrine
(also called *methylamphetamine hydrochloride*) (chemical dependency
and pharmacology)], and *meth*
[methyl (chemistry, laboratory, and
pharmacology)]} {not an abbreviation}

METHb
methemoglobin (hematology and laboratory)

MeTHF
methyltetrahydrofolic acid (chemistry)

met hgb
methemoglobin (hematology and laboratory)

methyl-CCNU
methyl-1-(-2-chloroethyl)-3-cyclohexyl-
1-nitrosourea [also called *nitrosourea*,
and *semustine*] (chemotherapy, oncology, and pharmacology)

methyl-GAG
methyl-glyoxal bisguanylhydrazone (chemotherapy, oncology, and pharmacology)

m et n
mane et nocte [morning and night]
(pharmacology)

m. et n.
mane et nocte [morning and night]
(pharmacology)

METS
metabolic equivalents [multiples of resting oxygen uptake] (laboratory)

mets
metastases (laboratory, oncology, and pathology) {pronounced "metz"}

m et sig
misce et signa [mix and write a label] (pharmacology)

m. et sig.
misce et signa [mix and write a label] (pharmacology)

Metz
Metzenbaum [instruments] (surgery) {pronounced "metz"}

"metz"
{pronunciation of *METS* [metabolic equivalents (laboratory)], *mets* [metastases (laboratory, oncology, and pathology)], and *Metz* [Metzenbaum (instruments) (surgery)]} {not an abbreviation}

MEV
million electron volts (electricity and measurement)

MeV
megaelectron volt (electricity and measurement)
megavolt (electricity and measurement)
megavoltage (electricity and measurement)

Mev
megavolt (electricity and measurement)
megavoltage (electricity and measurement)

Mev.
million electron volts (electricity and measurement)

mev
million electron volts (electricity and measurement)

Mex.
Mexican [national origin]

MF
medium frequency (measurement)
5-methyltetrahydrofolate (laboratory)
microflocculation (laboratory)
microscopic factor (laboratory)
midcavity forceps (obstetrics and surgery)
mitogenic factor (laboratory)
mitomycin-C and 5-fluorouracil (chemotherapy, oncology, and pharmacology)
mitotic figure (laboratory)
multiplying factor (laboratory)
mycosis fungoides (laboratory)
myelin figure (laboratory)
myocardial fibrosis (cardiovascular)
myofibrillar (laboratory)

M/F
male-to-female [ratio] (statistics)

M & F
male and female
mother and father

Mf
microfilaria(e) (laboratory)

mF
millifarad (measurement)

mf
microfilaria(e) (laboratory)
millifarad (measurement)

MFA
methyl fluoracetate (chemistry)
monofluoroacetate (chemistry)

MFAT
multifocal atrial tachycardia (cardiovascular)

MFB
metallic foreign body (emergency medicine)

m-FC
membrane fecal coli [broth] (gastroenterology and laboratory)

MFCC
Marriage, Family, and Child Counselor
(psychiatry)

MFCM
Master, Faculty of Community Medicine
(education)

MFD
mid-forceps delivery (obstetrics)
minimum fatal dose (pharmacology and
radiation therapy)

M.F.D.
minimum fatal dose (pharmacology and
radiation therapy)

mfd
microfarad (measurement)

MFEM
maximal forced expiratory maneuver
(respiratory)

MFG
modified heat degraded gelatin (laboratory)

mfg
manufactured
manufacturing

MFH
malignant fibrous histiocytoma (laboratory)
membrane-free hemolysate (hematology
and laboratory)

MFHom
Member of the Faculty of Homeopathy
(homeopathic medicine)

MFID
multielectrode flame ionization detector
(physics)

m flac
membrana flaccida [also called *pars
flaccida membranae tympani* and
Shrapnell's membrane] (otorhinolaryngology)

m. flac.
membrana flaccida [also called *pars

flaccida membranae tympani and
Shrapnell's membrane] (otorhinolaryngology)

MFOM
Master, Faculty of Occupational Medicine (education and occupational
medicine)

MFP
monofluorophosphate (chemistry)
myofascial pain (neurology)

MFR
mid-forceps rotation (obstetrics)
mucus flow rate (otorhinolaryngology)

mfr
manufacturer

M:F ratio
male-to-female ratio (statistics)

MF sol
merthiolate-formaldehyde [stock] solution (laboratory)

MFSS
Medical Field Service School [Army]
(armed forces and education)

MFST
Medical Field Service Technician
(armed forces)

MFT
muscle function test (neurology)

m ft
mistura fiat [let a mixture be made]
(pharmacology)

m. ft.
mistura fiat [let a mixture be made]
(pharmacology)

MFTVP
Motor-Free Test of Visual Perception
(psychiatry)

MFW
multiple fragment wounds (armed forces
and emergency medicine)

MG
Marcus Gunn [pupil] (ophthalmology)
margin
menopausal gonadotropin (endocrinology, gynecology, and laboratory)
mesiogingival (dentistry)
methylglucoside (chemistry)
Michaelis-Gutmann [bodies] (urology)
milligram [equal to ⅟₆₀ grain] (measurement)
monoglyceride (chemistry and laboratory)
muscle group (neurology and orthopedics)
myasthenia gravis (neurology)

Mg
magnesium (chemistry, laboratory, and
pharmacology)

mg
milligram [equal to ⅟₆₀ grain] (measurement)

mg%
milligram percent [also called *milligrams per 100 cubic centimeters,
milligrams per 100 milliliters,* or *milligrams per deciliter*] (measurement)

μmg
micromilligram (measurement)

mμg
millimicrogram [also called *nanogram*]
(measurement)

MGA
melengestrol acetate [a progestin and
antineoplastic] (chemotherapy, gynecology, oncology, and pharmacology)

MGBG
methyl-glyoxal bisguanylhydrazone [also
called *methyl-GAG*] (chemotherapy,
oncology, and pharmacology)

MGC
minimal glomerular change (nephrology)

MGD
mixed gonadal dysgenesis (endocrinology and genetics)

mgd
million gallons per day (measurement)

mg/dl
milligram per deciliter (measurement)

MGDS
Member in Dental Surgery (dentistry)

mg-el
milligram-element [radioactive] (measurement, radiation therapy, and radiology)

MGF
maternal grandfather
mother's grandfather

mgf
maternal grandfather

MGGH
methylglyoxal guanylhydrazone (chemistry)

MGH
Massachusetts General Hospital (administration)
monoglyceride hydrolase (chemistry)

mgh
milligram-hour [radioactivity] (measurement, radiation therapy, and radiology)

mg-hr
milligram-hour [radioactivity] (measurement, radiation therapy, and radiology)

MGM
maternal grandmother
mother's grandmother

mgm
maternal grandmother
milligram (measurement)

MGN
membranous glomerulonephritis (nephrology)

MGP
marginal granulocyte pool (hematology and laboratory)

MGR
modified gain ratio (rehabilitation)
murmurs, gallops, or rubs (cardiovascular)

mgtis
meningitis (neurology)

MGUS
monoclonal gammopathies of undetermined significance (immunology)

MGW
magnesium sulfate, glycerine, water [enema] (gastroenterology and pharmacology)

M-GXT
multistage graded exercise test (cardiovascular)

MH
malignant histiocytosis (oncology)
malignant hyperpyrexia (emergency medicine)
malignant hyperthermia (emergency medicine)
mammotropic hormone [also called *prolactin*] (endocrinology, gynecology, and laboratory)
marital history
Master Herbalist
medical history
melanophore hormone (chemistry)
menstrual history (gynecology and obstetrics)
mental health (psychiatry)
murine hepatitis [of mice] (veterinary medicine)

M.H.
multiple handicapped (genetics, psychiatry, and rehabilitation)

M/H
microcytic/hypochromic [anemia] (hematology)

M-H
Mueller-Hinton [agar] (laboratory)

mH
millihenry (measurement)

MHA
Mental Health Association (psychiatry)
methemalbumin (laboratory)
microangiopathic hemolytic anemia (hematology)
microhemagglutination [test for syphilis] (gynecology, infectious diseases, laboratory, and urology)
mixed hemadsorption (laboratory)

MHA-TP
microhemagglutination—*Treponema pallidum* (laboratory)

MHB
maximum hospital benefit
methemoglobin (laboratory)

MHb
methemoglobin (laboratory)
myohemoglobin (laboratory)

MHBSS
modified Hank's balanced salt solution (pharmacology)

MHC
major histocompatibility complex (genetics)
Mental Health Care [British] (psychiatry)
mental health clinic (psychiatry)

mhcp
mean horizontal candlepower (electricity and measurement)

m.h.c.p.
mean horizontal candlepower (electricity and measurement)

MHCS
Mental Hygiene Consultation Service (psychiatry)

MHCU
Mental Health Care Unit (psychiatry)

MHD
magnetohydrodynamics (physics)
maintenance hemodialysis (nephrology)
mean hemolytic dose (radiation therapy)
Medical Holding Detachment
Mental Health Department (psychiatry)
Mental Health Digest (psychiatry and publishing)
minimum hemolytic dose

M.H.D.
minimum hemolytic dose

MHDU
medical hemodialysis unit (nephrology)

mHg
An error in several editions of DOR-LAND'S ILLUSTRATED MEDICAL DICTIONARY—should be mmHg [millimeters of mercury].

MHI
Mental Health Institute (psychiatry)

MHLC
Multidimensional Health Locus of Control [diagnostic scale] (administration)

MHLS
metabolic heat load simulator (laboratory)

MH/MR
mental health and mental retardation (neurology and psychiatry)

MHN
massive hepatic necrosis (gastroenterology)

MHP
Mental Health Project (psychiatry)
1-mercuri-2-hydroxypropane (chemistry)

MHPE
3-methoxy-4-hydroxyphenylethanol (chemistry)

MHPE Conj
3-methoxy-4-hydroxyphenylethanol conjugate (chemistry)

MHPG
methoxyhydrophenylglycol [also called *3-methoxy-4-hydroxyphenylglycol*] (chemistry)

MHPG Conj
methoxyhydrophenylglycol conjugate [also called *3-methoxy-4-hydroxyphenylglycol conjugate*] (chemistry)

MHR
major histocompatibility region (genetics)
maximal heart rate (cardiovascular)
maximum heart rate (cardiovascular)
methemoglobin reductase (hematology and laboratory)

MHRI
Mental Health Research Institute [University of Michigan] (psychiatry and research)

MHS
major histocompatibility system (genetics)
malignant hypothermia susceptible [patients] (emergency medicine)
maximum Histalog stimulation (gastroenterology)

MHST
multiphasic health screen test

MHVD
Merek's herpesvirus disease [of chickens] (veterinary medicine)

MH virus
murine hepatitis virus [of mice] (veterinary medicine)

MHW
medial heel wedge (orthopedics and physical therapy)

M. Hx.
medical history

MHyg
Master of Hygiene (education)

MHz
megahertz [1 million cycles per second] (measurement)

mHz
megahertz [1 million cycles per second] (measurement)

MI
maturation index (laboratory)
medical illustration (art and publishing)
medical illustrator (art and publishing)
medical inspection
melanophore index (chemistry)
menstrual induction (gynecology)
mental institution (psychiatry)
mercaptoimidazole (pharmacology)
mesioincisal (dentistry)
metabolic index (laboratory)
Michigan [Postal Service state designation]
migration inhibition
mitotic index (laboratory)
mitral incompetence (cardiovascular)
mitral insufficiency (cardiovascular)
myocardial infarction (cardiovascular)
myo-inositol (chemistry and dietary)

MIA
medically indigent adult (administration and insurance)
missing in action (armed forces)

MIBiol
Member of the Institute of Biology (biology)

MIBK
methyl isobutyl ketone (laboratory)

MIBT
methyl isatin-betathiosemicarbasone (chemistry)

MIC
maternal and infant care (neonatology and obstetrics)
Medical Interfraternity Conference
microcytosis (laboratory)
microscopic (laboratory)
microscopic findings in centrifugal urinary sediment (laboratory)
microscopy (laboratory)
minimal inhibitory concentration (laboratory, pharmacology, and radiation therapy)
minimal isorrheic concentration (laboratory, pharmacology, and radiation therapy)
minimum inhibitory concentration (laboratory, pharmacology, and radiation therapy)

MICN
medical intensive care nurse (nursing)
mobile intensive care nurse (emergency medicine and nursing)

mic pan
mica panis [bread crumb]

mic. pan.
mica panis [bread crumb]

MIC-RN
Mobile Intensive Care Registered Nurse (emergency medicine and nursing)

micro
microscopic (laboratory) {pronounced "my-crow"}
microscopy (laboratory) {pronounced "my-crow"}

micro-
{not an abbreviation} [one-millionth or prefix for 10^{-6}] (measurement) {pronounced "my-crow"}

microbiol
microbiological (microbiology)
microbiology

micromicro-
{not an abbreviation} [prefix for 10^{-12}] (measurement) {obsolete, now called *pico-*}

MICU
Medical Intensive Care Unit {pronounced "mik-u"}
Mobile Intensive Care Unit (emergency medicine) {pronounced "mik-u"}

MID
maximum inhibiting duration (laboratory, pharmacology, and radiation therapy)
mesioincisodistal (dentistry)
minimal infective dose (pharmacology and radiation therapy)
minimal inhibiting dose (pharmacology and radiation therapy)

M.I.D.
minimum infective dose (pharmacology and radiation therapy)

mid
middle

middle/3
middle third [of long bones] (orthopedics)

midnoc
midnight

mid sag
midsagittal (anatomy)

MIF
macrophage-inhibiting factor (hematology and laboratory)
melanocyte-stimulating hormone inhibiting factor (endocrinology and laboratory)
melanocyte-stimulating hormone release-inhibiting factor (endocrinology and laboratory)
merthiolate-iodine-formaldehyde (pharmacology)
midinspiratory flow (respiratory)
migration-inhibiting factor [test] (allergy and laboratory)
migration-inhibition factor [test] (allergy and laboratory)

migration-inhibitory factor [test for macrophages] (allergy and laboratory)
mixed immunofluorescence (laboratory)

MIFA
mitomycin-C, 5-fluorouracil, and Adriamycin (chemotherapy, oncology, and pharmacology)

MIFR
maximal inspiratory flow rate (respiratory)

MIg
membrane immunoglobulin (immunology and laboratory)
malaria immunoglobulin (immunology, infectious diseases, laboratory, and respiratory)
measles immunoglobulin (immunology, infectious diseases, laboratory, and pediatrics)

MIH
Master of Industrial Health (education)
melanocyte-stimulating hormone-inhibitory hormone (endocrinology and laboratory)
migraine with interparoxysmal headache (neurology)
minimal intermittent [dosage of] heparin (cardiovascular and pharmacology)

MI insuf
mitral insufficiency (cardiovascular)

MIKA
minor karyotypic abnormalities (genetics)

"mik-u"
{pronunciation of *MICU* [Medical Intensive Care Unit and Mobile Intensive Care Unit (emergency medicine)]} {not an abbreviation}

mil
military (armed forces)

milliliter (measurement) [slang] {pronounced "mill"}
one-thousandth [0.001] (measurement)

"mill"
{pronunciation of *mil* [milliliter (slang)]} (measurement) {not an abbreviation}

"mill-E"
{pronunciation of *milli-* [prefix for 10^{-3} (not an abbreviation)]} (measurement) {not an abbreviation}

milli-
{not an abbreviation} [prefix for 10^{-3}] (measurement) {pronounced "mill-E"}

milli IU/ml
milli-International Unit per milliliter (measurement)

MIMS
Medical Information Management System
Medical Inventory Management System
Monthly Index of Medical Specialties

MIN
medial interlaminar nucleus (neurology and orthopedics)
minimum

min
mineral (chemistry, dietary, and pharmacology)
minimal
minimum
minimum [a minim] (measurement)
minor
minute (measurement)

MINA
monoisonitrosoacetone (chemistry)

"min-E"
{pronunciation of *mini-* [prefix denoting small size (not an abbreviation)]} {not an abbreviation}

mini-
{not an abbreviation} [prefix denoting small size] {pronounced "min-E"}

MINIA
monkey intranuclear inclusion agent (laboratory)

MInstSP
Member Institution of Sewage Purification (ecology)

MIO
minimal identifiable odor
motility indol ornithine [medium] (laboratory)

M.I.O.
minimal identifiable odor

MIP
maximum inspiratory pressure (respiratory)
mean intravascular pressure (cardiovascular)
middle interphalangeal joint (orthopedics and podiatry)

MIPS
myocardial isotopic perfusion scan (cardiovascular and radiology)

MIRD
Medical Internal Radiation Dose (radiology and radiation therapy)

MIRP
myocardial infarction rehabilitation program (cardiovascular and rehabilitation)

MIRU
myocardial infarction research unit (cardiovascular and research)

Mis. Astig.
mixed astigmatism (ophthalmology)

misc
miscarriage (obstetrics)
miscellaneous

misce
{not an abbreviation} [Latin word for *mix*] (pharmacology)

MISO
misonidazole [an antiprotozoal] (pharmacology)

MIST
Medical Information Service by Telephone

mist
mistura [mixture] (pharmacology)

mist.
mistura [mixture] (pharmacology)

MIT
Massachusetts Institute of Technology (education)
miracidial immobilization test (laboratory)
mono-iodotyrosine (endocrinology and laboratory)

mit
mitte [send]

mit.
mitte [send]

Mith
mithramycin (chemotherapy, oncology, and pharmacology)

mit insuf
mitral insufficiency (cardiovascular)

Mito
mitomycin-C (chemotherapy, oncology, and pharmacology)

MITO-C
mitomycin-C (chemotherapy, oncology, and pharmacology)

mit sang
mitte sanguinem [bleed]

mit. sang.
mitte sanguinem [bleed]

mitt
mitte [send]

mitte sang
mitte sanguineum [bleed]

mitt tal
mitte tales [send such]

mIU
milli-International Unit (measurement)

mix mon
mixed monitor (obstetrics)

mixt
mixture (pharmacology)

MJ
marijuana [also called *Mary Jane*] (chemical dependency and pharmacology)

M-J
Mead Johnson [company] (pharmacology)

MJL
medial joint line (orthopedics)

MJT
Mead Johnson tube (surgery)

MJI
Masters and Johnson Institute (gynecology, obstetrics, psychiatry, research, and urology)

MK
Merck [company] (pharmacology)
monkey kidney [cell culture] (laboratory)

MK-421
{not an abbreviation} [an experimental diuretic made by Merck] (pharmacology)

MKB
megakaryoblast (hematology and laboratory)

mkg
meter kilogram (measurement)

M.K.S.
meter-kilogram-second [system] (measurement)

mks
meter-kilogram-second (measurement)

MKV
killed-measles virus (laboratory and pharmacology)

ML
Licentiate in Medicine (education)
Licentiate in Midwifery (education and obstetrics)
lingual margin (dentistry)
malignant lymphoma (oncology and pathology)
mesiolingual (dentistry)
middle lobe [of lung] (respiratory)
midlife
midline (anatomy)
milliliter (measurement)

M.L.
Licentiate in Medicine (education)
midline (anatomy)

M:L
monocyte-lymphocyte [ratio] (hematology and laboratory)

M-L
Martin-Lewis [medium] (laboratory)

Ml
milliliter (measurement)

mL
millilambert (measurement)
milliliter (measurement)

ml
milliliter (measurement)

MLA
Medical Library Association (library science)
mentolaeva anterior [left mentoanterior position] (obstetrics)
mesiolabial (dentistry)
monocytic leukemia, acute (hematology)

M.L.A.
mentolaeva anterior [left mentoanterior position] (obstetrics)

MLa
mesiolabial (dentistry)

MLAI
mesiolabioincisal (dentistry)

MLaI
mesiolabioincisal (dentistry)

MLAP
mean left atrial pressure (cardiovascular)
mesiolabiopulpal (dentistry)

MLaP
mesiolabiopulpal (dentistry)

MLB
monaural loudness balance (otorhinolaryngology)

MLC
minimal lethal concentration (pharmacology and radiation therapy)
mixed leukocyte culture (laboratory)
mixed lymphocyte culture (laboratory)
multilamellar cytosome (laboratory)
myelomonocytic leukemia, chronic (hematology)

MLCO
Member of the London College of Osteopathy (osteopathic medicine)

MLD
median lethal dose (pharmacology and radiation therapy)
metachromatic leukodystrophy (genetics, hematology, and neurology)
minimal lethal dose (pharmacology and radiation therapy)

M.L.D.
median lethal dose (pharmacology and radiation therapy)
minimum lethal dose (pharmacology and radiation therapy)

MLD 50
median lethal dose [of radiation] (radiation therapy)

MLD$_{50}$
median lethal dose [of radiation] (radiation therapy)

MLE
midline episiotomy (obstetrics)

M leprae
Mycobacterium leprae [the bacterial cause of leprosy] (dermatology, infectious diseases, and laboratory)

MLF
median longitudinal fasciculus (neurology and ophthalmology)

MLI
mesiolinguoincisal (dentistry)

M lines
{not an abbreviation} (radiology)

MLK
Martin Luther King, Junior, Hospital (administration)

MLNS
mucocutaneous lymph node syndrome [also called *Kawasaki's disease*] (dermatology, ophthalmology, otorhinolaryngology, and pediatrics)

MLO
mesiolinguo-occlusal (dentistry)

MLP
mentolaeva posterior [left mentoposterior position] (obstetrics)
mesiolinguopulpal (dentistry)

M.L.P.
mentolaeva posterior [left mentoposterior position] (obstetrics)

MLR
mixed lymphocyte reaction (hematology and laboratory)

M:L ratio
maltase-to-lactase ratio (laboratory)

MLS
mean life span (oncology)
median life span (oncology)
median longitudinal section (laboratory and pathology)
myelomonocytic leukemia, subacute (hematology)

MLT
median lethal time [of radiation] (radiation therapy)
Medical Laboratory Technician (library science)
mentolaeva transversa [left mentotransverse position] (obstetrics)

M.L.T.
mentolaeva transversa [left mentotransverse position] (obstetrics)

MLT (AMT)
Medical Laboratory Technician (American Medical Technologists) (laboratory)

M.L.T. (ASCP)
Medical Laboratory Technician (American Society of Clinical Pathologists) (laboratory and pathology)

MLV
Moloney's leukemogenic virus (laboratory)
mouse leukemia cells (laboratory)
multilaminar vesicles (laboratory)
murine leukemic virus [of mice] (veterinary medicine)

MLVSS
mixed liquor volatile suspended solids (chemistry)

MM
Major Medical (insurance)
malignant melanoma (dermatology and oncology)
Marshall-Marchetti [operation] (gynecology, surgery, and urology)
medial malleolus (orthopedics)
millimeter (measurement)
mixed monitor [external tocotransducer

and internal scalp electrode] (neonatology and obstetrics)
mucous membrane (gastroenterology, otorhinolaryngology, and urology)
multiple myeloma (oncology)
murmurs (cardiovascular)
muscles (neurology and orthopedics)
muscularis mucosa (anatomy, neurology, orthopedics, and surgery)
myeloid metaplasia (hematology)
{not an abbreviation} [measurement of creatine phosphokinase (CPK) isoenzyme MM band of skeletal muscles] (cardiovascular and laboratory)

M.M.
mucous membranes (gastroenterology, otorhinolaryngology, and urology)

M & M
milk and molasses (dietary)
morbidity and mortality (statistics)

mM
millimole (measurement)

mm
methylmalonyl [coenzyme A mutase] (laboratory)
millimeter (measurement)
mucous membrane (gastroenterology, otorhinolaryngology, and urology)
murmur (cardiovascular)
muscles (neurology and orthopedics)

mm³
cubic millimeter (measurement)

μmm
micromillimeter [also called *nanometer*] (measurement)

MMA
medical materials account (armed forces)
methylmalonic acid (laboratory)

MMATP
methadone maintenance and aftercare treatment program (chemical dependency and pharmacology)

MMC
migrating myoelectric complexes (neurology)
minimal medullary concentration (orthopedics)
mitomycin C (chemotherapy, oncology, and pharmacology)

MMD
mass median diameter [of particles] (physics)
minimal morbidostatic dose (radiation therapy)
mean narrow dose (radiation therapy)

MMDA
myristicin [also called *glyceryl trimyristate*] (chemical dependency) {slang}

MMECT
multiple monitor electroconvulsive therapy (psychiatry)

MMED
Master of Medicine (education)

MMEF
maximal midexpiratory flow (respiratory)
maximum midexpiratory flow (respiratory)

MMEFR
maximum midexpiratory flow rate (respiratory)

MMF
maximum midexpiratory flow [rate] (respiratory)
mean maximum flow (respiratory)
Member of the Medical Faculty (education)

MMFR
maximum midexpiratory flow rate (respiratory)
maximum midflow rate (radiology)

MNR
marrow neutrophil reserve (hematology and laboratory)

MnSSEPS
median nerve somatosensory evoked potentials (neurology)

MNTB
medial nucleus of the trapezoid body (neurology and otorhinolaryngology)

MNU
methylnitrosourea (chemotherapy, oncology, and pharmacology)

MO
manually operated
Master of Obstetrics (education and obstetrics)
Master of Osteopathy (education and osteopathic medicine)
medial oblique [view] (radiology)
Medical Officer (armed forces)
mesio-occlusal (dentistry)
mineral oil (pharmacology)
minute output [of heart] (cardiovascular)
Missouri [Postal Service state designation]
molecular orbit (chemistry)
mono-oxygenase (laboratory)
month
no evidence of distal metastasis (oncology and pathology)

M.O.
Medical Officer (armed forces)

MO$_2$
myocardial oxygen [consumption] (cardiovascular)

Mo
mode
molybdenum (chemistry)

Mo.
month

mo
month
mother

MOA
mechanism of action

MOAB
monoclonal antibody

MOAD
methotrexate, vincristine, L-asparaginase, and dexamethasone (chemotherapy, oncology, and pharmacology)

MOB
medical office building
nitrogen mustard, vincristine, and bleomycin (chemotherapy, oncology, and pharmacology)

mob
mobilization

MOB-III
vincristine, bleomycin, and methotrexate (chemotherapy, oncology, and pharmacology)
vincristine, bleomycin, and mitomycin-C (chemotherapy, oncology, and pharmacology)

mobil
mobility

MOC
maximum oxygen consumption (respiratory)

MOCA
methotrexate, Oncovin, Cytoxan, and Adriamycin (chemotherapy, oncology, and pharmacology)

MOD
maturity-onset diabetes (endocrinology)
Medical Officer of the Day (administration)
Medical Officer on Duty (administration)
medicine, osteopathy, and dentistry
mesio-occlusodistal (dentistry)
moderate

mod
modality (physical therapy)
moderate

mode DDD
{not an abbreviation} [a pacemaker
mode] (cardiovascular)

mode DVI
{not an abbreviation} [a pacemaker
mode] (cardiovascular)

mode VVI
{not an abbreviation} [a pacemaker
mode] (cardiovascular)

MODM
mature-onset diabetes mellitus (endocrinology)
maturity-onset diabetes mellitus (endocrinology)

mod praesc
modo praescripto [as directed, in the
manner prescribed] (pharmacology)

mod. praesc.
modo praescripto [as directed, in the
manner prescribed] (pharmacology)

MODY
maturity-onset diabetes of the youth
(endocrinology)

MOF
marine oxidation/fermentation [me-
dium] (laboratory)
methotrexate, Oncovin [vincristine], and
5-fluorouracil (chemotherapy, oncology, and pharmacology)
methyl-CCNU [MeCCNU or semustine],
vincristine, and 5-fluorouracil (chemotherapy, oncology, and pharmacology)
multiple organ failure

MOF-STREP
methyl-CCNU [MeCCNU or semustine],
vincristine, 5-fluorouracil, and streptozocin (chemotherapy, oncology, and
pharmacology)

MO & G
Master of Obstetrics and Gynecology

(education, gynecology, and obstetrics)

MOH
Medical Officer of Health (administration)

M.O.H.
Medical Officer of Health (administration)

mol
mole (measurement)
molecular (chemistry)
molecule (chemistry)

μmol
micromole (measurement)

molc
molar concentration (chemistry and
physics)

μmole
micromole (measurement)

moll
mollis [soft]

mol/l
molecules per liter (measurement)

Mol. wt.
molecular weight (chemistry)

mol wt
molecular weight (chemistry)

MOM
milk of magnesia (gastroenterology and
pharmacology) {pronounced "mom"}

"mom"
{pronunciation of *MOM* [milk of magne-
sia]} (gastroenterology and pharmacology) {not an abbreviation}

MOMA
3-methyoxy-4-hydroxymandelic acid
[also called *methoxyhydroxyman-
delic acid*] (laboratory)

Mon
mongolian [as in the Mongol nationality or as in Down's syndrome] (genetics, national origin, and neurology)

mon
monocyte (laboratory)

MONO
mononucleosis, infectious (infectious diseases) {pronounced "mon-oh"}

Mono
monocyte (laboratory) {pronounced "mon-oh"}
mononucleosis (infectious diseases) {pronounced "mon-oh"}

mono
monocyte (laboratory) {pronounced "mon-oh"}
mononucleosis (infectious diseases) {pronounced "mon-oh"}

"mon-oh"
{pronunciation of *MONO, Mono* and *mono* [monocyte and mononucleosis] (infectious disease and laboratory) {not an abbreviation}

"mon-ohs"
{pronunciation of *monos* [monocytes]} (laboratory) {not an abbreviation}

monos
monocytes (laboratory) {pronounced "mon-ohs"}

MOOW
Medical Officer of the Watch (armed forces)

MOP
medical outpatient
mother of pearl (oceanography)
nitrogen mustard, Oncovin, and prednisone (chemotherapy, oncology, and pharmacology) {pronounced "mop"}
nitrogen mustard, Oncovin, and procarbazine (chemotherapy, oncology, and pharmacology) {pronounced "mop"}

"mop"
{pronunciation of *MOP* [nitrogen mus-

tard, Oncovin, and prednisone or nitrogen mustard, Oncovin, and procarbazine] and *MOPP* [mechlorethamine (Mustargen or nitrogen mustard), Oncovin (vincristine), procarbazine, and prednisone or methotrexate, Oncomycin, prednisone, and procarbazine or Mustine, Oncovin (vincristine), procarbazine, and prednisone]} (chemotherapy, oncology, and pharmacology) {not an abbreviation}

MOP-BAP
nitrogen mustard, vincristine, procarbazine, prednisone, Adriamycin, and bleomycin (chemotherapy, oncology, and pharmacology)

MOPP
mechlorethamine [Mustargen or nitrogen mustard], Oncovin [vincristine], procarbazine, and prednisone (chemotherapy, oncology, and pharmacology) {pronounced "mop"}
methotrexate, Oncomycin, prednisone, and procarbazine (chemotherapy, oncology, and pharmacology) {pronounced "mop"}
Mustine, Oncovin [vincristine], procarbazine, and prednisone (chemotherapy, oncology, and pharmacology) {pronounced "mop"}

MOPP/ABVD
mechlorethamine, vincristine, procarbazine, prednisone, doxorubicin, bleomycin, vinblastine, and dacarbazine (chemotherapy, oncology, and pharmacology)

MOPP-LO BLEO
mechlorethamine [Mustargen], Oncovin [vincristine], procarbazine, prednisone, and bleomycin (chemotherapy, oncology, and pharmacology)

MOPV
monovalent oral poliovirus vaccine (infectious diseases, neurology, and pharmacology)

MOR
Medical Officer Report [Navy] (armed
forces)
morphine (chemical dependency and
pharmacology)

MORC
Medical Officers Reserve Corps (armed
forces)

M.O.R.C.
Medical Officers Reserve Corps (armed
forces)

mor dict
more dicto [in the manner directed]
(pharmacology)

mor. dict.
more dicto [in the manner directed]
(pharmacology)

MORE
Management of Radiographic Environ-
ments (radiology)

morph
morphine (chemical dependency and
pharmacology) {slang}
morphological (laboratory and pathology)
morphology (laboratory and pathology)

mor sol
more solito [in the usual manner] (pharmacology)

mor. sol.
more solito [in the usual manner] (pharmacology)

mortal
mortality (statistics)

mos
months

MOSFET
metal oxide semiconductor field effect
transistor (electronics)

MOsm
milliosmole (measurement)

mOsm
milliosmole (measurement)

mosm
milliosmole (measurement)

mOsmol
milliosmole (measurement)

MOTT
mycobacteria other than tubercle [bacil-
lus] (laboratory)

MOUS
multiple occurrences of unexplained
symptoms

M-OVAL
macrovalocytes (laboratory)

MOX
moxalactam [an antibiotic; also called
Moxam] (pharmacology)

MP
mean pressure (cardiovascular)
medical payment (insurance)
melphalan [L-phenylalanine mustard]
and prednisone (chemotherapy, oncology, and pharmacology)
Member of Parliament (government)
menstrual period (gynecology)
mentum posterior (obstetrics)
mercaptopurine (chemotherapy, oncology, and pharmacology)
mesiopulpal (dentistry)
metacarpophalangeal (orthopedics)
metatarsophalangeal (orthopedics and
podiatry)
methylprednisolone sodium succinate
(allergy, hematology, oncology, ophthalmology, pharmacology, and rheumatology)
metropolitan police (law)
middle phalanx (orthopedics)
military police (armed forces)
military policeman (armed forces)
monophosphate (laboratory)
mouth pressure (dentistry and otorhinolaryngology)
mucopolysaccharide (cardiovascular,

genetics, neurology, ophthalmology, and orthopedics)
mucopurulent (laboratory)
multiparous (gynecology and obstetrics)
mycoplasmal pneumonia (respiratory)
myeloma protein (laboratory, oncology, and orthopedics)

M.P.
metacarpophalangeal (orthopedics)

6MP
6-mercaptopurine (chemotherapy, oncology, and pharmacology)

6-MP
6-mercaptopurine (chemotherapy, oncology, and pharmacology)

mp
melting point (chemistry)
modo prescripto [as directed] (pharmacology)
myeloma protein (laboratory, oncology, and orthopedics)

MPA
main pulmonary artery (cardiovascular and respiratory)
Medical Procurement Agency (administration)
medroxyprogesterone acetate [also called *Depo-Provera*] (endocrinology, gynecology, and pharmacology)
methylprednisolone acetate (allergy, hematology, oncology, ophthalmology, pharmacology, and rheumatology)

MPA
megapascal (measurement)

MPAP
mean pulmonary artery pressure (cardiovascular)

MPB
male pattern baldness (dermatology and endocrinology)

MPC
marine protein concentrate (laboratory)
maximum permissible concentration (radiation therapy and radiology)

meperidine, promethazine, and chlorpromazine (pharmacology)
minimal mycoplasmacidal concentration (laboratory)
minimum protoacidal contamination
myeloblastpromyelocyte compartment (hematology and laboratory)

MPCU
maximum permissible concentration of unidentified radionucleotides (radiation therapy and radiology)

MPD
maximum permissible dose (radiation therapy and radiology)
multiple personality disorder (psychiatry)
myofascial pain dysfunction (neurology)

MPDS
myofascial pain dysfunction syndrome (neurology)

MPE
maximum possible error

MPEH
methylphenylethylhydantoin (laboratory)

M period
{not an abbreviation} [the period of active mitosis] (chemistry, genetics, and laboratory)

MPG
miles per gallon (measurement)

mpg
miles per gallon (measurement)

MPGM
monophosphoglycerate mutase (laboratory)

MPGN
membranoproliferative glomerulonephritis [also called *membranous proliferative glomerulonephritis*] (nephrology)

mesangioproliferative glomerulonephritis (nephrology)

MPH
Master of Public Health (education)
methylphenidate (neurology, pharmacology, and psychiatry)
miles per hour (measurement)
milk protein hydrolysate (laboratory)

M.P.H.
Master of Public Health (education)

mph
miles per hour (measurement)

MPharm
Master in Pharmacy (education and pharmacology)

M phase
phase of mitosis (laboratory)

MPHR
maximum predicted heart rate (cardiovascular)

MPhysA
Member of the Physiotherapists' Association [British] (physical therapy and rehabilitation)

M.Phys.A.
Member of the Physiotherapists' Association [British] (physical therapy and rehabilitation)

MPI
maximum permitted intake (dietary)
maximum point of impulse (cardiovascular)
Medi-Physica, Incorporated [radiopharmaceutical company] (manufacturing, pharmacology, and radiology)
multiphasic personality inventory (psychiatry)
myocardial perfusion imaging (cardiovascular and radiology)

MPJ
metacarpophalangeal joint (orthopedics)
metatarsophalangeal joint (orthopedics and podiatry)

MPL
maximum permissible level [also called *maximum permissible limit*] (radiation therapy and radiology)
melphalan (chemotherapy, oncology, and pharmacology)
mesiopulpolingual (dentistry)

MPLa
mesiopulpolabial (dentistry)

MPL + PRED
melphalan and prednisone (chemotherapy, oncology, and pharmacology)

MPL + PRED(MP)
melphalan and prednisone (chemotherapy, oncology, and pharmacology)

MPM
malignant papillary mesothelioma (oncology)
multipurpose meal (dietary)

MPN
most probable number

MPO
maximum power output
myeloperoxidase [an enzyme] (laboratory)

MPP
massive periretinal proliferation (ophthalmology)
maximum perfusion pressure (cardiovascular)
Medical Personnel Pool (administration)
mercaptopyrazidopyrimidine (chemistry)

MPPT
methylprednisolone pulse therapy (allergy, hematology, oncology, ophthalmology, pharmacology, and rheumatology)

MPR
marrow production rate (hematology and laboratory)

MPS
Member of the Pharmaceutical Society
(pharmacology)
Michigan Picture Stories (psychiatry)
Microbial Profile System (laboratory)
mononuclear phagocyte system (laboratory)
movement produced stimuli (neurology)
mucopolysaccharide (cardiovascular,
genetics, laboratory, neurology, ophthalmology, and orthopedics)
mucopolysaccharidosis (cardiovascular,
genetics, neurology, ophthalmology,
and orthopedics)
multiphasic screening (laboratory)

MPS IV
mucopolysaccharidosis IV [also called
Morquio-Brailsford disease, Morquio-Brailsford syndrome, and *Morquio's syndrome*] (cardiovascular, genetics, neurology, ophthalmology, and orthopedics)

MPSMT
Merrill-Palmer Scale of Mental Tests
(psychiatry)

MPsyMed
Master of Psychological Medicine (education and psychology)

MPT
morphine provocative test (gastroenterology and laboratory)

MPTR↓
motor, pain, touch, reflex deficit (neurology)

MPU
Medical Practitioners Union [British]

M.P.U.
Medical Practitioners Union [British]

MPV
mean platelet volume (hematology and
laboratory)
metatarsus primus varus (orthopedics
and podiatry)

MR
magnetic resonance (radiology)

may repeat (pharmacology)
measles-rubella [vaccine] (pharmacology)
medial rectus [muscle] (ophthalmology)
medical record (medical records)
medical records [department] (medical
records)
mental retardation (genetics, neurology,
and psychiatry)
mentally retarded (genetics, neurology,
and psychiatry)
metabolic rate (laboratory)
methyl red (chemistry)
mitral reflux (cardiovascular)
mitral regurgitation (cardiovascular)
mortality rate (statistics)
mortality ratio (statistics)
motivation research (psychiatry and research)
muscle relaxant (neurology, orthopedics, and pharmacology)

M.R.
mentally retarded (genetics, neurology,
and psychiatry)
mental retardation (genetics, neurology,
and psychiatry)

M & R
measure and record

MR x 1
may repeat once (pharmacology)
may repeat times one (pharmacology)

Mr
master
mister

mR
milliroentgen (measurement and radiology)

mr
milliroentgen (measurement and radiology)

MRA
Medical Record Administrator (medical
records)

M.R.A.
Medical Record Administrator (medical records)

MRAA
Mental Retardation Association of America (genetics, neurology, and psychiatry)

MRACGP
Member of the Royal Australasian College of General Practice

MRACO
Member of the Royal Australasian College of Ophthalmologists (ophthalmology)

MRACP
Member of the Royal Australasian College of Physicians

M.R.A.C.P.
Member of the Royal Australasian College of Physicians

MRACR
Member of the Royal Australasian College of Radiologists (radiology)

MRad
Master of Radiology (education and radiology)

mrad
millirad (measurement and radiation therapy)

MRAN
medical resident admitting note (medical records)

MRANZCP
Member of the Royal Australian and New Zealand College of Psychiatrists (psychiatry)

MRAP
mean right atrial pressure (cardiovascular)

MRBC
monkey red blood cells (laboratory)

MRBF
mean renal blood flow (nephrology)

MRC
Medical Registration Council (administration)
Medical Research Council (research)
Medical Reserve Corps (armed forces)
methylrosaniline chloride [also called *crystal violet* and *gentian violet;* an anthelmitic, antibacterial, antifungal, and dye] (laboratory and pharmacology)

M.R.C.
Medical Reserve Corps (armed forces)

MRCGP
Member of the Royal College of General Practitioners

MRCI
Medical Registration Council of Ireland
Medical Research Council of Ireland (research)

MRCOG
Member of the Royal College of Obstetricians and Gynaecologists (gynecology and obstetrics)

MRCP
Member of the Royal College of Physicians

M.R.C.P.
Member of the Royal College of Physicians

MRCPA
Member of the Royal College of Pathologists of Australia (pathology)

MRCPath
Member of the Royal College of Pathologists (pathology)

MRCPE
Member of the Royal College of Physicians of Edinburgh

M.R.C.P.E.
Member of the Royal College of Physicians of Edinburgh

MRCP(Glasg)
Member of the Royal College of Physicians and Surgeons of Glasgow qua Physician

M.R.C.P.(Glasg.)
Member of the Royal College of Physicians and Surgeons of Glasgow qua Physician

MRCPI
Member of the Royal College of Physicians of Ireland

M.R.C.P.I.
Member of the Royal College of Physicians of Ireland

MRCPsych
Member of the Royal College of Psychiatrists (psychiatry)

MRCS
Member of the Royal College of Surgeons

M.R.C.S.
Member of the Royal College of Surgeons

MRCSE
Member of the Royal College of Surgeons of Edinburgh

M.R.C.S.E.
Member of the Royal College of Surgeons of Edinburgh

MRCSI
Member of the Royal College of Surgeons in Ireland

M.R.C.S.I.
Member of the Royal College of Surgeons in Ireland

MRCVS
Member of the Royal College of Veterinary Surgeons (veterinary medicine)

M.R.C.V.S.
Member of the Royal College of Veterinary Surgeons (veterinary medicine)

MRD
medical records department (medical records)
minimal residual disease
minimal reacting dose (radiation therapy)
minimum reaction dose (radiation therapy)

M.R.D.
minimum reacting dose (radiation therapy)

mrd
millirutherford (measurement)

MR-E
methemoglobin reductase (hematology and laboratory)

mrem
millirem [of radiation] (measurement and radiation therapy)
milliroentgen equivalent, man (measurement and radiation therapy)

mrep
milliroentgen equivalent, physical (measurement and radiation therapy)

MRF
melanocyte-stimulating hormone [MSH] releasing factor (laboratory)
melanophore-stimulating hormone [MSH] releasing factor (laboratory)
mesencephalic reticular formation (neurosurgery)
midbrain reticular formation (neurosurgery)
mitral regurgitation flow (cardiovascular)
müllerian regression factor (embryology, laboratory, and obstetrics)

MRFT
modified rapid fermentation test (laboratory)

MRG
murmurs, rubs, and gallops (cardiovascular)

MRH
melanocyte-stimulating hormone [MSH] releasing hormone (laboratory)
melanophore-stimulating hormone [MSH] releasing hormone (laboratory)

MRHA
mannose-resistant hemagglutination (laboratory)

mrhm
milliroentgen per hour at one meter (measurement and radiation therapy)

MRI
magnetic resonance imaging [scan and unit] (radiology)
Medical Research Institute (research)
Member of the Royal Institution
Mental Research Institute (psychiatry and research)
moderate renal insufficiency (nephrology)

MRIF
melanocyte-stimulating hormone [MSH] release inhibiting factor (laboratory)
melanophore-stimulating hormone [MSH] release inhibiting factor (laboratory)

MRIH
melanocyte-stimulating hormone release-inhibiting hormone (laboratory)

MRIPHH
Member of the Royal Institute of Public Health and Hygiene

MRL
Medical Record Librarian [now called *Medical Record Administrator*] (medical records)
Medical Research Laboratory [Navy and Air Force] (armed forces, laboratory, and research)
minimal response level (radiation therapy)

M.R.L.
Medical Record Librarian [now called *Medical Record Administrator*] (medical records)

MR MAX
{not an abbreviation} [a magnetic resonance system] (radiology)

mRNA
messenger ribonucleic acid (genetics and laboratory)

MRO
muscle receptor organ (neurology and orthopedics)

MROD
Medical Research and Operations Directorate [NASA] (aerospace medicine and research)

MRP
Medical Reimbursement Plan (insurance)
Members Retirement Plan [of the American Medical Association] (insurance)

MRR
marrow release rate (hematology and laboratory)

MRS
magnetic resonance spectroscopy (radiology)
Medical Receiving Station (emergency medicine)
methicillin-resistant *Staphylococcus [aureus]* (laboratory, orthopedics, and rheumatology)
mistress
multiple representative sections (laboratory and pathology)

MRSH
Member of the Royal Society of Health
methicillin-resistant *Staphylococcus aureus* (laboratory, orthopedics, and rheumatology)

MRT
median recognition threshold
Medical Records Technician (medical records)
milk-ring test [also called *abortus Band ring test*] (laboratory and veterinary medicine)
muscle response test (neurology and orthopedics)

M.R.T.
Medical Records Technician (medical records)

MRU
Mass Radiographic Unit (radiology)
minimal reproductive units (bacteriology and laboratory)

MRV
minute respiratory volume (respiratory)
mixed respiratory vaccine (infectious diseases, pharmacology, and respiratory)

MRVP
mean right ventricular pressure (cardiovascular)
methyl red, Voges-Proskauer [medium] (laboratory)

MR-VP broth
{not an abbreviation} [used for the methyl red and Voges-Proskauer test] (laboratory)

MS
complex of substrate and activating metal ion (chemistry)
maladjustment score (psychiatry)
mass spectrometry (laboratory)
Master of Science (education)
Master of Surgery (education and surgery)
medical science
Medical Services [Navy] (armed forces)
medical student (education)
medical supplies (manufacturing and pharmacology)
Medical Survey (statistics)
mental status (neurology and psychiatry)
mentally retarded (genetics, neurology, and psychiatry)

minimal support
Mississippi [Postal Service state designation]
mitral stenosis (cardiovascular)
Mobile Surgery [British]
modal sensitivity
molar solution (chemistry)
Mongolian spot (dermatology)
morphine sulfate (chemical dependency and pharmacology)
motile sperm (laboratory and urology)
mucosubstance (laboratory)
multiple sclerosis (neurology)
muscle shortening (orthopedics and surgery)
muscle strength (neurology and orthopedics)
musculoskeletal (orthopedics)

M.S.
Master of Surgery (education and surgery)
mental status (neurology and psychiatry)
multiple sclerosis (neurology)

M & S
microculture and sensitivity (laboratory)

MS-222
tricaine methane sulphonate (chemistry)

Ms
manuscript (publishing)
miss
mistress
musculoskeletal (orthopedics)

ms
manuscript (publishing)
millisecond (measurement)
mitral stenosis (cardiovascular)

MSA
mannitol salt agar [plate] (laboratory)
Medical Services Administration (administration)
mine safety appliance (industrial medicine and manufacturing)
multiplication-stimulating activity (laboratory)

MSAA
multiple sclerosis-associated agent (laboratory and neurology)

MSAF
meconium stained amniotic fluid (neonatology and obstetrics)

MSAFP
maternal serum alpha fetoprotein (laboratory and obstetrics)

MSB
Martin's Scarlet Blue
mid-small bowel (gastroenterology)
most significant bit (mathematics)

MsB
Master of Science in Bacteriology (bacteriology and education)

MSBLA
mouse-specific B lymphocyte antigen (laboratory)

MSC
Medical Service Corps (armed forces)
Medical Specialist Corps (armed forces)
Medical Staff Corps [British] (armed forces)

MSc
Master of Science (education)

MSCA
McCarthy Scales of Children's Abilities (psychiatry)

MSCC
midstream clean catch [urine sample] (laboratory)

MScD
Doctor of Medical Science (education
Doctor of Science in Medicine (education)
Master of Dental Science (dentistry and education)

MSCE
monitored self-care evaluation (occupational therapy)

MScMed
Master of Medical Science (education)

MScN
Master of Science in Nursing (education and nursing)

mscp
mean spherical candle power (electricity and measurement)

MSD
Merck, Sharp, and Dohme [company] (pharmacology)
most significant digit (mathematics)

MSDC
Mass Spectrometry Data Centre [United Kingdom] (laboratory)

MSE
mental status examination (neurology and psychiatry)
medical support equipment

mse
mean square error (mathematics)

MSEA
Medical Society Executives Association (administration)

msec
millisecond (measurement)

MSER
mean systolic ejection rate (cardiovascular)

MSES
medical school environmental stress (education, neurology, and psychiatry)

MSET
multistage exercise test (cardiovascular)

MSF
macrophage spreading factor (laboratory)

MSG
massage (physical therapy and rehabilitation)
methysergide [a serotonin antagonist] (neurology and pharmacology)
monosodium glutamate (chemistry, dietary, laboratory, and neurology)

MSH
medical self-help (rehabilitation)
melanocyte-stimulating hormone (laboratory)
melanophore-stimulating hormone [intermedin] (laboratory)

α-MSH
alpha-melanocyte-stimulating hormone (laboratory)

β-MSH
beta-melanocyte stimulating hormone (laboratory)

MSH-IF
melanocyte-stimulating hormone inhibiting factor (laboratory)
melanophore-stimulating hormone [intermedin] inhibiting factor (laboratory)

MSHy
Master of Science in Hygiene (education)

MSI
medium-scale integration

MS I
Medical Student-I [first year] (education)

MS II
Medical Student-II [second year] (education)

MS III
Medical Student-III [third year] (education)

MS in Rad
Master of Science in Radiology (education and radiology)

MSIR
{not an abbreviation} [a brand name for a morphine sulfate preparation] (pharmacology)

MS IV
Medical Student-IV [fourth year] (education)

MSK
medullary sponge kidney (nephrology)
musculoskeletal (orthopedics)

MSKCC
Memorial Sloan-Kettering Cancer Center (administration, oncology, and research)

MSKP
Medical Sciences Knowledge Profile (education)

MSL
midsternal line (anatomy)

M.S.L.
midsternal line (anatomy)

MSLA
mouse-specific lymphocyte antigen (laboratory)

MSLT
multiple sleep latency test (neurology)

MSM
Master of Medical Science (education)
mineral salts medium (laboratory)
medial superior olive [of the brain] (neurosurgery)

MSN
Master of Science in Nursing (education and nursing)
mildly subnormal (laboratory)

MSP
mouse serum protein (allergy and laboratory)

MSPGN
mesangial proliferative glomerulonephritis (nephrology)

MSPH
Master of Science in Public Health (education)

MSPhar
Master of Science in Pharmacy (education and pharmacology)

MSPS
myocardial stress perfusion scintigraphy (cardiovascular and radiology)

MSR
Member of the Society of Radiographers (radiology)
muscle stretch reflexes (neurology and orthopedics)

MSRG
Member of the Society for Remedial Gymnasts (sports medicine)

MSRPP
multidimensional scale for rating psychiatric patients (psychiatry)

MSS
Marital Satisfaction Scale (psychiatry)
massage (physical therapy and rehabilitation)
Medical Service School [Air Force] (armed forces and education)
Medical Superintendents' Society (administration)
mental status schedule (neurology and psychiatry)
minor surgery suite (surgery)
motion sickness susceptibility (gastroenterology, neurology, and otorhinolaryngology)   .
mucus-stimulating substance (laboratory)
muscular subaortic stenosis (cardiovascular)

Mss
manuscripts (publishing)

MSSc
Master of Sanitary Science (ecology and education)

MSSE
Master of Science in Sanitary Engineering (ecology and education)

MSSR
Medical Society for the Study of Radiesthesia (research)

MSSVD
Medical Society for the Study of Venereal Diseases (gynecology, infectious diseases, research, and urology)

MST
mean survival time (oncology)
mean swell time [botulism test] (laboratory)

MSTA
{not an abbreviation} [brand name of a mumps skin test antigen] (infectious diseases, laboratory, and pharmacology)

MSTh
mesothorium (chemistry, oncology, and radiation therapy)

MSU
maple syrup urine (laboratory and urology)
medical studies unit (research)
midstream urine [specimen] (laboratory)
monosodium urate (laboratory)

MSUD
maple syrup urine disease (urology)

MSurg
Master of Surgery (education and surgery)

MSV
maximal sustained level of ventilation (respiratory)
Moloney's sarcoma virus [of mice] (labo-

ratory, oncology, research, and veterinary medicine)
murine sarcoma virus [of mice] (laboratory, oncology, research, and veterinary medicine)

MSW
Master of Social Welfare (education and social services)
Master of Social Work (education and social services)
Medical Social Worker (social services)
multiple stab wounds (emergency medicine)

MSWYE
modified seawater yeast extract [agar] (laboratory)

MT
empty
malaria therapy (infectious diseases and respiratory)
malignant teratoma (oncology)
mammary tumor (gynecology and oncology)
mammary tumor [of mice] (oncology, research, and veterinary medicine)
maximal therapy
Medical Technologist (laboratory)
medical transcriptionist (medical records)
membrana tympani [tympanic membrane] (otorhinolaryngology)
metatarsal (orthopedics and podiatry)
methoxytyramine (chemistry)
methyltyrosine (endocrinology and laboratory)
microtome [an instrument] (laboratory and pathology)
microtubule (laboratory)
middle turbinate (otorhinolaryngology)
Montana [Postal Service state designation]
more than
muscles and tendons (orthopedics)
music therapy (rehabilitation)

M.T.
medical transcriptionist (medical records)

M-T
macroglobulin-trypsin [complex] (laboratory)

3-MT
3-methoxytyramine (chemistry)

MT6
mercaptomerin (pharmacology)

MTA
Medical Technical Assistant (laboratory)
metatarsus adductus (orthopedics and podiatry)
myoclonic twitch activity (neurology)

MT (AMT)
Medical Technologist (American Medical Technologists) (laboratory)

MT (ASCP)
Registered Medical Technologist (American Society of Clinical Pathologists) (laboratory and pathology)

MT(ASCP)SBB
Medical Technologist (American Society of Clinical Pathologists) Specialist in Blood Bank [Technology] (hematology, laboratory, and pathology)

MT bar
metatarsal bar (orthopedics and podiatry)

MTBE
methyl tert-butyl ether [to liquefy cholesterol gallstones] (gastroenterology and pharmacology)

MTBF
mean time between failures (statistics)

MTC
medical test cabinet
Medical Training Center (education)
medullary thyroid carcinoma (endocrinology and oncology)
mitomycin-C (chemotherapy, oncology, and pharmacology)

⁹⁹ᵐTc
technetium pertechnetate (radiology)

⁹⁹ᵐTcMAA
technetium 99 macroaggregated albumin (radiology)

⁹⁹ᵐTc-PIPIDA scan
technetium pertechnetate/N-para-isopropylacetanilide-iminodiacetic acid scan (radiology)

MTCS
Madelian Thomas Completion Stories (psychiatry)

⁹⁹ᵐTc-SC
technetium pertechnetate-sulfur colloid (radiology)

MTD
maximal tolerated dose (radiation therapy)
Midwife Teacher's Diploma (education and obstetrics)
Monroe Tidal drainage (urology)

mtd
mitte tales doses [send such doses] (pharmacology)

m.t.d.
mitte tales doses [send such doses] (pharmacology)

MTDDA
Minnesota Test for Differential Diagnosis of Aphasia (neurology and speech and language therapy)

MTDT
modified tone decay test (neurology and orthopedics)

M.T.E.-5
{not an abbreviation} [a multielectrolyte concentrate] (pharmacology)

MTF
maximum terminal flow
Medical Treatment Faculty
modulation transfer function (radiology)

MTH
metharbital [an anticonvulsant] (neurology and pharmacology)
mithramycin (chemotherapy, oncology, and pharmacology)

MTHF
methyltetrahydrofolic acid (laboratory)

MTI
malignant teratoma intermediate (oncology)
minimum time interval

MTJ
midtarsal joint (orthopedics and podiatry)

MTLP
metabolic toxemia of late pregnancy (obstetrics)

MTM
modified Thayer-Martin [medium] (laboratory)

MTO
Medical Transport Officer

MTOC
microtubule organizing center (laboratory)
mitotic organizing center (laboratory)

MTP
metatarsophalangeal [joint] (orthopedics and podiatry)
microtubule protein (laboratory)

MTR
mass, tenderness, rebound [on abdominal examination] (gastroenterology)
Meinicke turbidity reaction (laboratory)
Mental Treatment Rules (psychiatry)

MTS
moderate tactile stimulus (neurology)
Monosyllable, Trochee, Spondee Test [of speech discrimination] (otorhinolaryngology and speech and language therapy)

MTT
malignant trophoblastic teratoma (oncology)
mean transit time [of blood through heart and lungs] (cardiovascular and respiratory)
monotetrazolium (laboratory)

MTU
malignant teratoma undifferentiated (oncology)
methylthiouracil (endocrinology, laboratory, and pharmacology)

M tuberc
Mycobacterium tuberculosis (infectious diseases, laboratory, and respiratory)

M. tuberculosis
Mycobacterium tuberculosis (infectious diseases, laboratory, and respiratory)

MTV
mammary tumor virus [of mice] (oncology, research, and veterinary medicine)
metatarsus varus (orthopedics and podiatry)
Music Television [cable music television station]

MTX
methotrexate (chemotherapy, oncology, and pharmacology)

MTx
methotrexate (chemotherapy, oncology, and pharmacology)

MTX + MP
methotrexate and mercaptopurine (chemotherapy, oncology, and pharmacology)

MTX + MP + CTX
methotrexate, mercaptopurine, and Cytoxan [cyclophosphamide] (chemotherapy, oncology, and pharmacology)

MU
million units (measurement)
Montevideo unit [measure of length and strength of contractions] (obstetrics)

mouse unit [referring to gonadotropins] (laboratory)

4-MU
4-methylumbelliferone [an antispasmodic] (pharmacology)

Mu
Mache unit [referring to radium emanations] (radiation therapy and radiology)

M.u.
Mache unit [referring to radium emanations] (radiation therapy and radiology)

Mu.
muscle (neurology and orthopedics)

mU
milliunit (measurement)

mu
micron (measurement)
milliunit (measurement)

m.u.
mouse unit [referring to gonadotropins] (laboratory)

MUC
maximum urinary concentration (laboratory and urology)

muc
mucilago [mucilage] (pharmacology)

MUGA
multigated angiogram (cardiovascular and radiology) {pronounced "mug-ah"}
multiple gate acquisition analysis [scan] (cardiovascular and radiology) {pronounced "mug-ah"}
multiple gated acquisition [blood pool radionuclide scan] (cardiovascular and radiology) {pronounced "mug-ah"}

"mug-ah"
{pronunciation of *MUGA* [multigated angiogram, multiple gate acquisition analysis (scan) *or* multiple gated acquisition (blood pool radionuclide scan)]} (cardiovascular and radiology) {not an abbreviation}

MU-GAL
methylumbelliferyl-β-galactosidase

MUGX
multiple gated acquisition exercise [scan] (cardiovascular and radiology)

"mull-tea"
{pronunciation of *MULTI* [multiple]} {not an abbreviation}

"mull-tea-vitz"
{pronunciation of *multivits* [multivitamins]} (pharmacology) {not an abbreviation}

"mull-tip"
{pronunciation of *multip* [multipara and multiparous]} (gynecology and obstetrics) {not an abbreviation}

mult
multiple

MULTI
multiple {pronounced "mull-tea"}

multip
multipara (gynecology and obstetrics) {pronounced "mull-tip"}
multiparous (gynecology and obstetrics) {pronounced "mull-tip"}

multivits
multivitamins (pharmacology) {pronounced "mull-tea-vitz"}

MuLV
murine leukemia virus [of mice] (research and veterinary medicine)

MUMPS
Massachusetts General Hospital Utility Multi-Programming System

MUO
myocardiopathy of unknown origin (cardiovascular)

MUP
motor unit potential (neurology)
mouse urine protein (allergy and laboratory)

MurNAc
N-acetylmuramate (laboratory)

MURC
measurable undesirable respiratory contaminants (laboratory and respiratory)

musc
muscle (orthopedics)
muscular (orthopedics)

MUST
medical unit, self-contained, transportable (emergency medicine)

MUU
mouse uterine unit (laboratory and measurement)

MUWU
mouse uterine weight unit (laboratory and measurement)

MV
Medicus Veterinarius [veterinary physician] (veterinary medicine)
megavolt (electricity and measurement)
microvilli (laboratory)
microwave (physics)
minute volume (respiratory)
mitral valve [image on transesophageal echocardiogram] (cardiovascular)
mixed venous [blood] (cardiovascular, hematology, and laboratory)

M.V.
Medicus Veterinarius [veterinary physician] (veterinary medicine)

Mv
mendelevium (chemistry)

mV
millivolt (electricity and measurement)

mv
millivolt (electricity and measurement)

MVA
malignant ventricular arrhythmias (cardiovascular)
mitral valve area (cardiovascular)
motor vehicle accident (emergency medicine)

M-VAC
methotrexate, vinblastine, doxorubicin, and cisplatin (chemotherapy, oncology, and pharmacology)

MVB
mixed venous blood (cardiovascular, hematology, and laboratory)
multivesicular body (laboratory)

MVC
maximum vital capacity (respiratory)
maximal voluntary contraction (neurology)
myocardial vascular capacity (cardiovascular)

MVD
Doctor of Veterinary Medicine (veterinary medicine)

MVE
mitral valve echo (cardiovascular)
Murray Valley encephalitis (neurology)

MV grad
mitral valve gradient (cardiovascular)

MVH
methotrexate, VP-16, and hexamethylmelamine (chemotherapy, oncology, and pharmacology)

MVI
multiple vitamin infusion (pharmacology)
multivitamins intravenously (pharmacology)
{not an abbreviation} [brand name for parenteral multivitamins] (pharmacology)

MVI 12
{not an abbreviation} [brand name for parenteral multivitamins] (pharmacology)

MVLS
mandibular vestibulolingual sulcoplasty (neurosurgery)
Meecham Verbal Language Scale (speech and language therapy)

MVM
microvillous membrane (laboratory)

MVMT
movement

MVO$_2$
myocardial oxygen consumption (cardiovascular)
myocardial oxygen ventilation [rate] (cardiovascular)

MVP
mitral valve prolapse (cardiovascular)
most valuable player (sports medicine)

MVPD-26
methotrexate, citrovorum factor, VM-26, procarbazine, and dexamethasone (chemotherapy, oncology, and pharmacology)

MVPP
Mustine, vinblastine, procarbazine, and prednisone (chemotherapy, oncology, and pharmacology)
nitrogen mustard, vinblastine [Velban], procarbazine, and prednisone (chemotherapy, oncology, and pharmacology)

MVPS
mitral valve prolapse syndrome (cardiovascular)

MVR
massive vitreous retraction (ophthalmology)
massive vitreous retractor [blade] (ophthalmology)
maximum ventilation rate (respiratory)

mitral valve regurgitation (cardiovascular)

mitral valve replacement (cardiovascular)

MVR blade
massive vitreous retractor blade (ophthalmology)

MVRI
mixed vaccine, respiratory infections (infectious diseases, pharmacology, and respiratory)

MVS
mitral valve stenosis (cardiovascular)

MVT
maximal ventilation time (respiratory)

MVV
maximum voluntary ventilation (respiratory)
maximum voluntary volume (respiratory)
mixed vespid venom (emergency medicine, laboratory, and pharmacology)

MVV$_1$
maximal ventilatory volume (respiratory)

MVV$_x$
maximal voluntary ventilation in a specified time period [The symbol "X" is replaced with a numerical qualifier— MVV60 = MVV performed at 60 breaths per minute.] (respiratory)

MW
microwave (physics)
molecular weight (chemistry)

mW
milliwatt (electricity and measurement)

mw
microwave (physics)

MWD
microwave diathermy (physical therapy)

MWS
Mikity-Wilson syndrome (neonatology and respiratory)

MX
matrix

Mx
maxwell [unit of magnetic force; now called *weber*] (physics) {obsolete}
Medex [a training program for physicians' assistants] (education)

mx
management (administration)
mixture (pharmacology)

MY
myxedematous (endocrinology)

My
myopia (ophthalmology)

my
mayer [unit of heat capacity] (orthopedics and rheumatology)

"my-ah-low"
{pronunciation of *myelo* [myelocyte]} (laboratory) {not an abbreviation}

Myco
Mycobacterium [a bacterium] (laboratory) {pronounced "my-co"}
Mycoplasma [a bacterium] (laboratory) {pronounced "my-co"}

"my-co"
{pronunciation of *Myco* [*Mycobacterium* or *Mycoplasma*; both are bacteria]} (laboratory) {not an abbreviation}

Mycol
mycology [the study of fungi] (laboratory)

"my-crow"
{pronunciation of *micro* and *micro-* [microscopic, microscopy, one-millionth, and prefix for 10^{-6}]} (laboratory and measurement) {not an abbreviation}

MYEL
multiple myeloma (hematology and oncology)

Myel
myelocyte (laboratory)

myel
myelin (laboratory)
myelinated (anatomy, laboratory, and neurology)

myelo
myelocyte (laboratory) {pronounced "my-ah-low"}

MyG
myasthenia gravis (neurology)

MYOC-A
myocarditis, pericarditis (cardiovascular)

MYOGLB
myoglobin (hematology and laboratory)

myop
myopia (ophthalmology)

MYS
myasthenic syndrome (neurology)

MYSOLN
Mysoline [an anticonvulsant] (neurology and pharmacology)

MYTGC
Miller-Yoder Test of Grammatical Comprehension (speech and language therapy)

MZ
mantle zone (neurology and pathology)
monozygotic (genetics)

MZA
monozygotic twins raised apart (genetics)

MZT
monozygotic twins raised together (genetics)

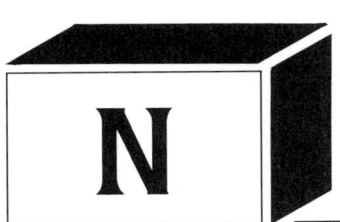

ν
nu [thirteenth letter of the Greek alphabet]

N
asparagine (chemistry and laboratory)
nasal (otorhinolaryngology)
negative
Negro [color or race]
Negroid [color or race]
Neisseria (laboratory)
nerve (neurology)
neurologist (neurology)
neurology
neuropathy (neurology)
neutron number (physics)
never
newton (physics)
nicotinamide [also called *niacinamide;* a B complex vitamin] (laboratory and pharmacology)
nitrogen (chemistry)
no
Nocardia [a bacteria] (laboratory)
nodule(s) [a small mass of tissue] (multiple specialties)
nonmalignant [referring to tumors] (pathology)
Nonne [a globulin test; also called *Ross-Jones test*] (laboratory)
normal [referring to solutions or to structure and function of organs]
not
NPH [a type of insulin] (endocrinology and pharmacology)
nu [thirteenth letter of the Greek alphabet]
number
number of molecules (chemistry)
population size (statistics)
refractive index (chemistry)
size of sample (statistics)
unit for fast neutrons (physics)
unit of neutron dosage (physics)
{not an abbreviation} [symbol for an antigenic determinant of erythrocytes in blood typing] (hematology and laboratory)

N.
normal

N₂
molecular nitrogen (chemistry)

N3
cyclophosphamide, vincristine, trifluorothymidine, and papaverine (chemotherapy, oncology, and pharmacology)

5′-N
5′-nucleotidase (chemistry, genetics, and laboratory)

¹⁵N
radioactive nitrogen (chemistry)

n
haploid chromosome number [2n equals diploid number] (genetics and laboratory)
index of refraction (chemistry)
nano- [prefix for 10^{-9}] (measurement)
naris [nostril] (otorhinolaryngology)
nasal (otorhinolaryngology)
natus [born]
nerve (neurology)
neuter (gynecology, urology, and veterinary medicine)
neutron (physics)
neutron dosage [unit of] (physics)
normal
nostril (otorhinolaryngology)
number
number density of molecule (chemistry)
number of observations (statistics)
sample size (statistics)
size of sample (statistics)
{not an abbreviation} [symbol for index of refraction] (chemistry)

n.
{not an abbreviation} [symbol for normal] (chemistry)

n.
nerve (neurology)

5n
pentaploidy [state of having five sets of chromosomes] (genetics and laboratory)

7n
heptaploidy [state of having seven sets of chromosomes] (genetics and laboratory)

8n
octaploidy [state of having eight sets of chromosomes] (genetics and laboratory)

NA
Narcotics Anonymous (chemical dependency and psychiatry)
neuraminidase [also called *sialidase*; an enzyme] (laboratory)
neutralizing antibody (laboratory)
neutrophil antibody (laboratory)
nicotinic acid (chemistry, laboratory, and pharmacology)
no abnormality
Nomina Anatomica [a compilation of anatomical nomenclature] (anatomy)
noradrenalin(e) [also called *norepinephrine*] (cardiovascular and pharmacology)
not admitted
not applicable
not available
nucleic acid (genetics and laboratory)
nucleus ambiguus (laboratory and neurology)
numerical aperature (chemistry and laboratory)
nurse anesthetist (anesthesiology and nursing)
nurse's aide (nursing)
nursing assistant (nursing)
Nursing Auxiliary [British] (nursing)

N.A.
numerical aperture (chemistry and laboratory)
nursing assistant (nursing)

N/A
no alternative
not applicable

Na
Avogadro's number (chemistry)
natrium [sodium] (chemistry, laboratory, and pharmacology)

Na+
natrium [sodium] (chemistry, laboratory, and pharmacology)

^{24}Na
radioactive sodium (chemistry)

NAA
naphthaleneacetic acid (laboratory)
neuron activation analysis (neurology)
nicotinic acid amide (chemistry, laboratory, and pharmacology)
no apparent abnormalities

NAACLS
National Accrediting Agency for Clinical Laboratory Sciences (government and laboratory)

N.A.A.C.L.S.
National Accrediting Agency for Clinical Laboratory Sciences (government and laboratory)

NAACOG
Nurses Association of the American College of Obstetricians and Gynecologists (nursing and obstetrics)

NAACP
National Association for the Advancement of Colored People
neoplasia, allergy, Addison's disease, collagen vascular disease, and parasites

NAAFA
National Association to Aid Fat Americans (dietary)

NAAP
N-acetyl-4-amino-phenazone (chemistry and pharmacology)

NAB
non-A, non-B [hepatitis] (gastroenterology, infectious diseases, and laboratory)

novarsenobenzene [also called *neoarsphenamine*; formerly used as an antisyphilitic] (pharmacology)

NABP
National Association of Boards of Pharmacy (pharmacology)

NaBr
sodium bromide (neurology and pharmacology)

NABS
normoactive bowel sounds (gastroenterology)

NABSP
National Association of Blue Shield Plans (insurance)

NAC
N-acetyl-L-cysteine (laboratory)

National Asthma Center (respiratory)

nitrogen mustard, Adriamycin, and lomustine [CCNU] (chemotherapy, oncology, and pharmacology)

Noise Advisory Council (ecology and industrial medicine)

NACD
not acidified (laboratory)

NACDS
North American Clinical Dermatologic Society (dermatology)

NACED
National Advisory Council on the Employment of the Disabled (government and rehabilitation)

NaCl
sodium chloride [salt] (chemistry, dietary, laboratory, and pharmacology)

NACOR
National Advisory Committee on Radiation (radiology)

N.A.C.O.R.
National Advisory Committee on Radiation (radiology)

NACT
National Alliance of Cardiovascular Technologists (cardiovascular)

NAD
nicotinamide-adenine dinucleotide [also called *codehydrogenase I, coenzyme I (CoI), dihydroenzyme I,* and, formerly, *diphosphopyridine nucleotide (DPN)*] (genetics and laboratory)

no active disease

no acute distress

no apparent distress

no appreciable disease

normal axis deviation (cardiovascular)

nothing abnormal detected

nothing abnormal discovered

N.A.D.
no appreciable disease

NAD+
nicotinamide-adenine dinucleotide [oxidized form] (laboratory)

NADA
New Animal Drug Applications (pharmacology, research, and veterinary medicine)

NADH
nicotinamide-adenine dinucleotide [reduced form] [formerly called *diphosphopyridine nucleotide, reduced*] (laboratory)

NADP
nicotinamide-adenine-dinucleotide phosphate [also called *codehydrogenase II, coenzyme II (CoII), triphosphopyridine nucleotide (TPN),* and *Warburg's coenzyme*] (genetics and laboratory)

NADP+
nicotinamide-adenine-dinucleotide phosphate [oxidized form] (laboratory)

NADPH
nicotinamide-adenine-dinucleotide phosphate [reduced form] [formerly called *triphosphopyridine nucleotide, reduced*] (laboratory)

NAEMT
National Association of Emergency Medical Technicians (emergency medicine)

NAF
National Amputation Foundation (orthopedics and rehabilitation)
National Ataxia Foundation (neurology)

NaF
sodium fluoride (chemistry, dentistry, pharmacology, and water treatment)

NAG
narrow angle glaucoma (ophthalmology)
nonagglutinating (laboratory)

NAH
Nevada Association for the Handicapped (rehabilitation)

NAHCS
National Association of Health Career Schools (education)

NAHG
National Association of Humanistic Gerontology (geriatrics)

NAHI
National Athletic Health Institute (sports medicine)

NAHPA
National Association of Hospital Purchasing Agents (administration and manufacturing)

NAHSA
National Association for Hearing and Speech Action (otorhinolaryngology and speech and language therapy)

NAHSE
National Association of Health Services Executives (administration)

NAHSR
National Association of Human Services Technologists

NAHU
National Association of Health Underwriters (insurance)

NAI
nonaccidental injury (emergency medicine)

NA I
Nursing Assistant Level I (nursing)

NaI
sodium iodide (pharmacology)

NA II
Nursing Assistant Level II (nursing)

NA III
Nursing Assistant Level III (nursing)

NA IV
Nursing Assistant Level IV (nursing)

Na & K
sodium and potassium [urine test] (laboratory)

Na & KSP
sodium and potassium spot [urine test] (laboratory)

NAM
natural actomyosins (laboratory)

NAMCS
National Ambulatory Medical Care Survey (administration and statistics)

NAME
National Association of Medical Examiners (pathology)

N.A.M.E.
National Association of Medical Examiners (pathology)

NAMH
National Association of Mental Health (psychiatry)

N.A.M.H.
National Association of Mental Health (psychiatry)

NAMRU
Navy Medical Reserve Unit (armed forces)

NAMS
National Ambient Air Monitoring Stations (ecology and meteorology)
Nurses and Army Medical Specialists (armed forces and nursing)

NAMT
National Association for Music Therapy (psychiatry and rehabilitation)

NANA
N-acetyl neuraminic acid (laboratory)

NANB
non-A, non-B [hepatitis] (gastroenterology and infectious diseases)

NANBH
non-A, non-B hepatitis (gastroenterology and infectious diseases)

nano-
{not an abbreviation} [prefix for 10^{-9}] (measurement) {pronounced "nan-oh"}

"nan-oh"
{pronunciation of *nano-* [prefix for 10^{-9} {not an abbreviation}]} (measurement) {not an abbreviation}

NAON
National Association of Orthopaedic Nurses (nursing and orthopedics)

NAOO
National Association of Optometrists and Opticians (ophthalmology)

NAOP
National Alliance for Optional Parenthood (obstetrics)

NAOT
National Association of Orthopaedic Technologists (orthopedics)

NAP
nasion pogonion [angle of convexity] (anatomy)
neutrophil alkaline phosphatase (laboratory)
nucleic acid acid phosphorus (laboratory)
nucleic acid phosphorus (laboratory)

NAPA
N-acetyl-p-aminophenol [also called *acetaminophen* and *paracetamol*] (laboratory and pharmacology) {pronounced "nap-ah"}
N-acetyl procainamide (cardiovascular and pharmacology) {pronounced "nap-ah"}
N-acetylated procainamide (cardiovascular and pharmacology) {pronounced "nap-ah"}

"nap-ah"
{pronunciation of *NAPA* [*N*-acetyl-p-aminophenol (also called *acetaminophen* and *paracetamol*; laboratory and pharmacology), *N*-acetyl procainamide (cardiovascular and pharmacology), and *N*-acetylated procainamide (cardiovascular and pharmacology)]} {not an abbreviation}

NAPCA
National Air Pollution Control Administration (ecology)

Na Pent
sodium Pentothal [brand name for thiopental sodium] (anesthesiology and pharmacology)

NAPH
naphthyl (chemistry and pharmacology)

NAPN
National Association of Physicians' Nurses (nursing)

NAPNAP
National Association of Pediatric Nurses Associates and Practitioners (nursing and pediatrics)

NAPNE
National Association for Practical Nurse Education (education and nursing)

NAPNES
National Association for Practical Nurse Education and Services (education and nursing)

N.A.P.N.E.S.
National Association for Practical Nurse Education and Services (education and nursing)

NAPPH
National Association of Private Psychiatric Hospitals (psychiatry)

NAPT
National Association for the Prevention of Tuberculosis (infectious diseases and respiratory)

NAR
nasal airway resistance (otorhinolaryngology)

NARA
Narcotics Addict Rehabilitation Act (chemical dependency and government)
National Association of Recovered Alcoholics (chemical dependency and psychiatry)

NARAL
National Abortion Rights Action League (gynecology and obstetrics)

NARC
narcotic (chemical dependency and pharmacology)
narcotics officer [slang for law enforcement officer] (chemical dependency) {pronounced "nark"}

narcotism (chemical dependency)
National Association for Retarded Children (genetics, pediatrics, and psychiatry)

Narc
narcotic (chemical dependency and pharmacology)
narcotism (chemical dependency)

narc
narcotics officer [slang for law enforcement officer] (chemical dependency) {pronounced "nark"}

narco
narcolepsy (neurology)
narcotics hospital (chemical dependency and psychiatry)
narcotics officer [slang] (chemical dependency) {pronounced "nark-oh"}
narcotics treatment center (chemical dependency)

NARD
National Association of Retail Druggists (pharmacology)

Na$_{reab}$
sodium reabsorption rate (laboratory)

NARF
National Association for Rehabilitation Facilities (rehabilitation)

"nark"
{pronunciation of NARC and narc [narcotics officer (slang for law enforcement officer)]} (chemical dependency) {not an abbreviation}

"nark-oh"
{pronunciation of narco [narcotics officer (slang)]} (chemical dependency) {not an abbreviation}

NARMC
Naval Aerospace and Regional Medical Center (armed forces and aerospace medicine)

NARMH
National Association for Rural Mental Health (psychiatry)

NARS
National Acupuncture Research Society (acupuncture and research)

NAS
nasal (otorhinolaryngology)
National Academy of Sciences
National Association of Sanitarians
neonatal abstinence syndrome (neonatology and obstetrics)
no added salt (dietary)

N.A.S.
National Academy of Sciences

NASA
National Aeronautics and Space Administration (aerospace medicine and government)

NASE
National Association for the Study of Epilepsy (neurology)

N.A.S.E.
National Association for the Study of Epilepsy (neurology)

NASEAN
National Association for State Enrolled Assistant Nurses (nursing)

NASL
nasal (otorhinolaryngology)

NASM
Naval Aviation School of Medicine (armed forces and education)

NASMV
National Association on Standard Medical Vocabulary (education)

NAS-NRC
National Academy of Sciences-National Research Council (research)

N.A.S.-N.R.C.
National Academy of Sciences-National Research Council (research)

Na-Spt
sodium spot [urine test] (laboratory)

NASULGC
National Association of State Universities and Land Grant Colleges (education)

NASW
National Association of Social Workers (social services)

NAT
N-acetyltransferase (laboratory)
natal (neonatology and obstetrics)
no action taken

Nat
national
native
natural

nat.
national
native
natural

N.A.T.A.
National Athletic Trainers Association (sports medicine)

Natr
natrium [sodium] (chemistry, laboratory, and pharmacology)

NATTS
National Association of Trade and Technical Schools (education)

NB
newborn (neonatology and obstetrics)
needle biopsy (pathology and surgery)
nitrous oxide-barbiturate (anesthesiology and pharmacology)
no bowel movement (gastroenterology)
normal bowel movement (gastroenterology)
nota bene [note well, take notice]

N.B.
newborn (neonatology and obstetrics)

Nb
niobium [formerly called *columbium*] (chemistry)

nb
nota bene [note well]

n.b.
nota bene [note well]

NBA
National Basketball Association (sports medicine)
non-weight-bearing ambulation (orthopedics, physical therapy, and rehabilitation)

NBC
nonbattle casualty (armed forces)

NBI
no bone injury (emergency medicine and orthopedics)
nonbattle injury (armed forces)

NBM
no bowel movement (gastroenterology)
normal bowel movement (gastroenterology)
nothing by mouth (dietary)

NBME
National Board of Medical Examiners (pathology)

N.B.M.E.
National Board of Medical Examiners (pathology)

NBN
narrow band nerve (neurology and orthopedics)
newborn nursery (neonatology)

NBO
nonbed occupancy

NBOT
National Board of Orthopaedic Technologists (orthopedics)

NBRT
National Board for Respiratory Therapy (respiratory)

NBS
National Bureau of Standards (measurement)
no bacteria seen (laboratory)
normal blood serum (hematology and laboratory)
normal bowel sounds (gastroenterology)
normal burro serum (laboratory)

N.B.S.
National Bureau of Standards (measurement)

NBT
nitroblue tetrazolium [test] (laboratory)

NBTE
nonbacterial thrombotic endocarditis (cardiovascular)

NBTNF
newborn, term, normal female (neonatology and obstetrics)

NBTNM
newborn, term, normal male (neonatology and obstetrics)

NBTS
National Blood Transfusion Service (hematology)

NBT test
nitro blue tetrazolium [dye] test (laboratory)

NBW
normal birth weight (neonatology)

NC
nasal cannula (otorhinolaryngology and respiratory)
neural crest (anatomy and neurology)
neurocirculatory (cardiovascular, neurology, and orthopedics)
neurologic check (neurology)
nitrocellulose [also called *pyroxylin*] (laboratory)
no casualty (armed forces and emergency medicine)
no change

no complaint(s)
noise criterion (otorhinolaryngology)
noncompliance (pharmacology)
noncompliant (pharmacology)
noncontributory
normocephalic [on physical examination] (anatomy and neurology)
North Carolina [Postal Service state designation]
nose cone
not completed
not cultured (laboratory)
Nurse Corps (nursing)

N/C
nasal cannula [oxygen administration] (respiratory)
neurocirculatory (cardiovascular, neurology, and orthopedics)
no complaints

nc
nanocurie [also called *millimicrocurie*] (radiation therapy)
no change
no charge

n/c
no change
no complaint

NCA
National Certification Agency for Medical Laboratory Personnel (government and laboratory)
National Council on Aging (geriatrics)
National Council on Alcoholism (chemical dependency)
neurocirculatory asthenia (neurology)
nonspecific cross-reacting antigen (laboratory)

N.C.A.
National Council on Alcoholism (chemical dependency)

NCAE
National Center for Alcohol Education (chemical dependency and education)

NCAMI
National Committee Against Mental Illness (psychiatry)

N.C.A.M.L.P.
National Certification Agency for Medical Laboratory Personnel (government and laboratory)

N-CAP
Nurses Coalition for Action in Politics (nursing)

NCAS
neocarzinostatin [also called *zinostatin*] (chemotherapy, oncology, and pharmacology)

NCAT
normocephalic and atraumatic [on head examination] (anatomy and neurology)

NC/AT
normocephalic and atraumatic [on head examination] (anatomy and neurology)

NCB
no code blue [for terminal cases] (cardiovascular and respiratory)

NCCDC
National Center for Chronic Disease Control (research)

NCCDS
National Cooperative Crohn's Disease Study (gastroenterology and research)

NCCEA
Neurosensory Center Comprehensive Examination for Aphasia (neurology and speech and language therapy)

NCCIP
National Center for Clinical Infant Programs (neonatology)

N.C.C.L.S.
National Committee for Clinical Laboratory Standards (laboratory)

NCCLVP
National Coordinating Committee on

Large Volume Parenterals (gastroenterology)

NCCPA
National Committee on Certification of
Physician's Assistants

NCCU
Newborn Convalescent Care Unit (neonatology)

NCD
National Commission on Diabetes (endocrinology)
National Council on Drugs (chemical dependency and pharmacology)
normal childhood diseases (pediatrics)
normal childhood disorders (pediatrics)
not considered disabling
not considered disqualifying

NCDA
National Council on Drug Abuse (chemical dependency)

NDCD
National Communicable Disease Center
(infectious diseases)

NCE
new chemical entities (chemistry)
nonconvulsive epilepsy (neurology)

NCEHPHP
National Council on the Education of
Health Professionals in Health Promo-
tion (education)

NCES
National Center for Educational Statistics (education and statistics)

NCF
neutrophil chemotactic factor (laboratory)

NCFA
Narcolepsy and Catalepsy Foundation of
America (neurology)

NCGS
National Cooperative Gallstone Study
(gastroenterology and research)

NCHC
National Council of Health Centers (administration)

NCHCA
National Commission for Health Certify-
ing Agencies (administration)

N.C.H.C.A.
National Commission for Health Certify-
ing Agencies (administration)

NCHCT
National Center for Health Care Technology (administration)

N.C.H.L.S.
National Council of Health Laboratory
Services (laboratory)

NCHMHHSO
National Coalition of Hispanic Mental
Health and Human Services Organiza-
tions (psychiatry and social services)

NCHS
National Center for Health Statistics
(statistics)

NCHSR
National Center for Health Services Research (research)

NCI
naphthalene, creosote, iodoform (chemistry and pharmacology)
National Cancer Institute (oncology)

nCi
nanocurie (measurement and radiation
therapy)

nCi.
nanocurie (measurement and radiation
therapy)

NCIB
National Collection of Industrial Bacteria (bacteriology and industrial medicine)

NCJ
needle catheter jejunostomy (gastroenterology)

NCL
National Chemical Laboratory (chemistry and laboratory)
neuronal ceroid lipofuscinosis (genetics and neurology)

NCM
nailfold capillary microscope (laboratory)

NCME
Network for Continuing Medical Education (education)

NCMH
National Committee for Mental Health (psychiatry)

N.C.M.H.
National Committee for Mental Hygiene (psychiatry)

NCMHI
National Clearinghouse for Mental Health Information (Department of Health and Human Services) (psychiatry)

NCMI
National Committee against Mental Illness (psychiatry)

NCN
National Council of Nurses (nursing)

N.C.N.
National Council of Nurses (nursing)

NCNC
normochromic, normocytic [anemia] (hematology and laboratory)

NCNCA
normochromic, normocytic anemia (hematology and laboratory)

NCP
no caffeine or pepper (dietary)
noncollagen protein (laboratory)
nursing care plan (nursing)

NCPE
noncardiac pulmonary edema (cardiovascular and respiratory)

NCPR
no cardiopulmonary resuscitation [for terminal patients] (cardiovascular and respiratory)

NCR
nuclear-cytoplasmic ratio (laboratory)

N:C ratio
nuclear-cytoplasmic ratio (laboratory)

NCRE
National Council on Rehabilitation Education (education and rehabilitation)

NCRND
National Committee for Research in Neurological Diseases (neurology and research)

N.C.R.N.D.
National Committee for Research in Neurological Diseases (neurology and research)

NCRP
National Council on Radiation Protection (radiology)
National Committee on Radiation Protection and Measurements (measurement and radiology)

NCRPM
National Committee on Radiation Protection and Measurements (measurement and radiology)

NCRV
National Committee for Radiation Victims (radiology)

NCS
neocarzinostatin [also called *zinostatin*] (chemotherapy, oncology, and pharmacology)
nerve conduction studies (neurology)
no concentrated sweets (dietary)

NCSC
National Council on Senior Citizens (geriatrics)

NCSH
National Clearinghouse for Smoking and Health (chemical dependency and respiratory)

NCSN
National Council for School Nurses (education and nursing)

NCT
nerve conduction tests (neurology)
nerve conduction time (neurology)
neural crest tumor (neurology and neurosurgery)

NCTC
National Collection of Type Cultures (laboratory)

NCV
nerve conduction velocity (neurology and orthopedics)

ND
nasal deformity (otorhinolaryngology)
natural death (pathology)
Naval Dispensary (armed forces)
neonatal death (neonatology and pathology)
neoplastic disease (oncology)
nervous debility (neurology and psychiatry)
neurotic depression (psychiatry)
neutral density
Newcastle disease (respiratory and veterinary medicine)
New Drug (pharmacology)
new drugs (pharmacology)
no data
no disease
nondisabling
normal delivery (gynecology and obstetrics)
normal development (neonatology and pediatrics)
North Dakota [Postal Service state designation]
nose drops (otorhinolaryngology and pharmacology)
not detectable

not detected
not determined
not diagnosed
not done
Nursing Doctorate (education and nursing)

N & D
nodular and diffuse [lymphoma] (oncology)

Nd
neodymium (chemistry)
number of dissimilar [matches]

N_d
{not an abbreviation} [symbol for refractive index] (chemistry)

n_D
{not an abbreviation} [symbol for refractive index] (chemistry)

NDA
National Dental Association (dentistry)
new drug application (pharmacology)
no data available
no demonstrable antibodies (laboratory)
no detectable activity (laboratory)

N.D.A.
National Dental Association (dentistry)

NDC
National Dairy Council (dietary)
Naval Dental Clinic (armed forces and dentistry)
National Drug Code (pharmacology)

NDCR
National Drug Code Directory (pharmacology)

NDD
no dialysis days (nephrology)

NDDG
National Diabetes Data Group (endocrinology)

NDE
near death experience

NDEA
no deviation of electrical axis [on electrocardiogram] (cardiovascular)

NDF
new dosage form (pharmacology)
no disease found

NDGA
nordihydro-guaiaretic acid (laboratory)

NDH
Natural Disaster Hospital (emergency medicine)

NDI
nephrogenic diabetes insipidus (endocrinology and nephrology)

NDIR
nondispersive infrared analyzer (laboratory)

NDM
New Dimensions in Medicine (research)

NDMA
nitrosodimethylaniline (chemistry)

NDP
net dietary protein (dietary)

NDS
Naval Dental School (armed forces and dentistry)

NDSB
Narcotic Drugs Supervisory Board (chemical dependency)

NDSC
National Down Syndrome Congress (genetics)

NDSS
National Down Syndrome Society (genetics)

NDT
neurodevelopmental treatment (neurology)

nondestructive testing

NDTA
National Dental Technicians Association (dentistry)

NDTI
National Disease and Therapeutic Index

NDV
Newcastle disease virus (laboratory, respiratory, and veterinary medicine)

Nd. YAG
neodymium-yttrium-aluminum-garnet [laser] (neurosurgery and ophthalmology)

Nd:YAG laser
neodymium:yttrium-aluminum-garnet laser (neurosurgery and ophthalmology)

NE
National Emergency (emergency medicine and government)
Nebraska [Postal Service state designation]
nerve ending (neurology)
nerve excitability [test] (neurology)
neural excitation (neurology)
neurologic examination (neurology)
neurological examination (neurology)
no effect
nonelastic
norepinephrine (cardiovascular, chemistry, laboratory, and pharmacology)
northeast (direction)
not elevated (laboratory)
not enlarged
not evaluated
not examined

Ne
neon [a gas used in neon lights] (chemistry)

NEA
National Education Association (education)

nebul
nebula [a spray] (respiratory and pharmacology)

NEC
necrotizing enterocolitis (gastroenterology and pediatrics)
not elsewhere classifiable
not elsewhere classified

n.e.c.
not elsewhere classified

NECHI
Northeastern Consortium for Health Information (statistics)

NECP
New England College of Pharmacy (education and pharmacology)

NED
no evidence of disease
no expiration date (pharmacology)
normal equivalent deviation

"nee-ah"
{pronunciation of -*pnea* [suffix indicating relationship to breathing {not an abbreviation}]} (respiratory) {not an abbreviation}

"nee-mah"
{pronunciation of *nema* [nematode, threadworm]} (laboratory) {not an abbreviation}

"nee-oh"
{pronunciation of *neo*- [prefix referring to new, new form of, *or* recent {not an abbreviation}] and *pneo*- [prefix indicating relationship to the breath or breathing {not an abbreviation}]} (respiratory) {not an abbreviation}

NEEP
negative end-expiratory pressure (laboratory and respiratory)

"nef"
{pronunciation of *NEPH* [nephrology]} {not an abbreviation}

NEFA
nonesterified fatty acid (laboratory)

NEG
negative {pronounced "neg"}
nonenzymatic glycosylation (laboratory)

Neg.
negative {pronounced "neg"}

neg
negative {pronounced "neg"}
Negro [referring to color or race] {pronounced "neg"}
Negroid [referring to color or race] {pronounced "neg"}

"neg"
{pronunciation of *NEG* [negative], Neg. [negative], and *neg* [negative, Negro, and Negroid]} {not an abbreviation}

NegGram
{not an abbreviation} [trade name for preparation of *nalidixic acid*] (pharmacology)

NEHA
National Environmental Health Association (ecology)

NEHE
Nurses for Environmental Health Education (ecology, education, and nursing)

NEI
National Eye Institute (ophthalmology)

NEJM
New England Journal of Medicine (publishing)

NEM
N-ethylmaleimide (chemistry)

nem
Nährungs Einheit Milch [*Nährungsteinheit Milch*, nutritional milk unit] (dietary) {pronounced "nem"}

"nem"
{pronunciation of *nem* [*Nährungs Einheit Milch* (also called *Nährungsteinheit Milch* and *nutritional milk unit*)]} (dietary) {not an abbreviation}

NEMA
National Eclectic Medical Association

N.E.M.A.
National Eclectic Medical Association

nema
nematode [threadworm] (laboratory) {pronounced "nee-mah"}

NEMCH
New England Medical Center Hospitals (administration)

NEMD
nonspecific esophageal motility disorder (gastroenterology)
nonspecific esophageal motor dysfunction (gastroenterology)

NEO
neonatology

neo
negative expiratory pressure (respiratory)
neoarsphenamine [also called *novarsenobenzene;* formerly used as an antisyphilitic] (pharmacology)

neo-
{not an abbreviation} [prefix referring to new, new form of, or recent] {pronounced "nee-oh"}

NEP
negative expiratory pressure (respiratory)
nephrology

NEPD
no evidence of pulmonary disease (respiratory)

NEPH
nephrology {pronounced "nef"}

NER
no evidence of recurrence

NERD
no evidence of recurrent disease

NERHL
Northeastern Radiological Health Laboratory (radiology)

nerv
nervous (neurology and psychiatry)

NES
not elsewhere specified

NESP
Nurse Education Support Program (education and nursing)

NET
nasoendotracheal tube (anesthesiology, otorhinolaryngology, and respiratory)
norethisterone [also called *norethindrone;* a progestin] (gynecology, obstetrics, and pharmacology)

n et m
nocte et mane [night and morning]

n. et m.
nocte et mane [night and morning]

ne tr s num
ne tradas sine nummo [do not deliver unless paid]

neu
neurilemma (neurology)

neur.
neurology {pronounced "nur"}

NEUR-A
neurogenic battery acute (neurology and urology)

NEURO
neurologic (neurology) {pronounced "nur-oh"}
neurology {pronounced "nur-oh"}

Neuro
neurology {pronounced "nur-oh"}

neuro
neurologic (neurology) {pronounced
    "nur-oh"}
neurology {pronounced "nur-oh"}

NEUROL
neurologic (neurology)
neurology

Neurol
neurologic (neurology)
neurology

Neuropath
neuropathologist (neurology) {pro-
    nounced "nur-oh-path"}
neuropathology (neurology) {pro-
    nounced "nur-oh-path"}

Neuro-Surg
neurosurgeon (neurology and neurosur-
    gery) {pronounced "nur-oh-surge"}
neurosurgery (neurology and neurosur-
    gery) {pronounced "nur-oh-surge"}

neurosurg
neurosurgeon (neurology and neurosur-
    gery) {pronounced "nur-oh-surge"}
neurosurgery (neurology and neurosur-
    gery) {pronounced "nur-oh-surge"}

neut
neuter (gynecology, urology, and veteri-
    nary medicine)
neutral

Neutra-Phos-K
{not an abbreviation} [trade name for a
    preparation of *potassium phosphate*]
    (pharmacology)

"new-mah"
{pronunciation of *pneuma*- [prefix indi-
    cating relationship to air or gas or to
    respiration {not an abbreviation}]}
    (chemistry, laboratory, and respira-
    tory) {not an abbreviation}

"new-mah-toe"
{pronunciation of *pneumato*- [prefix in-
    dicating relationship to air or gas or to
    respiration {not an abbreviation}]}
    (chemistry, laboratory, and respira-
    tory) {not an abbreviation}

NEX
nose to ear to xiphoid (anatomy)

NEY
neomycin egg yolk [agar] (laboratory)

NF
National Formulary [a book of official
    standards recognized by the Pure
    Food and Drugs Act of 1906 and up-
    dated every five years] (dietary and
    pharmacology)
Negro female [referring to gender and
    race]
nephritic factor (laboratory)
neurofibromatosis (neurology and rheu-
    matology)
neutral fraction (laboratory)
noise factor (otorhinolaryngology)
none found
nonfiltered (laboratory)
nonwhite female [referring to ethnic ori-
    gin and gender]
normal flow
not found

N.F.
National Formulary [a book of official
    standards recognized by the Pure
    Food and Drugs Act of 1906 and up-
    dated every 5 years] (dietary and
    pharmacology)

nF
nanofarad (measurement)

N factor
{not an abbreviation} (dietary and labo-
    ratory)

NFAR
no further action required

NFB
National Foundation for the Blind (oph-
    thalmology)
nonfermenting bacteria (laboratory)

NFC
National Fertility Center (gynecology, obstetrics, and urology)
nonfavorably considered

NFD
neurofibrillary degeneration (neurology)

NFIC
National Foundation for Ileitis and Colitis (gastroenterology)

NFID
National Foundation for Infectious Diseases (infectious diseases)

NFIP
National Foundation for Infantile Paralysis (neurology and pediatrics)

NFL
National Football League (sports medicine)
nerve fiber layer (neurology and neurosurgery)

NFLPN
National Federation for Licensed Practical Nurses (nursing)

N.F.L.P.N.
National Federation for Licensed Practical Nurses (nursing)

NFMD
National Foundation for Muscular Dystrophy (neurology)

NFME
National Fund for Medical Education (education)

NFND
National Foundation for Neuromuscular Diseases (neurology)

NFNID
National Foundation for Non-Invasive Diagnostics

NFPA
National Fire Protection Association (emergency medicine and government)

NFS
National Fertility Study (gynecology, obstetrics, and urology)

NFT
neurofibrillary tangle (neurology)

NFTD
normal full-term delivery (gynecology and obstetrics)

NFTSD
normal full-term spontaneous delivery (gynecology and obstetrics)

NFTT
nonorganic failure to thrive (neonatology and pediatrics)

NFW
nursed fairly well (dietary, neonatology, obstetrics, and pediatrics)

NG
nanogram [also called *millimicrogram*] (measurement)
nasogastric (gastroenterology)
new growth
nitroglycerin (cardiovascular, chemistry, and pharmacology)
no go
no good

N-G
nasogastric (gastroenterology)

ng
nanogram [also called *millimicrogram*] (measurement)
nasogastric (gastroenterology)

NGC
nucleus reticularis gigantocellularis (neurology)

NGF
nerve growth factor (laboratory and neurology)

n giv
not given

ngm
nanogram (measurement)

NGO
Nongovernmental Observer

NGR
narrow gauze roll (surgery)
nasogastric replacement (gastroenterology)

NGSA
nerve growth stimulating activity (laboratory and neurology)

NGT
nasogastric tube (gastroenterology)

N G tube
nasogastric tube (gastroenterology)

NGU
nongonococcal urethritis (gynecology and urology)

NH
Naval Hospital (armed forces)
New Hampshire [Postal Service state designation]
nodular histiocytic [lymphoma] (oncology)
nonhuman
nursing home (nursing)

NHA
National Health Association (administration)
National Hearing Association (otorhinolaryngology)
National Hemophilia Association (hematology)
nonspecific hepatocellular abnormality (gastroenterology and laboratory)

NHANES
National Health and Nutritional Examination Survey (dietary and statistics)

NHAS
National Hearing Aid Association (otorhinolaryngology)

NHBPCC
National High Blood Pressure Coordinating Committee (cardiovascular)

NHC
National Health Council
nonhistone chromosomal [protein] (genetics and laboratory)

N.H.C.
National Health Council

NHCU
Nursing Home Care Unit (nursing)

NHD
normal hair distribution (dermatology and endocrinology)

NHDS
National Hospital Discharge Survey (administration and statistics)

NHF
National Health Federation

NHG
normal human globulin (laboratory)

NHI
National Health Insurance (insurance)
National Heart Institute (cardiovascular)

N.H.I.
National Health Insurance (insurance)

NHL
National Hockey League (sports medicine)
nodular histiocytic lymphoma (oncology)
non-Hodgkin's lymphoma (oncology)

NHLBI
National Heart, Lung, and Blood Institute (cardiovascular, hematology, and respiratory)

NHLI
National Heart and Lung Institute (cardiovascular and respiratory)

NHMRC
National Health and Medical Research
Council (research)

N.H.M.R.C.
National Health and Medical Research
Council (research)

NHP
New Health Practitioners [Nurse Practitioners and Physician's Assistants]
(nursing)
normal human pooled plasma (hematology and laboratory)
nursing home placement

NHPF
National Health Policy Forum (administration)

NHRC
National Health Research Center (research)

NHS
National Health Service [British]
normal horse serum (laboratory)
normal human serum (hematology and
laboratory)
pooled native human serum (hematology and laboratory)

N.H.S.
National Health Service [British]

NHSAS
National Health Service Audit Staff
[British]

NHSM
no hepatosplenomegaly [on physical ex-
amination] (gastroenterology)

NHSR
National Hospital Service Reserve

NH2-terminal
{not an abbreviation} [also called *N*-ter-
minal] (laboratory)

NI
first cranial nerve (neurology)
neurological improvement (neurology)
no improvement

no information
Noise Index (otorhinolaryngology)
not identified (laboratory)
not indicated (laboratory)
not isolated (laboratory)

Ni
nickel (chemistry)

NIA
National Institute of Aging (geriatrics)
nephelometric inhibition assay (laboratory)
no information available
Nutrition Institute of America (dietary)

NIAAA
National Institute on Alcohol Abuse and
Alcoholism (chemical dependency)

NIADDK
National Institute of Arthritis, Diabetes,
and Digestive and Kidney Diseases
(endocrinology, gastroenterology, nephrology, orthopedics, rheumatology,
and urology)

NIAID
National Institute of Allergy and Infectious Diseases (allergy and infectious
diseases)

NIAL
not in active labor (obstetrics)

NIAMD
National Institute of Arthritis and Metabolic Diseases (internal medicine, orthopedics, and rheumatology)

NIB
National Institute for the Blind (ophthalmology)

NIBS
Nippon Institute of Biological Sciences
(biology)

NIBSC
National Institute for Biological Stan-

dards and Control (biology and measurement)

NIC
neonatal intensive care (neonatology)
newborn intensive care (neonatology)
noninvasive carotid [study] (cardiovascular)

Nic.
nicotinyl alcohol [also called *nicotinic
alcohol*] (cardiovascular and pharmacology)

NICC
neonatal intensive care center (neonatology)

NICE
noninvasive carotid examination (cardiovascular)
noninvasive cerebrovascular examination (cardiovascular)

NICHHD
National Institute of Child Health and
Human Development (pediatrics)

NICM
National Institute of Comparative Medicine

NICU
neonatal intensive care unit (neonatology)
newborn intensive care unit (neonatology)
neurological intensive care unit (neurology)

NID
noninsulin-dependent [diabetes] (endocrinology)

NIDA
National Institute on Drug Abuse (chemical dependency)

NIDD
noninsulin-dependent diabetes (endocrinology)

NIDDM
noninsulin-dependent diabetes mellitus
(endocrinology)

NIDM
National Institute for Disaster Mobilization (emergency medicine)
noninsulin-dependent diabetes mellitus
(endocrinology)

NIDR
National Institute of Dental Research
(dentistry and research)

NIEHS
National Institute of Environmental
Health Sciences (ecology)

NIF
negative inspiratory force (respiratory)

N.I.F.
negative inspiratory force (respiratory)

nig
niger [black]

"nigh-tro"
{pronunciation of *NITRO* and *Nitro* [ni-
troglycerin (cardiovascular, chemistry, and pharmacology) and sodium
nitroprusside (cardiovascular and
pharmacology)]} {not an abbreviation}

NIGMS
National Institute of General Medical
Sciences

NIH
National Institutes of Health [in Bethesda, Maryland]
{not an abbreviation} [agar medium for
sterility testing, also called *sterility
test culture*] (gynecology, laboratory,
obstetrics, and urology)

NIH 204
{not an abbreviation} [an antimalarial
drug] (infectious diseases, pharmacology, and respiratory)

NIHL
noise-induced hearing loss (otorhinolaryngology)

NIHM
National Institute of Mental Health (psychiatry)

NIHR
National Institute of Handicapped Research (neurology, orthopedics, rehabilitation, and research)

NIHS
National Institute of Hypertension Studies (cardiovascular)

NII
second cranial nerve (neurology)

NIIC
National Injury Information Clearinghouse (emergency medicine and statistics)

NIII
third cranial nerve (neurology)

NIIP
National Institute of Industrial Psychology (industrial medicine and psychology)

NIIS
National Institute of Infant Services (neonatology and pediatrics)

nil
{not an abbreviation} [Latin word for none or nothing]

NIL disease
nothing in light disease [nephrotic syndrome] (nephrology)

"nim-foe"
{pronunciation of *nympho* [nymphomaniac]} (psychiatry) {not an abbreviation}

NIMH
National Institute of Mental Health (psychiatry)

NIMP
National Intern Matching Program (education)

NIMR
National Institute for Medical Research (research)

NINCDS
National Institute of Neurological and Communicable Diseases and Stroke (infectious diseases and neurology)

NINDB
National Institute of Neurological Diseases and Blindness [part of the National Institutes of Health] (neurology and ophthalmology)

NINDS
National Institute of Neurological Diseases and Stroke (cardiovascular and neurology)

NINVS
noninvasive neurovascular studies (cardiovascular and neurology)

NIOSH
National Institute of Occupational Safety and Health (industrial medicine)

NIP
mononitroiodophenyl (laboratory)
negative inspiratory pressure (respiratory)
nipple (gynecology, neonatology, obstetrics, and pediatrics)

NIPE
noninvasive peripheral [vascular] evaluation (cardiovascular)
noninvasive peripheral [vascular] examination (cardiovascular)

NIRMP
National Intern and Resident Matching Program (education)

NIRNS
National Institute for Research in Nuclear Science (nuclear medicine, physics, and research)

NIROS-SCOPE
Near Infrared Oxygen Sufficiency Scope [monitors oxygen delivery to brain during surgery] (surgery)

NIT
National Intelligence Test (psychiatry)

NITRO
nitroglycerin (cardiovascular, chemistry, and pharmacology) {pronounced "nigh-tro"}
sodium nitroprusside (cardiovascular and pharmacology) {pronounced "nigh-tro"}

Nitro
nitroglycerin (cardiovascular, chemistry, and pharmacology) {pronounced "nigh-tro"}
sodium nitroprusside (cardiovascular and pharmacology) {pronounced "nigh-tro"}

NIV
fourth cranial nerve (neurology)
nodule-inducing virus (laboratory)

NIX
ninth cranial nerve (neurology)

NJ
nasojejunal (gastroenterology)
New Jersey [Postal Service state designation]

NJ feeding
nasojejunal feeding (gastroenterology)

NJUP
New Jersey Utilization Program (administration)

NK
natural killer [cells] (laboratory)
no ketones (laboratory)
Nomenklatur Kommission (German) [Commission on Nomenclature] (education and research)

none known
not known

NKA
no known allergies (allergy and general medicine)

NKC
natural killer cells (laboratory)

NK cells
natural killer cells (laboratory)

NKDA
no known drug allergies (allergy and general medicine)

NKH
nonketotic hyperglycemia (endocrinology)
nonketotic hyperosmotic (laboratory)

NKHS
nonketotic hyperosmolar syndrome (laboratory)

NKMA
no known medication allergies (allergy and general medicine)

NL
nasolacrimal (ophthalmology and otorhinolaryngology)
nodular lymphoma (oncology and pathology)
normal
normal limits

Nl.
normal

nl
nanoliter [also called *millimicroliter*] (measurement)
non licet [it is not permitted]
non liquet [it is not clear]
normal
normal limits

NLA
National Leukemia Association (hematology and oncology)
neuroleptanalgesia (neurology)

NLD
nasolacrimal duct (ophthalmology and otorhinolaryngology)
necrobiosis lipoidica diabeticorum [a dermatosis usually occurring in diabetics] (dermatology and endocrinology)

NL duct
nasolacrimal duct (ophthalmology and otorhinolaryngology)

Nle
norleucine (laboratory)

NLEF
National Lupus Erythematosus Association (rheumatology)

NLF
nasolabial fold (dentistry, neurology, otorhinolaryngology, and plastic surgery)

N lines
{not an abbreviation} (radiology)

NLM
National Library of Medicine (library sciences)
noise level monitor (otorhinolaryngology)

N.L.M.
National Library of Medicine (library sciences)

NLN
National League for Nursing (nursing)
no longer needed

N.L.N.
National League for Nursing (nursing)

NLNE
National League for Nursing Education (education and nursing)

NLP
neurolinguistic programming (neurology, rehabilitation, and speech and language therapy)
no light perception (neurology and ophthalmology)
nodular liquifying panniculitis (dermatology)
normal light perception (neurology and ophthalmology)

NLT
normal lymphocyte transfer [test] (laboratory)
not later than
not less than

nlt
not less than

NM
Negro male [referring to gender and race]
neuromotor (neurology and orthopedics)
neuromuscular (neurology and orthopedics)
New Mexico [Postal Service state designation]
nictitating membrane (ophthalmology and veterinary medicine)
night and morning
nitrogen mustard (chemotherapy, oncology, and pharmacology)
nodular melanoma (dermatology and oncology)
nodular mixed [lymphoma] (oncology)
nonmotile (laboratory)
nonwhite male [referring to ethnic origin and gender]
normetadrenalin(e) (laboratory)
not measurable (laboratory)
not measured (laboratory)
not mentioned
nuclear medicine (nuclear medicine and radiology)

Nm
nux moschata [nutmeg] (dietary and pharmacology)

Nm
newton-meter (measurement)

nM
nanomolar [also called *millimicromolar*]
(measurement)

nm
nanometer [also called *millimicron*]
(measurement)
nonmetallic (chemistry)
nux moschata [nutmeg] (dietary and
pharmacology)

NMA
National Malaria Association (infectious
diseases and respiratory)
National Medical Association
neurogenic muscular atrophy (neurology)

N.M.A.
National Malaria Association (infectious
diseases and respiratory)
National Medical Association

NMAC
National Medical Audiovisual Center
(ophthalmology and otorhinolaryngology)

NMC
National Medical Care
Naval Medical Center (armed forces)

NMD
normal muscle development (neurology
and orthopedics)

NME
National Medical Enterprises, Incorporated

NMF
National Medical Fellowships
National Migraine Foundation (neurology)
nonmigrating fraction [referring to sper-
matozoa] (laboratory and urology)

NMI
no middle initial [referring to a person's
name]

NMJ
neuromuscular junction (neurology and
orthopedics)

NML
National Medical Library (library science)
nodular mixed lymphoma (oncology)

NMN
nicotinamide mononucleotide (laboratory)
normetanephrine (laboratory)

NMNA
National Male Nurse Association (nursing)

NMNRU
National Medical Neuropsychiatric Research Unit (neurology, psychiatry,
and research)

nmol
nanomole [also called *millimicromole*]
(measurement)

nmole
nanomole [also called *millimicromole*]
(measurement)

NMP
Naval Medical Publication (armed forces
and publishing)
normal menstrual period (gynecology)

NMR
nictitating membrane response (ophthalmology and veterinary medicine)
nuclear magnetic resonance [scanning
and spectroscopy, same as magnetic
resonance imaging (MRI)] (nuclear
medicine and radiology)

NMRDC
Naval Medical Research and Development Command (armed forces and research)

NMRI
National Medical Research Institute (research)
Naval Medical Research Institute (armed forces and research)

NMRL
Naval Medical Research Laboratory (armed forces and research)

NMRU
Naval Medical Research Unit (armed forces and research)

NMS
Naval Medical School (armed forces and education)
neuroleptic malignant syndrome (neurology and psychiatry)
neuromuscular stimulator (neurology and orthopedics)
nonmedical science [category] (education)

NMSS
National Multiple Sclerosis Society (neurology)

N.M.S.S.
National Multiple Sclerosis Society (neurology)

NMT
no more than (pharmacology)
Nuclear Medicine Technologist (nuclear medicine and radiology)
Nuclear Medicine Technology (nuclear medicine and radiology)
neuromuscular tension (neurology)

NMTCB
Nuclear Medicine Technology Certification Board

NMU
neuromuscular unit (neurology)

NN
neonatal (neonatology)
nurse's notes (medical records and nursing)

N/N
normocytic/normochromic [anemia] (hematology and laboratory)
nurse's notes (medical records and nursing)

N:N
{not an abbreviation} [indicates the presence of the azo group] (chemistry)

nn
nervi [nerves] (neurology)
nomen novum [new name]

NNA
normochromic, normocytic anemia (hematology and laboratory)

NNC
National Nutrition Consortium (dietary)

NND
neonatal death (neonatology and statistics)
New and Nonofficial Drugs (pharmacology)

N.N.D.
New and Nonofficial Drugs (pharmacology)

NNDC
National Naval Dental Center (armed forces and dentistry)

NNE
neonatal necrotizing enterocolitis (gastroenterology and neonatology)

NNEB
National Nursery Examination Board (neonatology)

NNI
noise and number index (otorhinolaryngology)

NNM
Nicolle-Novy-MacNeal [bacteriological culture medium] (laboratory)

NNMC
National Naval Medical Center (armed forces)

N.N.M.C.
National Naval Medical Center (armed forces)

N.N.N. culture
{not an abbreviation} [a culture medium] (laboratory)

NNO
no new orders (medical records and nursing)

N-N orders
nurse to nurse orders (medical records and nursing)

n nov
nomen novum [new name]

NNP
neonatal nurse practitioner (neonatology and nursing)
nerve net pulse (neurology)

NNR
New and Nonofficial Remedies (pharmacology)
new nonofficial remedies (pharmacology)

NNU
net nitrogen utilization (laboratory and respiratory)

NO
narcotics officer (chemical dependency and law)
nitric oxide (chemistry)
none obtained
number

N₂O
nitrous oxide [an anesthetic] (anesthesiology)

No
nobelium (chemistry)
number
numero [to the number of]

No.
number
numero [to the number of]

no
number
numero [to the number of]

no.
number

NOA
National Optometric Association (ophthalmology)
nurse obstetric assistant (nursing and obstetrics)

NOAPP
National Organization of Adolescent Pregnancy and Parenting (obstetrics and pediatrics)

NOC
nocte [at night] (pharmacology)

Noc
nocturia (urology)

noc
nocte [at night] (pharmacology)
nocturia (urology)

NOCT
nocte [at night] (pharmacology)

noct
nocte [at night] (pharmacology)
noctis [night, nocturnal, *nox*]
nocturnal

noct maneq
nocte maneque [at night and in the morning] (pharmacology)

NOD
nondefinitive pattern (laboratory)
notify of death (administration)

NOEL
no observed effect level [of a toxin] (chemistry and laboratory)

NOF
National Osteopathic Foundation (osteopathic medicine)

NOGM
no gammopathy detected (laboratory)

NOLDAR
Noludar [a hypnotic] (pharmacology)

NOM
normal extraocular movements (ophthalmology)

nom dub
nomen dubium [a doubtful name]

NOMI
nonocclusive mesenteric infarction (cardiovascular and gastroenterology)

nom nov
nomen novum [new name]

nom nud
nomen nudum [a name without designa-
tion]

non-A, non-B
{not an abbreviation} [non-A, non-B hep-
atitis] (gastroenterology and infectious diseases)

NOND
none detected (laboratory)

NONE
none seen (laboratory)

NONF
nonfasting (laboratory)

NON-REM
nonrapid eye movement [sleep] (neurology)

non-REM
nonrapid eye movement [sleep] (neurology)

non rep
non repetatur [do not repeat, no refill]
(pharmacology)

non repetat
non repetatur [do not repeat, no refill]
(pharmacology)

NONS
nonspecific (laboratory)

non-vis
nonvisualization {pronounced "non-viz"}
nonvisualized {pronounced "non-viz"}
nonvisualizing {pronounced "non-viz"}

"non-viz"
{pronunciation of *non-vis* [nonvisu-
alization, nonvisualized, and nonvi-
sualizing} {not an abbreviation}

$N_2O:O_2$
nitrous oxide to oxygen ratio (anesthesiology, laboratory, and respiratory)

NOOB
not out of bed

NOP
not otherwise provided for

NOPHN
National Organization for Public Health
Nursing (nursing)

N.O.P.H.N.
National Organization for Public Health
Nursing (nursing)

NOR
noradrenaline [also called *norepinephrine*] (endocrinology, laboratory, and
neurology)
nortriptyline [an antidepressant] (neurology, pharmacology, and psychiatry)
nucleolar organizing region (chemistry,
genetics, and laboratory)

Noradr
noradrenaline [also called *norepinephrine*] (endocrinology, laboratory, and
neurology)

NORC
National Opinion Research Center (research)
normal curve (laboratory)

NORD
this part of package not ordered (laboratory)

"nor-ep-E"
{pronunciation of *NOR-EPI* [norepinephrine]} (endocrinology, laboratory, and neurology) {not an abbreviation}

NOR-EPI
norepinephrine (endocrinology, laboratory, and neurology) {pronounced "nor-ep-E"}

norleu
norleucine (laboratory and neurology)

NORM
normal {pronounced "norm"}

norm
normal {pronounced "norm"}
{not an abbreviation} [a word denoting a fixed or ideal standard] (statistics)

"norm"
{pronunciation of *NORM* and *norm* [normal]} {not an abbreviation}

NORML
normal

NOS
not otherwise specified

NOSIE
Nurse Observation Scale for Inpatient Evaluation (nursing)

NOSTA
Naval Ophthalmic Support and Training Activity (armed forces and ophthalmology)

NOTB
National Ophthalmic Treatment Board [British] (ophthalmology)

N.O.T.B.
National Ophthalmic Treatment Board [British] (ophthalmology)

nov
novum [new]

nov n
novum nomen [new name]

NOVS
National Office of Vital Statistics (statistics)

nov sp
novum species [new species]

NP
nasal prongs [for administration of oxygen] (respiratory)
nasopharyngeal (otorhinolaryngology)
nasopharynx (otorhinolaryngology)
near point
neuropathology (neurology and neuropathology)
neurophysin (endocrinology, laboratory, and neurology)
neuropsychiatric (neurology, neuropsychiatry, and psychiatry)
neuropsychiatry (neurology, neuropsychiatry, and psychiatry)
newly presented
nitrogen-phosphorus (laboratory)
no pain
nonpracticing
normal plasma (hematology and laboratory)
normal pressure
not perceptible
not performed
not practiced
not pregnant (gynecology, obstetrics, and radiology)
not present
nucleoplasmic [index] (laboratory)
nucleoprotein (laboratory)
nucleoside phosphorylase (laboratory)
nucleus pulposus (neurology and orthopedics)
Nurse Practitioner (nursing)

nursed poorly (neonatology and obstetrics)
nursing procedure (nursing)

N.P.
Nurse Practitioner (nursing)

Np
neper [unit] (physics)
neptunium (chemistry)
neurophysin (endocrinology, laboratory, and neurology)

np
nomen proprium [proper name (label with)] (pharmacology)

NPA
National Pharmaceutical Association (pharmacology)
National Pituitary Agency (endocrinology and neurology)
near-point accommodation (ophthalmology)

NPB
nodal premature beat (cardiovascular)

NPC
nasopharyngeal carcinoma (oncology and otorhinolaryngology)
near point of convergence (ophthalmology)
no previous complaint
nodal premature contractions (cardiovascular)
nonpatient contact

N.P.C.
near point of convergence (ophthalmology)
nonproductive cough (respiratory and respiratory therapy)

NPCa
nasopharyngeal carcinoma (oncology and otorhinolaryngology)

NPCC
National Poison Control Center (chemistry, emergency medicine, and research)

NPCP
National Prostatic Cancer Project (oncology and urology)

NPD
natriuretic plasma dialysate (laboratory and nephrology)
Niemann-Pick disease (neurology)
nitrogen-phosphorus detector (laboratory)

NP detector
nitrogen-phosphorus detector (laboratory)

NPDL
nodular poorly differentiated lymphocytic (oncology and pathology)

NPDR
nonproliferative diabetic retinopathy (endocrinology and ophthalmology)

NPEV
nonpolio enterovirus (infectious diseases and laboratory)

NPF
National Parkinson Foundation (neurology)
National Pharmaceutical Foundation (pharmacology)
National Psoriasis Foundation (dermatology)

NPFT
Neurotic Personality Factor Test (psychiatry)

NPH
isophane [a neutral protamine Hagedorn insulin] (endocrinology and pharmacology)
neutral protamine Hagedorn [insulin] (endocrinology and pharmacology)
no previous history
normal pressure hydrocephalus (neurology)
{not an abbreviation} [brand name for a preparation of insulin isophane sus-

NPH insulin
neutral protamine Hagedorn insulin (endocrinology and pharmacology)

pension] (endocrinology and pharmacology)

NPHS
Northwick Park Heart Study (cardiovascular)

NPHWA
National Presbyterian Health and Welfare Association

NPhx
nasopharynx (otorhinolaryngology)

NPI
Neuropsychiatric Institute (neurology, neuropsychiatry, and psychiatry)
no present illness

NPL
National Physical Laboratory (laboratory)
neoproteolipid (laboratory)
nodular poorly differentiated lymphoma (oncology and pathology)

NPN
nonprotein nitrogen (laboratory)

NPO
non per os [*nil per os,* nothing by mouth, *nulla per os*]

N.P.O.
non per os [*nil per os,* nothing by mouth, *nulla per os*]

npo
non per os [*nil per os,* nothing by mouth, *nulla per os*]

n.p.o.
non per os [*nil per os,* nothing by mouth, *nulla per os*]

NPO/HS
nulla per os hora somni [nothing by mouth at bedtime]

NPOS
nitrite positive (laboratory)

4-NPP
4-nitrophenylphosphate (chemistry)

NPR
net protein ratio (laboratory)

NPRL
Naval Prosthetics Research Laboratory (armed forces, orthopedics, rehabilitation, and research)

NPT
neoprecipitin test (laboratory)
neopyrithiamine hydrochloride (chemistry)
nocturnal penile tumescence [monitor] (urology)
normal pressure and temperature

NPU
net protein utilization (laboratory)

NPV
nucleopolyhedrosis virus (laboratory)

NR
neutral red [a dye] (chemistry and laboratory)
no radiation (neurology, radiation therapy, and radiology)
no refill [in prescriptions] (pharmacology)
no report
no response (neurology)
nodal rhythm (cardiovascular)
non repetatur [do not repeat] (pharmacology)
nonreactive (neurology)
nonrebreathing (respiratory)
nonresponsive (neurology)
normal
normal range
normal record
not readable
not recorded
not resolved
nurse (nursing)
Nursing Representative (nursing)

nutritive ratio (dietary)
Reynold's number (cardiovascular and laboratory)

nr
near

n.r.
non repetatur [not to be repeated] (pharmacology)

NRA
National Rifle Association (emergency medicine and sports medicine)
nucleus raphe alatus (neurology)
nucleus retroambigualis (neurology)

NRBC
National Rare Blood Club (hematology)
nucleated red blood cell (hematology and laboratory)

NRbc
nucleated red blood cell [mass] (hematology and laboratory)

NRBS
nonrebreathing system (respiratory)

NRC
National Research Council (research)
normal retinal correspondence (ophthalmology)
Nuclear Regulatory Commission (government, nuclear medicine, radiation therapy, radiology, and research)

N.R.C.
National Research Council (research)
normal retinal correspondence (ophthalmology)
Nuclear Regulatory Commission (government, nuclear medicine, radiation therapy, radiology, and research)

NRCA
National Rehabilitation Counseling Association (rehabilitation)

N.R.C.C.
National Registry in Clinical Chemistry (chemistry)

NRD
nonrenal death (statistics)

NRDC
National Respiratory Disease Conference (respiratory)

NRDL
Naval Radiological Defense Laboratory (armed forces, laboratory, and radiology)

NREM
nonrapid eye movement [sleep] (neurology)

NREMS
nonrapid eye movement sleep (neurology)

NREMT
National Registry of Emergency Medical Technicians (emergency medicine)

NREMT-P
National Registry of Emergency Medical Technicians—Paramedics (emergency medicine)

NRF
Neurosciences Research Foundation (neurology and research)

NRH
nodular regenerative hyperplasia [of liver] (gastroenterology)

NRK
normal rat kidney (research)

N.R.M.
National Registry of Microbiologists (microbiology)

NRR
note, record, report (medical records and nursing)

NRRL
Northern Regional Research Laboratory (laboratory and research)

NRS
Nevada Revised Statute (law)
normal rabbit serum (laboratory)
normal reference serum (laboratory)

N.R.S.C.C.
National Reference System in Clinical
Chemistry (chemistry)

NRSFPS
National Reporting System for Family
Planning Services (gynecology, obstet-
rics, social services, and statistics)

nrsg
nursing

NRT
neuromuscular re-education techniques
(neurology and rehabilitation)

NS
natural sciences
nephrosclerosis (nephrology)
nephrotic syndrome (nephrology)
nervous system (neurology)
neurological survey (neurology)
neurosecretory (laboratory and neurology)
neurosurgeon (neurology and neurosurgery)
neurosurgery (neurology and neurosurgery)
neurosyphilis (gynecology, infectious
diseases, neurology, and urology)
neurotic score (psychiatry)
no sample (laboratory)
no specimen (laboratory)
nonspecific
nonstimulation
nonsymptomatic
normal saline [solution] (pharmacology
and surgery)
normal serum (hematology and laboratory)
not seen
not significant
not sufficient
nuclear sclerosis (ophthalmology)
nylon suture (surgery)

N.S.
normal saline [solution] (pharmacology
and surgery)

N/S
normal saline [solution] (pharmacology
and surgery)

Ns
nerves (neurology)

ns
nanosecond (measurement)
no sequelae
no specimen (laboratory)
not significant
nursing services (nursing)
Nursing Sister [British Royal Navy]
(armed forces and nursing)
nylon suture (surgery)

NSA
National Security Agency (government)
Neurological Society of America (neurology)
no salt added (cardiovascular, dietary,
and nephrology)
no serious abnormality
no significant abnormality
normal serum albumin (laboratory)

N.S.A.
Neurological Society of America (neurology)

nsa
no salt added (cardiovascular, dietary,
and nephrology)
no significant abnormalities

NSABP
National Surgical Adjuvant Breast and
Bowel Project (gastroenterology, gy-
necology, and surgery)
National Surgical Adjuvant Breast Pro-
ject (gynecology and surgery)

NSAIA
nonsteroidal anti-inflammatory agent
(gastroenterology, orthopedics, pharmacology, and rheumatology)

NSAID
nonsteroidal anti-inflammatory drug
(gastroenterology, orthopedics, phar-

macology, and rheumatology) {pro-
nounced "en-said" or "N-said"}

"N-said"
{pronunciation of *NSAID* [nonsteroidal
anti-inflammatory drug]} (gastroenterology, orthopedics, pharmacology,
and rheumatology) {not an abbrevia-
tion}

NSAID's
nonsteroidal anti-inflammatory drugs
(gastroenterology, orthopedics, pharmacology, and rheumatology) {pro-
nounced "N-saydz"}

NSAM
Naval School of Aviation Medicine
(aerospace medicine, armed forces,
and education)

"N-saydz"
{pronunciation of *NSAID's* [nonsteroidal
anti-inflammatory drugs]} (gastroenterology, orthopedics, pharmacology,
and rheumatology) {not an abbrevia-
tion}

NSC
National Security Council (government)
neurosecretory cells (laboratory and
neurology)
no significant change
nonservice connected (armed forces and
Veterans Administration)
not service connected (armed forces and
Veterans Administration)

NSCC
National Society for Crippled Children
(orthopedics, pediatrics, rehabilitation, research, and social services)

N.S.C.C.
National Society for Crippled Children
(orthopedics, pediatrics, rehabilitation, research, and social services)

NSCD
nonservice connected disability (armed
forces and Veterans Administration)

NSCLC
non-small-cell lung cancer (oncology and
respiratory)

NSCPT
National Society for Cardiopulmonary
Technology (cardiovascular and respi-
ratory)

NSCTI
National Society for Cardiopulmonary
Technology, Incorporated (cardiovas-
cular and respiratory)

NSD
no significant defect
no significant deficiency
no significant deviation
no significant difference
no significant disease
nominal single dose (pharmacology and
radiation therapy)
nominal standard dose (pharmacology
and radiation therapy)
normal spontaneous delivery (gynecology and obstetrics)

NSDA
nonsteroid dependent asthmatic (respiratory)

NSDP
National Society of Dental Prosthetists
(dentistry)

NSE
neuron-specific enolase [an enzyme]
(laboratory)

nsec
nanosecond (measurement)

NSF
National Science Foundation
nodular subepidermal fibrosis (dermatology)

N.S.F.
National Science Foundation

NSFTD
normal spontaneous full-term delivery (gynecology and obstetrics)

NSG
neurosecretory granules (laboratory and neurology)
nursing

nsg
nursing

NSGCTT
nonseminomatous germ cell tumor of the testis (urology)

Nsg Sta
nursing station (nursing)

NSH
National Society for Histotechnology (histology, laboratory and pathology)

N.S.H.
National Society for Histotechnology (histology, laboratory and pathology)

NSI
negative self-image (psychiatry)
Neurosciences Institute (neurology)

NSILA
nonsuppressible insulin-like activity (endocrinology and laboratory)

NS-ILA
nonsuppressible insulin-like activity (endocrinology and laboratory)

NSM
neurosecretory material (laboratory and neurology)
neurosecretory motoneuron (laboratory and neurology)
nutrient sporulation medium [agar] (laboratory)

NSMR
National Society for Medical Research (research)

N.S.M.R.
National Society for Medical Research (research)

NSN
nephrotoxic serum nephritis (nephrology)
nicotine-stimulated neurophysin (endocrinology, laboratory, and neurology)

Nsn
number of similar negative [matches] (laboratory)

NSNA
National Student Nurse Association (education and nursing)

N.S.N.A.
National Student Nurse Association (education and nursing)

NSND
nonsymptomatic, nondisabling
normal saline nose drop(s) (otorhinolaryngology and pharmacology)

NSO
Neosporin ointment [a topical antibiotic] (dermatology, ophthalmology, and pharmacology)

NSP
National Stuttering Project (speech and language therapy)
neuron-specific protein (laboratory and neurology)
nutritional support panel (dietary)

Nsp
number of similar positive [matches] (laboratory)

NSPB
National Society for the Prevention of Blindness (ophthalmology)

N.S.P.B.
National Society for the Prevention of Blindness (ophthalmology)

NSPE
specimen unobtainable (laboratory)

NSPR
National Society of Patient Representation

NSPVT
nonsustained polymorphic ventricular tachycardia (cardiovascular)

NSQ
Neuroticism Scale Questionnaire (psychiatry)
not sufficient quantity (laboratory)

NSR
nasoseptal reconstruction (otorhinolaryngology)
nasoseptal repair (otorhinolaryngology)
nonspecific reaction (laboratory)
normal sinus rhythm (cardiovascular)
not seen regularly

NSRR
normal sinus rate and rhythm (cardiovascular)

NSS
normal saline solution (pharmacology and surgery)
not statistically significant (statistics)

1/2 NSS
one-half normal saline solution (pharmacology and surgery)

½ NSS
one-half normal saline solution (pharmacology and surgery)

NSSP
normal size, shape, and position [on examination] (anatomy)

NSSPAVAF
normal size, shape, and position, anteverted, and anteflexed [uterus on examination] (anatomy and gynecology)

NSST
nonspecific ST segment changes [on electroencephalogram] (cardiovascular)
Northwestern Syntax Screening Test (speech and language therapy)

NSSTT
nonspecific ST and T [wave on electrocardiogram] (cardiovascular)

NST
nonstress test [for fetal monitoring] (obstetrics)
normal sphincter tone (gastroenterology)
not sooner than
nutritional support team (dietary)

NSU
nonspecific urethritis (gynecology and urology)

NSurg
neurosurgery (neurology and neurosurgery)

NSV
nonspecific vaginitis (gynecology)

NSVD
normal spontaneous vaginal delivery (gynecology and obstetrics)

NSVT
nonsustained ventricular tachycardia (cardiovascular)

NSY
nursery (neonatology and pediatrics)

Nsy
nursery (neonatology and pediatrics)

NT
nasotracheal (otorhinolaryngology)
neotetrazolium (laboratory)
nephrostomy tube (nephrology)
neurotensin (laboratory)
neutralization test (laboratory)
neutralizing
no test
nontender
nontypable (laboratory)
normotensive (cardiovascular)
nortriptyline [an antidepressant] (neurology, pharmacology, and psychiatry)
not tender
not tested

N.T.
nasotracheal (otorhinolaryngology, respiratory, and respiratory therapy)
Nurse Technician (nursing)

N & T
nose and throat (otorhinolaryngology)

N+T
nose and throat (otorhinolaryngology)

5'-NT
5'-nucleotidase [an enzyme] (laboratory)

Nt
neutralization (laboratory)

NTA
National Tuberculosis Association (infectious diseases and respiratory)
nitrilotriacetic acid (chemistry)
Nurse Training Act (nursing)

N.T.A.
National Tuberculosis Association (infectious diseases and respiratory)

NTAB
nephrotoxic antibody (laboratory and nephrology)

N/TBC
nontuberculous (infectious diseases, laboratory, and respiratory)

NTC
neurotrauma center (emergency medicine and neurology)

NTD
neural tube defect (neurology)
nitroblue tetrazolium dye [test] (allergy and laboratory)
5'-nucleotidase [an enzyme] (laboratory)

NTE
not to exceed (pharmacology)

N-terminal
{not an abbreviation} (genetics)

NTF
normal throat flora (laboratory and otorhinolaryngology)

NTG
nitroglycerin (cardiovascular, chemistry, and pharmacology)
nontoxic goiter (endocrinology)
nontreatment group (research)

N.T.G.
nitroglycerin (cardiovascular, chemistry, and pharmacology)

NTGO
nitroglycerin ointment (cardiovascular and pharmacology)

NTG SL
nitroglycerin sublingual(ly) (cardiovascular and pharmacology)

NTIS
National Technical Information Service [previously *Clearinghouse for Federal Scientific and Technical Information*] (government)

NTLI
neurotensin-like immunoreactivity (laboratory)

NTMB
nontuberculous mycobacterium [a bacterium] (laboratory)

NTMNG
nontoxic, multinodular goiter

NTMI
nontransmural myocardial infarction (cardiovascular)

NTN
nephrotoxic nephritis (nephrology)

NTP
National Toxicology Program (toxicology)
Nitrol paste (cardiovascular and pharmacology)

normal temperature and pressure
nucleoside triphosphate (laboratory)
5′-nucleotidase [an enzyme] (laboratory)
sodium nitroprusside [an antihypertensive and reagent] (cardiovascular, laboratory, and pharmacology)

N.T.P.
normal temperature and pressure

NTR
nutrition (dietary)

NTRC
National Toxins Research Center (research and toxicology)

NTRDA
National Tuberculosis and Respiratory Disease Association (infectious diseases and respiratory)

NTRS
National Therapeutic Recreation Society (rehabilitation)

NTS
nasotracheal suction (neonatology, otorhinolaryngology, and respiratory)
nucleus tractus solitarii (neurology and otorhinolaryngology)

NTSB
National Transportation Safety Board (government)

NTT
nasotracheal tube (anesthesiology, otorhinolaryngology, respiratory, and surgery)

NT (T)
nasotracheal (tube) (anesthesiology, otorhinolaryngology, respiratory, and surgery)

NTU
Navy Toxicology Unit (armed forces and toxicology)

NU
name unknown
neurology

nU
nanounit (measurement)

NUBC
National Uniform Billing Committee (administration and insurance)

nuc
nucleated (laboratory)

nucl
nucleus (laboratory)

NUD
nonulcer dyspepsia (gastroenterology)

NUG
necrotizing ulcerative gingivitis (dentistry and otorhinolaryngology)

NUI
National University of Ireland (education)

NuKO
{not an abbreviation} [an orthosis] (orthopedics)

nullip
nullipara (gynecology and obstetrics) {pronounced "null-ip"}

"null-ip"
{pronunciation of *nullip* [nullipara]} (gynecology and obstetrics) {not an abbreviation}

NUMBR
number

nu/nu mouse
{not an abbreviation} (research)

"nur"
{pronunciation of *neur.* [neurology]} {not an abbreviation}

"nur-oh"
{pronunciation of *NEURO, Neuro,* and *neuro* [neurologic and neurology]} {not an abbreviation}

"nur-oh-path"
{pronunciation of Neuropath [neuropathologist or neuropathology]} (neurology) {not an abbreviation}

"nur-oh-surge"
{pronunciation of *Neuro-Surg* and *neurosurg* [neurosurgeon and neurosurgery]} {not an abbreviation}

NURSE
Nurses Underrepresented in Social Equality (nursing)

NUV
near ultraviolet (chemistry)

NV
fifth cranial nerve (neurology)
negative variation
neurovascular (cardiovascular, neurology, and orthopedics)
Nevada [Postal Service state designation]
next visit
nonvaccinated (immunology and pediatrics)
nonvenereal (gynecology, infectious diseases, and urology)
nonveteran (armed forces)
nonvolatile (chemistry)

N.V.
nerve and vein (cardiovascular, neurology, orthopedics, and surgery)

N & V
nausea and vomiting (gastroenterology)

N/V
nausea and vomiting (gastroenterology)
nausea and/or vomiting (gastroenterology)

Nv
naked vision (ophthalmology)

NVA
near visual acuity (ophthalmology)

NVD
nausea, vomiting, and diarrhea (gastroenterology)

nausea, vomiting, or diarrhea (gastroenterology)
neck vein distention (cardiovascular)
neovascularization of the disc (ophthalmology)
neurovesical dysfunction (neurology)
Newcastle virus disease (laboratory, respiratory, and veterinary medicine)
no venereal disease (gynecology, infectious diseases, and urology)
nonvalvular [heart] disease (cardiovascular)

NVE
neovascular edema (ophthalmology)
neovascularization elsewhere (cardiovascular)

NVG
neovascular glaucoma (ophthalmology)

NVI
sixth cranial nerve (neurology)

NVII
seventh cranial nerve (neurology)

NVIII
eighth cranial nerve (neurology)

NVM
nonvolatile matter (chemistry)

NVS
neurological vital signs (neurology)

NVSS
normal variant short stature (endocrinology and pediatrics)

N.V.T.
nerve, vein, and tendon (cardiovascular, neurology, orthopedics, and surgery)

NW
naked weight (measurement)
northwest (direction)

NWA
National Wrestling Alliance (sports medicine)

NWB
no weight-bearing (orthopedics and physical therapy)
non-weight-bearing (orthopedics and physical therapy)

NWF
National War Formulary (armed forces and government)

NX
tenth cranial nerve (neurology)

nx
nourishment (dietary)

NXI
eleventh cranial nerve (neurology)

NXII
twelfth cranial nerve (neurology)

NY
New York [Postal Service state designation]

NYAM
New York Academy of Medicine

NYAS
New York Academy of Science

NYBC
New York Blood Center (hematology)

NYC
New York City (government)

NYD
not yet diagnosed

N.Y.D.
not yet diagnosed

NYHA
New York Heart Association [classifications I, II, III, and IV] (cardiovascular)

nympho
nymphomaniac (psychiatry) {pronounced "nim-foe"}

NYP
not yet published (publishing)

nyst
nystagmus (neurology and ophthalmology)

NZB
New Zealand black [mouse] (research)

NZW
New Zealand white [mouse] (research)

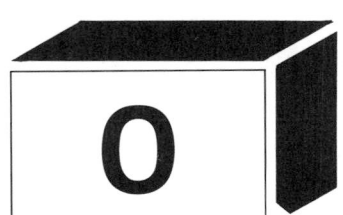

Ω
omega [twenty-fourth letter of the Greek alphabet]
ohm (electricity and measurement)

O
omicron [fifteenth letter of the Greek alphabet]

O
absence of sex chromosome (genetics and laboratory)
none
nonmotile (laboratory)
objective [findings on physical examination]
obstetrics (obstetrics)
obvious
occiput (anatomy, neurology, and obstetrics)
occlusal (dentistry and otorhinolaryngology)
octarius [pint] (measurement)
oculus [eye] (ophthalmology)
often
ohm (electricity and measurement)
ohne Hauch [German symbol referring to a nonmobile type of micro-organism] (laboratory)
old
open
opening
opening [of an electric circuit] (electricity)
operon (genetics)
opium (chemical dependency and pharmacology)
oral (dentistry and otorhinolaryngology)
orally (dentistry and otorhinolaryngology)
orange
orbit (ophthalmology and otorhinolaryngology)
orderly
other
oxygen (chemistry, laboratory, and respiratory)

respirations [on anesthesia chart] (anesthesiology and respiratory)
without film (bacteriology and laboratory)
zero
{not an abbreviation} [referring to suture material size] (surgery)
{not an abbreviation} [chemical symbol for oxygen] (chemistry)

O
{not an abbreviation} [symbol for the nonmotile strain of an organism and its surface antigen] (laboratory)

O.
none
nonmotile organism (laboratory)
obstetrics (obstetrics)
occiput (anatomy, neurology, and obstetrics)
occlusal (dentistry and otorhinolaryngology)
octarius [pint] (measurement)
oculus [eye] (ophthalmology)
opening
operator (surgery)
operon (genetics)
opium (chemical dependency and pharmacology)
oral (dentistry and otorhinolaryngology)
orange
orderly
oxygen (chemistry, laboratory, and respiratory)
respirations [on anesthesia record] (anesthesiology and respiratory)

O
none

O₂
molecular oxygen (chemistry, laboratory, and respiratory)

oxygen [diatomic molecule] (chemistry, laboratory, and respiratory)
{not an abbreviation} [symbol for both eyes] (ophthalmology)

o
orally (dentistry and otorhinolaryngology)

o
omicron [fifteenth letter of the Greek alphabet]

o-
{not an abbreviation} [chemical symbol for *ortho-* (prefix in chemical compounds)] (chemistry)

ō
negative
none
without

OA
occipital artery (cardiovascular and neurology)
occiput anterior [position] (obstetrics)
old age (geriatrics)
opiate analgesia (pharmacology)
oral alimentation (dietary and gastroenterology)
osteoarthritis (orthopedics and rheumatology)
Overeaters Anonymous (dietary)
oxalic acid (chemistry, laboratory, and pharmacology)

O & A
observation and assessment

OAA
Old Age Assistance (geriatrics, government, and social services)
Opticians Association of America (ophthalmology)
oxaloacetic acid (chemistry)

OAAD
ovarian ascorbic acid depletion [test] (gynecology and laboratory)

OAB
Old Age Benefits (geriatrics, government, and social services)

OAD
obstructive airway disease (respiratory)

OADC
oleic acid, albumin, dextrose, catalase [medium] (laboratory)

OAF
open air factor
osteoclast activating factor (laboratory and orthopedics)

OAP
Office of Adolescent Pregnancy (obstetrics, pediatrics, and social services)
Old Age Pension (geriatrics, government, and social services)
old age pensioner (geriatrics)
Oncovin [vincristine], ARA-C [cytarabine or cytosine arabinoside], and prednisone (chemotherapy, oncology, and pharmacology)
ophthalmic artery pressure (ophthalmology)
osteoarthropathy (orthopedics)
oxygen at atmospheric pressure (respiratory)

OAP-BLEO
Oncovin [vincristine], ARA-C [cytarabine or cytosine arabinoside], prednisone, and bleomycin (chemotherapy, oncology, and pharmacology)

OAR
other administrative reasons (administration)

OAS
Old Age Security (geriatrics, government, and social services)

OASDHI
Old Age, Survivors, Disability and Health Insurance [Program] (geriatrics, government, and social services)

OASI
Old Age and Survivors Insurance (geriatrics, government, and social services)

OASP
organic acid soluble phosphorus (chemistry and laboratory)

OAV
oculoauriculovertebral dysplasia (neurology, ophthalmology, and otorhinolaryngology)

OAWO
opening abductory wedge osteotomy (orthopedics)

OB
objective benefit
obstetrical (obstetrics)
obstetrician (obstetrics)
obstetrics [also used to refer to both gynecology and obstetrics] (obstetrics) {pronounced "oh-be"}
occult bleeding (gastroenterology and hematology)
occult blood (gastroenterology, laboratory, and urology)

O.B.
obstetrics (obstetrics)

O & B
opium and belladonna (chemical dependency and pharmacology)

OB+
occult blood positive (gastroenterology, laboratory, and urology)

OB(+)
occult blood positive (gastroenterology, laboratory, and urology)

Ob
obstetrics (obstetrics) {pronounced "oh-be"}

ob
obiit [he died, she died]

ob.
obiit [he died, she died]

OBD
organic brain disease (neurology and psychiatry)

OBE
Office of Biological Education (biology and education)
Order of the British Empire (government)
out-of-body experience (parapsychology)

OBECALP
{not an abbreviation} [placebo capsule or tablet. It is *placebo* spelled backward.] (pharmacology)

OBG
obstetrician-gynecologist (gynecology and obstetrics)
obstetrics and gynecology (gynecology and obstetrics)

OB-GYN
obstetrics and gynecology (gynecology and obstetrics) {pronounced "oh-be-gee-why-N" or "oh-be-guy-nee"}

obj
object
objective

OBL
oblique

obl
oblique

OBN
occult blood negative (gastroenterology, laboratory, and urology)

OBP
occult blood positive (gastroenterology, laboratory, and urology)
ova, blood, and parasites (gastroenterology and laboratory)

OBS
obstetrical service (obstetrics)
obstetrics (obstetrics)

organic brain syndrome (neurology and psychiatry)

O.B.S.
organic brain syndrome (neurology and psychiatry)

Obs
observed
observer
obsolete

obs
observation
observe
obsolete
obstetrician (obstetrics)
obstetrics

OBSC
field obscured (laboratory)

OBST
obstetrics

Obst
obstetrician (obstetrics)
obstetrics

obst
obstetrician (obstetrics)
obstetrics
obstruction

OBUS
Obstetrical Ultrasound System (obstetrics and radiology)

OC
obstetrical conjugate (obstetrics)
occlusocervical (dentistry)
office call
on call
only child (pediatrics)
oral care (dentistry and otorhinolaryngology)
oral contraceptive (endocrinology, gynecology, obstetrics, and pharmacology)
original claim (insurance)
over-the-counter [drug] (pharmacology)
oxygen consumed (respiratory)

O & C
onset and course [of a disease or injury]

OCA
oculocutaneous albinism (dermatology, genetics, and ophthalmology)
Oncovin [vincristine], cyclophosphamide, and Adriamycin [doxorubicin] (chemotherapy, oncology, and pharmacology)

O₂ cap
oxygen capacity (respiratory)

OCC
occasional

Occ
occasionally
occlusion (dentistry and otorhinolaryngology)

occ
occasional
occasionally
occipital (neurology)
occiput (anatomy, neurology, and obstetrics)
occlusion (dentistry and otorhinolaryngology)

OCC-BL
occult blood (gastroenterology, laboratory, and urology)

OCCC
open chest cardiac compression (cardiovascular)

OCCM
open chest cardiac massage (cardiovascular)

OccTh
occupational therapist (occupational therapy and rehabilitation)
occupational therapy (occupational therapy and rehabilitation)

Occup
occupation
occupational

occup
occupation
occupational

OCD
Office of Child Development (government, neonatology, and pediatrics)
Office of Civil Defense (government)
osteochondritis dissecans (orthopedics)
ovarian cholesterol depletion [test] (cardiovascular, gastroenterology, and laboratory)

OCG
oral cholecystogram (gastroenterology, radiology, and surgery)

OCHAMPUS
Office of the Civilian Health and Medical Program for the Uniformed Services (insurance)

OCL
Orthopedic Casting Laboratory (orthopedics)

OCN
oculomotor nucleus (neurology and ophthalmology)

OCP
oral contraceptive pill (endocrinology, gynecology, obstetrics, and pharmacology)
ova, cysts, parasites (gastroenterology and laboratory)

OCR
Office of Civil Rights (government)
optical character reader (computer science)
optical character recognition (computer science)

OCS
open canalicular system [of platelets] (hematology and laboratory)
outpatient clinic substation (administration)

OCT
optimal cutting temperature [a medium] (laboratory)
ornithine carbamoyltransferase [also called *ornithine transcarbamylase*] (gastroenterology and laboratory)
oxytocin challenge test (laboratory and obstetrics)

Octup
octuplus [eight-fold]

octup
octuplus [eight-fold]

OCU
observation care unit

oculo-
{not an abbreviation} [prefix referring to the eye] (ophthalmology) {pronounced "oc-U-low"}

"oc-U-low"
{pronunciation of *oculo-* [prefix referring to the eye]} (ophthalmology) {not an abbreviation}

OCV
ordinary conversational voice (otorhinolaryngology and speech and language therapy)

OD
Doctor of Optometry (education and ophthalmology)
drug overdose (chemical dependency, emergency medicine, pharmacology, and psychiatry)
occupational disease (occupational medicine)
ocular density (ophthalmology)
oculus dexter [right eye] (ophthalmology)
officer of the day (administration and armed forces)
on duty (administration and armed forces)
once a day [Note: This is considered a dangerous usage.]
once daily [Note: This is considered a dangerous usage.]
open drop
optical density [also called *absorbance*] (chemistry and laboratory)

originally derived
out-of-date
outside diameter (measurement)
overdose [drug overdose] (chemical dependency, emergency medicine, pharmacology, and psychiatry)

O.D.
Doctor of Optometry (education and ophthalmology)
oculus dexter [right eye] (ophthalmology)
overdose [drug overdose] (chemical dependency, emergency medicine, pharmacology, and psychiatry)
outside diameter (measurement)

O/D
overdose [drug overdose] (chemical dependency, emergency medicine, pharmacology, and psychiatry)

△ OD 450
deviation of optical density at 450 [also called *absorbance*] (chemistry and laboratory)

od
omni die [daily, every day, once daily] (pharmacology) [Note: *This is considered a dangerous usage.*]
overdose [drug overdose] (chemical dependency, emergency medicine, pharmacology, and psychiatry)
{not an abbreviation} [the influence supposedly exerted upon the nervous system by mesmerism] (neurology and psychiatry) {obsolete}

o.d.
omni die [daily, every day, once daily] (pharmacology) [Note: *This is considered a dangerous usage.*]
overdose [drug overdose] (chemical dependency, emergency medicine, pharmacology, and psychiatry)

ODA
occipito-dextra anterior [right occipitoanterior position (obstetrics)

O.D.A.
occipito-dextra anterior [right occipitoanterior position] (obstetrics)

ODAP
Oncovin [vincristine], dianhydrogalactitol, Adriamycin [doxorubicin], and cis-platinum (chemotherapy, oncology, and pharmacology)

ODB
opiate-directed behavior (pharmacology and psychiatry)

ODD
oculodentodigital dysplasia (genetics, ophthalmology, orthopedics, and otorhinolaryngology)

OD'd
overdosed (chemical dependency, emergency medicine, pharmacology, and psychiatry) {pronounced "oh-deed"}

"oh-deed"
{pronunciation of *OD'd* [overdosed]} (chemical dependency, emergency medicine, pharmacology, and psychiatry) {not an abbreviation}

ODM
ophthalmodynamometry (measurement and ophthalmology)

ODMC
Office for Dependents Medical Care (government and social services)

Odont
odontology (dentistry)

odonto-
{not an abbreviation} [prefix referring to the relationship to a tooth or teeth] (dentistry and otorhinolaryngology) {pronounced "oh-don-toe"}

odoram
odoramentum [a perfume] (pharmacology)

odorat
odoratus [odorous, smelling, perfuming]

ODP
occipito-dextra posterior [right occipitoposterior position] (obstetrics)

O.D.P.
occipito-dextra posterior [right occipitoposterior position] (obstetrics)

ODQ
opponens digiti quinti [muscle] (neurology and orthopedics)

ODT
occipito-dextra transversa [right occipitotransverse position] (obstetrics)

O.D.T.
occipito-dextra transversa [right occipitotransverse position] (obstetrics)

-odynia
{not an abbreviation} [a suffix referring
to pain]

odyno-
{not an abbreviation} [a prefix referring
to pain] {pronounced "oh-die-no"}

OE
on examination
otitis externa (otorhinolaryngology)

O & E
observation and evaluation
observation and examination

Oe
oersted [unit of magnetizing force] (measurement and physics)

OEE
outer enamel epithelium (dentistry)

OEF
oil emersion field (laboratory)

OEM
open-end marriage (psychiatry and social services)

OEO
Office of Economic Opportunity (government)

OER
osmotic erythrocyte enrichment (hematology and laboratory)
oxygen enhancement ratio (laboratory
and respiratory)

OES
Olympus Endoscopy System (gastroenterology)
optical emission spectroscopy (laboratory)

oesoph
oesophagus [also called *esophagus*]
(gastroenterology)

OF
occipitofrontal [also called *occipital-
frontal* (diameter)] (neonatology and
pediatrics)
orbitofrontal (neurology and orthopedics)
osmotic fragility [test] (laboratory)
osteitis fibrosa (orthopedics)
Ovenstone factor (laboratory)

O/F
oxidation/fermentation [medium] (laboratory)

Of
official (administration and government)

OFC
occipital-frontal circumference [also
called *occipitofrontal circumference*]
(neonatology and pediatrics)

OFD
object-film distance (radiology)
oral-facial-digital (genetics)

Off
official (administration and government)

OG
obstetrics and gynecology (gynecology
and obstetrics)
occlusogingival (dentistry)
optic ganglion (neurology and ophthalmology)

orange green [stain] (laboratory)
orogastric [feeding] (dietary and gastro-enterology)

O & G
obstetrics and gynecology (gynecology and obstetrics)

OGD
old granulomatus disease (radiology, pulmonary)

OGF
orogastric feeding (dietary and gastroenterology)
ovarian growth factor (endocrinology, gynecology, and laboratory)

OGM
outgrowth medium (laboratory)

O GRA
Salmonella O Group A [a bacterium] (bacteriology and laboratory)

O GRB
Salmonella O Group B [a bacterium] (bacteriology and laboratory)

O GRC
Salmonella O Group C [a bacterium] (bacteriology and laboratory)

O GRD
Salmonella O Group D [a bacterium] (bacteriology and laboratory)

OGS
oxogenic steroid (endocrinology, gynecology, laboratory, and pharmacology)

OGTT
oral glucose tolerance test (endocrinology and laboratory)

OH
hydroxycorticosteroid (endocrinology, gynecology, laboratory, and pharmacology)
occupational health (occupational medicine)
occupational history
Ohio [Postal Service state designation]

omni hora [every hour] (pharmacology)
open heart [surgery] (cardiovascular and surgery)
oral hygiene (dentistry)
osteopathic hospital (administration and osteopathic medicine)
outpatient hospital (administration)

17 OH
17-hydroxycorticosteroids (endocrinology, gynecology, laboratory, and pharmacology)

o.h.
omni hora [every hour] (pharmacology)

OHA
oral hypoglycemic agent (endocrinology and pharmacology)

"oh-are"
{pronunciation of *OR* and *O.R.* [operating room]} (surgery) {not an abbreviation}

"oh-are-tek"
{pronunciation of *OR tech* [operating room technician]} (surgery) {not an abbreviation}

"oh-be"
{pronunciation of *OB* and *Ob* [obstetrics]} (obstetrics) {not an abbreviation}

"oh-be-gee-why-N"
{pronunciation of *OB-GYN* [obstetrics and gynecology]} (gynecology and obstetrics) {not an abbreviation}

"oh-be-guy-nee"
{pronunciation of *OB-GYN* [obstetrics and gynecology]} (gynecology and obstetrics) {not an abbreviation}

OHC
hydroxycholecalciferol [a form of vitamin D] (chemistry, dietary, gastroenterology, laboratory, and pharmacology)
occupational health center (occupational therapy)
outer hair cell (laboratory)

25-OHC
25-hydroxycholecalciferol [a form of vitamin D] (chemistry, dietary, gastroenterology, laboratory, and pharmacology)

OHCS
hydroxycorticosteroid (endocrinology, gynecology, laboratory, and pharmacology)

17-OHCS
17-hydroxycorticosteroid (endocrinology, gynecology, laboratory, and pharmacology)

17-OHCs
17-hydroxycorticosteroids (endocrinology, gynecology, laboratory, and pharmacology)

OHD
hydroxycholecalciferol [also called *activated vitamin D*] (chemistry, dietary, gastroenterology, laboratory, and pharmacology)
Office of Human Development [part of Department of Health and Human Services] (government)
organic heart disease (cardiovascular)

OHDA
hydroxydopamine [also called *oxidopamine*] (laboratory and neurology)

"oh-die-no"
{pronunciation of *odyno-* [a prefix referring to pain {not an abbreviation}]} {not an abbreviation}

OH-DOC
hydroxydeoxycorticosterone (endocrinology and laboratory)

18-OH-DOC
18-hydroxydeoxycorticosterone (endocrinology and laboratory)

"oh-don-toe"
{pronunciation of *odonto-* [prefix referring to the relationship to a tooth or teeth {not an abbreviation}]} (dentistry

and otorhinolaryngology) {not an abbreviation}

OHF
Omsk hemorrhagic fever (infectious diseases and respiratory)

OHFA
hydroxy fatty acid (laboratory)

OHG
oral hypoglycemic (endocrinology and pharmacology)

OHI
Occupational Health Institute (occupational medicine)
ocular hypertension indicator (cardiovascular and ophthalmology)

OHIAA
hydroxyindolacetic acid (laboratory and oncology)

OH-IAA
hydroxyindolacetic acid (laboratory and oncology)

5OHIAA
5-hydroxyindolacetic acid (laboratory and oncology)

OHIP
Ontario Health Insurance Plan [Canada] (insurance)

"oh-moe"
{pronunciation of *omo-* [prefix indicating relationship to the shoulder {not an abbreviation}]} (neurology and orthopedics) {not an abbreviation}

OHN
occupational health nurse (nursing and occupational medicine)

"oh-nigh-row"
{pronunciation of *oneiro-* [prefix indicating relationship to a dream {not an ab-

breviation}]} (psychiatry) {not an abbreviation}

"oh-oh"
{pronunciation of *oo-* [prefix indicating relationship to an egg or ovum {not an abbreviation}]} (gynecology and obstetrics) {not an abbreviation}

OHP
oxygen high pressure [for hyperbaric oxygen therapy] (neurology, respiratory, and sports medicine)
oxygen under high pressure [for hyperbaric oxygen therapy] (neurology, respiratory, and sports medicine)
oxygen under hyperbaric pressure [for hyperbaric oxygen therapy] (neurology, respiratory, and sports medicine)

17-OHP
17-hydroxyprogesterone (endocrinology, gynecology, and pharmacology)

"oh-piz-tho"
{pronunciation of *opistho-* [prefix meaning backwards or indicating relationship to the back {not an abbreviation}]} (neurology and orthopedics) {not an abbreviation}

OHR
Office of Health Research [part of the Environmental Protection Agency] (ecology, government, and research)

OHRR
open heart recovery room (cardiovascular and surgery)

OHS
obesity hypoventilation syndrome (respiratory)
open heart surgery (cardiovascular and surgery)

"oh-sha"
{pronunciation of *OSHA* [Occupational Safety and Health Act or Administration]} (government and occupational medicine) {not an abbreviation}

"oh-sis"
{pronunciation of *-osis* [suffix indicating

a process {not an abbreviation}]} {not an abbreviation}

OHSU
Oregon Health Sciences University Hospital (administration and education)

"oh-tea"
{pronunciation of *OT* [occupational therapy]} (occupational therapy) {not an abbreviation}

"oh-toe"
{pronunciation of *OTO* and *oto* [otolaryngology and otology (otorhinolaryngology)] and *oto-* [prefix indicating relationship to the ear {not an abbreviation} (otorhinolaryngology)]} {not an abbreviation}]

"oh-two-sat"
{pronunciation of *O₂ sat* [oxygen saturation]} (chemistry, laboratory, and respiratory) {not an abbreviation}

"oh-vaa"
{pronunciation of *ovi-* [prefix indicating relationship to an egg or an ovum {not an abbreviation}]} (gynecology, laboratory, and obstetrics) {not an abbreviation}

"oh-vaar-E-oh"
{pronunciation of *ovario-* [prefix indicating relationship to the ovary {not an abbreviation}]} (gynecology and obstetrics) {not an abbreviation}

"oh-vo"
{pronunciation of *ovo-* [prefix indicating relationship to an egg or an ovum {not an abbreviation}]} (gynecology, laboratory, and obstetrics) {not an abbreviation}

OI
opsonic index (laboratory and research)
orgasmic impairment (gynecology and urology)
orientation inventory (neurology and psychiatry)

osteogenesis imperfecta (genetics, neonatology, orthopedics, and pediatrics)
oxygen income (respiratory)
oxygen index (cardiovascular, laboratory, and respiratory)
oxygen intact (respiratory)

OID
organism identification number (laboratory)

OIF
oil-immersion field (laboratory)
Osteogenic Imperfecta Foundation (genetics, neonatology, orthopedics, and pediatrics)

OIH
orthoiodohippurate (chemistry, nuclear medicine, and radiology)
ovulation-inducing hormone (endocrinology, gynecology, and laboratory)

OIHA
orthoiodohippuric acid (chemistry, nuclear medicine, and radiology)

OINT
ointment (pharmacology)

oint
ointment (pharmacology)

OIP
organizing interstitial pneumonia (respiratory)

OIR
Office of International Research [a part of the National Institutes of Health] (government and research)

OIRD
object-to-image receptor distance (radiology)

OIT
organic integrity test (psychiatry)

OJ
orange juice [*Note: This is considered a dangerous usage.*]
orthoplast jacket (orthopedics)

oj
orange juice [*Note: This is considered a dangerous usage.*]

OK
okay [all right, approved, correct]
Oklahoma [Postal Service state designation]

OKAN
optokinetic after nystagmus (neurology and ophthalmology)

OKN
optokinetic nystagmus (neurology and ophthalmology)

OL
oculus laevus [left eye] (ophthalmology)

O.L.
oculus laevus [left eye] (ophthalmology)

OI
oleum [oil] (pharmacology)

o.l.
oculus laevus [left eye] (ophthalmology)

-ol
{not an abbreviation} [a suffix indicating that a substance is an alcohol or phenol] (chemistry and pharmacology)

OLA
occipitolaeva anterior [left occipitoanterior position] (obstetrics)

O.L.A.
occipitolaeva anterior [left occipitoanterior position] (obstetrics)

"oh-lee-oh"
{pronunciation of *oleo* [oleomargarine]} (dietary) {not an abbreviation}

"oh-lee-oh-vit-ah-min-dee-three"
{pronunciation of *oleovitamin D₃* [7-dehydrocholesterol, activated (a vitamin)]} (chemistry and dietary) {not an abbreviation}

"oh-lee-oh-vit-ah-min-dee-two"
{pronunciation of *oleovitamin D₂* [calciferol (a vitamin)]} (chemistry and dietary) {not an abbreviation}

oleo
oleomargarine (dietary) {pronounced "oh-lee-oh"}

oleovitamin D₂
calciferol [a vitamin] (chemistry and dietary) {pronounced "oh-lee-oh-vit-ah-min-dee-two"}

oleovitamin D₃
7-dehydrocholesterol, activated [a vitamin] (chemistry and dietary) {pronounced "oh-lee-oh-vit-ah-min-dee-three"}

olf
olfactory (otorhinolaryngology)

OLH
ovine lactogenic hormone (endocrinology and laboratory)
ovine leuteinizing hormone (endocrinology and laboratory)

oLH
ovine leuteinizing hormone (endocrinology and laboratory)

oligo-
{not an abbreviation} [a prefix meaning *few, little,* or *scanty*} {pronounced "all-ah-go"}

O lines
{not an abbreviation} (radiology)

Ol oliv
oleum olivae [olive oil] (pharmacology)

OLP
abnormal lipoprotein (cardiovascular, gastroenterology, and laboratory)

occipitolaeva posterior [left occipitoposterior position] (obstetrics)

O.L.P.
occipitolaeva posterior [left occipitoposterior position] (obstetrics)

Ol res
oleoresin (chemistry, laboratory, and pharmacology)

ol. res.
oleoresin (chemistry, laboratory, and pharmacology)

OLT
occipitolaeva transversa [left occipitotransverse position] (obstetrics)

O.L.T.
occipitolaeva transversa [left occipitotransverse position] (obstetrics)

OL&T
owners, landlords, and tenants

OM
obtuse marginal [artery] (cardiovascular)
occipitomental [diameter of head] (neonatology and pediatrics)
occupational medicine
Ochsner-Mahorner [echocardiogram] (cardiovascular)
omni mane [every morning] (pharmacology) [*Note: This is considered a dangerous usage.*]
Opticalman [Navy] (armed forces and ophthalmology)
osteomalacia (orthopedics)
osteomyelitis (infectious diseases and orthopedics)
otitis media (otorhinolaryngology)
ovulation method [of birth control] (gynecology and obstetrics)

OM-1
first obtuse marginal [coronary artery] (cardiovascular)

OM-2
second obtuse marginal [coronary artery] (cardiovascular)

om
omni mane [every morning] (pharmacology) [*Note: This is considered a dangerous usage.*]

o.m.
omni mane [every morning] (pharmacology) [*Note: This is considered a dangerous usage.*]

OMA
Operation Medicare Alert (government and insurance)

-oma
{not an abbreviation} [a suffix indicating a neoplasm or tumor] (oncology and pathology) {Pronunciation varies with the root word to which the suffix is attached.}

OMAD
Oncovin [vincristine], methotrexate, citrovorum factor, Adriamycin [doxorubicin], and actinomycin-D (chemotherapy, oncology, and pharmacology)

OMCA
otitis media, catarrhal, acute (otorhinolaryngology)

OMD
ocular muscular dystrophy (neurology and ophthalmology)

OME
Office of the Medical Examiner (government and pathology)
otitis media with effusion (otorhinolaryngology)

OMI
old myocardial infarction (cardiovascular)

OMN BIH
omni bihora [every two hours] (pharmacology)

omn bih
omni bihora [every two hours] (pharmacology)

omn. bih.
omni bihora [every two hours] (pharmacology)

omn h
omni hora [every hour] (pharmacology)

OMN HOR
omni hora [every hour] (pharmacology)

omn hor
omni hora [every hour] (pharmacology)

omn. hor.
omni hora [every hour] (pharmacology)

omn 2 hor
omni secunda hora [every two hours] (pharmacology)

omn man
omni mane [every morning] (pharmacology)

OMN NOCT
omni nocte [every night] (pharmacology)

omn noct
omni nocte [every night] (pharmacology)

omn. noct.
omni nocte [every night] (pharmacology)

omn quad hor
omni quadrante hora [every quarter of an hour] (pharmacology)

omo-
{not an abbreviation} [prefix indicating relationship to the shoulder] (neurology and orthopedics) {pronounced "oh-moe"}

OMPA

octamethyl pyrophosphoramide [a systemic insecticide for plants] (chemistry)

otitis media, purulent, acute (otorhinolaryngology)

OM QUAR HOR

omni quarta hora [every quarter of an hour] (pharmacology)

om quar hor

omni quarta hora [every quarter of an hour] (pharmacology)

om. quar. hor.

omni quarta hora [every quarter of an hour] (pharmacology)

OMR

operative mortality rate (statistics and surgery)

OM & S

osteopathic medicine and surgery (osteopathic medicine and surgery)

OMSC

otitis media, secretory, chronic (otorhinolaryngology)

otitis media, suppurative, chronic (otorhinolaryngology)

OMT

Ophthalmic Medical Assistant (ophthalmology)

ON

office nurse (nursing)

omni nocte [every night] (pharmacology) [*Note: This is considered a dangerous usage.*]

optic nerve (neurology and ophthalmology)

Ortho-Novum (endocrinology, gynecology, and pharmacology)

orthopedic nurse (nursing and orthopedics)

overnight

on

omni nocte [every night] (pharmacology) [*Note: This is considered a dangerous usage.*]

o.n.

omni nocte [every night] (pharmacology) [*Note: This is considered a dangerous usage.*]

ONC

oncology (oncology)

Orthopedic Nursing Certificate (education, nursing, and orthopedics)

over-the-needle catheter (cardiovascular, surgery, and radiology)

ONCG-A

oncogenic virus battery—acute (laboratory and oncology)

ONCO

oncology (oncology) {pronounced "onco"}

onco

oncology (oncology) {pronounced "onco"}

onco-

{not an abbreviation} [prefix indicating relationship to a mass, swelling, or tumor] (oncology and pathology) {pronounced "on-co"}

"on-co"

{pronunciation of *ONCO* and *onco* [oncology (oncology)] and *onco-* [prefix indicating relationship to a mass, swelling, or tumor {not an abbreviation} (oncology and pathology)]} {not an abbreviation}

OND

Ophthalmic Nursing Diploma (education, nursing, and ophthalmology)

other neurological disorders (neurology)

ONDS

Oriental nocturnal death syndrome (neurology)

O'Neal

O'Neal, Jones and Feldman [manufacturer] (pharmacology)

ONEG
O negative [blood type] (hematology and laboratory)

"on-eh-ko"
{pronunciation of *onycho-* [prefix indicating relationship to the nails {not an abbreviation}]} (dermatology, orthopedics, and podiatry) {not an abbreviation}

oneiro-
{not an abbreviation} [prefix indicating relationship to a dream] (psychiatry) {pronounced "oh-nigh-row"}

"on-ik"
{pronunciation of *onych-* [prefix indicating relationship to the nails {not an abbreviation}]} (dermatology, orthopedics, and podiatry) {not an abbreviation}

ONP
operating nursing procedure (nursing and surgery)
ortho-nitrophenyl (laboratory)

ONPG
ortho-nitropheyl-beta-galactosidase [also called *o-nitrophenyl-beta-galactoside*] (laboratory)

ONP-GAL
ortho-nitropheyl-beta-galactosidase (laboratory)

ONS
Oncology Nursing Society (nursing and oncology)

ONTG
oral nitroglycerin (cardiovascular and pharmacology)

ONTR
orders not to resuscitate (cardiovascular, oncology, and respiratory)

onych-
{not an abbreviation} [prefix indicating relationship to the nails] (dermatology, orthopedics, and podiatry) {pronounced "on-ik"}

onycho-
{not an abbreviation} [prefix indicating relationship to the nails] (dermatology, orthopedics, and podiatry) {pronounced "on-eh-ko"]

OO
oophorectomized (gynecology)
oophorectomy (gynecology)

oo-
{not an abbreviation} [prefix indicating relationship to an egg or ovum] (gynecology and obstetrics) {pronounced "oh-oh"}

OOB
out of bed
out-of-body [experience] (parapsychology)

O.O.B.
out of bed

OOBBRP
out of bed with bathroom privileges

OOC
out of control

OOLR
ophthalmology, otology, laryngology, rhinology (ophthalmology and otorhinolaryngology)

OOP
out on pass
out of pelvis (obstetrics)
out of plaster (orthopedics and radiology)

oophor-
{not an abbreviation} [prefix indicating relationship to the ovary] (gynecology and obstetrics) {pronounced "ou-for" or "ou-ou-for"}

oophoro-
{not an abbreviation} [prefix indicating relationship to the ovary] (gynecology

and obstetrics) {pronounced "ou-for-oh" or "ou-ou-for-oh"}

OOR
out of room

OOT
out of town

OP
occiput posterior [position] (obstetrics)
open
opening pressure [of lumbar puncture]
  (neurology)
operation (surgery) {pronounced "op"}
operative procedure (surgery)
ophthalmology (ophthalmology)
oropharynx (otorhinolaryngology)
osmotic pressure (laboratory)
osteoporosis (orthopedics)
other than psychotic (psychiatry)
outpatient
overproof
ovine prolactin (laboratory)

O.P.
opening pressure [of lumbar puncture]
  (neurology)
outpatient

O & P
ova and parasites (laboratory)

Op
operation (surgery)
outpatient

op
operation (surgery) {pronounced "op"}
opposite
opus [work]

"op"
{pronunciation of *OP* and *op* [operation]} (surgery) {not an abbreviation}

OPAL
Oncovin [vincristine], Adriamycin, L-asparaginase, and prednisone (chemotherapy, oncology, and pharmacology)

OPB
outpatient basis

OPC
outpatient clinic (administration)
oxypneumocardiogram (cardiovascular)

OPCA
olivopontocerebellar atrophy (neurology)

op cit
opus citatum [in the work cited] {pronounced "op-sit"}

op. cit.
opus citatum [in the work cited] {pronounced "op-sit"}

OP code
operation code (surgery)

OPD
optical path difference (ophthalmology)
otopalatodigital (otolaryngology, radiology)
outpatient department (administration)
outpatient dispensary (administration)

O,p'-DDD
ortho,para'-dichloro-diphenyldichloroethane [also called *mitotane* and *o,p'-dichloro-diphenyldichlorethane*] (chemotherapy, oncology, and pharmacology)

o,p'-DDD
ortho,para'-dichloro-diphenyldichloroethane [also called *mitotane* and *o,p'-dichloro-diphenyldichlorethane*] (chemotherapy, oncology, and pharmacology)

OpDent
operative dentistry (dentistry and surgery)

OPE
orbiting primate experiment (aerospace medicine and research)

OPG
ocular plethysmography [also called *oculoplethysmography* and *ophthal-*

ORAN
orange (laboratory)

ORANS
Oak Ridge Analytical Systems

orchi-
{not an abbreviation} [prefix indicating relationship to the testes] (urology) {pronounced "or-key"}

orchido-
{not an abbreviation} [prefix indicating relationship to the testes] (urology) {pronounced "or-key-doe"}

orchio-
{not an abbreviation} [prefix indicating relationship to the testes] (urology) {pronounced "or-key-oh"}

ORD
optical rotary dispersion (laboratory)

Ord
orderly

ORDA
Office of Recombinant DNA Activities (genetics and research)

OREF
Orthopedic Research and Education Foundation (education, orthopedics, and research)

O.R.E.F.
Orthopedic Research and Education Foundation (education, orthopedics, and research)

OR enema
oil retention enema (gastroenterology and pharmacology)

org
organic
organism (laboratory)
organization

organiz
organization
organizational

organo-
{not an abbreviation} [prefix indicating relationship to an organ] {pronounced "or-gan-oh"}

"or-gan-oh"
{pronunciation of *organo-* [prefix indicating relationship to an organ {not an abbreviation}]} {not an abbreviation}

ORIF
open reduction and internal fixation [also called *open reduction, internal fixation,* or *open reduction with internal fixation*] (orthopedics)

orig
origin
original
originating

OrJ
orange juice (dietary)

"or-key"
{pronunciation of *orchi-* [prefix indicating relationship to the testes {not an abbreviation}]} (urology) {not an abbreviation}

"or-key-doe"
{pronunciation of *orchido-* [prefix indicating relationship to the testes {not an abbreviation}]} (urology) {not an abbreviation}

"or-key-oh"
{pronunciation of *orchio-* [prefix indicating relationship to the testes {not an abbreviation}]} (urology) {not an abbreviation}

ORL
otorhinolaryngology

orl
otorhinolaryngology

ORN
operating room nurse (nursing and surgery)

orthopedic nurse (nursing and orthopedics)

Orn
ornithine (laboratory)

ORNL
Oak Ridge National Laboratory

ORO
Orapouche [an arbovirus] (laboratory)

oro-
{not an abbreviation} [prefix indicating relationship to the mouth] (dentistry and otorhinolaryngology) {pronounced "or-oh"}

"or-oh"
{pronunciation of *oro-* [prefix indicating relationship to the mouth {not an abbreviation}] (dentistry and otorhinolaryngology) and *orrho-* [prefix indicating relationship to serum {not an abbreviation}]} {not an abbreviation}

ORP
oxidation-reduction potential (laboratory)

orrho-
{not an abbreviation} [prefix indicating relationship to serum] {pronounced "or-oh"}

ORS
oral surgeon (dentistry and oral surgery)
Orthopedic Research Society (orthopedics and research)
orthopedic surgeon (orthopedics and surgery)
orthopedic surgery (orthopedics and surgery)

O.R.S.
Orthopedic Research Society (orthopedics and research)

ORT
operating room technician (surgery)
oral rehydration therapy

OR tech
operating room technician (surgery) {pronounced "oh-are-tek"}

ORTH
orthopedics

orth
orthopedics

ORTHO
orthopedics {pronounced "or-tho"}

Ortho
orthopedics {pronounced "or-tho"}

ortho
orthodontics (dentistry) {pronounced "or-tho"}
orthodontist (dentistry)
orthopedics {pronounced "or-tho"}

ortho-
{not an abbreviation} [prefix indicating correct, normal, or straight] (chemistry, dentistry, and orthopedics) {pronounced "or-tho"}

"or-tho"
{pronunciation of *ORTHO, Ortho,* and *ortho* [orthopedics] (orthopedics), *ortho* [orthodontics] (dentistry), and *ortho-* [prefix indicating correct, normal, or straight {not an abbreviation}] (chemistry, dentistry, and orthopedics)} {not an abbreviation}

orthop
orthopnea (respiratory) {pronounced "or-thop"}

"or-thop"
{pronunciation of *orthop* [orthopnea]} (respiratory) {not an abbreviation}

ortho, para' - DDD
ortho,para'-dichloro-diphenyldichlorethane [also called *mitotane* and *o,p'-dichloro-diphenyldichlorethane*] (chemotherapy, oncology, and pharmacology)

orthopod
orthopedist [orthopedic physician] (orthopedics) {pronounced "or-tho-pod"}

"or-tho-pod"
{pronunciation of *orthopod* [orthopedist
(orthopedic physician)]} (orthopedics)
{not an abbreviation}

OS
by mouth (pharmacology)
occupational safety (government and occupational medicine)
oculus sinister [left eye] (ophthalmology)
opening snap (cardiovascular)
oral surgery (dentistry and oral surgery)
orthopedic surgery (orthopedics and
surgery)
orthopedics
Osgood-Schlatter [disease] (orthopedics)
osteogenic sarcoma (oncology and orthopedics)
osteosarcoma (oncology and orthopedics)
osteosclerosis (orthopedics)

O.S.
oculus sinister [left eye] (ophthalmology)

Os
osmium (chemistry)

os
oculus sinister [left eye] (ophthalmology)
{not an abbreviation} [Latin word for an
opening, mouth, or bone] (gastroenterology, orthopedics, otorhinolaryngology, and podiatry)

o.s.
oculus sinister [left eye] (ophthalmology)

OSA
obstructive sleep apnea (neurology, otorhinolaryngology, and respiratory)
Office of Services to the Aging (geriatrics and government)
Optical Society of America (ophthalmology)

O.S.A.
Optical Society of America (ophthalmology)

O₂ sat
oxygen saturation (chemistry, laboratory, and respiratory) {pronounced
"oh-two-sat"}

oscheo-
{not an abbreviation} [prefix indicating
relationship to the scrotum] (urology)
{pronounced "os-key-oh"}

oscillo-
{not an abbreviation} [prefix indicating
relationship to oscillation] {pro-
nounced "os-cil-oh" or "os-l-low"}

"os-cil-oh"
{pronunciation of *oscillo-* [prefix indicating relationship to oscillation {not an
abbreviation}]} {not an abbreviation}

OSD
overside drainage

-ose
{not an abbreviation} [suffix indicating
the substance is a carbohydrate]
(chemistry, dietary, and laboratory)
{pronounced "osz"}

OSF
outer spiral fibers [of the cochlea] (otorhinolaryngology)

OSH
Occupational Safety and Health [Act or
Administration] (government and oc-
cupational medicine)

OSHA
Occupational Safety and Health Act
(government and occupational medicine) {pronounced "oh-sha"}
Occupational Safety and Health Administration (occupational medicine and
government) {pronounced "oh-sha"}

"os-l-low"
{pronunciation of *oscillo-* [prefix indicating relationship to oscillation {not an
abbreviation}]} {not an abbreviation}

-osis
{not an abbreviation} [suffix indicating a process] {pronounced "oh-sis"}

"os-key-oh"
{pronunciation of *oscheo-* [prefix indicating relationship to the scrotum {not an abbreviation}]} (urology) {not an abbreviation}

OSM
osmolality (laboratory)
oxygen saturation meter (laboratory and respiratory)

μOSM
microosmole (measurement)

Osm
osmole (measurement)

osM
osmolar (laboratory)

osm
osmotic (laboratory)

OSMED
otospondylomegaepiphyseal dystrophy (ortho, radiology)

Osmo
osmole (measurement)

osmo-
{not an abbreviation} [prefix indicating relationship to odors or indicating relationship to an impulse or to osmosis] (chemistry, laboratory, and otorhinolaryngology) {pronounced "oz-moe"}

osmol
osmole (measurement)

OSM S
osmolarity serum (laboratory)

OSM U
osmolarity urine (laboratory)

OSN
off service note

OSRD
Office of Scientific Research and Development (United States of America government) (government and research)

O.S.R.D.
Office of Scientific Research and Development (United States of America government) (government and research)

OSS
Office of Space Science (aerospace medicine, government, and research)
Office of Strategic Services (United States of America government) (government)
osseous (orthopedics and pathology)

OS-SPT
osmolality urine-spot [test] (laboratory)

OST
object sorting test (psychiatry)
Office of Science and Technology (United States of America government) (government and research)

Ost
osteotomy (orthopedics)

"os-tea-oh"
{pronunciation of *Osteo* and *osteo* [osteomyelitis, osteopath, osteopathy (orthopedics)] and *osteo-* [prefix indicating relationship to a bone or the bones (dentistry, neurology, orthopedics, and podiatry) {not an abbreviation}]} {not an abbreviation}

Osteo
osteomyelitis (orthopedics) {pronounced "os-tea-oh"}
osteopath {pronounced "os-tea-oh"}
osteopathy (orthopedics) {pronounced "os-tea-oh"}

osteo
osteomyelitis (orthopedics) {pronounced "os-tea-oh"}

osteopath (osteopathic medicine) {pronounced "os-tea-oh"}

osteopathy (osteopathic medicine) {pronounced "os-tea-oh"}

osteo-

{not an abbreviation} [prefix indicating relationship to a bone or the bones] (dentistry, neurology, orthopedics, and podiatry) {pronounced "os-tea-oh"}

osteopath

{not an abbreviation} (osteopathic medicine)

OStJ

Officer of the Order of Saint John of Jerusalem

"os-toe-me"

{pronunciation of *ostomy* [a word referring to any operation in which an artificial opening is created between two hollow organs or between one or more such viscera and the abdominal wall {not an abbreviation}] (gastroenterology and surgery)} {not an abbreviation}

ostomy

{not an abbreviation} [refers to any operation in which an artificial opening is created between two hollow organs or between one or more such viscera and the abdominal wall] (gastroenterology and surgery) {pronounced "os-toe-me"}

OSTS

Office of State Technical Services (government)

OSUK

Ophthalmological Society of the United Kingdom (ophthalmology)

O.S.U.K.

Ophthalmological Society of the United Kingdom (ophthalmology)

"osz"

{pronunciation of -*ose* [suffix indicating the substance is a carbohydrate {not

an abbreviation}]} (chemistry, dietary, and laboratory) {not an abbreviation}

OT

objective test (psychology)

occlusion time (cardiovascular and surgery)

occupational therapist (occupational therapy and rehabilitation)

Occupational Therapist (occupational therapy and rehabilitation)

occupational therapy (occupational therapy and rehabilitation) {pronounced "oh-tea"}

old term (anatomy)

old terminology

old tuberculin (infectious diseases, pharmacology, and respiratory)

olfactory threshold (otorhinolaryngology)

orotracheal (anesthesiology and otorhinolaryngology)

Otis Test (psychiatry)

otolaryngology (otorhinolaryngology)

otology (otorhinolaryngology)

serum glutamine oxaloacetate transaminase [SGOT] (cardiology, gastroenterology, and laboratory)

O.T.

occupational therapy (occupational therapy and rehabilition)

O/T

oral temperature (measurement)

Ot

otolaryngologist (otorhinolaryngology)

otolaryngology (otorhinolaryngology)

OTA

Office of Technology Assessment (United States of America government) (government)

orthotoluidine arsenite [test for blood in urine] (laboratory and urology)

OTC

ornithine transcarbamylase (laboratory)

over-the-counter [referring to nonprescription drugs] (pharmacology)

oxytetracycline (pharmacology)

otc
over-the-counter [referring to nonprescription drugs] (pharmacology)

OTD
organ tolerance dose (radiology)
oral temperature device (measurement)
out the door

OTF
oral transfer factor (laboratory)

OTH
other

OTM
orthotoluidine manganese sulfate (laboratory)

OTO
otolaryngology (otorhinolaryngology)
  {pronounced "oh-toe"}
otology (otorhinolaryngology) {pro-
  nounced "oh-toe"}

oto
otolaryngology (otorhinolaryngology)
  {pronounced "oh-toe"}
otology (otorhinolaryngology) {pro-
  nounced "oh-toe"}

oto-
{not an abbreviation} [prefix indicating
  relationship to the ear] (otorhinolaryngology) {pronounced "oh-toe"}

OTOL
otology (otorhinolaryngology)

Otol
otologist (otorhinolaryngology)
otology (otorhinolaryngology)

otol
otologist (otorhinolaryngology)
otology (otorhinolaryngology)

otolar
otolaryngology (otorhinolaryngology)

OTR
Occupational Therapist, Registered [also
  called *Registered Occupational Ther-*

apist] (occupational therapy and rehabilitation)
Ovarian Tumor Registry (gynecology
  and oncology)

OTReg
Occupational Therapist Registered [Can-
  ada] (occupational therapy and rehabilitation)

OTS
orotracheal suction (otorhinolaryngology and respiratory)

OTSC
Office of the Surgeon General (government)

OTT
orotracheal tube (respiratory)

OT (T)
orotracheal (tube) (respiratory)

OU
observation unit
oculi unitas [both eyes together] (ophthalmology)
oculus uterque [each eye] (ophthalmology)

O.U.
oculi unitas [both eyes together] (ophthalmology)
oculus uterque [each eye] (ophthalmology)

o.u.
oculi unitas [both eyes together] (ophthalmology)
oculus uterque [each eye] (ophthalmology)

"ou-for-oh"
{pronunciation of *oophoro-* [prefix indicating relationship to the ovary {not
  an abbreviation}]} (gynecology and obstetrics) {not an abbreviation}

"ou-ou-for"

{pronunciation of *oophor-* [prefix indicating relationship to the ovary {not an abbreviation}]} (gynecology and obstetrics) {not an abbreviation}

"ou-ou-for-oh"

{pronunciation of *oophoro-* [prefix indicating relationship to the ovary {not an abbreviation}]} (gynecology and obstetrics) {not an abbreviation}

OURQ

outer upper right quadrant (anatomy)

OV

office visit
ovalbumin (laboratory)
ovary (gynecology and obstetrics)
overventilation [also called *hyperventilation*] (respiratory)
ovulating (gynecology and obstetrics)
ovum [egg] (gynecology, laboratory, and obstetrics)

O_2V

oxygen ventilation equivalent (laboratory and respiratory)

Ov

ovary (gynecology)
ovum [egg] (gynecology, laboratory, and obstetrics)

ov

ovum [egg] (gynecology, laboratory, and obstetrics)

OVAL

ovalocytes (laboratory)

OVALO

ovalocytosis (laboratory)

ovario-

{not an abbreviation} [prefix indicating relationship to the ovary] (gynecology and obstetrics) {pronounced "oh-vaar-E-oh"}

OVD

occlusal vertical dimension (dentistry)

ovi-

{not an abbreviation} [prefix indicating relationship to an egg or an ovum] (gynecology, laboratory, and obstetrics) {pronounced "oh-vaa"}

OVLT

organum vasculosum of the lamina terminalis (neurology)

ovo-

{not an abbreviation} [prefix indicating relationship to an egg or an ovum] (gynecology, laboratory, and obstetrics) {pronounced "oh-vo"}

OVR

Office of Vocational Rehabilitation (rehabilitation)

OVX

ovariectomized (gynecology)

OW

open wedge [osteotomy] (orthopedics)
ordinary welfare
out-of-wedlock (gynecology, neonatology, pediatrics, psychiatry, and obstetrics)

O/W

oil in water [referring to emulsions] (pharmacology)
oil-water [ratio] (laboratory)

OWA

organics-in-water analyser (laboratory)

OWLS

Oxford Word and Language Service [in England] (grammar)

OX

oxacillin (pharmacology)
oxymel [honey, water, and vinegar] (pharmacology)

OX2

Proteus vulgaris antigen Ox-2 (gastroenterology, laboratory, nephrology,

ophthalmology, otorhinolaryngology,
respiratory, and urology)

OX19
Proteus vulgaris antigen Ox-19 (gastroenterology, laboratory, nephrology,
ophthalmology, otorhinolaryngology,
respiratory, and urology)

ox
oxymel [honey, water, and vinegar]
(pharmacology)

"ox-E"
{pronunciation of *oxy-* [prefix - (a)
meaning *quick, sharp,* or *sour* and
(b) indicating the presence of oxygen
in a compound {not an abbreviation}]}
(chemistry, laboratory, and respiratory) {not an abbreviation}

OXK
Proteus vulgaris antigen Ox-K (gastroenterology, laboratory, nephrology,
ophthalmology, otorhinolaryngology,
respiratory, and urology)

OXLAT
oxalate (laboratory)

OXY
oxygen (chemistry, laboratory, and respiratory)
oxytocin (laboratory, obstetrics, and
pharmacology)

oxy-
{not an abbreviation} [prefix - (a) meaning *quick, sharp,* or *sour* and (b) indicating the presence of oxygen in a
compound] (chemistry, laboratory,
and respiratory) {pronounced "ox-E"}

oz
ounce (measurement)

oz.
ounce (measurement)

"oz-moe"
{pronunciation of *osmo-* [prefix indicating relationship to odors or indicating
relationship to an impulse or to osmosis {not an abbreviation}]} (chemistry,
laboratory, and otorhinolaryngology)
{not an abbreviation}

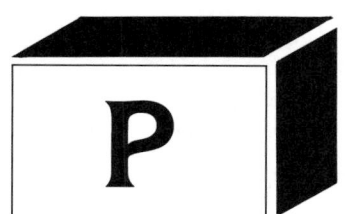

P

π
pi [sixteenth letter of the Greek alphabet]

Φ
phi [twenty-first letter of the Greek alphabet]

φ
phi [twenty-first letter of the Greek alphabet]

P
page
pain
para [followed by an Arabic or Roman numeral] (gynecology and obstetrics)
parity (obstetrics)
part
parte [part]
partial pressure (laboratory and respiratory)
partial tension (laboratory and respiratory)
passive (orthopedics and rehabilitation)
Pasteurella [a bacteria] (laboratory)
pater [father]
paternally contributing (genetics)
patient
per [by]
percentile (measurement)
perceptual speed (rehabilitation and speech and language therapy)
percussion (respiratory)
perforation (otorhinolaryngology)
Perfusionist (cardiovascular and hematology)
peripheral
peyote [illicit drug] (chemical dependency, chemistry, pharmacology, and psychiatry)
pharmacopoeia (pharmacology)
phenolphthalein [a cathartic and pH indicator] (laboratory and pharmacology)
phenylalanine [an amino acid] (laboratory)

phosphate (chemistry, laboratory, and pharmacology)
phosphorus (chemistry, laboratory, and pharmacology)
physiology
pink
pint (measurement)
placebo (pharmacology)
plan
plasma (hematology and laboratory)
Plasmodium [the malarial parasite] (gastroenterology, infectious diseases, and laboratory)
pole (chemistry)
pondere [by weight]
poise [unit of dynamic viscosity] (measurement and physics)
poison (chemistry, laboratory, and pharmacology)
polymyxin [an antibiotic] (pharmacology)
pondus [weight] (measurement)
population (statistics)
porcelain (dentistry)
porphyrin (dermatology, gastroenterology, genetics, hematology, laboratory, and neurology)
position
positive
post [after]
post [surgery laboratory work] (laboratory and surgery)
posterior
postpartum (gynecology and obstetrics)
prednisone [an anti-inflammatory] (pharmacology)
premolar (dentistry)
presbyopia (ophthalmology)
president
pressure (measurement)
pressure [in blood or gas] (laboratory and respiratory)
primary
primipara (gynecology and obstetrics)

611

primitive [referring to hemoglobin] (hematology and laboratory)
probability (statistics)
product (laboratory)
prolactin (endocrinology, gynecology, laboratory, and obstetrics)
proline [an amino acid] (genetics and laboratory)
propionic (bacteriology and laboratory)
protein (dietary, laboratory, and pharmacology)
Proteus [a bacterium] (laboratory)
proximum [near]
psychiatrist (psychiatry)
psychiatry
pugillus [handful] (measurement)
pulse (cardiovascular)
punctum proximum [near point (of vision)] (ophthalmology)
pupil (ophthalmology)
{not an abbreviation} [chemical symbol for phosphorus] (chemistry, laboratory, and pharmacology)

P.

near point (ophthalmology)
partial pressure (laboratory and respiratory)
Pasteurella [a bacterium] (laboratory)
percentile (measurement)
percussion (respiratory)
peyote [illicit drug] (chemical dependency, chemistry, pharmacology, and psychiatry)
pharmacopeia (pharmacology)
plasma (hematology and laboratory)
Plasmodium [the malarial parasite] (gastroenterology, infectious diseases, and laboratory)
poise [unit of dynamic viscosity] (measurement and physics)
polarization (laboratory)
pondere [by weight] (pharmacology)
population (statistics)
position
posterior
postpartum (gynecology and obstetrics)
premolar (dentistry)
presbyopia (ophthalmology)
pressure (measurement)
primipara (gynecology and obstetrics)
probability (statistics)
proline [an amino acid] (genetics and laboratory)

protein (chemistry, dietary, laboratory, and pharmacology)
Proteus [a bacteria] (laboratory)
proximum [near]
psychiatry
pugillus [handful] (pharmacology)
pulse (cardiovascular)
pupil (ophthalmology)

P#

para [followed by an Arabic or Roman numeral] (gynecology and obstetrics)

P̄

after

P₁

first parental generation [also called *parental generation*] (genetics)
first pulmonic heart sound [also called *pulmonic first sound*] (cardiovascular)

P2

second pulmonic heart sound [also called *pulmonic second sound*] (cardiovascular)

P₂

second pulmonic heart sound [also called *pulmonic second sound*] (cardiovascular)

P-2

second pulmonic heart sound [also called *pulmonic second sound*] (cardiovascular)

P/3

proximal third [of bone] (orthopedics)

P 32

radioactive phosphorus (chemistry, nuclear medicine, and radiology)

P³²

radioactive phosphorus (chemistry, nuclear medicine, and radiology)

³²P
radioactive phosphate [also called *radio-phosphate*] (chemistry, nuclear medicine, radiation therapy, and radiology)

P-50
oxygen half-saturation pressure of hemoglobin (hematology, laboratory, and respiratory)

P-55
hydroxypregnanedione (endocrinology and laboratory)

P231
radioactive phosphorus (chemistry, nuclear medicine, and radiology)

⁻P
high-energy phosphate band (chemistry)

p
momentum (physics)
page
papilla [referring to optic papilla] (ophthalmology)
para- [prefix meaning abnormal, accessory to, apart from, beside, beyond, near, or resembling or, in organic chemistry, indicating a 1,4-substituted benzene ring]
physiologic (physiology)
pico- [prefix for 10^{-12}] (measurement)
pint (measurement)
post [after]
probability (statistics)
proton (chemistry and physics)
pulse (cardiovascular)
pupil (ophthalmology)
sample proportion
{not an abbreviation} [frequency of more common allele of a pair] (genetics)
{not an abbreviation} [symbol for the short arm of a chromosome] (genetics)

p
mean gas pressure (laboratory and respiratory)
[*Note: This abbreviation is subscripted.*]

p.
parte [part]

pater [father]
per [by]
pondere [by weight] (measurement)
pondus [weight] (measurement)
post [after]
proximum [near]
pugillus [handful] (measurement)
punctum proximum [near point (of vision)] (ophthalmology)

p-
para- [in organic chemistry, a prefix indicating a 1,4-substituted benzene ring] (chemistry)

p 1
para 1 [unipara, having borne one child] (gynecology and obstetrics)

p 2
para 2 [bipara, having borne two children] (gynecology and obstetrics)

p 3
para 3 [tripara, having borne three children] (gynecology and obstetrics)

PA
Paleopathology Association (pathology)
paralysis agitans (neurology)
paranoia (psychiatry)
pathology
Pennsylvania [Postal Service state designation]
per annum [by year]
percentage activity (measurement)
periapical (anatomy)
pernicious anemia (hematology)
phakic-aphakic (ophthalmology)
phenol alcohol (chemistry and pharmacology)
phosphatidic acid (laboratory)
phosphoarginine (laboratory)
photoallergenic [response] (allergy and dermatology)
physician assistant
Physician's Assistant
pituitary-adrenal (endocrinology)
plasma aldosterone (endocrinology and laboratory)

plasminogen activator (cardiovascular and pharmacology)
platelet adhesiveness (hematology and laboratory)
polyarteritis (cardiovascular and rheumatology)
posterior-anterior [chest x-ray projection; also called *posteroanterior*] (radiology and respiratory)
prealbumin (laboratory)
pregnancy-associated (obstetrics)
presents again
primary amenorrhea (gynecology)
primary anemia (hematology)
prior to admission
proactivator (hematology and laboratory)
professional association
prolonged action (pharmacology)
proprietary association
psychiatric aide (psychiatry)
psychoanalyst (psychiatry)
psychogenic aspermia (psychiatry and urology)
pulmonary artery (cardiovascular and respiratory)
pulmonary atresia (respiratory)
pulpoaxial (dentistry)
pyrrolizidine alkaloid (chemistry)

P.A.
pernicious anemia (hematology)
Physician's Assistant

P-A
posterior-anterior [chest x-ray projection; also called *posteroanterior*] (radiology and respiratory)

P$_A$
alveolar pressure (laboratory and respiratory)
partial pressure in arterial blood (laboratory and respiratory)

P & A
percussion and auscultation (respiratory)

P$_2$ = A$_2$
second pulmonary sound equals second aortic sound (cardiovascular)

P$_2$ > A$_2$
second pulmonary sound greater than second aortic sound (cardiovascular)

P$_2$ < A$_2$
second pulmonary sound less than second aortic sound (cardiovascular)

Pa
pascal (measurement)
protactinium [chemical symbol for] (chemistry)

p.a.
per annum [yearly]

PAA
phenylacetic acid (genetics and laboratory)
pyridineacetic acid (chemistry)

3-PAA
3-pyridineacetic acid (chemistry)

P(A-a)O$_2$
alveolar-arterial pressure difference [previously A-aDO$_2$] (laboratory and respiratory)

P(A-awo)
pressure gradient from alveolus to airway opening (laboratory and respiratory)

PAB
para-aminobenzoic [acid] (chemistry and pharmacology)
premature atrial beat (cardiovascular)
purple agar base [medium] (laboratory)

PABA
para-aminobenzoic acid (chemistry, dermatology, and pharmacology) {pronounced "pah-ba"}

PAC
papular acrodermatitis of childhood (dermatology and pediatrics)
parent-adult-child [in transactional analysis] (psychiatry)

phenacetin [acetophenetidin], aspirin, caffeine (pharmacology)

Platinol [cis-platinum], Adriamycin, and cyclophosphamide (chemotherapy, oncology, and pharmacology)

Political Action Committee (government and politics)

premature atrial contraction [also called *premature auricular contraction*] (cardiovascular)

PACC
protein A immobilized in collodion charcoal

PACE
cis-platinum, Adriamycin, cyclophosphamide, and vindesine (chemotherapy, oncology, and pharmacology)

personalized aerobics for cardiovascular enhancement (cardiovascular and rehabilitation)

PACH
pipers to after coming head (obstetrics)

pachy-
{not an abbreviation} [prefix meaning *thick*] {pronounced "pak-E"}

PA$_{CO2}$
alveolar carbon dioxide pressure [in blood gases] (laboratory and respiratory)

alveolar carbon dioxide tension [in blood gases] (laboratory and respiratory)

PaCO$_2$
arterial carbon dioxide pressure [in blood gases] (laboratory and respiratory)

arterial carbon dioxide tension [in blood gases] (laboratory and respiratory)

PACP
pulmonary artery counter-pulsation (cardiovascular and respiratory)

PACS
picture archiving and communications systems (radiology)

PACT
Philadelphia Association for Clinical Trials (pharmacology and research)

PAD
percutaneous abscess drainage (surgery)

percutaneous automated diskectomy (neurology and orthopedics)

peripheral arterial disease (cardiovascular)

phonological acquisition device

phenacetin, aspirin, desoxyephedrine [methylamphetamine] (pharmacology)

primary affective disorder (psychiatry)

psychoaffective disorder (psychiatry)

pulsatile assist device (cardiovascular)

PADP
pulmonary artery diastolic pressure (cardiovascular and respiratory)

PAE
partes aequales [in equal parts] (pharmacology)

pae
partes aequales [in equal parts] (pharmacology)

p. ae.
partes aequales [in equal parts] (pharmacology)

paed
paediatrics [pediatrics]

PAF
paroxysmal atrial fibrillation [also called *paroxysmal auricular fibrillation*] (cardiovascular)

platelet activating factor (hematology and laboratory)

platelet aggregation factor (hematology and laboratory)

pseudoamniotic fluid (obstetrics)

pulmonary arteriovenous fistula (cardiovascular and respiratory)

PA & F
percussion, auscultation, and fremitus (respiratory)

PAFIB
paroxysmal atrial fibrillation (cardiovascular)

PAG
pariaqueductal grey matter (neurology)
polyacrylamide gel [electrophoresis] (laboratory)

PAGE
polyacrylamide gel electrophoresis (laboratory)
Program for Automated Gated Evaluation (cardiovascular and research)

PAGMK
primary African green monkey kidney (research)

PAH
para-aminohippurate [clearance test] (laboratory and urology)
para-aminohippuric [acid] (laboratory and urology)
polycyclic aromatic hydrocarbon (chemistry)
pulmonary artery hypertension (cardiovascular and respiratory)
pulmonary artery hypotension (cardiovascular and respiratory)

PAHA
para-aminohippuric acid (laboratory and urology)

"pah-ba"
{pronunciation of *PABA* [para-aminobenzoic acid]} (chemistry, dermatology, and pharmacology)

PAHO
Pan-American Health Organization

P.A.H.O.
Pan-American Health Organization

"pah-row"
{pronunciation of *pero-* [prefix meaning *deformed* or *maimed* {not an abbreviation}]} {not an abbreviation}

"pah-sah"
{pronunciation of *PASA* [proximal artic-

ular set angle]} (orthopedics and podiatry) {not an abbreviation}

PAIgG
platelet-associated immunoglobulin G (hematology, immunology, and laboratory)

"pair-ah"
{pronunciation of *Para* [not an abbreviation but referring to a formula indicating the number of pregnancies, abortions or miscarriages, and living children (gynecology and obstetrics)]; *Para.* [number of pregnancies (gynecology and obstetrics)]; *para* [para {a woman who has given birth to a living child (not an abbreviation)} (gynecology and obstetrics), paraplegia (neurology), and paracentesis (surgery)]; and *para.* [paracentesis (surgery) and paraplegia and paraplegic (neurology)]} {not an abbreviation}

"pair-ah-ate"
{pronunciation of *para VIII* [octipara, having borne eight children {not an abbreviation}]} (obstetrics)

"pair-ah-oh"
{pronunciation of *Para 0* [same as *nullipara* {not an abbreviation}]} (gynecology and obstetrics) {not an abbreviation}

"pair-ah-one"
{pronunciation of *Para I* [unipara (having borne one child) {not an abbreviation}]} (gynecology and obstetrics) {not an abbreviation}

"pair-ah-two"
{pronunciation of *Para II* [bipara (having borne two children) {not an abbreviation}]} (gynecology and obstetrics) {not an abbreviation}

"pair-ah-three"
{pronunciation of *Para III* [tripara (having borne three children) {not an ab-

breviation}]} (gynecology and obstetrics) {not an abbreviation}

"pair-E"
{pronunciation of *peri-* [prefix meaning *around* {not an abbreviation}]} {not an abbreviation}

"pair-E-oh"
{pronunciation of *perio* [periodontist]} (dentistry) {not an abbreviation}

"pair-N"
{pronunciation of *paren* [parentheses]} (grammar) {not an abbreviation}

PAIVS
pulmonary atresia with intact ventricular septum (cardiovascular)

"pak-E"
{pronunciation of *pachy-* [prefix meaning *thick* {not an abbreviation}]} {not an abbreviation}

PAL
pathology laboratory [test] (laboratory and pathology)
posterior axillary line (anatomy)

"pal-ah-toe"
{pronunciation of *palato-* [prefix indicating relationship to the palate {not an abbreviation}]} (dentistry and otorhinolaryngology) {not an abbreviation}

palato-
{not an abbreviation} [prefix indicating relationship to the palate] (dentistry and otorhinolaryngology) {pronounced "pal-ah-toe"}

"pale-E"
{pronunciation of *pali-* [prefix meaning *again* {not an abbreviation}]} {not an abbreviation}

"pale-E-oh"
{pronunciation of *paleo-* [prefix meaning *old* {not an abbreviation}]} {not an abbreviation}

"pale-in"
{pronunciation of *palin-* [prefix meaning

old {not an abbreviation}]} {not an abbreviation}

paleo-
{not an abbreviation} [prefix meaning *old*] {pronounced "pale-E-oh"}

pali-
{not an abbreviation} [prefix meaning *again*] {pronounced "pale-E"}

palin-
{not an abbreviation} [prefix meaning *again*] {pronounced "pale-in"}

Pa line
pulmonary artery line (cardiovascular)

PALN
para-aortic lymph node (anatomy, cardiovascular, and surgery)

palp
palpable
palpate
palpated
palpitation (cardiovascular)

palpi
palpitation (cardiovascular)

PALS
Paired Associate Learning Subtest (speech and language therapy)

PAM
penicillin aluminum monostearate [also called *crystalline penicillin G in two percent (2%) aluminum monostearate*] (pharmacology)
L-phenylalanine mustard [also called *Alkeran* and *melphalan*] (chemotherapy, oncology, and pharmacology)
potential acuity meter (ophthalmology)
pralidoxime chloride (pharmacology)
primary amoebic meningoencephalitis (infectious diseases and neurology)
pulmonary alveolar macrophages (laboratory)
pulmonary alveolar microlithiasis (respiratory)

2-pyridine aldoxime methiodide (pharmacology)

2-PAM
pralidoxime (pharmacology)

pam
pamphlet (education and publishing)

PAN
periarteritis nodosa (cardiovascular and rheumatology)
periodic alternating nystagmus (neurology and ophthalmology)
peroxyacetyl nitrate (chemistry)
peroxyacylnitrate (chemistry)
polyarteritis nodosa (cardiovascular and rheumatology)
positional alcohol nystagmus (neurology and ophthalmology)

pan-
{not an abbreviation} [prefix meaning *all*] {pronounced "pan"}

"pan"
{pronunciation of *pan-* [prefix meaning *all* {not an abbreviation}]} {not an abbreviation}

pancreatico-
{not an abbreviation} [prefix indicating relationship to the pancreatic duct] (gastroenterology and surgery) {pronounced "pan-kree-at-ah-ko"}

pancreato-
{not an abbreviation} [prefix indicating relationship to the pancreas] (gastroenterology and surgery) {pronounced "pan-kree-at-oh"}

P. and A.
Protection and Advocacy Office (social services)

"pan-kree-at-ah-ko"
{pronunciation of *pancreatico-* [prefix indicating relationship to the pancreatic duct {not an abbreviation}]} (gastroenterology and surgery) {not an abbreviation}

"pan-kree-at-oh"
{pronunciation of *pancreato-* [prefix indicating relationship to the pancreas {not an abbreviation}]} (gastroenterology and surgery) {not an abbreviation}

PA$_{N2O}$
mean alveolar nitrous oxide tension (laboratory and respiratory)

PANS
puromycin aminonucleoside [an antibiotic] (pharmacology)

pant-
{not an abbreviation} [prefix meaning *all* or *the whole*] {pronounced "pant"}

"pant"
{pronunciation of *pant-* [prefix meaning *all* or *the whole* {not an abbreviation}]} {not an abbreviation}

panto-
{not an abbreviation} [prefix meaning *all* or *the whole*] {pronounced "pan-toe"}

"pan-toe"
{pronunciation of *panto-* [prefix meaning *all* or *the whole* {not an abbreviation}]} {not an abbreviation}

PAO
peak acid output (laboratory)

PA$_O$
pulmonary artery occlusion [pressure] [wedge pressure] (cardiovascular)

PA$_{O2}$
alveolar oxygen pressure [in blood gases] (laboratory and respiratory)
alveolar oxygen tension [in blood gases] (laboratory and respiratory)

PaO₂
arterial partial pressure of oxygen (laboratory and respiratory)

Pa$_{O2}$
arterial partial pressure of oxygen (laboratory and respiratory)

pAO$_2$
oxygen pressure in the aorta (laboratory and respiratory)
oxygen pressure on room air (laboratory and respiratory)

PAOD
peripheral arterial occlusive disease (cardiovascular)
peripheral arteriosclerotic occlusive disease (cardiovascular)

PAOP
pulmonary artery occlusion pressure (cardiovascular)

PAP
Papanicolaou [diagnosis, smear, stain, or test] (gynecology, laboratory, obstetrics, and pathology) {pronounced "pap"}
peak airway pressure (respiratory) {pronounced "pap"}
peroxidase-antiperoxidase [enzymes] (laboratory)
positive airway pressure (respiratory) {pronounced "pap"}
primary atypical pneumonia (respiratory)
prostatic acid phosphatase (laboratory, oncology, and urology)
pulmonary alveolar proteinosis (respiratory)
pulmonary artery pressure (cardiovascular) {pronounced "pap"}

Pap
Papanicolaou [diagnosis, smear, stain, or test] (gynecology, laboratory, obstetrics, and pathology) {pronounced "pap"}

pap
{not an abbreviation} [any soft food] (dietary and gastroenterology) {pronounced "pap"}

"pap"
{pronunciation of *PAP* [peak airway pressure (respiratory), positive airway pressure (respiratory), and pulmonary artery pressure (cardiovascular)], *PAP* and *Pap* [Papanicolaou (diagnosis, smear, stain, or test)] (gynecology, laboratory, obstetrics, and pathology), and *pap* [any soft food (dietary and gastroenterology) {not an abbreviation}]} {not an abbreviation}

"pap-oh-va"
{pronunciation of *papova* [papillomavirus, polyomavirus, vacuolative virus (an acronym for this group of DNA viruses)]} (dermatology and laboratory)

papova
papillomavirus, polyomavirus, vacuolative virus [acronym for this group of DNA viruses] (dermatology and laboratory) {pronounced "pap-oh-va"}

PAPP
pappenheimer bodies (hematology and laboratory)
para-aminopropiophenone
pregnancy-associated plasma protein (laboratory and obstetrics)

PAPS
phosphoadenosine diphosphosulfate [also called *3'-phosphoadenosine-5'-phosphosulfate* and *phosphoadenosyl-phosphosulfate*] (laboratory)

PA/PS
pulmonary atresia/pulmonary stenosis (cardiovascular and respiratory)

Pap smear
Papanicolaou smear (gynecology, laboratory, obstetrics, and pathology) {pronounced "pap smear"}

"pap smear"
{pronunciation of *Pap smear* [Papanicolaou smear]} (gynecology, laboratory, obstetrics, and pathology)

PAP technique
peroxidase-antiperoxidase technique

part. vic.
partitis vicibus [in divided doses] (pharmacology)

PARU
postanesthetic recovery unit (anesthesiology and surgery)

parv
parvus [small]

parv.
parvus [small]

PAS
para-aminosalicylic [acid; also called *Pamisyl*] (pharmacology)
periodic acid-Schiff [method, reaction, reagent, stain, technique, or test] (gastroenterology, laboratory, and rheumatology)
peripheral anterior synechia (ophthalmology)
Professional Activities Study [of the Commission on Professional and Hospital Activities] (administration)
progressive accumulated stress (psychiatry)
pulmonary artery stenosis (cardiovascular)

PASA
para-aminosalicylic acid (pharmacology)
proximal articular set angle (orthopedics and podiatry) {pronounced "pah-sah"}

PAS-C
para-aminosalicylic acid crystallized with ascorbic acid (pharmacology)

PASD
after diastase digestion (laboratory)

P'ase
alkaline phosphatase (laboratory)

Pas Ex
passive exercise (physical therapy and rehabilitation)

PASM
periodic acid-silver methenamine (laboratory)

pass
passive (neurology, orthopedics, psychiatry, and rehabilitation)

PAS stain
periodic acid-Schiff stain (gastroenterology, laboratory, and rheumatology)

PAST
periodic acid-Schiff technique (laboratory)

Past
Pasteurella [a bacterium] (laboratory)

Past.
Pasteurella [a bacterium] (laboratory)

PAT
paroxysmal atrial tachycardia [also called *paroxysmal auricular tachycardia*] (cardiovascular) {pronounced "pat"}
patient
percent acceleration time (measurement)
preadmission testing (laboratory)
pregnancy at term (obstetrics)
psychoacoustic testing (otorhinolaryngology and psychiatry)

P.A.T.
paroxysmal atrial tachycardia [also called *paroxysmal auricular tachycardia*] (cardiovascular) {pronounced "pat"}

pat
patent
patented (government)

"pat"
{pronunciation of *PAT* and *P.A.T.* [paroxysmal atrial tachycardia (also called *paroxysmal auricular tachycardia*)]} (cardiovascular) {not an abbreviation}

PATCO
prednisone, vincristine, thioguanine, cytosine arabinoside, and cyclophospha-

mide (chemotherapy, oncology, and pharmacology)

PATE

Psychodynamic and Therapeutic Education (education and psychiatry)

pulmonary artery thromboembolectomy (cardiovascular)

PATH

pathology {pronounced "path"}

pituitary adrenotropic hormone (endocrinology and laboratory)

Path

pathogenic (pathology) {pronounced "path"}

pathological (pathology) {pronounced "path"}

pathologist (pathology) {pronounced "path"}

pathology {pronounced "path"}

path

pathogenic (pathology) {pronounced "path"}

pathological (pathology) {pronounced "path"}

pathologist (pathology) {pronounced "path"}

pathology {pronounced "path"}

"path"

{pronunciation of *PATH* [pathology] and *Path* and *path* [pathogenic, pathological, pathologist, and pathology (pathology)]} {not an abbreviation}

"path-E"

{pronunciation of -*pathy* [suffix indicating relationship to a disease or morbid condition {not an abbreviation}]} {not an abbreviation}

patho-

{not an abbreviation} [prefix indicating relationship to a disease] {pronounced "path-oh"}

"path-oh"

{pronunciation of *patho*- [prefix indicating relationship to a disease {not an abbreviation}]} {not an abbreviation}

-pathy

{not an abbreviation} [suffix indicating a disease or morbid condition] {pronounced "path-E"}

pat med

patent medicine (pharmacology)

PAT/TM

patient's time

"pause"

{pronunciation of *POS* and *pos* [positive]} {not an abbreviation}

PAVe

procarbazine, Alkeran, and Velban (chemotherapy, oncology, and pharmacology)

PAW

peak airway pressure (laboratory and respiratory)

pulmonary artery wedge [pressure] (cardiovascular and laboratory)

Paw

pressure in the airway [level to be specified] (laboratory and respiratory)

Pawo

pressure at the airway opening (laboratory and respiratory)

PAWP

pulmonary arterial wedge pressure (cardiovascular and laboratory)

PB

paraffin bath (orthopedics, physical therapy, and rehabilitation)

peroneus brevis [muscle] (orthopedics)

phenobarbital [also called *phenobarbitone*] (pharmacology)

phonetically balanced [referring to word lists] (speech and language therapy)

piggyback [intravenous administration] (pharmacology)

powder bed

powder board

pressure breathing (respiratory)

protein binding (laboratory)
protein-bound (laboratory)

P.B.
Pharmacopoeia Britannica [British
Pharmacopoeia] (pharmacology)

P & B
phenobarbital and belladonna (pharmacology)

Pb
phenobarbital (pharmacology)
plumbum [lead] (chemistry and laboratory)
presbyopia (ophthalmology)

PBA
percutaneous bladder aspiration (urology)
phenylboronate agarose (laboratory)
polyclonal B-cell activities (laboratory)
Pressure Breathing Assister (respiratory)
pulbobuccoaxial (dentistry)

P$_{BA}$
brachial arterial pressure (cardiovascular)

PBB
polybromated biphenyls (chemistry)

PBBH
Peter Bent Brigham Hospital [Boston]
(administration)

PBBs
polybromated biphenyls (chemistry)

PBC
peripheral blood cells (hematology and laboratory)
point of basal convergence (ophthalmology)
prebed care
primary biliary cirrhosis (gastroenterology)

PBD
percutaneous biliary drainage (gastroenterology and surgery)

PBE
Perlsucht Bacillen-Emulsion [a form of

tuberculin] (infectious diseases, pharmacology, and respiratory)

PBF
pulmonary blood flow (cardiovascular
and respiratory)

PB-Fe
protein-bound iron (laboratory)

PBG
porphobilinogen [qualitative in urine]
(genetics, hematology, and laboratory)

PGB-QN
porphobilinogen—quantitative (genetics, hematology, and laboratory)

PBI
partial bony impaction (orthopedics and
radiology)
penile-brachial index (cardiovascular
and urology)
phenformin [an oral hypoglycemic
agent] (endocrinology and pharmacology) {obsolete}
protein-bound iodine (laboratory)

P.B.I.
protein-bound iodine (laboratory)

PB^{131}I
protein-bound radioactive iodine (nuclear medicine and radiology)

PBK
phosphorylase b kinase [an enzyme]
(laboratory)

PB (K)
phonetically balanced (kindergarten)
(education and speech and language
therapy)

PBL
peripheral blood leukocyte (hematology
and laboratory)
peripheral blood lymphocyte (hematology and laboratory)

PBLI
premature birth, live infant (neonatology and obstetrics)

PBM
peripheral blood mononuclear [cell] (hematology and laboratory)

PBMC
peripheral blood mononuclear cell (hematology and laboratory)

PBME
Physiology and Biomedical Engineering [Program] (engineering and physiology)

PBMNC
peripheral blood mononuclear cell (hematology and laboratory)

PBN
paralytic brachial neuritis (neurology)
polymyxin B sulfate, bacitracin, and neomycin [a combination of antibacterials] (pharmacology)

PBO
penicillin in beeswax [an antibiotic] (pharmacology)
placebo (pharmacology)

PBP
peak blood pressure (cardiovascular)
penicillin-binding protein (laboratory)
purified Brucella protein (laboratory)

PBPE
Population Biology/Physiological Ecology (biology and ecology)

Pb-RBC
lead red blood count [for lead poisoning] (laboratory)

PBS
phosphate-buffered normal saline (pharmacology)
phosphate-buffered sodium (pharmacology)
Public Broadcasting Station (television)

Pbs
pressure at the body surface (laboratory and respiratory)

PBSP
prognostically bad signs during pregnancy (obstetrics)

PBT$_4$
protein-bound thyroxine (endocrinology and laboratory)

PBV
predicted blood volume (cardiovascular)
pulmonary blood volume (cardiovascular and respiratory)

PBW
posterior bite-wing (dentistry)

PBZ
phenoxybenzamine [an antihypertensive] (cardiovascular and pharmacology)
phenylbutazone (pharmacology and rheumatology)
Pyribenzamine [brand name for a preparation of *tripelennamine*] (allergy and pharmacology)
{not an abbreviation} [brand name for a preparation of *tripelennamine*] (allergy and pharmacology)

PC
packed cells (hematology)
palmitoyl carnitine (pharmacology)
paper chromatography (laboratory)
parent cells (laboratory)
percent (measurement)
pentose cycle (laboratory)
Pharmacy Corps (pharmacology)
phosphate cycle (laboratory)
phosphatidyl choline [also called *lecithin*] (pharmacology)
phosphocreatine (pharmacology)
phosphorylcholine (pharmacology)
Physicians Corporation
plasmacytoma (hematology and oncology)
platelet concentrate (hematology and pharmacology)

P.C.

platelet concentration (hematology and laboratory)

platelet count (hematology and laboratory)

pneumotaxic center (respiratory)

pondus civile [avoirdupois weight] (measurement)

portacaval (cardiovascular)

post cibos [after meals] (pharmacology)

postcoital (gynecology, obstetrics, and urology)

posterior circumflex [artery] (cardiovascular)

posterior chamber (ophthalmology)

precordium (cardiovascular)

precaution category (psychiatry)

premature contraction [of heart] (cardiovascular)

present complaint

printed circuit (computer science)

professional corporation (business)

Prosthetics Center (orthopedics, rehabilitation, and research)

pseudoconditioning control (psychiatry)

Psychodevelopment Checklist (psychiatry)

pubococcygeus [muscle] (gynecology, neurology, orthopedics, and urology)

pulmonary capillary (cardiovascular and respiratory)

pulmonic closure (cardiovascular)

pure clairvoyance (parapsychology)

pyruvate carboxylase (laboratory)

P.C.

pondus civile [avoirdupois weight] (measurement)

Pc

packed cells (hematology)

pc

percent (measurement)

picocurie [also called *micromicrocurie*] (measurement, radiation therapy, and radiology)

pondus civile [avoirdupois weight] (measurement)

post cibos [after meals] (pharmacology)

post cibum [after food] (pharmacology)

pc.

picocurie (measurement, radiation therapy, and radiology)

p.c.

pondus civile [avoirdupois weight] (measurement)

post cibos [after meals] (pharmacology)

post cibum [after food] (pharmacology)

p̄c

post cibos [after meals] (pharmacology)

PCA

passive cutaneous anaphylaxis (allergy and research)

patient care aide (nursing)

patient care assistant (nursing)

patient-controlled analgesia [system] (neurology and pharmacology)

perchloric acid (chemistry)

percutaneous carotid arteriogram (cardiovascular and radiology)

phenylcarboxylic acid (chemistry)

porous-coated anatomic [prosthesis] (orthopedics)

posterior cerebral artery (cardiovascular and neurology)

posterior communicating artery (cardiovascular and neurology)

President's Council on Aging (geriatrics and government)

procoagulation activity (hematology and laboratory)

P.C.A.

{not an abbreviation} [a porous coated anatomic total hip replacement system by Howmedica] (orthopedics)

PCB

pancuronium bromide [a muscle relaxant] (anesthesiology, pharmacology, and respiratory)

paracervical block (anesthesiology, gynecology, and obstetrics)

polychlorinated biphenyl(s) (chemistry)

postcoital bleeding (gynecology)

procarbazine (chemotherapy, oncology, and pharmacology)

PcB

near point convergence to the intercentral base line (ophthalmology)

PCBs
polychlorinated biphenyls (chemistry)

PCC
personal care clinic (administration)
pheochromocytoma (endocrinology and oncology)
phosphate carrier compound (laboratory)
Poison Control Center (emergency medicine)
premature chromosome condensation (genetics)
primary care clinic (administration)
prothrombin-complex concentration (hematology and laboratory)

P.C.C.
Poison Control Center (emergency medicine)

PCc
periscopic concave (ophthalmology)

P.Cc.
periscopic concave (ophthalmology)

PCCU
post-coronary care unit (cardiovascular)

PCD
phosphate-citrate-dextrose (laboratory)
plasma cell dyscrasia (hematology)
polycystic disease (gynecology, nephrology, and obstetrics)
posterior corneal deposits (ophthalmology)
pulmonary clearance delay (respiratory)

PCDUS
plasma cell dyscrasia of unknown significance (hematology)

PCE
cis-platinum, cyclophosphamide, and vindesine (chemotherapy, oncology, and pharmacology)
polymer-coated erythromycin [an antibiotic] (pharmacology)
pseudocholinesterase (laboratory)
pulmocutaneous exchange (respiratory)

PCEN
paracentesis fluid (laboratory and surgery)

PCF
pharyngoconjunctival fever (ophthalmology and otorhinolaryngology)
posterior cranial fossa (anatomy and neurology)
prothrombin conversion factor (hematology and laboratory)

PCG
paracervical ganglion (neurology)
phonocardiogram (cardiovascular)
pubococcygeus [muscle] (gynecology, neurology, orthopedics, and urology)

pcg
picogram (measurement)

PCH
paroxysmal cold hemoglobinuria (laboratory and urology)

PC HE
pseudocholinesterase [an enzyme] (laboratory)

PCI
prophylactic cranial irradiation (neurology, oncology, and radiation therapy)

pCi
picocurie (measurement, radiation therapy, and radiology)

PCIC
Poison Control Information Center (emergency medicine)

P.C.I.C.
Poison Control Information Center (emergency medicine)

PCIOL
posterior chamber intraocular lens (ophthalmology)

PCKD
polycystic kidney disease (nephrology)

PCL
persistent corpus luteum (gynecology)
posterior chamber lens (ophthalmology)
posterior cruciate ligament (orthopedics)

PCM
protein-calorie malnutrition (dietary)
protein-carboxyl methylase (laboratory)

p-CMB
para-chloromercuribenzoate [an organic
  mercury compound] (laboratory)

PCMO
Principal Clinical Medical Officer [Brit-
  ish]
Principal Colonial Medical Officer [Brit-
  ish]

P.C.M.O.
Principal Colonial Medical Officer [Brit-
  ish]

PCMU
physico-chemical measurements unit
  [British] (measurement)

PCMX
chloroxylenol [an antibacterial and dis-
  infectant] (dermatology and pharmacology)

PCN
penicillin [an antibiotic] [*Note: This is
  considered a dangerous abbreviation.*] (pharmacology)
percutaneous nephrostomy (nephrology
  and surgery)
pregnenolone carbonitril (pharmacology
  and rheumatology)
Primary Care Nursing (nursing)

pcn
penicillin [an antibiotic] [*Note: This is
  considered a dangerous abbreviation.*] (pharmacology)

PCNV
Provisional Committee on Nomenclature
  of Viruses (virology)

PCO
patient complains of

polycystic ovary (gynecology and obstetrics)

P$_{CO}$
carbon monoxide tension (laboratory
  and respiratory)

PCO$_2$
carbon dioxide partial pressure [in blood
  gases] (laboratory and respiratory)
carbon dioxide pressure [in blood gases]
  (laboratory and respiratory)
carbon dioxide tension [in blood gases]
  (laboratory and respiratory)

Pco$_2$
carbon dioxide pressure [in blood gases]
  (laboratory and respiratory)
carbon dioxide tension [in blood gases]
  (laboratory and respiratory)

pCO$_2$
carbon dioxide concentration [in blood
  gases] (laboratory and respiratory)
carbon dioxide partial pressure [in blood
  gases] (laboratory and respiratory)
carbon dioxide pressure [in blood gases]
  (laboratory and respiratory)
carbon dioxide tension [in blood gases]
  (laboratory and respiratory)

*p*CO$_2$
carbon dioxide pressure [in blood gases]
  (laboratory and respiratory)
carbon dioxide tension [in blood gases]
  (laboratory and respiratory)

PCOB
Permanent Central Opium Board [Ge-
  neva] (chemical dependency and psychiatry)

PCOD
polycystic ovary disease (gynecology
  and obstetrics)

PCON
platelet concentration (hematology and
  laboratory)

PCOS
polycystic ovary syndrome (gynecology and obstetrics)

PCP
parachlorophenol [an antibacterial and topical anti-infective] (pharmacology)
Patient Care Publications (publishing)
pentachlorophenate [a topical antibacterial] (pharmacology)
pentachlorophenol [a toxic wood preservative] (chemistry)
peripheral coronary pressure (cardiovascular)
phencyclidine palmitate (chemistry)
phencyclidine pill [an illicit psychedelic drug, phencyclidine hydrochloride] (chemical dependency, pharmacology, psychiatry, and veterinary medicine) [*Note: This is not the abbreviation of phencyclidine piperdine which is a misnaming of phencyclidine from its chemical name of 1-(1-phenylcyclohexyl)piperdine.*]
pneumocystic pneumonia (respiratory)
Pneumocystis carinii pneumonia [found frequently in patients with acquired immunodeficiency syndrome (AIDS)] (immunology, laboratory, and respiratory)
pneumocystis pneumonia [found frequently in patients with acquired immunodeficiency syndrome (AIDS)] (immunology, laboratory, and respiratory)
primary care physician
principal care provider [to care for the patient] (hospice care, rehabilitation, and social services)
pulmonary capillary pressure (cardiovascular and respiratory)

PCPA
para-chlorophenylalanine [also called *fenclonine*; a serotonin inhibitor] (pharmacology)

pcpn
precipitation

PCPT
perception

pcpt
perception

PCR
personal care residence (rehabilitation and social services)
protein catabolic rate (laboratory)

P$_{cr}$
plasma creatinine (laboratory and nephrology)

PCS
palliative care service (oncology)
Patterns of Care Study (research)
portacaval shunt (cardiovascular and gastroenterology)
primary cancer site (oncology)

Pcs.
preconscious (anesthesiology and neurology)

pcs
preconscious (anesthesiology and neurology)

PCSM
percutaneous stone manipulation (nephrology, surgery, and urology)

PCT
plasmacrit test [for syphilis] (gynecology, infectious disease, laboratory, and urology)
plasmacytoma (hematology and oncology)
porcine calcitonin (orthopedics and pharmacology)
porphyria cutanea tarda (dermatology, gastroenterology, genetics, and neurology)
portacaval transposition (cardiovascular and gastroenterology)
postcoital test (gynecology, laboratory, and urology)
prothrombin consumption time (hematology and laboratory)
proximal convoluted tubule [of a nephron] (nephrology)

pct
percent (measurement)

PCU
pain control unit (neurology)
post-coronary care unit (cardiovascular)

PCV
packed cell volume (hematology and
laboratory)
parietal cell vagotomy (gastroenterology
and surgery)
polycythemia vera (hematology)
procarbazine, lomustine [CCNU], and
vincristine (chemotherapy, oncology,
and pharmacology)

PCV-M
myeloid metaplasia with polycythemia
vera (hematology)

PCW
pulmonary capillary wedge [position or
pressure] (cardiovascular)

PCWP
pulmonary capillary wedge pressure
(cardiovascular)

PCx
periscopic convex (ophthalmology)

P.Cx.
periscopic convex (ophthalmology)

PCXR
portable chest x-ray (radiology)

PCZ
procarbazine (chemotherapy, oncology,
and pharmacology)
prochlorperazine [an antiemetic] (gastroenterology and pharmacology)

PD
Doctor of Pharmacy (education and
pharmacology)
Dublin Pharmacopoeia [Ireland] (pharmacology)
papilla diameter (measurement)
paralyzing dose (pharmacology)
Parke-Davis [pharmaceutical company]
(pharmacology)
parkinsonism dementia (neurology)

Parkinson's disease (neurology)
pars distalis [a part of the pituitary
gland] (endocrinology and neurosurgery)
patent ductus (cardiovascular, neonatology, and pediatrics)
pediatrics
percutaneous drain (surgery)
peritoneal dialysis (nephrology)
phenyldichlorarsine
phosphate dehydrogenase (laboratory)
phosphate dextrose [media] (laboratory)
plasma defect (hematology)
poorly differentiated (oncology)
porphobilinogen deaminase [an enzyme]
(dermatology, gastroenterology, genetics, laboratory, and neurology)
postnasal drainage (otorhinolaryngology)
postural drainage (respiratory)
potential difference (neurology)
pressor dose (cardiovascular and pharmacology)
prism diopter (measurement and ophthalmology)
progression of a disease
psychopathic deviate (psychiatry)
psychotic depression (psychiatry)
psychotic deviate (psychiatry)
pulmonary disease (respiratory)
pulpodistal (dentistry)
pupillary distance [also called *interpu-
pillary distance*] (ophthalmology and
plastic surgery)

P.D.
Doctor of Pharmacy (education and
pharmacology)
preventive dentistry (dentistry)
pupillary distance [also called *interpu-
pillary distance*] (ophthalmology and
plastic surgery)

P/D
packs per day [of cigarettes] (cardiovascular, oncology, and respiratory)

P-D
Parke-Davis [pharmaceutical company]
(pharmacology)

Pd
palladium (chemistry)

pd
papilla diameter (measurement)
per diem [by the day]
prism diopter (ophthalmology)
pupillary distance [also called *interpu-pillary distance*] (ophthalmology and plastic surgery)

p.d.
papilla diameter (measurement)
per diem [by the day]
prism diopter (ophthalmology)
pupillary distance [also called *interpu-pillary distance*] (ophthalmology and plastic surgery)

PDA
patent ductus arteriosus (cardiovascular, neonatology, and pediatrics)
pediatric allergy (allergy and pediatrics)
posterior descending artery (cardiovascular)
predialyzed human albumin (laboratory)
posterior descending artery (cardiovascular)
principal diagonal artery (cardiovascular)

PDAB
para-dimethylaminobenzaldehyde [used in a reagent] (laboratory)

PDB
para-dichlorobenzene
phosphorus-dissolving bacteria (laboratory)

PDC
pediatric cardiology (cardiovascular and pediatrics)
pediatrics-cardiology (cardiovascular and pediatrics)
penta-decylcatechol
preliminary diagnostic clinic (administration)
private diagnostic clinic (administration)
Psychodevelopment Checklist (psychiatry)

PD & C
postural drainage and clapping (respiratory)

PDD
platinum diamminodichloride [also called *cisplatin* and *cis-platinum*] (chemotherapy, oncology, and pharmacology)
pyridoxine-deficient diet (dietary)

P.D.D.S.
Parasitic Disease Drug Service (parasitology and pharmacology)

PDE
paroxysmal dyspnea on exertion (cardiovascular and respiratory)
phosphodiesterase [an enzyme] (genetics and laboratory)
pulsed Doppler echocardiography (cardiovascular)

PDF
Parkinson's Disease Foundation (neurology)

PDFC
premature dead female child (gynecology and obstetrics)

PDFG
platelet-derived growth factor (endocrinology, laboratory, and pharmacology)

PDG
phosphogluconate dehydrogenase (laboratory)

6-PDG
6-phosphogluconate dehydrogenase (laboratory)

PDGA
pteroyldiglutamic acid [a vitamin of the B complex] (laboratory)

PDGF
platelet-derived growth factor (endocri-

nology, laboratory, and pharmacology)

PDH
packaged disaster hospital (emergency medicine)
past dental history (dentistry)
phosphate dehydrogenase (laboratory)
pyruvate dehydrogenase (laboratory and neurology)

PDHC
pyruvate dehydrogenase complex (laboratory and neurology)

PDI
Psychomotor Development Index (neurology and psychiatry)

P-diol
pregnanediol (gynecology, laboratory, and obstetrics) {pronounced "pea-di-all"}

PDL
poorly differentiated lymphocytic (hematology, laboratory, oncology, and pathology)

PDL
pudendal (gynecology and urology)

pdl
pudendal (gynecology and urology)

PDL-D
poorly differentiated lymphocytic—diffuse (hematology, laboratory, oncology, and pathology)

PDLL
poorly differentiated lymphocytic lymphoma (hematology, laboratory, oncology, and pathology)

PDL-N
poorly differentiated lymphocytic—nodular (hematology, laboratory, oncology, and pathology)

PDMC
premature dead male child (gynecology and obstetrics)

PDMS
Patient Data Management Systems (medical records)

PDN
prednisone [an anti-inflammatory] (orthopedics, pharmacology, and rheumatology)
private duty nurse (nursing)

PDP
piperidino-pyrimidine (laboratory)

PD & P
postural drainage and percussion (respiratory)

P.D. & P.
postural drainage and percussion (respiratory)

PDQ
Physician's Data Query (oncology)
pretty darn quick [at once, immediately, pretty damn quick] (slang)

PDR
pediatric-radiology (pediatrics and radiology)
Physicians' Desk Reference (pharmacology and publishing)
proliferative diabetic retinopathy (endocrinology and ophthalmology)

pdr
powder (pharmacology)

PDS
pain dysfunction syndrome (neurology)
paroxysmal depolarizing shift (cardiovascular)
patient data system (pharmacology)
pediatric surgery (pediatrics and surgery)
peritoneal dialysis system (nephrology)
polydioxanone suture (surgery)
predialyzed human serum (laboratory)
primary dependence study (chemical dependency)

PdS
psychiatric deviate, subtle (psychiatry)

PDGXT
predischarge graded exercise test (cardiovascular)

PDT
photodynamic therapy (ophthalmology)

PDU
pulsed Doppler ultrasonography (radiology)

PDUR
Predischarge Utilization Review [Program] (medical records)

PDWHF
platelet-derived wound healing factor (hematology and laboratory)

PDX
probable diagnosis

PE
Edinburgh Pharmacopoeia (pharmacology)
paper electrophoresis (laboratory)
pediatrics
pericardial effusion (cardiovascular)
phakoemulsification (ophthalmology)
pharyngoesophageal (gastroenterology and otorhinolaryngology)
phenylephrine [an adrenergic] (pharmacology)
phosphatidylethanolamine (laboratory)
photoelectric effect (physics)
photographic effect
physical education (education and rehabilitation)
physical evaluation
physical examination
physical exercise (physical therapy and rehabilitation)
Physiological Ecology (ecology and physiology)
pleural effusion (cardiovascular and respiratory)
pneumatic equalization [tube] (otorhinolaryngology)
polyethylene [suture (surgery) or tube (otorhinolaryngology)]
potential energy (physics)

powdered extract (pharmacology)
practical exercise (physical therapy and rehabilitation)
pressure equalization [tube] (otorhinolaryngology)
pressure equalizing [tube] (otorhinolaryngology)
probable error (laboratory)
pulmonary edema (cardiovascular and respiratory)
pulmonary embolism (cardiovascular and respiratory)
pulmonary embolus (cardiovascular and respiratory)

P.E.
protein electrophoresis (laboratory)

P_1E_1
{not an abbreviation} [brand name for a preparation of one percent epinephrine and one percent pilocarpine ophthalmic solution] (ophthalmology and pharmacology)

PE-50
{not an abbreviation} [a type of polyethylene cannula] (surgery)

Pe
pressure on expiration (laboratory and respiratory)

PEA
phenethyl alcohol [blood agar] (laboratory)

"pea-case"
{pronunciation of *PKase* [protein kinase]} (laboratory) {not an abbreviation}

"pea-dee-ah"
{pronunciation of *pedia-* [prefix indicating relationship to a child {not an abbreviation}]} (pediatrics) {not an abbreviation}

"pea-di-all"
{pronunciation of *P-diol* [pregnanediol]} (gynecology, laboratory, and obstetrics) {not an abbreviation}

"pea-dough"
{pronunciation of *pedo-* [prefix indicating relationship to a child {not an abbreviation}]} (pediatrics) {not an abbreviation}
{pronunciation of *pedo-*} [prefix indicating relationship to a foot {not an abbreviation}]} (orthopedics and podiatry) {not an abbreviation}

"pea-ko"
{pronunciation of *pico-* [prefix for 10^{-12} {not an abbreviation}]} (measurement) {formerly *micromicro-*} {not an abbreviation}

"pea-low"
{pronunciation of *pelo-* [prefix indicating relationship to mud {not an abbreviation}]} {not an abbreviation}

"pea-nee-ah"
{pronunciation of *-penia* [suffix indicating an abnormal reduction in number of the word root element {not an abbreviation}]} {not an abbreviation}

"pea-pull-mon-alley"
{pronunciation of *P. pulmonale* [pulmonary pulmonale]} (cardiovascular) {not an abbreviation}

PEARL
pupils equal and react to light (neurology and ophthalmology)

"pea-tace"
{pronunciation of *p'tase* [phosphatase]} (laboratory) {not an abbreviation}

PEB
Physical Evaluation Board (armed forces)

P.E.B.
Physical Evaluation Board (armed forces)

PEBG
phenethylbiguanide [also called *phenformin*; an oral hypoglycemic agent] (endocrinology and pharmacology) {obsolete}

PEC
patient evaluation center (administration)
peritoneal exudate cells (laboratory)
pyogenic exotoxin C (laboratory)

PECHO
prostatic echogram (urology and radiology)

"peck-may-jor"
{pronunciation of *pec major* [pectoralis major (muscle)]} (anatomy and surgery) {not an abbreviation}

"peck-mine-or"
{pronunciation of *pec minor* [pectoralis minor (muscle)]} (anatomy and surgery) {not an abbreviation}

pec major
pectoralis major [muscle] (anatomy and surgery) {pronounced "peck-may-jor"}

pec minor
pectoralis minor [muscle] (anatomy and surgery) {pronounced "peck-mine-or"}

$PECO_2$
mixed expired carbon dioxide tension (laboratory and respiratory)

PED
pediatrics

PEd
physical education (education and rehabilitation)

PEDG
phenformin [a hypoglycemic agent] (endocrinology and pharmacology) {obsolete}

pedia-
{not an abbreviation} [prefix indicating relationship to a child] (pediatrics) {pronounced "pea-dee-ah"}

pedo-
{not an abbreviation} [prefix indicating

relationship to a child] (pediatrics)
{pronounced "pea-dough"}
{not an abbreviation} [prefix indicating
relationship to a foot] (orthopedics
and podiatry) {pronounced "pea-
dough"}

PEDS
pediatrics {pronounced "peeds"}

PeDS
Pediatric Drug Surveillance [Program]
(chemical dependency, pediatrics, and
psychiatry)

Peds
pediatrics {pronounced "peeds"}

peds
pediatrics {pronounced "peeds"}

"pee-co"
{pronunciation of *pico-* [prefix for 10^{-12}]}
(measurement) {not an abbreviation}

"peeds"
{pronunciation of *PEDS*, *Peds*, and *peds*
[pediatrics]} {not an abbreviation}

PEEP
positive end-expiratory pressure (laboratory and respiratory) {pronounced
"peep"}

P.E.E.P.
positive end-expiratory pressure (laboratory and respiratory) {pronounced
"peep"}

"peep"
{pronunciation of *PEEP* and *P.E.E.P.*
[positive end-expiratory pressure]}
(laboratory and respiratory) {not an
abbreviation}

PEF
peak expiratory flow [highest forced expiratory flow measured with a peak
flow meter] (laboratory and respiratory)
Psychiatric Evaluation Form (psychiatry)

PEFR
peak expiratory flow rate (laboratory
and respiratory)

P.E.F.R.
peak expiratory flow rate (laboratory
and respiratory)

PEFR/PIFR
peak expiratory flow/peak inspiratory
flow rate (laboratory and respiratory)

PEFSR
partial expiratory flow—static recoil
curve (laboratory and respiratory)

PEFV
partial expiratory flow volume (laboratory and respiratory)

PEG
percutaneous endoscopic gastrostomy
[for feeding tube placement] (gastroenterology and surgery)
pneumoencephalogram (neurology and
radiology)
pneumoencephalography (neurology
and radiology)
polyethylene glycol (pharmacology)

"peh-trol"
{pronunciation of *petrol* [petroleum]}
(chemistry and pharmacology) {not an
abbreviation}

PEI
phosphate excretion index (laboratory)
phosphorus excretion index (laboratory)
physical efficiency index (rehabilitation)

PEL
peritoneal exudate lymphocyte(s) (laboratory)

PELG
Pelger Muet anomaly (laboratory)

pelo-
{not an abbreviation} [prefix indicating
relationship to mud] {pronounced
"pea-low"}

PEM
prescription-event monitoring (pharmacology)
primary enrichment medium (laboratory)
probable error of measurement (laboratory)
pulmonary embolus (cardiovascular and respiratory)

PEMF
pulsing electromagnetic field [method of treating fractures] (orthopedics)

PEMS
Physical, Emotional, Mental Safety

PEN
parenteral and enteral nutrition (dietary and gastroenterology)
penicillin [*Note: This is considered a dangerous abbreviation.*] (pharmacology) {pronounced "pen"}

Pen
penicillin [*Note: This is considered a dangerous abbreviation.*] (pharmacology) {pronounced "pen"}

pen
penetrating (ophthalmology)

"pen"
{pronunciation of *PEN* and *Pen* [penicillin]} (pharmacology) [*Note: This is considered a dangerous abbreviation.*] {not an abbreviation}

PENG
photoelectric nystagmography (neurology and ophthalmology)

pen G
penicillin G [an antibiotic] {pronounced "pen-gee"} (pharmacology)

"pen-gee"
{pronunciation of *pen G* [penicillin G; an antibiotic] (pharmacology) {not an abbreviation}

-penia
{not an abbreviation} [suffix indicating an abnormal reduction in number of

the word root element] {pronounced "pea-nee-ah"}

penic
penicillin [*Note: This is considered a dangerous abbreviation.*] (pharmacology)

penic cam
penicillum camelinum [camel's-hair brush]

PEN-O
Penner serotype-O (laboratory)

PENS
percutaneous epidural nerve stimulator (neurology) {pronounced "penz"}

PENT
pentothal [also called *thiopentone sodium*] (anesthesiology and pharmacology) {pronounced "pent"}

Pent
pentothal [also called *thiopentone sodium*] (anesthesiology and pharmacology) {pronounced "pent"}

pent
pentothal [also called *thiopentone sodium*] (anesthesiology and pharmacology) {pronounced "pent"}

pent-
{not an abbreviation} [prefix meaning *five*] {pronounced "pent"}

"pent"
{pronunciation of *PENT, Pent,* and *pent* [pentothal (also called *thiopentone sodium*) (anesthesiology and laboratory)] and *pent-* [prefix meaning five {not an abbreviation}]} {not an abbreviation}

penta-
{not an abbreviation} [prefix meaning *five*] {pronounced "pent-ah"}

"pent-ah"
{pronunciation of *penta-* [prefix meaning *five* {not an abbreviation}]} {not an abbreviation}

Pen-V
{not an abbreviation} [trade mark for a preparation of penicillin V, an antibiotic] (pharmacology) {pronounced "pen-vee"}

Pen-Vee
{not an abbreviation} [trade mark for a preparation of penicillin V, an antibiotic] (pharmacology) {pronounced "pen-vee"}

"pen-vee"
{pronunciation of *Pen-V* and *Pen-Vee* [trade marks for preparations of penicillin V, antibiotics {not abbreviations}]} (pharmacology) {not an abbreviation}

Pen-Vee K
{not an abbreviation} [trade mark for a preparation of penicillin V potassium, an antibiotic] (pharmacology) {pronounced "pen-vee-kay"}

"pen-vee-kay"
{pronunciation of *Pen-Vee K* [trade mark for a preparation of penicillin V potassium; an antibiotic {not an abbreviation}] and *Pen VK* [a preparation of penicillin V potassium; an antibiotic}]} (pharmacology) {not an abbreviation}

Pen VK
penicillin V potassium [an antibiotic] (pharmacology) {pronounced "pen-vee-kay"}

"penz"
{pronunciation of *PENS* [percutaneous epidural nerve stimulator]} (neurology) {not an abbreviation}

PEO
progressive external ophthalmoplegia (neurology and ophthalmology)

PEP
cyclophosphamide, VM-26, and prednis-

olone (chemotherapy, oncology, and pharmacology)
phosphoenolpyruvate [an enzyme] (gastroenterology and laboratory)
physiological evaluation of primates (physiology, research, and veterinary medicine)
polyestradiol phosphate (chemotherapy, oncology, and pharmacology)
pre-ejection period (cardiovascular)
protein electrophoresis (laboratory)
Psychiatric Evaluation Profile (psychiatry)

P.E.P.
Pulmonary Education Program (education, nursing, and respiratory)

PEPCK
phosphoenolpyruvate carboxykinase [an enzyme] (gastroenterology and laboratory)

PEP/EP
pre-ejection period to ejection period (cardiovascular)

PEPI
pre-ejection period index (cardiovascular)

PEPP
positive expiratory pressure plateau (laboratory and respiratory)

PEPR
precision encoder and pattern recognizer (chemistry and laboratory)

PER
for each
pediatric emergency room (emergency medicine and pediatrics)
protein efficiency ratio (laboratory)
{not an abbreviation} [Latin word for *by* or *through*; should be lowercase letters]

Per
permission

per
perineal (anatomy, gastroenterology, gynecology, obstetrics, surgery, and urology)
periodic
person
{not an abbreviation} [Latin word for *by* or *through*]

per an.
per annum [by year]

percs
Percodan [also called *oxycodone*] (chemical dependency and pharmacology) {slang} {pronounced "perks"}

PERCUSS
percussion (respiratory)

Perf.
perforation (otorhinolaryngology)

perf
perforated
perforating
perforation

PERI
peritoneal fluid (laboratory and surgery)

peri
perineal (anatomy, gastroenterology, gynecology, obstetrics, surgery, and urology)

peri-
{not an abbreviation} [prefix meaning *around*] {pronounced "pair-E"}

periap
periapical (radiology and respiratory)

PERI/M
perimortem

perio
periodontist (dentistry) {pronounced "pair-E-oh"}

PERK
prospective evaluation of radial keratotomy [protocol] (ophthalmology) {pronounced "perk"}

"perk"
{pronunciation of *PERK* [prospective evaluation of radial keratotomy (protocol)]} (ophthalmology) {not an abbreviation}

"perks"
{pronunciation of *percs* [Percodan; also called *oxycodone*] (chemical dependency and pharmacology) {slang} {not an abbreviation}

PERL
pupils equal and react(ive) to light (neurology and ophthalmology)
pupils equal, regular, and react(ive) to light (neurology and ophthalmology)

PERLA
pupils equal and react(ive) to light and accommodation (neurology and ophthalmology) {pronounced "per-la"}
pupils equal, regular, and react(ive) to light and accommodation (neurology and ophthalmology) {pronounced "per-la"}

"per-la"
{pronunciation of *PERLA* [pupils equal and react(ive) to light and accommodation; pupils equal, regular, and react(ive) to light and accommodation] and *PERRLA* [pupils equal, round, and react(ive) to light and accommodation; pupils equal, round, regular, and react(ive) to light and accommodation]} (neurology and ophthalmology) {not an abbreviation}

perm
permanent {pronounced "perm"}

"perm"
{pronunciation of *perm* [permanent]} {not an abbreviation}

pero-
{not an abbreviation} [prefix meaning *deformed* or *maimed*] {pronounced "pah-row"}

per op emet
peracta operatione emetici [when the action of the emetic is over]

per. op. emet.
peracta operatione emetici [when the action of the emetic is over]

per os
{not an abbreviation} [Latin meaning *by mouth*] (pharmacology)

PEROX
peroxidase stain (laboratory)

perp
perpendicular
perpetrator {pronounced "perp"} (law enforcement) (slang)

"perp"
{pronunciation of *perp* [perpetrator]} (law enforcement) {not an abbreviation} (slang)

perpad
perineal pad (gynecology, obstetrics, and urology) {pronounced "per-pad"}

"per-pad"
{pronunciation of *perpad* [perineal pad]} (gynecology, obstetrics, and urology) {not an abbreviation}

PERR
pattern-evoked retinal response (neurology and ophthalmology)

PERRL
pupils equal, round, and react(ive) to light (neurology and ophthalmology)
pupils equal, round, regular, and react(ive) to light (neurology and ophthalmology)

PERRLA
pupils equal, round, and react(ive) to light and accommodation (neurology and ophthalmology) {pronounced "per-la"}
pupils equal, round, regular, and react(ive) to light and accommodation (neurology and ophthalmology) {pronounced "per-la"}

PERRLA (DC)
pupils equal, round, and react(ive) to light and accommodation (directly and consensually) (neurology and ophthalmology)

pers
personal

PERT
program evaluation and review technique (administration) {pronounced "pert"}

pert
pertussis [also called *whooping cough*] (pediatrics and respiratory)

"pert"
{pronunciation of *PERT* [program evaluation and review technique]} (administration) {not an abbreviation}

PES
Physicians Equity Services
pre-excitation syndrome [also called *Wolff-Parkinson-White syndrome*] (cardiovascular)

Pes
esophageal pressure [used to estimate intrapleural pressure] (laboratory and respiratory)

pes
{not an abbreviation} [Latin word for the foot or the terminal organ of the leg or lower limb] (neurology, orthopedics, and podiatry) {pronounced "pez"}

PESS
pessus [pessary] (gynecology and urology) {pronounced "pez"}

PET
parent effectiveness training (psychiatry)
positron-emission tomography (radiology) {pronounced "pet"}
pre-eclamptic toxemia (obstetrics)

pressure equalization tubes (otorhinolaryngology)
pressure equalizing tubes (otorhinolaryngology)
psychiatry emergency team (emergency
medicine and psychiatry)

"pet"
{pronunciation of *PET* [positron-emis-
sion tomography]} (radiology) {not an
abbreviation}

"pet-ah-low"
{pronunciation of *petalo-* [a prefix indicating relationship to a leaf {not an
abbreviation}]} {not an abbreviation}

-petal
{not an abbreviation} [a suffix meaning
directed toward or moving toward]
{pronounced "pet-al"}

"pet-al"
{pronunciation of *-petal* [a suffix meaning directed toward or moving toward
{not an abbreviation}]} {not an abbre-
viation}

petalo-
{not an abbreviation} [a prefix indicating
relationship to a leaf] {pronounced
"pet-ah-low"}

PETN
pentaerythritol tetraniconitate [also
called *niceritrol*] (pharmacology)
pentaerythritol tetranitrate (chemistry
and pharmacology)

petr
petroleum (chemistry and pharmacology)

petrol
petroleum (chemistry and pharmacology) {pronounced "peh-trol"}
{not an abbreviation} [an English word
for petroleum] (chemistry and pharmacology)

PET scan
positron emission tomographic scan (radiology)

PETT
positron emission transaxial tomography
(radiology)
positron emission transverse tomography (radiology)

PETT scan
positron emission transaxial tomography
scan (radiology)

PEx
physical examination

"pex-E"
{pronunciation of *-pexy* [suffix meaning
fixation {not an abbreviation}]} {not an
abbreviation}

-pexy
{not an abbreviation} [suffix meaning fix-
ation] {pronounced "pex-E"}

"pez"
{pronunciation of *pes* [Latin word for
the foot or the terminal end of the leg
or lower limb (neurology, orthopedics,
and podiatry) {not an abbreviation}]
and *PESS* [pessary, *pessus* (gynecology and urology)]} {not an abbrevia-
tion}

PF
L-phenylalanine mustard and 5-fluoro-
uracil (chemotherapy, oncology, and
pharmacology)
parafascicular nucleus (neurosurgery)
peak factor
peak flow (respiratory)
peritoneal fluid (gastroenterology and
surgery)
permeability factor (laboratory)
personality factor (psychiatry)
personality profile (speech and language
therapy)
phenylalanine and methotrexate (chemotherapy, oncology, and pharmacology)
picture frustration [study] (psychiatry)
plantar flexion (neurology, orthopedics,
and podiatry)

platelet factor (hematology and laboratory)
posterior fontanelle (anatomy and neonatology)
power factor
protection factor
pulmonary factor (respiratory)
Purkinje fibers (cardiovascular)

P/F
pass-fail [system] (education)

Pf
Pfeifferella [a former bacteria classification] (laboratory)

pF
picofarad (measurement)

PFA
para-fluorophenylalanine (laboratory)
profunda femoris artery (anatomy)

PF3a
platelet factor 3 availability (hematology)

PFAS
performic acid–Schiff [reaction] (laboratory)

PFB
pseudofolliculitis barbae (dermatology)

PFC
pelvic flexion contracture (orthopedics)
perfluorocarbon (chemistry)
persistent fetal circulation (cardiovascular and neonatology) {obsolete, now called *persistent pulmonary hypertension of the neonate (PPHN)*}
plaque-forming cell(s) (laboratory)

PFD
primary flash distillate

PFEAAC
posterior fossa extra-axial arachnoid cyst (ortho, radiology)

PFFD
proximal femoral focal deficiency (orthopedics)

PFIB
perfluoroisobutylene

PFK
phosphofructokinase [an enzyme] (laboratory)

PF joint
patellofemoral joint (orthopedics)

PFM
peak flow meter (respiratory)
porcelain fused to metal (dentistry)

PF nucleus
parafascicular nucleus (neurosurgery)

PFO
patent foramen ovale (cardiovascular and pediatrics)

PFP
platelet-free plasma (hematology and laboratory)

PFQ
personality factor questionnaire (psychiatry)

PFR
parotid flow rate (otorhinolaryngology)
peak flow rate [reading] (respiratory)
pulmonary flow rate (respiratory)

PFS
pulmonary function score (respiratory)

PFT
pancreatic function test (gastroenterology and laboratory)
parafascicular thalamotomy (neurosurgery)
phenylalanine mustard [melphalan], fluorouracil, tamoxifen (chemotherapy, oncology, and pharmacology)
posterior fossa tumor (neurosurgery)
pulmonary function test(s) (laboratory and respiratory)

P.F.T.
pulmonary function test(s) (laboratory and respiratory)

PFT's
pulmonary function tests (laboratory and respiratory)

PFU
plaque-forming unit (laboratory)
pock-forming unit(s) (laboratory)

PFV
physiological full value

PG
glycerate-3-phosphate (laboratory)
paralysie générale [general paralysis] (neurology)
paregoric [formerly called *tincture of opium*] (gastroenterology and pharmacology)
parental guidance (pediatrics and psychiatry)
Parental Guidance [motion picture rating]
Pharmacopoeia Germanica [German Pharmacopoeia] (pharmacology)
phosphatidylglycerol [test used to determine fetal lung maturity] (laboratory, neonatology, and obstetrics)
phosphogluconate (laboratory)
pituitary gonadotropin (endocrinology and laboratory)
plasma glucose (laboratory)
plasma triglyceride (laboratory)
polygalacturonate (laboratory)
postgraduate (education)
pregnanediol glucuronide (gynecology, laboratory, and obstetrics)
pregnant (obstetrics)
prostaglandin (laboratory, endocrinology, and pharmacology)
pyoderma gangrenosum (dermatology)

P.G.
Pharmacopoeia Germanica [German Pharmacopoeia] (pharmacology)

P & G
Procter and Gamble [pharmaceutical company] (pharmacology)

6-PG
6-phosphogluconate (laboratory)

Pg
pregnant (obstetrics)

pg
page
picogram [also called *microgamma* and *micromicrogram*] (measurement, radiation therapy, and radiology)

PGA
Professional Golfers Association (sports medicine)
prostaglandin A (endocrinology, laboratory, and pharmacology)
pteroylglutamic acid [also called *folic acid*] (pharmacology)

P.G.A.
pteroylglutamic acid [also called *folic acid*] (pharmacology)

PGA₁
prostaglandin A_1 (endocrinology and laboratory)

PGA₂
prostaglandin A_2 (endocrinology and laboratory)

3PGA
3-phosphoglycerate (laboratory)

PGA₃
prostaglandin A_3 (endocrinology and laboratory)

PGB
prostaglandin B (endocrinology and laboratory)

PGB₁
prostaglandin B_1 (endocrinology and laboratory)

PGB₂
prostaglandin B_2 (endocrinology and laboratory)

PGB$_3$
prostaglandin B$_3$ (endocrinology and laboratory)

PGC
primordial germ cell (embryology and laboratory)

PGC$_1$
prostaglandin C$_1$ (endocrinology and laboratory)

PGC$_2$
prostaglandin C$_2$ (endocrinology and laboratory)

PGC$_3$
prostaglandin C$_3$ (endocrinology and laboratory)

PGD
phosphogluconate dehydrogenase (laboratory)
phosphogluconic dehydrogenase (laboratory)
phosphoglyceraldehyde dehydrogenase (laboratory)
prostaglandin D (endocrinology and laboratory)

PGD$_1$
prostaglandin D$_1$ (endocrinology and laboratory)

PGD$_2$
prostaglandin D$_2$ (endocrinology and laboratory)

PGD$_3$
prostaglandin D$_3$ (endocrinology and laboratory)

PGDF
Pilot Guide Dog Foundation (ophthalmology and rehabilitation)

PGDH
phosphogluconate dehydrogenase (laboratory)

PGDR
plasma-glucose disappearance rate (laboratory)

PGE
platelet granule extract (hematology and laboratory)
prostaglandin E [also called *dinoprostone*] (endocrinology, laboratory, and pharmacology)

PGE$_1$
prostaglandin E$_1$ [also called *alprostadil*] (endocrinology, laboratory, and pediatric cardiology)

PGE$_2$
prostaglandin E$_2$ [also called *dinoprostone*] (endocrinology, laboratory, and pharmacology)

PGE$_3$
prostaglandin E$_3$ (endocrinology and laboratory)

PGF
paternal grandfather (genetics)
prostaglandin F [also called *dinoprost*] (endocrinology, laboratory, and pharmacology)

PGF$_1$
prostaglandin F$_1$ (endocrinology and laboratory)

PGF$_{1\alpha}$
prostaglandin F$_1$ alpha (endocrinology and laboratory)

PGF$_2$
prostaglandin F$_2$ [a labor inducer] (endocrinology, obstetrics, and pharmacology)

PGF$_{2\alpha}$
prostaglandin F$_2$ alpha [also called *dinoprost*] (endocrinology, laboratory, and pharmacology)

PGF$_3$
prostaglandin F$_3$ (endocrinology and laboratory)

pgf
paternal grandfather (genetics)

PGFM
prostaglandin F and its metabolite [dihydroketoprostaglandin] (endocrinology and laboratory)

PGG$_2$
prostaglandin G$_2$ (endocrinology and laboratory)

PGH
pituitary growth hormone (endocrinology, laboratory, pediatrics, and pharmacology)
plasma growth hormone (endocrinology and laboratory)
prostaglandin H (endocrinology and laboratory)

PGH$_2$
prostaglandin H$_2$ (endocrinology and laboratory)

PGI
phosphoglucoisomerase [also called *phosphoglucose isomerase*] (laboratory)
potassium, glucose, and insulin (pharmacology)

PGI$_2$
prostaglandin I$_2$ [also called *prostacyclin*] (endocrinology, laboratory, and pharmacology)

PGK
phosphoglycerate kinase (laboratory)

PGL
persistent generalized lymphadenopathy (internal medicine)
phosphoglycolipid (laboratory)

PGM
paternal grandmother (genetics)
phosphoglucomutase (laboratory)

pgm
paternal grandmother (genetics)

PGN
proliferative glomerulonephritis (nephrology)

PGO
ponto-geniculo-occipital (anatomy and neurology)

PGP
post–gamma proteinuria (nephrology and urology)

PGR
psychogalvanic response (psychiatry)

PgR
progesterone receptor (laboratory and oncology)

P-GRN
progranulocytes (hematology and laboratory)

PGS
plant growth substance (chemistry)

PGTR
plasma glucose tolerance rate (endocrinology and laboratory)

PGU
postgonococcal urethritis (gynecology, infectious disease, and urology)

PGUT
phosphogalactose-uridyl transferase (laboratory)

PGYE
peptone, glucose yeast extract [medium] (laboratory)

PH
past history
personal history
pharmacopeia (pharmacology)
phenyl (chemistry and laboratory)
poor health
porta hepatis (gastroenterology)
previous history
prostatic hypertrophy (urology)
public health (government)
pulmonary hypertension (cardiovascular and respiratory)
purpura hyperglobulinemia (laboratory)

P.H.
physically handicapped (neurology, orthopedics, and rehabilitation)

Ph
pharmacopoeia (pharmacology)
phenyl (chemistry and laboratory)
phosphate (laboratory)

Ph.
pharmacopeia (pharmacology)

Ph'
Philadelphia chromosome (genetics)

Ph¹
Philadelphia chromosome (genetics)

pH
{not an abbreviation} [symbol for expression of hydrogen ion concentration, referring to the acid/base balance; also called *negative logarithm of hydrogen ion concentration*] (chemistry and laboratory)

pH₁
isoelectric point (chemistry and laboratory)

ph
phial (pharmacology)
pinhole (ophthalmology)

PHA
arterial pH [hydrogen ion concentration] (laboratory and respiratory)
passive hemagglutination (laboratory)
peripheral hyperalimentation [solution] (dietary, gastroenterology, and pharmacology)
phenylalanine [an amino acid] (laboratory)
phytohemagglutinin (laboratory)
phytohemagglutinin antigen [a skin test for cellular based immunity] (immunology and laboratory)
pulse height analyzer (cardiovascular)

phaco-
{not an abbreviation} [prefix indicating relationship to a lens] {pronounced "fay-ko"}

phaeo
phaeochromocytoma [also called *pheochromocytoma*] (endocrinology and oncology) {pronounced "fee-oh"}

-phagia
{not an abbreviation} [suffix indicating a perversion of appetite] (gastroenterology) {pronounced "fay-gee-ah"}

phago-
{not an abbreviation} [prefix indicating relationship to consumption or eating by engulfing or ingestion] (gastroenterology) {pronounced "fay-go"}

-phagy
{not an abbreviation} [suffix indicating a perversion of appetite] {pronounced "fay-gee"}

phako-
{not an abbreviation} [prefix indicating relationship to a lens] {pronounced "fay-ko"}

phal
phalanges (orthopedics and podiatry)
phalanx (orthopedics and podiatry)

phallo-
{not an abbreviation} [prefix indicating relationship to the penis] (urology) {pronounced "fal-low"}

PHA-M
phytohemagglutinin M (laboratory)

phanero-
{not an abbreviation} [prefix meaning apparent or visible] {pronounced "fan-air-oh"}

Phar
pharmaceutical (pharmacology)
pharmacology

phar
pharmaceutical (pharmacology) {pronounced "far"}
pharmacology {pronounced "far"}

pharmacopoeia (pharmacology) {pronounced "far"}
pharmacy (pharmacology) {pronounced "far"}

PharB
Pharmaciae Baccalaureus [Bachelor of Pharmacy] (education and pharmacology)

Phar. B.
Pharmaciae Baccalaureus [Bachelor of Pharmacy] (education and pharmacology)

PharC
Pharmaceutical Chemist (pharmacology)

Phar. C.
Pharmaceutical Chemist (pharmacology)

PharD
Pharmaciae Doctor [Doctor of Pharmacy] (education and pharmacology)

Phar. D.
Pharmaciae Doctor [Doctor of Pharmacy] (education and pharmacology)

PharG
Graduate in Pharmacy (education and pharmacology)

Phar. G.
Graduate in Pharmacy (education and pharmacology)

PHARM
pharmacist (pharmacology) {pronounced "farm"}
pharmacy (pharmacology) {pronounced "farm"}

PharM
Pharmaciae Magister [Master of Pharmacy] (education and pharmacology)

Phar. M.
Pharmaciae Magister [Master of Pharmacy] (education and pharmacology)

pharm
pharmaceutical (pharmacology) {pronounced "farm"}

pharmacology {pronounced "farm"}
pharmacopoeia (pharmacology) {pronounced "farm"}
pharmacy (pharmacology) {pronounced "farm"}

pharmaco-
{not an abbreviation} [prefix indicating relationship to a drug or medicine] (pharmacology) {pronounced "farm-ah-ko"}

Pharm. D.
Doctor of Pharmacy (education and pharmacology)

pharyngo-
{not an abbreviation} [prefix indicating relationship to the pharynx] (otorhinolaryngology and respiratory) {pronounced "fair-in-go" or "fur-ing-go"}

PHB
Public Health Bibliography

PhB
Bachelor of Philosophy (education)
British Pharmacopoeia (pharmacology)

Ph.B.
British Pharmacopoeia (pharmacology)

PHBB
propylhydroxybenzyl benzimidazole (chemistry)

PHC
posthospital care
premolar aplasia, hyperhidrosis, and premature canities [syndrome] (dermatology and genetics)
primary hepatic carcinoma (gastroenterology and oncology)
primary hepatocellular carcinoma (gastroenterology and oncology)
proliferative helper cells (laboratory)

PhC
Pharmaceutical Chemist (pharmacology)

Ph.C.
Pharmaceutical Chemist (pharmacology)

Ph¹c
Philadelphia chromosome (genetics)

PhD
Pharmaciae Doctor [Doctor of Pharmacy] (education and pharmacology)
Philosophiae Doctor [Doctor of Philosophy] (education)

Ph.D.
Pharmaciae Doctor [Doctor of Pharmacy] (education and pharmacology)
Philosophiae Doctor [Doctor of Philosophy] (education)

PHE
postheparin esterase (laboratory)

Phe
phenylalanine [an amino acid] (genetics and laboratory)

PHEN
phenotype (laboratory)

phen-
{not an abbreviation} [prefix indicating: (1) a displaying or showing; (2) derived from or related to benzene or containing phenyl (chemistry)] {pronounced "fen"}

Pheno
phenobarbital (neurology and pharmacology)

pheno-
{not an abbreviation} [prefix indicating: (1) a displaying or showing; (2) derived from or related to benzene or containing phenyl (chemistry)] {pronounced "fen-oh"}

PHENOB
phenobarbital (neurology and pharmacology)

phenobarb
phenobarbital (neurology and pharmacology)

phenoxy-
{not an abbreviation} [prefix indicating the presence of OC_6H_5] (chemistry) {pronounced "fen-ox-E"}

PHENTH
phenothiazine (pharmacology and psychiatry)

PHENYL
phenylpropanol (pharmacology)

Pheo
pheochromocytoma [also called *phaeochromocytoma*] (endocrinology and oncology) {pronounced "fee-oh"}

pheo
pheochromocytoma [also called *phaeochromocytoma*] (endocrinology and oncology) {pronounced "fee-oh"}

pheo-
{not an abbreviation} [prefix indicating relationship to brown, dun, or dusky] {pronounced "fee-oh"}

PHF
paired helical filaments (laboratory and neurology)
Personal Hygiene Facility

PHFG
primary human fetal glia (laboratory)

PHG
phosphatidylglycerol [test used to determine fetal lung maturity] (laboratory, neonatology, and obstetrics)

PhG
Graduate in Pharmacy (education and pharmacology)
Pharmacopoeia Germanica [German Pharmacopeia] (pharmacology)

Ph.G.
Graduate in Pharmacy (education and pharmacology)
Pharmacopoeia Germanica [German Pharmacopeia] (pharmacology)

Phgly
phenylglycine (gastroenterology, neurology, and pharmacology)

PHH
posthemorrhagic hydrocephalus (neurology)

PHI
phosphohexose isomerase (laboratory)
physiological hyaluronidase inhibitor (laboratory)
Public Health Inspector (government)

P.H.I.
Public Health Inspector (government)

PhI
Pharmacopoeia Internationalis (pharmacology)

phial
phiala [bottle] (pharmacology)
{not an abbreviation} [English word for small vial or bottle] (pharmacology)

phial.
phiala [bottle] (pharmacology)

-philia
{not an abbreviation} [suffix indicating abnormal or notable attraction or fondness] (psychiatry) {pronounced "fill-E-ah"}

PHIM
posthypoxic intention myoclonus (neurology)

PHIS
Physically Handicapped in Science (rehabilitation)

PHK
platelet phosphohexokinase (laboratory)
postmortem human kidney [cells] (laboratory and nephrology)

PHL
Public Health Law (government)

PHLA
postheparin lipolytic activity (laboratory)

phleb-
{not an abbreviation} [prefix indicating relationship to a vein or veins] (cardiovascular and hematology) {pronounced "fleb"}

phlebo-
{not an abbreviation} [prefix indicating relationship to a vein or veins] (cardiovascular and hematology) {pronounced "flee-bow"}

phlogo-
{not an abbreviation} [prefix indicating relationship to inflammation] {pronounced "flow-go"}

PHLS
Public Health Laboratory Service [British] (laboratory)

P.H.L.S.
Public Health Laboratory Service [British] (laboratory)

PHLSB
Public Health Laboratory Service Board [British] (laboratory)

PHM
Pharmacist's Mate [in Navy] (armed forces and pharmacology)

PhM
Pharmaciae Magister [Master of Pharmacy] (education and pharmacology)

PHMDP
Pharmacist's Mate, Dental Prosthetic Technician [in Navy] (armed forces, dentistry, and pharmacology)

PhmG
Graduate in Pharmacy (education and pharmacology)

PHN
postherpetic neuralgia (dermatology, infectious disease, and neurology)
Public Health Nurse (government and nursing)

public health nursing (government and nursing)

PH$_2$O
partial pressure of water vapor (chemistry and laboratory)

-phobia
{not an abbreviation} [suffix indicating an abnormal dread or fear] (psychiatry) {pronounced "foe-be-ah"}

phon-
{not an abbreviation} [prefix indicating relationship to sound] (electronics, otorhinolaryngology, and speech and language therapy) {pronounced "fon"}

Phono
phonocardiogram (cardiovascular)

phono-
{not an abbreviation} [prefix indicating relationship to sound] (electronics, otorhinolaryngology, and speech and language therapy) {pronounced "foe-no"}

-phore
{not an abbreviation} [suffix indicating a carrier of the root word] {pronounced "for"}

-phoresis
{not an abbreviation} [suffix indicating transmission] {pronounced "for-E-sis"}

PHOS
phosphorus (chemistry and laboratory)

phos
phosphate (chemistry and laboratory) {pronounced "foss"}
phosphorus (chemistry and laboratory) {pronounced "foss"}

PHOS-S
phosphorus spot [urine test] (chemistry and laboratory)

phot-
{not an abbreviation} [prefix indicating relationship to light] {pronounced "foat"}

photo
photograph (photography)

photo-
{not an abbreviation} [prefix indicating relationship to light] {pronounced "foe-toe"}

PHP
postheparin phospholipase (laboratory)
postheparin plasma (laboratory)
prepaid health plan (insurance)
primary hyperparathyroidism (endocrinology)
pseudohypoparathyroidism (endocrinology)

PHPT
primary hyperparathyroidism (endocrinology)

PHPV
persistent hyperplastic primary vitreous (ophthalmology)

PHR
peak heart rate (cardiovascular)
Public Health Resorts (government)

phren-
{not an abbreviation} [prefix indicating relationship to the diaphragm or the mind] (neurology and respiratory) {pronounced "fren"}

PHRT protocol
procarbazine, hydroxyurea, radiotherapy protocol (chemotherapy, oncology, pharmacology, and radiation therapy)

PHS
posthypnotic suggestion (psychiatry)
Public Health Service (government)

P.H.S.
Public Health Service (government)

PHSP
Public Health Service Publications (government and publishing)

PhTD
Physical Therapy Doctor (physical therapy and rehabilitation)

PHTS
Psychiatric Home Treatment Service (psychiatry)

PHV
persistent hypertrophic vitreous (ophthalmology and pediatrics)

PHx
past history

Phx
pharynx (otorhinolaryngology)

PHY
pharyngitis (otorhinolaryngology)
physical

phyco-
{not an abbreviation} [prefix indicating relationship to algae or seaweed] (oceanography) {pronounced "fie-ko"}

phyllo-
{not an abbreviation} [prefix indicating relationship to leaves] {pronounced "fie-low" or "fill-oh"}

PHYS
physiological (physiology)
physiology

PhyS
physiological saline (pharmacology)

Phys
physician
physiology

phys
physical

phys dis
physical disability (rehabilitation)

PhysEd
physical education (education and rehabilitation) {pronounced "fizz-ed"}

phys ed
physical education (education and rehabilitation) {pronounced "fizz-ed"}

Physio.
physiologic (physiology)

physio
physiotherapist (physical therapy) {pronounced "fizz-E-oh"}
physiotherapy (physical therapy) {pronounced "fizz-E-oh"}

physio-
{not an abbreviation} [prefix indicating relationship to nature or indicating physical] {pronounced "fizz-E-oh"}

Physiol
physiological (physiology)
physiology

PhysMed
physical medicine (physical medicine) {pronounced "fizz-med"}

physo-
{not an abbreviation} [prefix indicating relationship to air or gas] {pronounced "fie-so"}

PhysTher
physical therapy (physical therapy and rehabilitation) {pronounced "fizz-ther"}

phyto-
{not an abbreviation} [prefix indicating relationship to a plant or plants] {pronounced "fie-toe"}

PI
pacing impulse (cardiovascular)
paranoid ideation (psychiatry)
patient's interests
performance intensity (rehabilitation)
perinatal injury (neonatology, obstetrics, and pediatrics)
peripheral iridectomy (ophthalmology)
personal injury
personality inventory (psychiatry)

Pharmacopoeia Internationalis (pharmacology)
phosphatidylinositol (laboratory)
physically impaired (rehabilitation)
pneumatosis intestinalis (gastroenterology)
poison ivy (dermatology)
ponderal index (measurement)
Porch Index (psychiatry and speech and language therapy)
pregnancy induced (obstetrics)
preinduction [examination] (armed forces)
present illness
primary infarction (cardiovascular)
proactive inhibition (psychiatry)
proinsulin (endocrinology and laboratory)
prolactin inhibitor (endocrinology and laboratory)
protamine insulin (endocrinology and pharmacology)
protean inhibitor (laboratory)
Protocol Internationale [International Protocol]
psychiatric institute (psychiatry)
pulmonary incompetence (respiratory)
pulmonary infarction (cardiovascular and respiratory)
pulmonary insufficiency (cardiovascular and respiratory)
{not an abbreviation} [a surgical stapler] (surgery)

P.I.
protamine insulin (endocrinology and pharmacology)
Protocol Internationale [International Protocol]

Pi
pressure of inspiration (respiratory)
pulmonary insufficiency (respiratory)

P$_i$
inorganic phosphate (chemistry)

Pi.
pressure of inspiration (respiratory)

pl
{not an abbreviation} [the pH of a solution at its isoelectric point] (chemistry and laboratory)

PIA
plasma insulin activity (laboratory)
Psychiatric Institute of America (psychiatry)

PIAT
Peabody Individual Achievement Test (psychiatry and speech and language therapy)

PIC
postinflammatory corticoid (laboratory)

PICA
Porch Index of Communicative Ability (psychiatry and speech and language therapy)
posterior inferior cerebellar artery (cardiovascular and neurology)
posterior inferior cerebral artery (cardiovascular and neurology)
posterior inferior communicating artery (cardiovascular and neurology)
posterior internal cerebral artery (cardiovascular and neurology)

pico-
{not an abbreviation} [prefix for 10^{-12}; formerly *micromicro-*] (measurement) {pronounced "pea-ko" or "pee-co"}

picro-
{not an abbreviation} [prefix meaning *bitter*] {pronounced "pik-row"}

PICU
pediatric intensive care unit (pediatrics)
pulmonary intensive care unit (respiratory)

PID
pelvic inflammatory disease (gynecology)
photoionization detector (chemistry and laboratory)
plasma-iron disappearance (laboratory)
prolapsed intervertebral disc [or disk] (neurology and orthopedics)

P.I.D.
pelvic inflammatory disease (gynecology)

PIDRA
portable insulin dosage-regulating apparatus (endocrinology and pharmacology)

PIDT
plasma-iron disappearance time (laboratory)

PIE
preimplantation embryo (gynecology and obstetrics)
pulmonary infiltrate with eosinophilia [syndrome] (respiratory)
pulmonary infiltration associated with eosinophilia (respiratory)
pulmonary interstitial edema (respiratory)
pulmonary interstitial emphysema (pediatrics and respiratory)

"pie-E-sis"
{pronunciation of -*piesis* [suffix meaning pressure {not an abbreviation}]} {not an abbreviation}

"pie-low"
{pronunciation of *pilo-* [prefix indicating relationship to hair or resembling or composed of hair {not an abbreviation}]} {not an abbreviation}

"pie-oh"
{pronunciation of *pio-* [prefix indicating relationship to fat {not an abbreviation}]} {not an abbreviation}

-piesis
{not an abbreviation} [suffix meaning pressure] {pronounced "pie-E-sis"}

PIF
peak inspiratory flow (laboratory and respiratory)
prolactin inhibiting factor (endocrinology and laboratory)
prolactin release-inhibiting factor (endocrinology and laboratory)
proliferation-inhibiting factor (laboratory)

P.I.F.
peak inspiratory force (laboratory and respiratory)

PIFR
peak inspiratory flow rate (laboratory and respiratory)

PIFT
platelet immunofluorescence test (hematology and laboratory)

pigm
pigmentum [paint]

PIH
pregnancy-induced hypertension (cardiovascular and obstetrics)
prolactin release-inhibiting hormone (endocrinology and laboratory)

PII
plasma inorganic iodine (chemistry and laboratory)
primary irritation indices

"pik-row"
{pronunciation of *picro-* [prefix meaning bitter {not an abbreviation}]} {not an abbreviation}

Pil.
pilula [pill] (pharmacology)
pilulae [pills] (pharmacology)

pil
pilula [pill] (pharmacology)
pilulae [pills] (pharmacology)

pil.
pilula [pill] (pharmacology)
pilulae [pills] (pharmacology)

pilo-
{not an abbreviation} [prefix indicating relationship to hair or resembling or composed of hair] {pronounced "pie-low"}

PIMCO
Physicians Insurance Medical Company
(insurance)

pimelo-
{not an abbreviation} [prefix indicating
relationship to fat] {pronounced "pim-
E-low"}

"pim-E-low"
{pronunciation of *pimelo-* [prefix indicating relationship to fat {not an ab-
breviation}]} {not an abbreviation}

ping
pinguis [fat, grease]

PINWOR
pinworm (gastroenterology and laboratory)

PIO
pemoline (neurology and pharmacology)

pio-
{not an abbreviation} [prefix indicating
relationship to fat] {pronounced "pie-
oh"}

PIP
6-mercaptopurine, vincristine, methotrexate, and citrovorum factor (chemotherapy, oncology, and pharmacology)
peak inspiratory pressure (laboratory
and respiratory)
piperacillin (pharmacology) [*Note: This
is considered a dangerous abbreviation as it may be mistaken for Pit*
(Pitocin or Pitressin).]
postinspiratory pressure (laboratory and
respiratory)
proximal interphalangeal [joint] (orthopedics and podiatry)
Psychotic Inpatient Profile (psychiatry)

P.I.P.
proximal interphalangeal [joint] (orthopedics and podiatry)

PIPIDA
N-para-isopropylacetanilide-iminodiace-
tic acid [scan] (radiology) [Note: *A*

^{99m}Tc-*PIPIDA scan is a technetium
PIPIDA scan.*]

PIPJ
proximal interphalangeal joint (orthopedics and podiatry)

PIR
postinhibitory rebound (neurology)

P-IRI
plasma immunoreactive insulin (endocrinology and laboratory)

PIRP
Provisional International Reference
Preparation

PIS
Provisional International Standard

PISA
phase invariant signature algorithm
(chemistry)

PIT
patellar inhibition test (neurology and
orthopedics)
picture identification test (psychiatry)
plasma iron turnover (hematology and
laboratory)

Pit
Pitocin (gynecology, obstetrics, and
pharmacology) [*Note: This is considered a dangerous abbreviation.*]
Pitressin (cardiovascular and pharmacology) [*Note: This is considered a dangerous abbreviation.*]

pit
pituitary [gland] (endocrinology)

PITR
plasma iron turnover rate (hematology
and laboratory)

PITS
parent-infant traumatic stress

PIV
parainfluenza virus (laboratory)
peripheral intravenous [line] (pharmacology)

PIVD
protruded intervertebral disc [or disk] (neurology and orthopedics)

pixel
picture element (computer science and radiology)

PJB
premature junctional beat (cardiovascular)

PJC
premature junctional contraction(s) (cardiovascular)

PJS
Peutz-Jeghers syndrome (gastroenterology and genetics)

PK
penetrating keratoplasty (ophthalmology)
Prausnitz-Künstner [reaction] (allergy, immunology, and laboratory)
psychokinesis (parapsychology)
pyruvate kinase [deficiency] (internal medicine and laboratory)

P$_K$
plasma potassium (laboratory)

pK
dissociation constant (chemistry and laboratory)
{not an abbreviation} [the negative logarithm of an ionization constant of an acid] (chemistry)

PKA
prokininogenase (laboratory)

pKa
negative log of dissociation constant (chemistry and laboratory)

PKase
protein kinase (laboratory) {pronounced "pea-case"}

PKD
polycystic kidney disease (nephrology)

PK reaction
Prausnitz-Künstner reaction (allergy, immunology, and laboratory)

PK test
Prausnitz-Künstner transfer test (allergy, immunology, and laboratory)

PKU
phenylketonuria (genetics, laboratory, neonatology, neurology, pediatrics, and psychiatry)

PKV
killed poliomyelitis vaccine (infectious diseases and laboratory)

pkV
peak kilovoltage (electricity and measurement)

PL
palm leaf reaction
perception of light [also called *light perception*] (neurology and ophthalmology)
peroneus longus [muscle] (orthopedics)
phospholipid (laboratory)
photoluminescence (laboratory)
place
placebo (pharmacology)
placental lactogen (endocrinology, laboratory, and obstetrics)
plantar (neurology and orthopedics)
plastic surgeon (plastic surgery)
plastic surgery
Public Law (government and law enforcement)
pulpolingual (dentistry)

P$_L$
pulmonary venous pressure (cardiovascular and respiratory)

transpulmonary pressure (cardiovascular and respiratory)

P.L.
perception of light [also called *light perception*] (neurology and ophthalmology)

PL1
programming language one (computer science)

Pl
plasma (hematology and laboratory)
Plasmodium [the malarial parasite] (infectious diseases)

pl
picoliter [also called *micromicroliter*] (measurement)
place
plastic surgery
plate
platelets (hematology and laboratory)
pleural (respiratory)
plural [meaning more than one]

pl.
place
plate
pleural (respiratory)
plural [meaning more than one]

PLA
phospholipase A (laboratory)
pulpolabial (dentistry)
pulpolinguoaxial (dentistry)

PLa
pulpolabial (dentistry)

plant-flex
plantar flexion (neurology and orthopedics)

PLAP
placental alkaline phosphatase (laboratory)

plasmo-
{not an abbreviation} [prefix indicating relationship to plasma or to the substance of a cell] (chemistry, hematol-

ogy, and laboratory) {pronounced "plaz-moe"}

-plast
{not an abbreviation} [suffix indicating any primitive living cell] (chemistry and laboratory) {pronounced "plast"}

"plast"
{pronunciation of *-plast* [suffix indicating any primitive living cell {not an abbreviation}]} (chemistry and laboratory) {not an abbreviation}

-plasty
{not an abbreviation} [suffix meaning the shaping or the surgical formation of] (surgery) {pronounced "plaz-tea"}

"plat-E"
{pronunciation of *platy-* [prefix meaning broad or flat {not an abbreviation}]} {not an abbreviation}

PLATL
platelets (hematology and laboratory)

platy-
{not an abbreviation} [prefix meaning broad or flat] {pronounced "plat-E"}

"plaz-moe"
{pronunciation of *plasmo-* [prefix indicating relationship to plasma or to the substance of a cell {not an abbreviation}]} (chemistry, hematology, and laboratory) {not an abbreviation}

"plaz-tea"
{pronunciation of *-plasty* [suffix meaning the shaping or the surgical formation of {not an abbreviation}]} (surgery) {not an abbreviation}

PLB
phospholipase B (laboratory)

PLC
proinsulin-like compound (endocrinology, laboratory, and pharmacology)

PLCL
polyclonal gammopathy identified (laboratory)

PL-CLP
platelet clumps (hematology and laboratory)

PLD
platelet defect (hematology and laboratory)
potentially lethal damage (radiology)
pregnancy, labor and delivery (obstetrics)

PLDD
poorly differentiated lymphoma, diffuse (oncology and pathology)

PL DYL
Placidyl [also called *ethchlorvynol*; a hypnotic and sedative] (pharmacology and psychiatry)

PLE
protein-losing enteropathy (gastroenterology)

"plea-gee-ah"
{pronunciation of *-plegia* [suffix meaning paralysis or a stroke {not an abbreviation}]} (neurology) {not an abbreviation}

"plea-oh"
{pronunciation of *pleo-* [prefix meaning more {not an abbreviation}]} {not an abbreviation}

PLED
periodic lateralized epileptiform discharge(s) (neurology) {pronounced "pled"}
periodic lateralizing epileptiform discharge(s) (neurology) {pronounced "pled"}

"pled"
{pronunciation of *PLED* [periodic lateralized epileptiform discharge(s) or periodic lateralizing epileptiform discharge(s)]} (neurology) {not an abbreviation}

PLED's
periodic lateralized epileptiform discharges (neurology) {pronounced "pleds"}
periodic lateralizing epileptiform discharges (neurology) {pronounced "pleds"}

"pleds"
{pronunciation of *PLED's* [periodic lateralized epileptiform discharges or periodic lateralizing epileptiform discharges]} (neurology) {not an abbreviation}

-plegia
{not an abbreviation} [suffix meaning paralysis or a stroke] (neurology) {pronounced "plea-gee-ah"}

pleo-
{not an abbreviation} [prefix meaning more] {pronounced "plea-oh"}

PLEU
pleural fluid (laboratory and respiratory)

pleur-
{not an abbreviation} [prefix indicating relationship to the pleura, to a rib, or to the side] {pronounced "plur"}

Pleur. Fl.
pleural fluid (laboratory and respiratory)

pleuro-
{not an abbreviation} [prefix indicating relationship to the pleura, to a rib, or to the side] {pronounced "plur-oh"}

PLEVA
pityriasis lichenoides et varioliformis acuta (dermatology)

"plex-E"
{pronunciation of *-plexy* [suffix meaning a seizure or stroke {not an abbreviation}]} (neurology) {not an abbreviation}

-plexy
{not an abbreviation} [suffix meaning a seizure or stroke] (neurology) {pronounced "plex-E"}

PLF
perilymphatic fistula (internal medicine)

PLFC
premature living female child (neonatology and obstetrics)

PLG
plasminogen [an enzyme] (hematology and laboratory)

PLGV
psittacosis-lymphogranuloma venereum (gynecology, infectious diseases, respiratory, urology, and veterinary medicine)

P-LGV
psittacosis-lymphogranuloma venereum (gynecology, infectious diseases, respiratory, urology, and veterinary medicine)

PLH
paroxysmal localized hyperhidrosis (dermatology)

PLIF
postlumbar interbody fusion (neurology and orthopedics)

P lines
{not an abbreviation} (radiology)

PLL
peripheral light loss (neurology and ophthalmology)
prolymphocytic leukemia (hematology and oncology)

PLM
polarized light microscopy (laboratory)

PLMC
premature living male child (neonatology and obstetrics)

PLMT
plasmacytoid lymphocyte(s) (hematology and laboratory)

PLN
pelvic lymph node (gynecology and surgery)
popliteal lymph node (orthopedics and surgery)
posterior lip nerve (neurology and otorhinolaryngology)

-ploid
{not an abbreviation} [suffix indicating in adjectives the condition of multiplication of chromosomes or in a noun a cell or individual having chromosome sets with multiplication] (chemistry, genetics, and laboratory) {pronounced "ploid"}

"ploid"
{pronunciation of -ploid [suffix indicating in adjectives the condition of multiplication of chromosomes or in a noun a cell or individual having chromosome sets with multiplication {not an abbreviation}]} (chemistry, genetics, and laboratory) {not an abbreviation}

PLP
pyridoxal phosphate (laboratory)

PLR
pronation/lateral rotation [fracture] (orthopedics)

PLR IV
pronation/lateral rotation IV [fracture] (orthopedics)

PLS
please
Preschool Language Scale [Zimmerman] (speech and language therapy)
primary lateral sclerosis (neurology)
prostaglandin-like substance (endocrinology and laboratory)

pls.
please

PLT
platelet (hematology and laboratory)
primed lymphocyte typing (hematology and laboratory)
psittacosis-lymphogranuloma venereum-trachoma [a group of organisms] (gynecology, infectious diseases, laboratory, otorhinolaryngology, respiratory, urology, and veterinary medicine)

PLT-G
giant platelet (hematology and laboratory)

Plts
platelets (hematology and laboratory)

plts
platelets (hematology and laboratory)

plumb
plumbum [lead] (chemistry and laboratory)

plumb.
plumbum [lead] (chemistry and laboratory)

"plur"
{pronunciation of *pleur-* [prefix indicating relationship to the pleura, to a rib, or to the side {not an abbreviation}]} (respiratory) {not an abbreviation}

"plur-oh"
{pronunciation of *pleuro-* [prefix indicating relationship to the pleura, to a rib, or to the side {not an abbreviation}]} (respiratory) {not an abbreviation}

PLV
live poliomyelitis vaccine (infectious diseases and pharmacology)
panleukopenia virus (hematology and laboratory)
phenylalanine-lysine-vasopressin (cardiovascular and pharmacology)
posterior left ventricle (cardiovascular)

plx
plexus (neurology)

P-LYM
prolymphocyte (hematology and laboratory)

PM
pacemaker (cardiovascular)
petit mal [epilepsy] (neurology)
photomultiplier tube (electronics)
physical medicine (physical medicine and rehabilitation)
poliomyelitis (infectious diseases, neurology, and orthopedics)
polymorphonuclear [leukocyte] (hematology and laboratory)
polymyositis (neurology, orthopedics, and rheumatology)
postmenopausal (gynecology)
post meridiem [after noon, evening, night]
post mortem [after death]
premolar (dentistry)
presents mainly
presystolic murmur (cardiovascular)
preventive medicine
primary motivation (psychiatry)
prostatic massage (urology)
pulpomesial (dentistry)

P.M.
post meridiem [after noon, evening, night]

Pm
promethium [a radioactive element previously called *florentium* and *illinium*] (chemistry)

pM
picomolar [also called *micromicromolar*] (measurement)

pm
picometer (measurement)
post meridiem [after noon, evening, night]

p.m.
post meridiem [after noon, evening, night]

PMA
papillary, marginal, attached [referring to gingiva] (dentistry)
para-methoxyamphetamine (pharmacology)
Pharmaceutical Manufacturers Association (pharmacology)
phosphomolybdic acid (laboratory)
premenstrual asthma (gynecology and respiratory)
prevalence of gingivitis [papillary, marginal, attached] (dentistry)
Primary Mental Abilities [test] (psychiatry)
Prinzmetal's angina (cardiovascular)
progressive muscular atrophy (neurology)
pyridylmercuric acetate (laboratory)

P.M.A.
Pharmaceutical Manufacturers Association (pharmacology)

PMax
peak inspiratory pressure (laboratory and respiratory)

PMB
cis-platinum, methotrexate, and bleomycin (chemotherapy, oncology, and pharmacology)
parahydroxymercuribenzoate [also called *p-mercuribenzoate* (chemistry and pharmacology)
polychrome methylene blue [dye] (laboratory)
polymorphonuclear basophil [leukocyte] (hematology and laboratory)
postmenopausal bleeding (gynecology)

P.M.B.
polymorphonuclear basophil leukocyte(s) (hematology and laboratory)

PMC
Pacific Medical Center (administration)
phenylmercuric chloride (chemistry)
pseudomembranous colitis (gastroenterology)

PMD
primary myocardial disease (cardiovascular)
private medical doctor

progressive muscular dystrophy (neurology)

P.M.D.
private medical doctor

PMd
private medical doctor
private physician

PM/DM
polymyositis/dermatomyositis (rheumatology)

PME
polymorphonuclear eosinophil(s) (hematology and laboratory)
postmenopausal estrogen (gynecology, laboratory, and pharmacology)

P.M.E.
polymorphonuclear eosinophil leukocyte(s) (hematology and laboratory)

PMF
L-phenylalanine mustard, 5-fluorouracil, and methotrexate (chemotherapy, oncology, and pharmacology)
progressive massive fibrosis (internal medicine)

PMH
past medical history

PMHR
predicted maximal heart rate (cardiovascular)

PMHx
past medical history

PMI
past medical illness
patient medication instruction(s) (pharmacology)
Patient Medication Instruction [sheets from the American Medical Association] (pharmacology)
phosphomannose isomerase (laboratory)
point of maximal impulse (cardiovascular)

point of maximum impulse (cardiovascular)

point of maximum intensity (cardiovascular)

posterior myocardial infarction (cardiovascular)

present medical illness

previous medical illness

P.M.I.

point of maximal impulse (cardiovascular)

PML

polymorphonuclear leukocyte(s) (hematology and laboratory)

posterior mitral leaflet (cardiovascular)

progressive multifocal leukoencephalopathy (neurology)

PMMA

polymethyl methacrylate (dentistry and orthopedics)

PMN

polymorphonuclear [leukocyte] (hematology and laboratory)

polymorphonuclear neutrophil(s) (hematology and laboratory)

P.M.N.

polymorphonuclear neutrophil [leukocyte(s)] (hematology and laboratory)

PMNG

polymorphonuclear granulocyte(s) (hematology and laboratory)

PMN's

polymorphonuclear neutrophil [leukocytes] (hematology and laboratory)

PMNL

polymorphonuclear leukocyte (hematology and laboratory)

PMNR

periadenitis mucosa necrotica recurrens (dentistry and otorhinolaryngology)

PMO

postmenopausal osteoporosis (gynecology and orthopedics)

Principal Medical Officer (administration)

pmole

picomole [also called *micromicromole*] (measurement)

P-MONO

promonocytes (laboratory)

PMP

pain management program (neurology)

past menstrual period (gynecology and obstetrics)

persistent mentoposterior [position] (obstetrics)

previous menstrual period (gynecology and obstetrics)

prior menstrual period (gynecology and obstetrics)

PMQ

phytylmenaquinone [also called *vitamin K*] (chemistry, laboratory, and pharmacology)

PMR

perinatal mortality rate (obstetrics, neonatology, and statistics)

physical medicine and rehabilitation

polymorphic reticulosis (ophthalmology)

polymyalgia rheumatica (rheumatology)

posteromedial release (orthopedics)

proportionate morbidity ratio (statistics)

proportionate mortality ratio (statistics)

protein magnetic resonance (laboratory)

PM & R

physical medicine and rehabilitation

P.M. & R.

physical medicine and rehabilitation

PMRAFNS

Princess Mary's Royal Air Force Nursing Service [British] (armed forces and nursing)

PMRS

physical medicine and rehabilitation service

PMS
chorionic gonadotropin in pregnant mare's serum (laboratory)

phenazine methosulfate (allergy, anesthesiology, gastroenterology, pharmacology, and respiratory)

poor miserable soul

postmenopausal syndrome (gynecology and psychiatry)

postmitochondrial supernatant (laboratory)

pregnant mare's serum (laboratory)

premenstrual syndrome (gynecology and psychiatry)

pureed, mechanical, soft [diet] (dietary)

PMSC
pluripotent myeloid stem cell (laboratory)

PMS diet
pureed, mechanical, soft diet (dietary)

PMSG
pregnant mare's serum gonadotropin (laboratory)

PMT
Porteus maze test (psychiatry)

premenstrual tension (gynecology and psychiatry)

PMTS
premenstrual tension syndrome (gynecology and psychiatry)

PMTT
pulmonary mean transit time (cardiovascular, laboratory, and respiratory)

PMV
prolapse of mitral valve (cardiovascular)

PMW
pacemaker wire(s) (cardiovascular)

PN
parenteral nutrition (dietary and gastroenterology)

perceived noise (otorhinolaryngology)

percussion note [on examination] (respiratory)

periarteritis nodosa (rheumatology)

peripheral nerve (neurology)

peripheral neuropathy (endocrinology, neurology, and orthopedics)

pneumonia (respiratory)

polyarteritis nodosa (rheumatology)

positional nystagmus (neurology and ophthalmology)

postnasal (otorhinolaryngology)

postnatal (neonatology, obstetrics, and pediatrics)

Practical Nurse (nursing)

progress note (medical records)

psychiatry-neurology (neurology and psychiatry)

psychoneurologist (neurology and psychiatry)

psychoneurotic [individual] (psychiatry)

pyelonephritis (nephrology)

P.N.
percussion note [on examination] (respiratory)

Practical Nurse (nursing)

P & N
psychiatry and neurology

P$_{N2}$
partial pressure of nitrogen (laboratory and respiratory)

Pn
pneumonia (respiratory)

PNA
Nomina Anatomica (Paris) [referring to anatomical nomenclature] (anatomy)

pentosenucleic acid [also called *ribonucleic acid* (RNA)] (genetics and laboratory)

PNa
plasma sodium (laboratory)

P$_{Na}$
plasma sodium (laboratory)

PNAS
prudent no salt added [diet] (cardiovascular and dietary)

PNAvQ
positive-negative ambivalent quotient (psychiatry)

PNB
premature nodal beat (cardiovascular)
prostatic needle biopsy (oncology and urology)

PNBT
para-nitro blue tetrazolium (laboratory)

PNC
penicillin (pharmacology) [*Note: This is considered a dangerous abbreviation.*]
peripheral nerve conduction (neurology)
pneumotaxic center (neurology and respiratory)
premature nodal contraction(s) (cardiovascular)
prenatal care (obstetrics)
prenatal clinic (obstetrics)
prenodal contraction (cardiovascular)
pseudonurse cells (laboratory and urology)

PND
paroxysmal nocturnal dyspnea (cardiovascular and respiratory)
postnasal drainage (otorhinolaryngology)
postnasal drip (otorhinolaryngology)

P.N.D.
paroxysmal nocturnal dyspnea (cardiovascular and respiratory)

pnd
pound (measurement)

PNE
Practical Nurse's Education (education and nursing)

-pnea
{not an abbreviation} [suffix indicating relationship to breathing] (respiratory) {pronounced "nee-ah"}

PNed
Nederlandsche Pharmacopee [Dutch pharmacopoeia] (pharmacology)

pneo-
{not an abbreviation} [prefix indicating relationship to the breath or breathing] (respiratory) {pronounced "nee-oh"}

PNET-MB
primitive neuroectodermal tumors—medulloblastoma (neonatology, neurology, and oncology)

pneu
pneumonia (respiratory)

pneuma-
{not an abbreviation} [prefix indicating relationship to air or gas or to respiration] (chemistry, laboratory, and respiratory) {pronounced "new-mah"}

pneumato-
{not an abbreviation} [prefix indicating relationship to air or gas or to respiration] (chemistry, laboratory, and respiratory) {pronounced "new-mah-toe"}

PNF
proprioceptive neuromuscular facilitation [reaction] (neurology and rehabilitation)

PNH
paroxysmal nocturnal hemoglobinuria (laboratory, nephrology, and urology)

PNI
peripheral nerve injury (neurology)
postnatal infection (neonatology, obstetrics, and pediatrics)
prognostic nutrition index (dietary)

PNK
polynucleotide kinase (laboratory)

PNMG
persistent neonatal myasthenia gravis (neonatology and neurology)

PNMT
phenylethanolamine-N-methyl transferase (laboratory)

PNO
Principal Nursing Officer (nursing)

PNP
para-nitrophenol (laboratory)
para-nitrophenyl (laboratory)
para-nitrophenyl-beta-galactosidase (laboratory)
Pediatric Nurse Practitioner (nursing and pediatrics)
peripheral neuropathy (neurology)
progressive nuclear palsy (neurology)
purine nucleotide phosphorylase (laboratory)

P-NP
para-nitrophenol (laboratory)

P.N.P.
peak negative pressure (laboratory and respiratory)
Pediatric Nurse Practitioner (nursing and pediatrics)

PNPG
para-nitrophenyl-beta-galactoside (laboratory)

PNPP
para-nitrophenylphosphate (laboratory)

PNPR
positive-negative pressure respiration (laboratory and respiratory)

P-NPS
para-nitrophenylsulfate (gastroenterology and pharmacology)

PNS
parasympathetic nervous system (neurology)
partial nonprogressing stroke (cardiovascular and neurology)
peripheral nerve stimulator (neurology)
peripheral nervous system (neurology)
practical nursing student (education and nursing)

PNSS
Pediatric Nutrition Surveillance System [Centers for Disease Control] (dietary and pediatrics)

PNT
patient
percutaneous nephrostomy tube (nephrology)

PNU
protein nitrogen unit (measurement)

PNV
prenatal vitamins (obstetrics and pharmacology)

Pnx
pneumothorax (cardiovascular and respiratory)

PO
partial pressure of oxygen (laboratory and respiratory)
parieto-occipital (neurology)
period of onset
per os [by mouth, orally] (pharmacology)
phone order
posterior
postoperative (surgery)

P-O
postoperative (surgery)

P.O.
per os [by mouth, orally] (pharmacology)

P & O
parasites and ova (gastroenterology and laboratory)

P/O
phone order

PO$_2$
partial pressure of oxygen [also called *partial tension of oxygen*] (laboratory and respiratory)

pO₂
oxygen pressure (laboratory and respiratory)
partial pressure of oxygen [also called *partial tension of oxygen*] (laboratory and respiratory)

po
per os [by mouth, orally] (pharmacology)

p.o.
per os [by mouth, orally] (pharmacology)

POA
pancreatic oncofetal antigen (gastroenterology and laboratory)
phalangeal osteoarthritis (orthopedics)
point of application
preoptic area (ophthalmology)
primary optic atrophy (ophthalmology)

POACH
prednisone, Oncovin [vincristine], cytosine arabinoside, cyclophosphamide, and Adriamycin (chemotherapy, oncology, and pharmacology)

POAG
primary open-angle glaucoma (ophthalmology)

POB
penicillin, oil beeswax [an antibiotic] (pharmacology)
phenoxybenzamine (cardiovascular and pharmacology)
place of birth (medical records)
prevention of blindness (ophthalmology)

POC
postoperative care (surgery)
products of conception (obstetrics) {pronounced "pock"}
purgeable organic carbon (chemistry)

POCA
Adriamycin, prednisone, cytosine arabinoside, and Oncovin [vincristine] (chemotherapy, oncology, and pharmacology)

POCC
procarbazine, Oncovin [vincristine], CCNU [CeeNU or lomustine], and cyclophosphamide [Cytoxan] (chemotherapy, oncology, and pharmacology)

pocill
pocillum [a small cup] (pharmacology)

"pock"
{pronunciation of *POC* [products of conception]} (obstetrics) {not an abbreviation}

pocul
poculum [cup] (pharmacology)

POD
perioxidase [also called *indirect oxidase*] (laboratory)
place of death (medical records)
podiatry
postoperative day [often followed by an Arabic numeral] (surgery)

pod-
{not an abbreviation} [prefix indicating relationship to the foot] (orthopedics and podiatry) {pronounced "pod"}

"pod"
{pronunciation of *pod-* [prefix indicating relationship to the foot {not an abbreviation}]} (orthopedics and podiatry) {not an abbreviation}

Pod.D.
Doctor of Podiatry (education and podiatry)

podo-
{not an abbreviation} [prefix indicating relationship to the foot] (orthopedics and podiatry) {pronounced "pod-oh"}

"pod-oh"
{pronunciation of *podo-* [prefix indicating relationship to the foot {not an abbreviation}]} (orthopedics and podiatry) {not an abbreviation}

PODx
postoperative diagnosis (surgery)

POE
postoperative endophthalmitis (ophthalmology and surgery)
postoperative exercise (rehabilitation and surgery)

"poe-lee-oh"
{pronunciation of *polio* [slang for *poliomyelitis*] and *polio-* [a prefix indicating relationship to the gray matter of the nervous system {not an abbreviation}]} (infectious diseases, neurology, and orthopedics) {not an abbreviation}

POEMS
plasma cell dyscrasia with polyneuropathy, organomegaly, endocrinopathy, monoclonal protein [M-protein], skin changes (dermatology, endocrinology, gastroenterology, and neurology) {pronounced "poems"}
polyneuropathy, organomegaly, endocrinopathy, monoclonal protein [M-protein], skin changes [syndrome] (dermatology, endocrinology, gastroenterology, and neurology) {pronounced "poems"}

"poems"
{pronunciation of *POEMS* [plasma cell dyscrasia with polyneuropathy, organomegaly, endocrinopathy, monoclonal protein (M-protein), skin changes or polyneuropathy, organomegaly, endocrinopathy, monoclonal protein (M-protein), skin changes (syndrome)]} (dermatology, endocrinology, gastroenterology, and neurology) {not an abbreviation}

POET
pulse oximeter/end tidal [carbon dioxide] (respiratory)

POF
pyruvate oxidation factor (laboratory)

PofE
portal of entry (surgery)
port of entry (immigration and surgery)

pOH
{not an abbreviation} [symbol referring to hydroxyl (OH) concentration or alkalinity of a solution] (chemistry and laboratory)

POHI
physically or otherwise health-impaired (rehabilitation)

POI
Personal Orientation Inventory (psychiatry)
poison (chemistry and laboratory)

poi
{not an abbreviation} [a Hawaiian food] (dietary) {pronounced "poi"}

"poi"
{pronunciation of *poi* [a Hawaiian food {not an abbreviation}]} (dietary) {not an abbreviation}

-poiesis
{not an abbreviation} [suffix meaning *formation*] {pronounced "poi-E-sis"}

"poi-E-sis"
{pronunciation of *-poiesis* [suffix meaning *formation* {not an abbreviation}]} {not an abbreviation}

POIK
poikilocytosis (hematology and laboratory)

poik
poikilocyte (hematology and laboratory)
poikilocytosis (hematology and laboratory)

"poi-kah-low"
{pronunciation of *poikilo-* [prefix meaning *irregular* or *varied* {not an abbreviation}]} {not an abbreviation}

poikilo-
{not an abbreviation} [prefix meaning *irregular* or *varied*] {pronounced "poi-kah-low"}

point A
{not an abbreviation} [also called *sub-spinale;* a radiographic cephalometric landmark] (neurology and radiology)

point Ar
{not an abbreviation} [also called *articulare;* a cephalometric landmark] (neurology)

point B
{not an abbreviation} [also called *submentale;* a radiographic cephalometric landmark] (neurology and radiology)

point Ba
{not an abbreviation} [also called *basion;* a cephalometric landmark] (neurology)

point Bo
Bolton point (neurology and radiology)

point Z
{not an abbreviation} (otorhinolaryngology)

pois
poison (chemistry and laboratory)

POL
premature onset of labor (obstetrics)

pol
polish (dentistry)
{not an abbreviation} [a gene of human T-cell lymphotropic virus III, associated with acquired immunodeficiency syndrome (AIDS)] (genetics, immunology, infectious diseases, laboratory, oncology, and research)

POLE
prednisolone, Oncovin [vincristine], and L-asparaginase (chemotherapy, oncology, and pharmacology)

polio
poliomyelitis (neurology) (slang) {pronounced "poe-lee-oh"}

polio-
{not an abbreviation} [a prefix indicating relationship to the gray matter of the nervous system] (neurology) {pronounced "poe-lee-oh"}

POLL
pollex [inch] (measurement)

poly
polyphagia (endocrinology and gastroenterology) {pronounced "poly"}
polydipsia (endocrinology and otorhinolaryngology) {pronounced "poly"}
polymorphonuclear leukocyte (hematology and laboratory) {pronounced "poly"}
polymorphonuclear neutrophil granulocyte (hematology and laboratory) {pronounced "poly"}
polyuria (endocrinology and urology) {pronounced "poly"}

poly-
{not an abbreviation} [prefix meaning *many* or *much*] {pronounced "poly"}

"poly"
{pronunciation of *poly* [polydysphagia (endocrinology and gastroenterology), polydipsia (endocrinology and otorhinolaryngology), polymorphonuclear leukocyte (hematology and laboratory), polymorphonuclear neutrophil granulocyte (hematology and laboratory), or polyuria (endocrinology and urology)] and *poly-* [prefix meaning many or much {not an abbreviation}]} {not an abbreviation}

poly(A)
polyadenylic acid (genetics and laboratory)

POLYC
polychromasia (hematology and laboratory)

"poly-morff"
{pronunciation of *polymorph* [polymorphonuclear (leukocyte)]} (hematology and laboratory) {not an abbreviation}

"poly-morffs"
{pronunciation of *polymorphs* [polymorphonuclear (leukocytes)]} (hematology and laboratory) {not an abbreviation}

polymorph
polymorphonuclear [leukocyte] (hematology and laboratory) {pronounced "poly-morff"}

polymorphs
polymorphonuclear [leukocytes] (hematology and laboratory) {pronounced "poly-morffs"}

POLYS
polymorphonuclear leukocytes (hematology and laboratory) {pronounced "polyz"}

%POLPS
percent of polymorphonuclear leukocytes (hematology and laboratory)

polys
polymorphonuclear leukocytes (hematology and laboratory) {pronounced "polyz"}

polys (segs)
polymorphonuclear segmented neutrophils (hematology and laboratory) {pronounced "polyz-segz"}

poly(U)
polyuridylic acid (genetics and laboratory)

"polyz"
{pronunciation of *POLYS* and *polys* [polymorphonuclear leukocytes]} (hematology and laboratory) {not an abbreviation}

"polyz-segz"
{pronunciation of *polys (segs)* [polymorphonuclear segmented neutrophils]} (hematology and laboratory) {not an abbreviation}

POMC
propriomelanocortin (pharmacology)

POMP
prednisolone, vincristine (Oncovin), methotrexate, and 6-mercaptopurine (chemotherapy, oncology, and pharmacology) {pronounced "pomp"}
prednisone, vincristine (Oncovin), methotrexate, and 6-mercaptopurine (chemotherapy, oncology, and pharmacology) {pronounced "pomp"}

POMP-24
6-mercaptopurine, Oncovin [vincristine], high-dose methotrexate, and prednisone (chemotherapy, oncology, and pharmacology) {pronounced "pomp-twen-tee-four"}

"pomp"
{pronunciation of *POMP* [prednisolone, vincristine (Oncovin), methotrexate, and 6-mercaptopurine or prednisone, vincristine (Oncovin), methotrexate, and 6-mercaptopurine]} (chemotherapy, oncology, and pharmacology) {not an abbreviation}

"pomp-twen-tee-four"
{pronunciation of *POMP-24* [6-mercaptopurine, Oncovin vincristine, high-dose methotrexate, and prednisone]} (chemotherapy, oncology, and pharmacology) {not an abbreviation}

POMR
problem-oriented medical record (medical records)

PON
particulate organic nitrogen (chemistry and laboratory)

pond
pondere [by weight] (pharmacology)

POOR
poor clot (hematology and laboratory)

"poorp"
{pronunciation of *PORP* [partial ossicular replacement prosthesis]} (otorhinolaryngology) {not an abbreviation}

"poo-vah"
{pronunciation of *PUVA* [psoralens and ultraviolet A (regimen or therapy for psoriasis)]} (dermatology) {not an abbreviation}

POP
paroxypropione (laboratory)
persistent occiputoposterior [also called *persistent occiput posterior (position)*] (obstetrics)
plasma oncotic pressure (hematology, laboratory, and oncology)
plasma osmotic pressure (hematology and laboratory)
plaster of paris (orthopedics) {pronounced "pop"}
popliteal (orthopedic, radiology)

P.O.P.
paroxypropione (laboratory)

POp
postoperative (surgery)

Pop
popliteal (cardiovascular, neurology, and orthopedics)
population (statistics)

pop
popliteal (cardiovascular, neurology, and orthopedics)
popular

"pop"
{pronunciation of *POP* [plaster of paris]} (orthopedics) {not an abbreviation}

poplit
popliteal (cardiovascular, neurology, and orthopedics)

POPOP
1,4-bis-(5-phenoxazole) benzene (laboratory)
p-bis[2-(5-phenyloxazolyl)]-benzene (laboratory)

POR
physician of record (administration and medical records)
problem-oriented record (medical records)

PORP
partial ossicular replacement prosthesis (otorhinolaryngology) {pronounced "poorp"}

PORPH
porphyrins (laboratory)

PORT
postoperative respiratory therapy (respiratory and surgery)

port
portable

POS
parosteal osteosarcoma (oncology and orthopedics)
polycystic ovarian syndrome (gynecology)
positive {pronounced "pause"}

pos
position
positive {pronounced "pause"}

POSC
Problem-Oriented System of Charting (medical records)

POSG
after glucose infusion started (laboratory)

POSM
patient-operated selector mechanism

Posmo
osmotic permeability (laboratory)

pos pr
positive pressure (respiratory)

POSS
possible
proximal over-shoulder strap (orthopedics)

poss
possible

post
posterior
post mortem [autopsy] (pathology)

postgangl
postganglionic (neurology and neurosurgery)

post-op
postoperative (surgery) {pronounced "post-op"}

"post-op"
{pronunciation of *post-op* [postoperative]} (surgery) {not an abbreviation}

POSTS
positive occipital sharp transients of sleep [on electroencephalogram] (neurology) {pronounced "posts"}

"posts"
{pronunciation of *POSTS* [positive occipital sharp transients of sleep (on electroencephalogram)]} (neurology) {not an abbreviation}

post. sag. D
posterior sagittal diameter (neurology and radiology)

post sing sed liq
post singulas sedes liquidas [after every loose stool] (gastroenterology and pharmacology)

post sing. sed. liq.
post singulas sedes liquidas [after every loose stool] (gastroenterology and pharmacology)

POT
potential (occupational therapy and rehabilitation)
potus [a drink] (pharmacology)

pot
potassa [also called *potassium hydrochloride*] (pharmacology)
potassium (chemistry, laboratory, and pharmacology)
potential (occupational therapy and rehabilitation)
potion (pharmacology)

{not an abbreviation} [slang for marijuana] (chemical dependency and law enforcement) [*Note: This is an illicit drug.*]

potass
potassium (chemistry, laboratory, and pharmacology)

POU
placenta, ovary, uterus (obstetrics)

POW
Powassan encephalitis (neurology)
prisoner of war (armed forces and psychiatry)

powd
powder (pharmacology)

POX-AC
pox battery, acute (laboratory)

PP
pancreatic polypeptide (endocrinology, gastroenterology, and laboratory)
paradoxical pulse (cardiovascular)
partial pressure (laboratory and respiratory)
pellagra preventive (dermatology, dietary, neurology, and psychiatry)
perfusion pressure (cardiovascular)
permanent partial [denture] (dentistry)
pink puffers [referring to emphysema] (respiratory)
pinpoint [pupils] (neurology and ophthalmology)
pin prick (neurology)
placental protein (laboratory and obstetrics)
Planned Parenthood (gynecology and obstetrics)
plasma protein (laboratory)
plethysmograph pressure (measurement)
Population Planning (government, gynecology, obstetrics, social services, and urology)
posterior pituitary (endocrinology and neurosurgery)

post partum [also called *postpartum*]
(gynecology and obstetrics)
postprandial (gastroenterology and laboratory)
private patient
private practice
prothrombin-proconvertin (hematology and laboratory)
protoporphyria (multiple specialties)
protoporphyrin (laboratory and multiple specialties)
proximal phalanx (orthopedics and podiatry)
pulse pressure (cardiovascular)
punctum proximum [near point of accommodation] (ophthalmology)
pyrophosphate (chemistry and radiology)

P & P
pins and plaster (orthopedics)
prothrombin and proconvertin [test] (hematology and laboratory)

pp
punctum proximum [near point of accommodation] (ophthalmology)

p.p.
punctum proximum [near point of accommodation] (ophthalmology)

p̅p̅
postprandial (gastroenterology)

PPA
phenylpropanolamine (allergy, gastroenterology, neurology, otorhinolaryngology, pharmacology, and respiratory)
phenylpyruvic acid (laboratory)
Pittsburgh pneumonia agent (laboratory and respiratory)
Population Planning Associates (gynecology, obstetrics, and urology)
postpartum amenorrhea (gynecology and obstetrics)

P$_{PA}$
pulmonary artery pressure (cardiovascular and respiratory)

PP & A
percussion, palpation, and auscultation (respiratory)

ppa
phiala prius agitate [the bottle having first been shaken] (pharmacology)

p.p.a.
phiala prius agitate [the bottle having first been shaken] (pharmacology)

pp & a
palpation, percussion, and auscultation (respiratory)

PPA pos
phenylpyruvic acid positive (laboratory)

PPB
parts per billion (measurement)
platelet-poor blood (hematology and laboratory)
positive pressure breathing (respiratory)

ppb
parts per billion (measurement)

PPBS
postprandial blood sugar (endocrinology and laboratory)

PPC
progressive patient care
proximal palmar crease (neurology and orthopedics)

PPCA
plasma prothrombin conversion accelerator (hematology and laboratory)

PPCF
plasma prothrombin conversion factor (hematology and laboratory)

P & P/CT
prothrombin and proconvertin control (hematology and laboratory)

PPD
packs per day [of cigarettes] (cardiovas-

cular, chemical dependency, and respiratory)

paraphenylenediamine [a dye] (laboratory)

percussion and postural drainage (respiratory)

permanent partial disability (neurology, orthopedics, and rehabilitation)

posterior polymorphous dystrophy (neurology)

postpartum day [often followed by an Arabic numeral] (obstetrics)

progressive perceptive deafness (otorhinolaryngology)

purified protein derivative [test for tuberculosis] (infectious diseases, laboratory, and respiratory)

P.P.D.
purified protein derivative [of tuberculin] (laboratory and respiratory)

P & PD
percussion and postural drainage (respiratory)

ppd
prepared

PPD-B
purified protein derivative, Battey [tuberculin] (laboratory and respiratory)

PPDC
Perfusion Program Directors Council (cardiovascular)

PPD-S
purified protein derivative, standard [tuberculin] (laboratory and respiratory)

PPE
porcine pancreatic elastase (laboratory)

PPF
pellagra preventive factor [also called *niacinamide*] (dermatology, dietary, laboratory, neurology, and psychiatry)

plasma protein fraction (laboratory)

P.P.F.
phagocytosis promoting factor (immunology and laboratory)

PPFA
Planned Parenthood Federation of America (gynecology, obstetrics, social services, and urology)

P.-P. factor
pellagra preventive factor [also called *niacinamide*] (dermatology, dietary, laboratory, neurology, and psychiatry)

PPG
pediatric pneumogram (pediatrics, radiology, and respiratory)

photoplethysmography (measurement)

ppg
picopicogram (measurement, radiation therapy, and radiology)

PPGF
polypeptide growth factor (endocrinology and laboratory)

PPH
postpartum hemorrhage (obstetrics)

primary pulmonary hypertension (cardiovascular and respiratory)

protocollagen proline hydroxylase (laboratory)

PPHN
persistent pulmonary hypertension of the neonate [formerly called *persistent fetal circulation (PFC)*] (cardiovascular neonatology, and respiratory)

PPHP
pseudo-pseudohypoparathyroidism (endocrinology)

PPI
patient package insert (pharmacology)

PPL
pars planus lensectomy (ophthalmology)

penicilloylpolylysine (allergy and laboratory) [Note: Used in skin testing to ascertain allergy to penicillin.]

protein-polysaccharide (laboratory)

Ppl
intrapleural pressure (laboratory and respiratory)

PPLO
pleuropneumonia-like organism(s) (laboratory and respiratory)

PPM
parts per million (measurement)
permanent pacemaker (cardiovascular)
phosphopentomutase (laboratory)
posterior papillary muscle [image on transesophageal echocardiography] (cardiovascular)

ppm
parts per million (measurement)
pulse per minute (measurement)

PPMD
posterior polymorphous dystrophy of the cornea (ophthalmology)

PPN
peripheral parenteral nutrition (dietary and gastroenterology)

PPNA
peak phrenic nerve activity (neurology)

PPNG
penicillinase-producing *Neisseria gonorrhoeae* (laboratory)

PPO
2,5-diphenyloxazole (laboratory)
platelet peroxidase (laboratory)
pleuropneumonia organism(s) (laboratory and respiratory)
preferred-provider organization (insurance)

PPP
passage, power, and passenger [evaluation of labor progress] (obstetrics)
pentose phosphate pathway (laboratory)
piss-poor protoplasm (laboratory) [slang]
platelet-poor plasma (hematology and laboratory)
polyphoretic phosphate (laboratory)
postpartum psychosis (obstetrics and psychiatry)

PPPBL
peripheral pulses palpable, both legs (cardiovascular and orthopedics)

PPPG
postprandial plasma glucose (endocrinology and laboratory)

PPPI
primary private practice income

PPR
Price precipitation reaction (laboratory)

PPROM
prolonged premature rupture of membranes (obstetrics)

PPRWP
poor precordial R-wave progression (cardiovascular)

PPS
pepsin A [an enzyme] (gastroenterology and laboratory)
Personal Preference Scale (psychiatry)
polyvalance pneumococcal polysaccharides [vaccine for patients with splenectomies] (gastroenterology, immunology, pharmacology, and surgery)
postpartum sterilization (gynecology and obstetrics)
postperfusion syndrome (cardiovascular)
postpump syndrome (cardiovascular)
Prausnitz-Kustner sclerosis [scleroderma] (rheumatology)

PPSB
prothrombin, proconvertin, Stuart factor, antihemophilic B factor (hematology and laboratory)

PPT
partial thromboplastin time (hematology and laboratory)
plant protease test (laboratory)

ppt
precipitate prepared (laboratory)
prepared

pptd
precipitated

PPTL
postpartum tubal ligation (gynecology
and obstetrics)

pptn
precipitation

P. pulmonale
pulmonary pulmonale (cardiovascular)
{pronounced "pea-pull-mon-alley"}

PPV
positive-pressure ventilation (respiratory)

PPVT
Peabody Picture Vocabulary Test (pediatrics, psychiatry, and speech and language therapy)

PQ
permeability quotient (laboratory)
pronator quadratus [muscle] (orthopedics)
pyrimethamine-quinine [antimalarial
therapy] (infectious diseases, pharmacology, and respiratory)

PQNS
protein, quantity not sufficient (laboratory)

PR
Panama red [type of marijuana] (chemical dependency and law enforcement)
[*Note: This is an illicit drug.*]
parallax and refraction (ophthalmology)
partial remission
partial response
patient relations
peer review (administration)
pelvic rock (orthopedics)
percentile rank (statistics)
perfusion rate (cardiovascular)
peripheral resistance (cardiovascular)
per rectum [through the rectum] (gastroenterology and pharmacology)
phenol red [also called *phenolsulphon-
phthalein*; used in tests of renal func-
tion] (chemistry, laboratory, and nephrology)

pityriasis rosea (dermatology)
posterior repair (gynecology and surgery)
predicted rate (cardiovascular and respiratory)
pregnancy rate (obstetrics)
pressoreceptor (laboratory)
pressure
prevention
proctologist (gastroenterology)
production rate (laboratory)
profile
progesterone receptor [assay] (gynecology, laboratory, and oncology)
progressive resistance
prolactin (laboratory)
prosthetic-group removing [enzyme]
(laboratory)
prosthion (dentistry)
protein (dietary and laboratory)
public relations (business)
Puerto Rican [national origin]
Puerto Rico [Postal Service designation]
pulmonic regurgitation (cardiovascular)
pulse rate (cardiovascular)
punctum remotum [far point of ac-
commodation] (ophthalmology)

P-R
Philips Roxane [pharmaceutical com-
pany] (pharmacology)
{not an abbreviation} [P-R interval on
electrocardiogram] (cardiovascular)

P & R
pelvic and rectal [examinations] (gastroenterology, gynecology, and obstetrics)
pulse and respiration (cardiovascular
and respiratory)

Pr
presbyopia (ophthalmology)
presentation
pressure (cardiovascular and respiratory)
prism (ophthalmology)
prolactin (laboratory)
propyl (chemistry and laboratory)

pr
pair
per rectum [through the rectum] (gastroenterology and pharmacology)
punctum remotum [far point of accommodation] (ophthalmology)

p.r.
per rectum [through the rectum] (gastroenterology and pharmacology)
punctum remotum [far point of accommodation] (ophthalmology)

PRA
plasma renin activity (laboratory)
progesterone receptor assay (endocrinology, gynecology, laboratory, oncology, and surgery)

prac
practice

PRACT
practitioner

pract
practical

prand
prandium [dinner]

PRAS
prereduced anaerobically sterilized [media] (laboratory)

PRAT
platelet radioactive antiglobulin test (hematology and laboratory)

p rat aetat
pro ratione aetatis [in proportion to age] (pharmacology)

p. rat. aetat.
pro ratione aetatis [in proportion to age] (pharmacology)

PRB
Personal Reaction Blank (psychiatry)
Prosthetics Research Board (orthopedics and research)

P.R.B.
Population Reference Bureau

Prosthetics Research Board (orthopedics and research)

PRBC
packed red blood cells (hematology)

PRBV
placental residual blood volume (obstetrics)

PRC
packed red cells (hematology)
plasma renin concentration (laboratory)

PRCA
pure red cell agenesis (hematology and laboratory)
pure red cell aplasia (hematology and laboratory)

PRD
partial reaction of degeneration (chemistry and laboratory)
postradiation dysplasia (oncology and radiation therapy)

PRE
photoreactivity (laboratory)
physical reconditioning exercises (orthopedics and rehabilitation)
progressive resistive exercise [also called *progressive resistance exercise*] (rehabilitation)

P.R.E.
progressive resistive exercise [also called *progressive resistance exercise*] (rehabilitation)

Pre
preliminary (laboratory and radiology)

pre
preliminary (laboratory and radiology)
preoperative(ly) (surgery) {pronounced "pre"}

"pre"
{pronunciation of *pre* [preoperative(ly)]} (surgery) {not an abbreviation}

p rec
per rectum [through the rectum] (gastroenterology and pharmacology)

precip
precipitate (laboratory)
precipitation

PRED
prednisone (pharmacology) {pronounced "pred"}

PreD$_3$
previtamin D$_3$ [a precursor to vitamin D$_3$ (cholecalciferol)] (laboratory)

pred
predicted
prednisone (pharmacology) {pronounced "pred"}

"pred"
{pronunciation of *PRED* and *pred* [prednisone]} *(pharmacology)* {not an abbreviation}

prefd
preferred

preg
pregnant (obstetrics)

pregang
preganglionic (neurology)

pregn
pregnant (obstetrics)

prelim
preliminary (laboratory and radiology) {pronounced "pre-lim"}

"pre-lim"
{pronunciation of *prelim* [preliminary]} (laboratory and radiology) {not an abbreviation}

prelim diag
preliminary diagnosis

prem
premature (neonatology, obstetrics, and pediatrics)

premature [infant] (neonatology, obstetrics, and pediatrics)

"pre-me"
{pronunciation of *premie* [premature (infant)]} (neonatology, obstetrics, and pediatrics) {not an abbreviation}

premie
premature [infant] (neonatology, obstetrics, and pediatrics) {pronounced "pre-me"}

preop
preoperative(ly) (surgery) {pronounced "pre-op"}

"pre-op"
{pronunciation of *preop* [preoperative(ly)]} (surgery) {not an abbreviation}

prep
preparation (pharmacology and surgery) {pronounced "prep"}
preparatory
prepare (surgery) {pronounced "prep"}
prepared (surgery) {pronounced "prep"}

"prep"
{pronunciation of *prep* [preparation (pharmacology and surgery), prepare (surgery), and prepared (surgery)]} {not an abbreviation}

prepd
prepared (surgery)

prepn
preparation (pharmacology and surgery)

prepped
prepared (surgery) {pronounced "prep-tah"}

"prep-tah"
{pronunciation of *prepped* [prepared]} (surgery) {not an abbreviation}

PRERLA
pupils round, equal, and reactive to light and accommodation (ophthalmology)

PRES
presence (laboratory)
present (laboratory)

PREs
progressive resistive exercises (orthopedics and rehabilitation)

preserv
preservation
preserve

Press
pressure

press
pressure {pronounced "press"}

"press"
{pronunciation of *press* [pressure]} {not an abbreviation}

prev
prevent
preventive
prevention
previous

PrevMed
preventive medicine

PREVMEDU
Preventive Medicine Unit

pre-voc
prevocational (education)

PRF
partial reinforcement
pontine reticular formation (neurology)
prolactin-releasing factor (laboratory)

PRFM
prolonged rupture of fetal membranes (obstetrics)

PRG
phleborrheogram (hematology and laboratory)
purge (pharmacology)

PRH
prolactin-releasing hormone (laboratory)

PRHBF
peak reactive hyperemia blood flow (cardiovascular)

PRI
phosphoriboseisomerase [an enzyme; also called *ribose-5-phosphate isomerase*] (laboratory)
P-R interval [on electrocardiogram] (cardiovascular)

PRIH
prolactin-releasing inhibiting hormone (laboratory)

PRIME
procarbazine, ifosfamide, and methotrexate (chemotherapy, oncology, and pharmacology)

"prime-ip"
{pronunciation of *primip* [primipara]} (obstetrics) {not an abbreviation}

primip
primipara (obstetrics) {pronounced "prime-ip"}

prim luc
prima luc [early in the morning]

prim m
primo mane [early in the morning]

PRIMP
primipara (obstetrics)

prin
principal

P-R interval
{not an abbreviation} [a portion of an electrocardiogram] (cardiovascular)

PRIST
paper radioimmunosorbent test (immu-

nology and laboratory) {pronounced "prist"}

"prist"
{pronunciation of *PRIST* [paper radioim-munosorbent test]} (immunology and laboratory) {not an abbreviation}

priv
private

PRL
prolactin (laboratory)

PRM
phosphoribomutase (laboratory)
photoreceptor membrane (laboratory)
premature rupture of membranes (obstetrics)
preventive medicine
Primary Reference Material (library science)

PRM-SDX
pyrimethamine-sulfadoxine (pharmacology)

PRN
Physicians Radio Network (communications)
pro re nata [as needed, as required, whenever necessary] (pharmacology)

prn
pro re nata [as needed, as required, whenever necessary] (pharmacology)

p.r.n.
pro re nata [as needed, as required, whenever necessary] (pharmacology)

PRO
pronation (neurology and orthopedics)
protein (dietary and laboratory)

P.R.O.
Peer Review Organization (administration)

Pro
proline [an amino acid] (laboratory)
pronation (neurology and orthopedics)
protein (dietary and laboratory)

prothrombin (hematology and laboratory)

Prob.
probable

prob
probability
probable
probably
problem

proc
procedure (surgery)
proceeding
process

PROCAN
Procan [also called *procainamide*] (cardiovascular and pharmacology)

Procarb
procarbazine (chemotherapy, oncology, and pharmacology) {pronounced "pro-carb"}

"pro-carb"
{pronunciation of *Procarb* [procarbazine]} (chemotherapy, oncology, and pharmacology) {not an abbreviation}

procs
proceedings

proct
proctologist (gastroenterology)
proctology (gastroenterology)

PROCTO
proctology (gastroenterology) {pronounced "prok-toe"}
proctoscopy (gastroenterology) {pronounced "prok-toe"}

procto
proctology (gastroenterology) {pronounced "prok-toe"}
proctoscopy (gastroenterology) {pronounced "prok-toe"}

prod
product
production (laboratory)

PRO EL
protein electrophoresis (laboratory)

Prof
professor (education)

prof
profession(al)

prog
progesterone (endocrinology, gynecology, laboratory, obstetrics, and pharmacology)
prognathism (dentistry and otorhinolaryngology)
prognosis
program
progress
progressive

progn
prognosis

prog note
progress note (medical records)

progr
progress

proj
project

"prok-toe"
{pronunciation of *PROCTO* and *procto* [proctology and proctoscopy]} (gastroenterology) {not an abbreviation}

PROLAC
prolactin (laboratory)

prolong
prolongatus [prolonged] {pronounced "pro-long"}

"pro-long"
{pronunciation of *prolong* [*prolongatus*, prolonged]} {not an abbreviation}

PROM
passive range of motion (neurology, or-

thopedics, and rehabilitation) {pronounced "prom"}
premature rupture of membranes (obstetrics) {pronounced "prom"}
prolonged rupture of membranes (obstetrics) {pronounced "prom"}

P-ROM
passive range of motion (neurology, orthopedics, and rehabilitation) {pronounced "prom"}

"prom"
{pronunciation of *PROM* and *P-ROM* [passive range of motion (neurology, orthopedics, and rehabilitation)] and *PROM* [premature rupture of membranes (obstetrics) and prolonged rupture of membranes (obstetrics)]} {not an abbreviation}

PRO-MACE
Adriamycin, cyclophosphamide, methotrexate, prednisone, and VP-16 (chemotherapy, oncology, and pharmacology) {pronounced "pro-mace"}

"pro-mace"
{pronunciation of *PRO-MACE* [Adriamycin, cyclophosphamide, methotrexate, prednisone, and VP-16]} (chemotherapy, oncology, and pharmacology) {not an abbreviation}

pron
pronation (orthopedics)

proph
prophylactic

prophy
prophylactic

pro rect
pro recto [by rectum] (gastroenterology and pharmacology)

pros
prostate (anatomy and urology)
prosthetic (orthopedics)

PROSO
protamine sulfate (cardiovascular, hematology, and laboratory)

prosth
prosthesis (orthopedics)

Prot
Protestant (religion)

prot
protein (chemistry, dietary, and laboratory)

protime
prothrombin time (hematology and laboratory) {pronounced "pro-time"}

pro time
prothrombin time (hematology and laboratory) {pronounced "pro-time"}

"pro-time"
{pronunciation of *protime* and *pro time* [prothrombin time]} (hematology and laboratory) {not an abbreviation}

PROTO
protoporphyrin (laboratory and multiple specialties)

prov
provisional [diagnosis]

PROVIMI
proteins, vitamins, and minerals (pharmacology)

prox
proximal

PRO-XAN
protein-xanthophyll (laboratory)

prox luc
proxima luce [the day before]

PRP
panretinal photocoagulation (endocrinology and ophthalmology)
pityriasis rubra pilaris (dermatology)
platelet-rich plasma (hematology and laboratory)

polymer of ribose phosphate (laboratory)
polyribose ribitol phosphate (laboratory)
pressure rate product
progressive rubella panencephalitis (infectious diseases and neurology)
proliferative retinopathy photocoagulation [laser] (ophthalmology)
Psychotic Reaction Profile (psychiatry)
pulse repetition frequency (respiratory)

PRPP
5-phosphoribosyl-1-pyrophosphate [also called *phosphoribosylpyrophosphate*] (laboratory)

PRRE
pupils round, regular, equal (neurology and ophthalmology)

PR-RSV
Prague strain Rous sarcoma virus (laboratory and oncology)

PRS
Personality Rating Scale (psychiatry)

PRSs
positive rolandic spikes (neurology)

PRT
pharmaceutical research and testing (pharmacology and research)
phosphoribosyl transferase (laboratory)

PRTH
prothrombin time (hematology and laboratory)

PRTH-C
prothrombin time control (hematology and laboratory)

PRU
peripheral resistance unit (cardiovascular)

PRV
polycythemia vera (hematology)

pseudorabies virus (infectious diseases and laboratory)

PRVEP
pattern reversal visual evoked potentials (neurology)

PRW
polymerized ragweed (allergy)

PRWP
poor R-wave progression [on electrocardiogram] (cardiovascular)

PRZF
pyrazofurin (chemotherapy, oncology, and pharmacology)

PS
chloropicrin [a gas] (armed forces and chemistry)
paradoxical sleep (neurology)
pathological stage (pathology)
patient's serum (laboratory)
pediatric surgery (pediatrics and surgery)
perceptual speed [test] (rehabilitation)
performance status (rehabilitation)
performing scale (rehabilitation)
periodic syndrome
phosphate saline [buffer] (laboratory)
phosphatidyl serine (laboratory)
photosystems
physical status
plastic surgery (plastic surgery)
point of symmetry
population sample (statistics)
Porter-Silber [chromogen] (endocrinology and laboratory)
postscript
postscriptum [postscript]
power supply
prescription (pharmacology)
psychiatric (psychiatry)
psychiatry
public school (education)
pulmonary [artery] stenosis (cardiovascular and respiratory)
pyloric stenosis (gastroenterology)
serum from a pregnant woman (laboratory and obstetrics)

P/S
polyunsaturated/saturated [fatty acid ratio] (cardiovascular and laboratory)

P.S.
postscript
postscriptum [postscript]

P & S
pain and suffering
paracentesis and suction (thoracic surgery)
Physicians and Surgeons

Ps
prescription [referring to drugs requiring a prescription] (pharmacology)
Pseudomonas [a bacterium] (laboratory)

ps
picosecond (measurement)
pseudo [a word meaning a sham or spurious] [slang]
pseudo- [a prefix meaning false or spurious]

p.s.
per second (measurement)

PSA
polyethylene sulfonic acid (chemistry)
prolonged sleep apnea (neurology)
prostate-specific antigen (endocrinology, laboratory, and urology)

PsA
psoriatic arthritis (orthopedics and rheumatology)

PSAn
psychoanalysis (psychiatry)
psychoanalyst (psychiatry)
psychoanalytic (psychiatry)
psychoanalytical (psychiatry)

PSB
phosphorus-solubilizing bacteria (laboratory)
protected specimen brush (laboratory and surgery)

PSC
Porter-Silber chromogen (endocrinology and laboratory)
posterior subcapsular cataract [extraction] (ophthalmology)
primary sclerosing cholangitis (gastroenterology)
pulse synchronized contractions (neurology)

PSCE
presurgical coagulation evaluation (hematology, laboratory, and surgery)

PSCP
posterior subcapsular cataractous plaque (ophthalmology)

PSD
peptone-starch-dextrose (laboratory)

PSE
point of subjective equality
portal systemic encephalopathy (gastroenterology and neurology)

psec
picosecond (measurement)

PSF
posterior spinal fusion (neurology and orthopedics)
pseudosarcomatous fasciitis (neurology and orthopedics)

PSG
peak systolic gradient (cardiovascular)
phosphate-saline-glucose [buffer] (laboratory)
polysomnogram (neurology)
presystolic gallop (cardiovascular)

PSGN
poststreptococcal glomerulonephritis (nephrology)

PSH
postspinal [anesthetic] headache (anesthesiology and neurology)

PSI
posterior sagittal index (neonatology and radiology)

pounds per square inch (measurement) {pronounced "sigh"}
Problem Solving Information [apparatus]
psychosomatic inventory (psychiatry)

PS I
American Society of Anesthesiologists' physical status patient classification for a healthy patient with localized pathological process (anesthesiology) [Note: Emergency operations are designated by an "E" after the classification.]

psi
pounds per square inch (measurement) {pronounced "sigh"}

p.s.i.
pounds per square inch (measurement) {pronounced "sigh"}

psia
pounds per square inch absolute (measurement)

psig
pounds per square inch gauge (measurement)

PS II
American Society of Anesthesiologists' physical status patient classification for a patient with mild to moderate systemic disease (anesthesiology) [Note: Emergency operations are designated by an "E" after the classification.]

PS III
American Society of Anesthesiologists' physical status patient classification for a patient with severe systemic disease limiting activity but not incapacitating (anesthesiology) [Note: Emergency operations are designated by an "E" after the classification.]

PSIL
preferred-frequency speech interference

level (otorhinolaryngology and speech and language therapy)

PSIS
posterior sacroiliac spine (anatomy and orthopedics)
posterior superior iliac spine [also called *posterosuperior iliac spine*] (anatomy and orthopedics)

PS IV
American Society of Anesthesiologists' physical status patient classification for a patient with incapacitating systemic disease (anesthesiology) [*Note: Emergency operations are designated by an "E" after the classification.*]

PSL
parasternal line (anatomy, cardiovascular, and respiratory)

PSL sol
potassium, sodium chloride, sodium lactate solution (pharmacology)

PSM
pansystolic murmur (cardiovascular)
presystolic murmur (cardiovascular)

PSMA
progressive spinal muscular atrophy (neurology and orthopedics)

PSMed
Psychosomatic Medicine

P sol
partly soluble (chemistry)

PSP
pace-setting potential (cardiovascular)
pancreatic spasmolytic peptide (gastroenterology and laboratory)
parathyroid secretory protein (endocrinology and laboratory)
periodic short pulse
Personal Security Preview (psychiatry)
phenolsulfonphthalein [also called *phenol red*; used in tests of renal function] (chemistry, laboratory, and nephrology)

positive spike pattern [on electroencephalograms] (neurology)
postsynaptic potential (neurosurgery)
progressive supranuclear palsy (neurology)
pseudopregnancy (gynecology and obstetrics)

P.S.P.
phenolsulfonphthalein [also called *phenol red*; used in tests of renal function] (chemistry, laboratory, and nephrology)

psp
posterior subcapsular plaque (ophthalmology)
postsynaptic potential (neurology)

PSR
extrahepatic portal systemic resistance (cardiovascular and gastroenterology)
pain sensitivity range (neurology)
pulmonary stretch receptors (laboratory and respiratory)

PSRBOW
premature spontaneous rupture of bag of waters (obstetrics)

PSR-BOW
premature spontaneous rupture of bag of waters (obstetrics)

PSRC
Plastic Surgery Research Council (plastic surgery and research)

PSRO
Professional Standards Review Organization (administration)

P.S.R.O.
Professional Standards Review Organization (administration)

PSS
physiological saline solution [0.9% sodium chloride] (pharmacology and surgery)

progressive systemic sclerosis [sclero-
derma] (rheumatology)
Psychiatric Services Section [of American Hospital Association] (psychiatry)

PST
paroxysmal supraventricular tachycardia (cardiovascular)
Pascal-Suttle Test (psychiatry)
penicillin, streptomycin, and tetracycline (pharmacology)
poststimulus time (neurology)

Pst
static transpulmonary pressure at a specific lung volume (laboratory and respiratory)

PSTN
Public Switch Telephone Network (communications)

PstTLC/TLC
coefficient of lung retraction expressed
per liter of total lung capacity (laboratory and respiratory)

P'STYL
Pronestyl [also called *procainamide*]
(cardiovascular and pharmacology)

PSU
postsurgical unit (surgery)

P-SURG
presurgery coagulation profile (hematology and surgery)

PSurg
plastic surgery

PSV
pressure support ventilation (respiratory)
psychological, social, and vocational
[adjustment factors] (psychiatry)

PS V
American Society of Anesthesiologists'
physical status patient classification
for a moribund patient not expected
to live (anesthesiology) [*Note: Emergency operations are designated by
an "E" after the classification.*]

PSVT
paroxysmal supraventricular tachycardia (cardiovascular)

PSW
Psychiatric Social Worker (psychiatry
and social services)

P.S.W.
Psychiatric Social Worker (psychiatry
and social services)

PSWT
Psychiatric Social Work Training [Brit-
ish] (psychiatry and social services)

Psy
psychiatry {pronounced "sigh"}

psych
psychology (psychology) {pronounced
"sighk"}

PSYCHEM
psychiatric chemistry (chemistry, pharmacology, and psychiatry) {pro-
nounced "sigh-kem"}

psychiat
psychiatric (psychiatry)
psychiatry

psycho
psychopath (psychiatry) {pronounced
"sigh-co"}

psychoan
psychoanalysis (psychiatry) {pro-
nounced "sigh-co-an"}

psychol
psychology (psychiatry) {pronounced
"sigh-call"}

psychopathol
psychopathological (psychiatry)
psychopathology (psychiatry)

psychophys
psychophysics (psychiatry) {pronounced
"sigh-co-fizz"}

psychophysiol
psychophysiology (psychiatry) {pro-
nounced "sigh-co-fizz"}

psychophysiol
psychophysiology (psychiatry)

PsychosMed
psychosomatic medicine (psychiatry)
{pronounced "sigh-coz-med"}

psychother
psychotherapy (psychiatry) {pronounced
"sigh-co-ther"}

psy-path
psychopath (psychiatry) {pronounced
"sigh-path"}
psychopathic (psychiatry) {pronounced
"sigh-path"}

psy-som
psychosomatic (psychiatry) {pro-
nounced "sigh-som"}

PT
parathyroid (endocrinology)
paroxysmal tachycardia (cardiovascular)
patient
permanent and total [disability] (government, neurology, and orthopedics)
pharmacy and therapeutics (pharmacology, physical therapy, and rehabilitation)
phenytoin (pharmacology)
phototoxicity
physical therapy
physical training (physical therapy and
sports medicine)
physiotherapy (physical therapy)
pine tar (chemistry, laboratory, and
pharmacology)
pint (measurement)
pneumothorax (respiratory)
polyvalent tolerance (laboratory)
posterior tibial [artery or pulse] (cardiovascular)
pronator teres [muscle] (orthopedics)
propylthiouracil (chemotherapy, oncology, and pharmacology)
prothrombin time (hematology and laboratory)
pulmonary tuberculosis (infectious diseases and respiratory)
pyramidal tract (neurology)

serum glutamic pyruvic transaminase
[SGPT] (cardiovascular, gastroenterology, and laboratory)

P.T.
Physical Therapist (physical therapy and
rehabilitation)
physical therapy

1 PT
one pint (measurement)

Pt
patient
platinum (chemistry)

pt
part
patient
perstetur [let it be continued] (pharmacology)
pint (measurement)
point

PTA
Parent Teacher Association (education)
percutaneous transluminal angioplasty
(cardiovascular)
persistent truncus arteriosus (cardiovascular, neonatology, and pediatrics)
phosphotungstic acid (laboratory)
physical therapy assistant (physical
therapy)
plasma thromboplastin antecedent [Fac-
tor XI] (hematology and laboratory)
posterior tibial [pulse] (cardiovascular
and orthopedics)
posttraumatic amnesia (psychiatry)
pretreatment anxiety (psychiatry)
prior to admission
prior to arrival
pure tone average (otorhinolaryngology)

P.T.A.
prior to admission

PT (A)
pure tone (average) (otorhinolaryngology)

PTAH
phosphotungstic acid hematoxylin (laboratory)

PTAP
purified [diphtheria] toxoid precipitated by aluminum phosphate (infectious diseases and pharmacology)

p'tase
phosphatase (laboratory) {pronounced "pea-tace"}

PTB
patellar tendon bearing [cast, orthosis, or prosthesis] (orthopedics)
prior to birth (neonatology and obstetrics)

PTBD
percutaneous transhepatic biliary drainage (gastroenterology)

PTBD-EF
percutaneous transhepatic biliary drainage - enteric feeding (dietary and gastroenterology)

PTC
percutaneous transhepatic cholangiogram (gastroenterology and radiology)
phenylthiocarbamide [also called *phenylthiourea*] (chemistry, genetics, and laboratory)
phenylthiocarbamoyl (laboratory)
pheochromocytoma, thyroid carcinoma [syndrome] (endocrinology, hematology, and oncology)
plasma thromboplastin component [also called *factor IX* and *Christmas factor*] (hematology and laboratory)
posterior trabeculae carneae (cardiovascular)
prothrombin complex (hematology and laboratory)

PTCA
percutaneous transluminal coronary angioplasty (cardiovascular and radiology)

PT-CT
prothrombin time control (hematology and laboratory)

PTC peptide
phenylthiocarbamoyl peptide (laboratory)

PTD
period to discharge
permanent total disability (neurology, orthopedics, and rehabilitation)
prior to discharge

Pt. Dhgtr.
patient's daughter

Pt. DTR
patient's daughter

PTE
parathyroid extract (endocrinology and pharmacology)
pretibial edema (cardiovascular and orthopedics)
proximal tibial epiphysis (orthopedics)
pulmonary thromboembolism (cardiovascular and respiratory)

PTED
pulmonary thromboembolic disease (cardiovascular and respiratory)

pt. ed.
patient education (education)

PteGlu
pterolyglutamic acid [also called *folic acid*] (chemistry, laboratory, and pharmacology)

PTEN
pentaerythritol tetranitrate [also called *niperyt, pentaerythrityl tetranitrate, penthrit,* and *pentrinitrol,* an explosive and a vasodilator] (cardiovascular, chemistry, and pharmacology)

PTF
plasma thromboplastin factor [also called *Factor X*] (hematology and laboratory)
proximal tubule fluid (laboratory)

PTFE
polytetrafluoroethylene [also called *polytef*; arterial graft material used for Impra grafts] (cardiovascular and surgery)

P.T.F.E.
polytetrafluoroethylene [also called *polytef*; arterial graft material used for Impra grafts] (cardiovascular and surgery)

PTG
teniposide (chemotherapy, oncology, and pharmacology)

PTH
parathyroid hormone [also called *parathormone*] (endocrinology and laboratory)
phenylthiohydantoin (neurology and pharmacology)
posttransfusion hepatitis (gastroenterology, hematology, and infectious diseases)

PTHS
parathyroid hormone secretion [rate] (endocrinology and laboratory)

PTI
persistent tolerant infection

PTL
perinatal telencephalic leukoencephalopathy (neonatology and neurology)
preterm labor (obstetrics)
sodium Pentothal (anesthesiology and pharmacology)

PTLD
prescribed tumor lethal dose (oncology and radiation therapy)

PTM
posttetanic potentiation (neurology)
posttransfusion mononucleosis (hematology and infectious diseases)

Ptm
transmural pressure pertaining to an airway or blood vessel (laboratory and respiratory)

PTMA
phenyltrimethylammonium (chemistry and pharmacology)

PTMDF
pupil, tension, media, disk, fundus (ophthalmology)

pTNM
classifications for postsurgical resection pathological staging of cancer (oncology) [*Note: The letters indicate postsurgical, tumor, nodes, and metastases.*]

PTO
Patent and Trademark Office (government)
Perlsucht-Tuberculin Original [also called *Spengler's tuberculin*] (infectious diseases, laboratory, pharmacology, and respiratory)
personal time off

P.T.O.
Perlsucht-Tuberculin Original [also called *Spengler's tuberculin*] (infectious diseases, laboratory, pharmacology, and respiratory)

PTP
posterior tibial pulse (cardiovascular and orthopedics)
posttetanic potentiation (neurology)
prior to program

P_{TP}
transpulmonary pressure (cardiovascular and respiratory)

Ptp
transpulmonary pressure (cardiovascular and respiratory)

PTPM
posttraumatic progressive myelopathy (neurology)

PTPN
peripheral [vein] total parenteral nutrition (dietary and gastroenterology)

PTR

peripheral total resistance (cardiovascular)

Perlsucht-Tuberculin Rest (infectious diseases, laboratory, pharmacology, and respiratory)

P.T.R.

Perlsucht-Tuberculin Rest (infectious diseases, laboratory, pharmacology, and respiratory)

PTS

para-toluenesulfonic acid (chemistry)

prior to surgery

PTSD

posttraumatic stress disorder (psychiatry)

PTT

partial thromboplastin time (hematology and laboratory)

particle transport time (laboratory)

patellar tendon transfer (orthopedics)

pulmonary transit time (respiratory)

PTT-CT

activated partial thromboplastin time, control (hematology and laboratory)

PTTH

prothoracicotropic hormone (entomology)

PTU

propylthiouracil (chemotherapy, oncology, and pharmacology)

6-PTU

6-propylthiouracil (chemotherapy, oncology, and pharmacology)

PTX

parathyroidectomy (endocrinology and surgery)

pneumothorax (cardiovascular and respiratory)

PTx

parathyroidectomy (endocrinology and surgery)

PTXA

parathyroidectomy and autotransplantation (endocrinology and surgery)

PTZ

pentylenetetrazol (neurology, pharmacology, and psychiatry)

PU

passed urine (urology)

peptic ulcer (gastroenterology)

per urethra (gynecology and urology)

pregnancy urine (laboratory, obstetrics, and urology)

prostatic urethra (anatomy and urology)

Pu

plutonium (chemistry)

purple

pub

public

published (publishing)

publisher (publishing)

PUBS

percutaneous umbilical blood sampling (neonatology)

PUD

peptic ulcer disease (gastroenterology)

pulmonary disease (respiratory)

P.U.D.

peptic ulcer disease (gastroenterology)

PuD

pulmonary disease (respiratory)

PUE

pyrexia of unknown etiology (internal medicine)

PUFA

polyunsaturated fatty acid (cardiovascular, chemistry, dietary, and laboratory)

PUH

pregnancy urine hormone (endocrinology, obstetrics, and urology)

PUL
percutaneous ultrasonic lithotripsy (nephrology, surgery, and urology)
pulmonary (respiratory) {pronounced "pull"}

pul
pulmonary (respiratory) {pronounced "pull"}

"pull"
{pronunciation of *PUL* and *pul* [pulmonary]} (respiratory) {not an abbreviation}

"pull-sas-pro-file"
{pronunciation of *PULSES profile* [physical condition, upper extremity function, lower extremity function, sensory and communication abilities, excretory control, social support]} [*Note: Scoring is 1 (total independence, 2 (symptomatology present but no impairment in the activities of daily living), 3 (impairment present and need for assistance from others), and 4 (total dependence).*] (neurology and rehabilitation)

pulm
pulmentum [gruel] (dietary)
pulmonary (respiratory)

PULSES profile
physical condition, upper extremity function, lower extremity function, sensory and communication abilities, excretory control, social support [*Note: Scoring is 1 (total independence, 2 (symptomatology present but no impairment in the activities of daily living), 3 (impairment present and need for assistance from others), and 4 (total dependence).*] (neurology and rehabilitation) {pronounced "pull-sas-pro-file"}

pulv
pulvis [powder] (pharmacology)

pulv gros
pulvis grossus [coarse powder] (pharmacology)

pulv subtil
pulvis subtilis [smooth powder] (pharmacology)

pulv tenu
pulvis tenuis [extremely fine powder] (pharmacology)

PUN
plasma urea nitrogen (laboratory)

PUNC
punctured

PUNL
percutaneous ultrasonic nephrolithotripsy (nephrology, radiology)

PUO
pyrexia of undetermined origin (internal medicine)
pyrexia of unknown origin (internal medicine)

PUPPP
pruritic urticarial papillary plaques of pregnancy (dermatology and obstetrics)

PUR
polyurethane (chemistry)

Purdue-F
Purdue-Frederick [pharmaceutical company] (pharmacology)

purg
purgative (pharmacology)
purgativus [cathartic, purgative] (pharmacology)

PUVA
psoralens and ultraviolet A [regimen or therapy for psoriasis] (dermatology) {pronounced "poo-vah"}

PV
paraventricular (cardiovascular)
paromomycin-vancomycin [blood agar] (laboratory)

peripheral vascular (cardiovascular, neurology, and orthopedics)
peripheral vein (cardiovascular)
peripheral vessels (cardiovascular)
per vaginam [through the vagina] (gynecology and obstetrics)
plasma volume (hematology and laboratory)
poliomyelitis vaccine (infectious diseases, immunology, neurology, pediatrics, and pharmacology)
polycythemia vera (hematology)
polyoma virus (laboratory and oncology)
portal vein (gastroenterology and cardiovascular)
postvoiding (urology)
pressure/volume
pulmonary vein (cardiovascular and respiratory)
pulmonic valve (cardiovascular)

P-V
Panton-Valentine [leukocidin] (bacteriology, hematology, and laboratory)
pressure-volume

P & V
percuss and vibrate (respiratory)
pyloroplasty and vagotomy (gastroenterology and surgery)

pv
per vaginam [through the vagina] (gynecology and obstetrics)

p.v.
per vaginam [through the vagina] (gynecology and obstetrics)

PVA
polyvinyl alcohol [fixative] (laboratory)

PVAS
postvasectomy [specimen] (laboratory and urology)

PVB
cis-platinum, vinblastine, and bleomycin (chemotherapy, oncology, and pharmacology)
premature ventricular beat (cardiovascular)

PVBS
possible vertebral-basilar system (cardiovascular and neurology)

PVC
polyvinyl chloride (chemistry)
postvoiding cystogram (radiology and urology)
premature ventricular contraction(s) (cardiovascular)
primary visual cortex (ophthalmology)
pulmonary venous congestion (cardiovascular and respiratory)

P.V.C.
premature ventricular contraction(s) (cardiovascular)

P_{VCO_2}
venous carbon dioxide pressure (laboratory and respiratory)

$PvCO_2$
venous carbon dioxide pressure (laboratory and respiratory)

PVC's
premature ventricular contractions (cardiovascular)

PVD
parent very disturbed (pediatrics)
percussion, vibration, and drainage (respiratory)
peripheral vascular disease (cardiovascular, endocrinology, and orthopedics)
posterior vitreous detachment (ophthalmology)
pulmonary vascular disease (cardiovascular and respiratory)

PVE
perivenous encephalomyelitis (neurology)
premature ventricular extrasystole (cardiovascular)
prosthetic valve endocarditis (cardiovascular)

PVEP
pattern visual evoked potential (neurology)

PVF
peripheral visual field (ophthalmology)
portal venous flow (cardiovascular and gastroenterology)
posterior vitreous face (ophthalmology)

PVH
preventricular hemorrhage (cardiovascular)

PVI
peripheral vascular insufficiency (cardiovascular, endocrinology, and orthopedics)
personal values inventory (psychiatry)

P Vivax
Plasmodium vivax [a malarial parasite] (entomology, infectious diseases, laboratory, and respiratory)

PVK
penicillin V potassium [an antibiotic] (pharmacology)

P-VL
Panton-Valentine leukocidin (bacteriology, hematology, and (laboratory)

PVM
pneumonia virus of mice (laboratory, respiratory, and veterinary medicine)
proteins, vitamins, minerals (dietary and pharmacology)

PVMed
preventative medicine

PVNPS
PostVietnam Psychiatric Syndrome (armed forces and psychiatry)

PVNS
pigmented villonodular synovitis (orthopedics)

PVO
peripheral vascular occlusion (cardiovascular, endocrinology, and orthopedics)

pulmonary venous occlusion (cardiovascular and respiratory)

PVOD
peripheral vascular occlusive disease (cardiovascular, endocrinology, and orthopedics)
pulmonary venous obstructive disease (cardiovascular and respiratory)

PVP
penicillin V potassium (pharmacology)
peripheral vein plasma (hematology and laboratory)
peripheral venous pressure (cardiovascular, endocrinology, and orthopedics)
polyvinylpyrrolidone [also called *povidone*] (pharmacology and surgery)
portal vein pressure (cardiovascular and gastroenterology)
technetium pyrophosphate [scan] (cardiovascular and radiology)

PVP-I
povidone-iodine (pharmacology and surgery)

PVR
peripheral vascular resistance (cardiovascular, endocrinology, and orthopedics)
postvoid residual [urine] (urology)
proliferative vitreoretinopathy (ophthalmology)
pulmonary vascular resistance (cardiovascular and respiratory)
pulse-volume recording (cardiovascular)

PVS
percussion, vibration, and suction (respiratory)
peripheral vascular surgery (cardiovascular and surgery)
peritoneovenous shunt (cardiovascular, gastroenterology, and neurology)
persistent vegetative state (neurology and psychiatry)
plexus visibility score (measurement)
premature ventricular systole (cardiovascular)

pulmonic valve stenosis [also called *pulmonary valvular stenosis*] (cardiovascular and respiratory)

PVT
paroxysmal ventricular tachycardia (cardiovascular)
portal vein thrombosis (cardiovascular, gastroenterology, and hematology)
pressure, volume, temperature
private

pvt
private

PW
plantar wart (orthopedics and podiatry)
posterior wall [myocardial infarction] (cardiovascular)
psychological warfare (armed forces and psychiatry)

Pw
progesterone withdrawal (endocrinology, gynecology, and obstetrics)
transthoracic pressure (laboratory and respiratory)

PWA
patient with acquired immunodeficiency syndrome [AIDS] (immunology)
person with acquired immunodeficiency syndrome [AIDS] (immunology)

P wave
{not an abbreviation} [a deflection on electrocardiogram] (cardiovascular)

PWB
partial weight-bearing (orthopedics and rehabilitation)

PWBC
peripheral white blood cell(s) (hematology and laboratory)

PWC
peak work capacity (cardiovascular)
physical work(ing) capacity (cardiovascular)

pwd
powder (pharmacology)

pwdr
powder (pharmacology)

PWI
posterior wall infarct (cardiovascular)

PWLV
posterior wall of left ventricle (cardiovascular)

PWM
pokeweed mitogen (laboratory)

PWP
pulmonary wedge pressure (cardiovascular and respiratory)

PWV
polistes wasp venom (laboratory)

PX
pancreatectomized (endocrinology, gastroenterology, and surgery)
physical examination

Px
past history
physical examination
pneumothorax (cardiovascular and respiratory)
prognosis

px
pneumothorax (cardiovascular and respiratory)

PXE
pseudoxanthoma elasticum (dermatology)

PXM
projection x-ray microscope (laboratory and radiology)

PY
pack years [of cigarette smoking] (cardiovascular, chemical dependency, and respiratory)

Py
phosphopyridoxal (laboratory)

PYA
psychoanalysis (psychiatry)

PYC
proteose-yeast castione [medium] (laboratory)

PyC
pyogenic culture (laboratory)

PYE
peptone yeast extract [medium] (laboratory)

PYG
peptone yeast extract glucose [medium] (laboratory)

PYGM
peptone-yeast glucose maltose [agar or broth] (laboratory)

PYM
psychosomatic medicine

PYP
pyrophosphate (chemistry)

Pyr
pyridine (chemistry and pharmacology)
pyruvate (laboratory)

PYRKIN
pyruvate kinase (hematology and laboratory)

PYKN
pyknocytes (hematology and laboratory)

PyrP
pyridoxamine phosphate [also called *pyridoxyl phosphate*] (laboratory)

PYRUV
pyruvate (laboratory)

PZ
pancreozymin [a hormone] (endocrinology, gastroenterology, and laboratory)

PZA
pyrazinamide [an antibacterial] (pharmacology)

PZ-CCK
pancreozymin-cholecystokinin (endocrinology, gastroenterology, and pharmacology)

PZI
protamine zinc insulin (endocrinology and pharmacology)

PZP
pregnancy zone protein (laboratory and obstetrics)

Q

blood volume (cardiovascular, hematology, laboratory, and respiratory)
cardiac output (cardiovascular)
clerical perception [on General Aptitude Test Battery] (business and education)
coenzyme Q [also called *ubiquinone*] (laboratory)
coulomb (measurement and physics)
glutamine (laboratory and nephrology)
perfusion (cardiovascular)
Quaalude [also called *methaqualone*] (chemical dependency, law enforcement, pharmacology, and psychiatry) {slang}
quantitative
quantity (measurement)
quantity [of electric charge or of heat] (physics)
quaque [each, every] (pharmacology)
quart (measurement)
quarter
quartile (statistics)
Queensland [fever; also called *query fever*] (dermatology and respiratory)
query [fever; also called *Queensland fever*] (dermatology and respiratory)
question
quinacrine [fluorescent method] (laboratory)
quinidine (pharmacology)
quinone [oxidizing agent] (laboratory)
quotient
volume of blood (cardiovascular, hematology, and laboratory)

Q.

coulomb [electric quantity] (measurement and physics)

Q̇

perfusion (cardiovascular)
rate of blood flow (cardiovascular)
time derivative (measurement)

Q°

every hour

Q′

every hour

Q_1

first [or lowest] quartile (statistics)

Q1°

every hour around the clock

Q_2

second quartile (statistics)

Q2°

every 2 hours
every 2 hours around the clock

Q2′

every 2 hours

Q_3

third quartile (statistics)

Q_6

ubiquinone-6 [also called *ubigquinone-Q_6*; a coenzyme] (cardiovascular and laboratory)

Q-6

ubiquinone-6 [also called *ubigquinone-Q_6*; a coenzyme] (cardiovascular and laboratory)

Q_9

ubichromanol-9
ubichromenol-9

Q_{10}

temperature coefficient (chemistry)
ubiquinone-50 [a coenzyme] (cardiovascular and laboratory)

Q-10
ubiquinone-50 [a coenzyme] (cardiovascular and laboratory)

q
electric charge (physics)
frequency of the rarer allele of a pair (genetics and laboratory)
quaque [each, every] (pharmacology)
quart (measurement)
quarter
{not an abbreviation} [refers to the long arm of a chromosome] (genetics and laboratory)

q.
quantity (measurement)
quaque [each, every] (pharmacology)

q°
every hour

q′
every hour

q2°
every 2 hours

q2′
every 2 hours

13q
{not an abbreviation} [13q-deletion syndrome is a genetic abnormality of chromosome 13] (genetics)

QA
quality assurance (manufacturing)

Qa
{not an abbreviation} [a series of loci] (genetics and laboratory)

QAC
quaternary ammonium compound (chemistry)

QAM
Quality Assurance Monitor (medical records)
quaque ante meridiem [every morning] (pharmacology)

Qa.m.
quaque ante meridiem [every morning] (pharmacology)

qam
quaque ante meridiem [every morning] (pharmacology)

q.a.m.
quaque ante meridiem [every morning] (pharmacology)

Q angle
Quatrefage's angle [also called *parietal angle*] (measurement and orthopedics)
{not an abbreviation} [found on testing quadriceps muscles and patellar tendon] (orthopedics)

QAP
quality assurance program (manufacturing)
quinine, Atabrine, pamaquine [treatment] (infectious diseases, pharmacology, and respiratory)

QAR
quality assurance reagent (cardiovascular and laboratory)
quantitative autoradiographic (radiology)

QARANC
Queen Alexandra's Royal Army Nursing Corps (armed forces and nursing)

QARNNS
Queen Alexandra's Royal Navy Nursing Service (armed forces and nursing)

QAS
quality assurance standards (manufacturing)

QAT
quality assurance technical [material] (manufacturing)

qhs
quaque hora somni [at bedtime, every night] (pharmacology)

q.h.s.
quaque hora somni [at bedtime, every night] (pharmacology)

QID
quater in die [four times a day] (pharmacology)

qid
quater in die [four times a day] (pharmacology)

q.i.d.
quater in die [four times a day] (pharmacology)

QIDN
Queen's Institute of District Nursing (nursing)

QIG
quantitative immunoglobulin (laboratory)

QIg
quantitative immunoglobulin (laboratory)

QISAM
queued indexed sequential access method (computer science)

QJ
quadriceps jerk (neurology and orthopedics)

QL
quantum libet [as much as desired, as much as you please] (pharmacology)

ql
quantum libet [as much as desired, as much as you please] (pharmacology)

q.l.
quantum libet [as much as desired, as much as you please] (pharmacology)

qlty
quality

QM
quaque mane [every morning] (pharmacology)

Qm
quaque mane [every morning] (pharmacology)

qm
quaque mane [every morning] (pharmacology)

q.m.
quaque mane [every morning] (pharmacology)

Q-M sign
Quénu-Muret sign (cardiovascular)

QMT
quantitative muscle testing (neurology and orthopedics)

QN
quaque nocte [once every night] (pharmacology)

Qn
quaque nocte [once every night] (pharmacology)

qn
quaque nocte [once every night] (pharmacology)

q.n.
quaque nocte [once every night] (pharmacology)

QNB
3-quinuclidinyl benzilate (cardiovascular, chemistry, gastroenterology, and pharmacology)

q. n hr.
every n hours [n being a variable] (pharmacology)

QNS
quantum non sufficiat [quantity not sufficient] (laboratory)
Queen's Nursing Sister (nursing)

q.n.s.
quantum non sufficiat [quantity not suf-
ficient] (laboratory)

QO
oxygen consumption (laboratory and
respiratory)

QO$_2$
oxygen consumption (laboratory and
respiratory)
oxygen quotient (laboratory and respiratory)

qO$_2$
oxygen quotient (laboratory and respiratory)

QOC
Quality of Contact

QOD
quaque other *die* [every other day]
(pharmacology)

Qod
quaque other *die* [every other day]
(pharmacology)

qod
quaque other *die* [every other day]
(pharmacology)

q.o.d.
quaque other *die* [every other day]
(pharmacology)

Q of C
quality of care

QOH
quaque other *hora* [every other hour]
(pharmacology)

qoh
quaque other *hora* [every other hour]
(pharmacology)

q.o.h.
quaque other *hora* [every other hour]
(pharmacology)

QON
quaque other *nocte* [every other night]
(pharmacology)

Qon
quaque other *nocte* [every other night]
(pharmacology)

qon
quaque other *nocte* [every other night]
(pharmacology)

q.o.n.
quaque other *nocte* [every other night]
(pharmacology)

QP
quadrant pain (gastroenterology)
qualified psychiatrist (psychiatry)
quanti-Pirquet [reaction] (laboratory and
respiratory)
quantum placeat [as much as you
please] (pharmacology)

Qp
pulmonary blood flow (cardiovascular
and respiratory)

qp
quantum placeat [as much as you
please] (pharmacology)

q.p.
quantum placeat [as much as you
please] (pharmacology)

QPC
quality of patient care (administration)
quadrigeminal plate cistern

Qpc
pulmonary capillary blood flow (cardiovascular and respiratory)

QPEEG
quantitative pharmaco-electroencepha-
lography (neurology)

QPM
quaque post meridiem [every night]
(pharmacology)

Qpm
quaque post meridiem [every night]
(pharmacology)

qpm
quaque post meridiem [every night]
(pharmacology)

q.p.m.
quaque post meridiem [every night]
(pharmacology)

Qp/Qs
{not an abbreviation} [left-to-right shunt ratio found on electrocardiography] (cardiovascular)

QPT
Quick prothrombin time (hematology and laboratory)

QPVT
Quick Picture Vocabulary Test (psychiatry and speech and language therapy)

QQ
quaque [also, each, every, *quoque*] (pharmacology)
quoque [also, each, every, *quaque*] (pharmacology)

qq
quaque [also, each, every, *quoque*] (pharmacology)
quoque [also, each, every, *quaque*] (pharmacology)

QQH
quaque quarta hora [every 4 hours] (pharmacology)

Qqh
quaque quarta hora [every 4 hours] (pharmacology)

qqh
quaque quarta hora [every 4 hours] (pharmacology)

q.q.h.
quaque quarta hora [every 4 hours] (pharmacology)

QQHOR
quaque hora [every hour] (pharmacology)

Qq. hor.
quaque hora [every hour] (pharmacology)

qq hor
quaque hora [every hour] (pharmacology)

QR
quadriradial (genetics and laboratory)
quantum rectum [quantity is correct] (pharmacology)
quick recovery
quinaldine red

Q.R.
Quick Recovery [Defibrillator] (cardiovascular)

qr
quadriradial (genetics and laboratory)
quarter
quarterly

Q-RB interval
{not an abbreviation} [a time wave interval on electrocardiograms] (cardiovascular)

QRS
{not an abbreviation} [a complex or segment on an electrocardiogram; often referred to as QRS interval] (cardiovascular)

QRS-ST
{not an abbreviation} [a segment on electrocardiograms] (cardiovascular)

QRS-T
{not an abbreviation} [a segment on electrocardiograms] (cardiovascular)

QRS-T interval
{not an abbreviation} [the duration of ventricular electrical activity on elec-

trocardiogram; also called *Q-T interval*] (cardiovascular)

QRZ
Quaddel Reaktion Zeit [wheal reaction time] (dermatology and laboratory)

QS
every shift (nursing)
quantum satis [sufficient quantity] (pharmacology)
quantum sufficit [as much as will suffice] (pharmacology)
quiet sleep (neurology)

QS2
total electromechanical systole (cardiovascular)

Q-S2
interval of time from beginning of QRS complex to beginning of second heart sound (cardiovascular)

qs
quantum satis [sufficient quantity] (pharmacology)
quantum sufficit [as much as will suffice] (pharmacology)

q.s.
quantum satis [sufficient quantity] (pharmacology)
quantum sufficit [as much as will suffice] (pharmacology)

QSAM
queued sequential access method (computer science)

Q̇san
anatomic shunt flow (laboratory and respiratory)

QSAR
quantitative structure-activity relationship (chemistry)

QSC
quasistatic compliance (measurement)

QS$_2$I
shortened electrochemical systole (cardiovascular)

Q̇sp
physiologic shunt flow [total venous admixture] (laboratory and respiratory)

QSPV
quasistatic pressure volume (measurement)

Qs/Qt
intrapulmonary shunt ratio (laboratory and respiratory)
right-to-left shunt ratio (laboratory and respiratory)

Q̇srel
relative shunt flow (laboratory and respiratory)

QSS
quantitative sacroiliac scintigraphy (orthopedics and radiology)

Q's sign
Quant's sign (orthopedics)

Q-S test
Queckenstedt-Stookey test (neurology)

Q SUFF
quantum sufficit [as much as will suffice] (pharmacology)

q suff
quantum sufficit [as much as will suffice] (pharmacology)

QT
blood volume quantity per unit of time (cardiovascular)
cardiac output (cardiovascular)
qualification test
Queckenstedt's test (neurology)
Quick Test (psychiatry)
Quick's test [for pregnancy (laboratory and obstetrics) or for prothrombin (hematology and laboratory)]
quiet

Q-T
{not an abbreviation} [refers to the Q-T interval (interval of time from beginning of QRS complex to end of T-

wave) electrocardiograms] (cardiovascular)

Qt
Quick's test [for pregnancy (laboratory and obstetrics) or for prothrombin (hematology and laboratory)]

qt
quart (measurement)
quiet

qt.
quantitative
quantity (measurement)
quart (measurement)
quiet

QTAM
queued telecommunications access method (computer science)

Q-T_c
corrected Q-T interval [on electrocardiograms] (cardiovascular)

qt. dx.
quantities duplex

Q-T interval
{not an abbreviation} [the duration of ventricular electrical activity on electrocardiogram; also called *QRS-T interval*] (cardiovascular)

quad
quadriceps [muscle] (neurology, orthopedics, and physical therapy) {pronounced "kwod"}
quadrilateral (orthopedics)
quadriplegia (neurology)
quadriplegic (neurology) {pronounced "kwod"}

quad atrophy
quadriceps atrophy (neurology and orthopedics)

quad ex
quadriceps exercise (orthopedics and rehabilitation)

quadrupl
quadruplicato [four times as much] (pharmacology)

quads
quadriceps (orthopedics)

qual
qualitative
quality

qual anal
qualitative analysis (laboratory)

QUALOD
Quaalude [also called *methaqualone*] (chemical dependency, law enforcement, pharmacology, and psychiatry)

quant
quantitative
quantity (measurement)

quant anal
quantitative analysis (laboratory)

quant suff
quantity sufficient (pharmacology)

quar
quarantine (infectious diseases)
quarterly

QUART
quadrantectomy, axillary dissection, and radiotherapy [treatment for breast cancer] (gynecology, oncology, and surgery) {pronounced "kwort"}

quart.
quarterly
quartus [fourth]

QUAT
quater [four times]
quattuor [four]

quat
quater [four times]
quattuor [four]

quer
querulous

quest.
question
questionable

QuF
Australian Queensland fever (dermatology and respiratory)

QUI
Queen's University of Ireland (education)

QUICHA
quantitative inhalation challenge apparatus (respiratory)

QUINID
quinidine (cardiovascular and pharmacology)

QUININ
quinine (infectious diseases, neurology, orthopedics, and pharmacology)

quinq
quinque [five]

QUINT
quintus [fifth]

quint
quintuplet (neonatology and obstetrics) {pronounced "kwint"}
quintus [fifth]

QUOTID
quotidie [daily] (pharmacology)

quotid
quotidie [daily] (pharmacology)

quor
quorum [of which]

quot
quotient
quoties [as often as necessary] (pharmacology)

QUOTID
quotidie [daily] (pharmacology)

quotid
quotidie [daily] (pharmacology)

quot op sit
quoties opus sit [as often as necessary] (pharmacology)

quot. o. s.
quoties opus sit [as often as necessary] (pharmacology)

QV
quantum vis [as much as you wish] (pharmacology)
quantum volueris [as much as you wish] (pharmacology)
quod vide [which see] (grammar)

qv
quantum vis [as much as you wish] (pharmacology)
quantum volueris [as much as you wish] (pharmacology)
quod vide [which see] (grammar)

q.v.
quantum vis [as much as you wish] (pharmacology)
quantum volueris [as much as you wish] (pharmacology)
quod vide [which see] (grammar)

Q-value
disintegration energy (physics)

QW
quality of working life

Q wave
{not an abbreviation} [an electrocardiographic wave] (cardiovascular)

QWERTY
{not an abbreviation} [standard keyboard arrangement] (business and education)

qwk
once a week [every week] (pharmacology)

q wk
once a week [every week] (pharmacology)

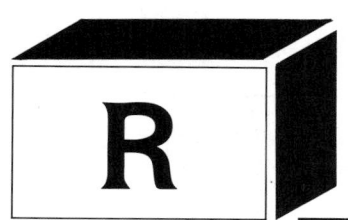

R

P
rho [seventeenth letter of the Greek alphabet]

ρ
rho [seventeenth letter of the Greek alphabet]

R
arginine [an amino acid] (laboratory)
Behnken's unit [of roentgen-ray exposure] (radiology)
organic radical [in chemical formulas] (chemistry, laboratory, and pharmacology)
race (nationality)
racemic (chemistry and laboratory)
radioactive mineral (chemistry, radiation therapy, and radiology)
Radiographer (radiology)
radiologist (radiology)
radiology
Rankine [temperature scale] (measurement)
rate
reaction (laboratory)
reading (rehabilitation and speech and language therapy)
Réaumur [temperature scale] (measurement)
recipe [take] (pharmacology)
rectal (gastroenterology and pharmacology)
rectum (gastroenterology)
rectus [muscle] (anatomy, gastroenterology, ophthalmology, and surgery)
registered trademark (business)
regression coefficient
regular
regular [insulin] (endocrinology and pharmacology)
regulator [gene] (genetics and laboratory)
Reiz [stimulus]
relapse
relaxed
remote

remotum [far]
repressor (genetics and laboratory)
resazurin [a pH indicator] (laboratory)
Resident
resistance
resistance [pressure per unit flow] (laboratory and respiratory)
resistant [referring to disease]
respiration(s) (respiratory)
response
rest [in cell cycles] (laboratory)
restricted
reverse Giemsa method (laboratory)
review
ribose (genetics and laboratory)
Rickettsia [a bacterium] (laboratory)
right
right eye (ophthalmology)
Rinne [test] (otorhinolaryngology)
roentgen (measurement and radiology)
roentgenologist (radiology)
roentgenology (radiology)
Rorschach [test] (psychiatry)
rough [referring to bacterial colonies] (laboratory)
rub (cardiovascular and respiratory)
{not an abbreviation} [any alkyl group of an alkane] (chemistry and laboratory)
{not an abbreviation} [indicates characteristic side chain in formulas of amino acids] (chemistry and laboratory)
{not an abbreviation} [symbol for a gas constant (8.315 joules)] (chemistry and laboratory)

R.
Behnken's unit [of roentgen-ray exposure] (radiology)
Rankine [temperature scale] (measurement)
Réaumur [temperature scale] (measurement)
rectus [muscle] (anatomy, gastroenterology, ophthalmology, and surgery)

remotum [far]
respiration (respiratory)
Rickettsia [a bacterium] (laboratory)
right
rough [referring to bacterial colonies] (laboratory)

(R)
rectal (gastroenterology and pharmacology)

+R
Rinne's test positive (otorhinolaryngology)

−R
Rinne's test negative (otorhinolaryngology)

μR
microroentgen (measurement, radiology and radiation therapy)

®
rectal (gastroenterology)
right

r
correlation coefficient (measurement and statistics)
radius [of a circle] (measurement)
resistance (electricity)
ribose (genetics and laboratory)
ring chromosome (genetics and laboratory)
roentgen (measurement and radiology)
sample correlation coefficient (measurement and statistics)

μr
microroentgen (measurement, radiation therapy, and radiology)

RA
radioactive (chemistry, radiation therapy, and radiology)
radioactivity (chemistry, radiation therapy, and radiology)
radiology
radium (chemistry, radiation therapy, and radiology)
ragweed antigen (allergies and laboratory)
Raynaud's [phenomenon] (neurology)

renal artery (cardiovascular and nephrology)
repeat action
residual air (respiratory)
rheumatoid arthritis (cardiovascular, infectious diseases, orthopedics, and rheumatology)
right angle [or angulation] (orthopedics)
right arm (neurology and orthopedics)
right atrial (cardiovascular)
right atrium (cardiovascular)
right auricle (cardiovascular)
robustrus archistriatalis [nucleus of brain] (neurosurgery)
Rokintansky-Aschoff [sinus of gallbladder] (anatomy, gastroenterology, and surgery)
room air (laboratory and respiratory)

R$_A$
airway resistance (respiratory)

R.A.
rescue ambulance (emergency medicine)

Ra
airway resistance (respiratory)
radium (chemistry, radiation therapy, and radiology)

Ra^{226}
radioactive radium (chemistry, radiation therapy, and radiology)

RAA
renin-angiotensin-aldosterone (cardiovascular, laboratory, and nephrology)
right atrial appendage (cardiovascular)

RAAMC
Royal Australian Army Medical Corps (armed forces)

RAB
Research Advisory Board (research)
rice, applesauce, and banana [diet] (dietary and gastroenterology)

remote afterload brachytherapy (radiology)

RABBI
Rapid Access Blood Bank Information (hematology and laboratory)

RAB diet
rice, applesauce, and banana diet (dietary and gastroenterology)

RABG
room air blood gases (laboratory and respiratory)

RABP
retinoic acid-binding protein (gastroenterology, laboratory, and oncology)

RAC
Recombinant RNA Advisory Committee (genetics and research)
Research Advisory Committee (research)
right atrial catheter (cardiovascular)

rac
racemic (chemistry and laboratory)

RA cell
rheumatoid arthritis cell (cardiovascular, infectious diseases, laboratory, orthopedics, and rheumatology)

RAD
radial (cardiovascular, neurology, and orthopedics)
radical (chemistry and laboratory)
radioactivity present in sample (laboratory)
radiology
reactive airway disease (respiratory)
right anterior descending
right axis deviation (cardiovascular)
roentgen administered dose (measurement, radiation therapy, and radiology) {pronounced "rad"}

RaD
radioactive lead [also called Pb^{210}] (chemistry, radiation therapy, and radiology)

Rad
radiotherapist (radiation therapy)
radiotherapy (radiation therapy)
radium (chemistry, radiation therapy, and radiology)

rad
radial (cardiovascular, neurology, and orthopedics)
radian (measurement)
radiation absorbed dose (measurement, radiation therapy, and radiology) {pronounced "rad"}
radical (chemistry and laboratory)
radius (measurement)
radix [root]

"rad"
{pronunciation of *RAD* [roentgen administered dose] and *rad* [radiation absorbed dose]} (measurement, radiation therapy, and radiology) {not an abbreviation}

RADA
radioactive (chemistry, radiation therapy, and radiology)
right acromiodorsoanterior [position] (obstetrics)
rosin amine-D-acetate (chemistry and pharmacology)

radar
radio detecting and ranging (armed forces and law enforcement) {pronounced "ray-dar"}

RADC
Royal Army Dental Corps (armed forces and dentistry)

RADIO
radiotherapy (radiation therapy) {pronounced "ray-dee-oh"}

radio-IEP
radioimmunoelectrophoresis (laboratory)

Radiol
radiologist (radiology)
radiology

RADISH
rheumatoid arthritis diffuse idiopathic
skeletal hyperostosis

RAD ISO VENO BILAT
radioactive isotopic venogram, bilateral
(cardiology, nuclear medicine, and radiology)

RADLCEN
radiological center (radiation therapy
and radiology)

RadLV
radiation leukemia virus (hematology,
laboratory, oncology, radiation therapy, and radiology)

RADP
right acromiodorsoposterior [position]
(obstetrics)

Rad Ther
radiation therapy

RADTS
rabbit antidog thymus serum (laboratory)

Rad. Ul.
radius-ulna (orthopedics)

rad-ul
radius-ulna (orthopedics)

RADWASTE
radioactive waste (chemistry, radiation
therapy, and radiology) {pronounced
"rad-waste"}

"rad-waste"
{pronunciation of *RADWASTE* [radio-
active waste] (chemistry, radiation
therapy, and radiology) {not an abbre-
viation}

RAE
right atrial enlargement (cardiovascular)

RAEB
refractory anemia, erythroblastic (hematology and laboratory)
refractory anemia with excess of blasto-

cytes [syndrome] (hematology and
laboratory)

RAEM
refractory anemia with excess myelo-
blasts (hematology and laboratory)

RAF
rheumatoid arthritis factor (cardiovascular, infectious diseases, laboratory,
orthopedics, and rheumatology)
Royal Air Force (armed forces)

RAFMS
Royal Air Force Medical Services
(armed forces)

RAG
room air gas (laboratory and respiratory)

Ragg
rheumatoid agglutinator (cardiovascular, infectious diseases, laboratory, orthopedics, and rheumatology)

RAH
right atrial hypertrophy (cardiovascular)

RAHC
Royal Alexandra Hospital for Children
(administration and pediatrics)

RAI
radioactive iodine [also called *radio-
iodine*] (endocrinology and radiology)

RAIU
radioactive iodine uptake (endocrinology and radiology)

RALT
routine admission laboratory tests (laboratory)

RAM
random access memory (computer sciences) {pronounced "ram"}

rapid alternating movements (neurology)

Research Aviation Medicine (aerospace medicine and research)

"ram"
{pronunciation of *RAM* [random access memory]} (computer sciences) {not an abbreviation}

RAMC
Royal Army Medical Corps (armed forces)

RAMT
rabbit antimouse thymocyte (laboratory)

RAN
resident's admission notes (medical records)

RAND
random [sample or specimen] (laboratory)

RAO
right anterior oblique [view] (cardiovascular and radiology)
right anterior occipital (neurology and radiology)

RAP
renal artery pressure (cardiovascular and nephrology)
right atrial pressure (cardiovascular)

RAPD
relative afferent pupillary defect (ophthalmology)

RAR
right arm recumbent [for blood pressure measurement] (cardiovascular)

rar
right arm reclining [for blood pressure measurement] (cardiovascular)
right arm recumbent [for blood pressure measurement] (cardiovascular)

RARLS
rabbit antirat lymphocyte serum (laboratory)

RAS
rasurae [filings, scrapings] (surgery)
renal artery stenosis (cardiovascular and nephrology)
reticular activating system (laboratory)
rheumatoid arthritis serum [factor] (cardiovascular, infectious diseases, laboratory, orthopedics, and rheumatology)

ras
rasurae [filings, scrapings] (surgery)

ras.
rasurae [filings, scrapings] (surgery)

RAST
radioallergosorbent test (allergy) {pronounced "rast" or "wrast"}

"rast"
{pronunciation of *RAST* [radioallergosorbent test]} (allergy) {not an abbreviation}

RAT
repeat action tablet (pharmacology)
right anterior thigh (anatomy and orthopedics)

RA test
rheumatoid arthritis test (cardiovascular, infectious diseases, laboratory, orthopedics, and rheumatology)

RATG
rabbit antithymocyte globulin (laboratory)

RATHAS
rat thymus antiserum (laboratory)

RATx
radiation therapy (oncology and radiation therapy)

RAV
Rous-associated virus (laboratory)

RAVC
Royal Army Veterinary Corps (armed forces and veterinary medicine)

RAW
airway resistance (respiratory)

R(AW)
airway resistance (respiratory)

Raw
airway resistance (laboratory and respiratory)

"ray-dar"
{pronunciation of radar [radio detecting and ranging]} (armed forces and law enforcement) {not an abbreviation}

"ray-dee-oh"
{pronunciation of *RADIO* [radiotherapy]} (radiation therapy) {not an abbreviation}

RAZ
razoxane (chemotherapy, oncology, and pharmacology)

RB
Rating Board [Veteran's Administration] (armed forces)
respiratory bronchiole (respiratory)
retrobulbar (anesthesiology and ophthalmology)
right bronchus (respiratory)
right buttock (anatomy)

R & B
right and below

Rb
rubidium (chemistry)

rb
rebreathing (respiratory)

RBA
rescue breathing apparatus (emergency medicine and respiratory)
right brachial artery (cardiovascular and orthopedics)
rose bengal antigen (laboratory)

RBB
right breast biopsy (gynecology and surgery)
right bundle-branch [block] (cardiovascular)

RBBB
right bundle-branch block (cardiovascular)

RBBsB
right bundle-branch system block (cardiovascular)

RBC
red blood cell(s) (hematology and laboratory)
red blood cell [count] (hematology and laboratory)
red blood corpuscle(s) (hematology and laboratory)
erythrocyte(s) (hematology and laboratory)

rbc
red blood cell(s) (hematology and laboratory)

RBCC
red blood cell cast (hematology and laboratory)

RBCD
right border of cardiac dullness [on percussion of the heart] (cardiovascular)

RBC FO
red blood cell fallout (hematology and laboratory)

RBC/hpf
red blood cells per high power field (hematology and laboratory)

rbc/hpf
red blood cells per high power field (hematology and laboratory)

RBCM
red blood cell mass (hematology and laboratory)

rbc's
red blood cells (hematology and laboratory)

RBCV
red blood cell volume (hematology and laboratory)

RBD
right border of dullness [on percussion of the heart] (cardiovascular)

RBE
relative biological effectiveness [of radiation] (oncology, radiation therapy, and radiology)

RBF
renal blood flow (cardiovascular and nephrology)

Rb Imp
rubber base impression (dentistry)

RBL
Reid's base line (anatomy, ophthalmology, and otorhinolaryngology)

RBN
retrobulbar neuritis (neurology and ophthalmology)

RBNA
Royal British Nurses Association (nursing)

RBOW
rupture(d) bag of water (obstetrics)

RBP
retinol-binding protein (laboratory)
riboflavine-binding protein (laboratory)

R.B.P.
resting blood pressure (cardiovascular)

RBS
random blood smear (hematology and laboratory)
random blood sugar (endocrinology and laboratory)

RBTC
Rational Behavior Therapy Center (psychiatry)

RBV
right brachial vein (cardiovascular and orthopedics)

RBZ
rubidazone [also called *zorubicin*] (chemotherapy, oncology, and pharmacology)

RC
reaction center (hematology and laboratory)
receptor-chemoeffector (laboratory)
red cell (hematology and laboratory)
red cell [casts] (hematology and laboratory)
red corpuscle (hematology and laboratory)
Red Cross (emergency medicine and social services)
referred care
respiration ceases (respiratory)
respiratory care (respiratory)
respiratory center (respiratory)
rest cure
retention catheter (surgery)
retrograde cystogram (radiology and urology)
Roman Catholic (religion)
root canal (dentistry)

R & C
Reed and Carnrick [company] (pharmacology)

R/C
reclining chair

Rc
response, conditioned (psychiatry and rehabilitation)

RCA
radionuclide cerebral angiogram (cardiovascular, neurology, and radiology)
red cell agglutination (hematology and laboratory)
right coronary artery (cardiovascular)

RCAF
Royal Canadian Air Force (armed forces)

RCAMC
Royal Canadian Army Medical Corps (armed forces)

rCBF
regional cerebral blood flow (cardiovascular and neurology)

RCBV
regional cerebral blood volume (cardiovascular and neurology)

RCC
radiochemical center (chemotherapy, oncology, pharmacology, radiation therapy, and radiology)
radiological control center (radiation therapy and radiology)
rape crisis center (gynecology, psychiatry, and social services)
receptor chemoeffector complex (laboratory)
red cell count (hematology and laboratory)
renal cell carcinoma (nephrology and oncology)
routine coronary care [orders] (cardiovascular)

RCCM
Regional Committee for Community Medicine [British] (administration and government)

RCD
relative cardiac dullness (cardiovascular)

RCDHS
rehabilitation and chronic disease hospital section (administration and rehabilitation)

RCF
red cell folate (hematology and laboratory)
relative centrifugal force (chemistry and laboratory)

RCFR
Red Cross Field Representative (emergency medicine and social services)

RCFS
reticulocyte cell-free system (hematology and laboratory)

RCG
radiocardiography (cardiovascular, radiology)

RCGP
Royal College of General Practitioners

RCHMS
Regional Committee for Hospital Medical Services (administration and government)

RCI
respiratory control index (respiratory)

RCITR
red cell iron turnover rate (hematology and laboratory)

RCM
radiographic contrast media (chemistry, pharmacology, and radiology)
red cell mass (hematology and laboratory)
reinforced clostridial medium (laboratory)
replacement culture medium (laboratory)
right costal margin (anatomy, cardiovascular, and respiratory)
Roux conditioned medium (laboratory)
Royal College of Midwives (obstetrics)

RCN
Royal College of Nursing (nursing)

RCO
aliphatic acyl radical (laboratory)

RCOG
Royal College of Obstetricians and Gynaecologists (gynecology and obstetrics)

R colony
rough colony [referring to bacterial colonies] (laboratory)

RCP
random chemistry profile (laboratory)
riboflavine carrier protein (laboratory)
Royal College of Physicians
Royal College of Psychiatrists (psychiatry)

RCPath
Royal College of Pathologists (pathology)

RCPM
Raven Coloured Progressive Matrices (psychiatry)

RCPsych
Royal College of Psychiatrists (psychiatry)

RCPSGlas
Royal College of Physicians and Surgeons, Glasgow

RCR
respiratory control ratio (respiratory)

R.C.R.A.
Resource Conservation and Recovery Act (ecology and government)

RCS
rabbit aorta-contracting substance (cardiovascular and laboratory)
reticulum cell sarcoma (laboratory and oncology)
Royal College of Science
Royal College of Surgeons

R.C.S.
Royal College of Surgeons

R/CS
repeat cesarean section (obstetrics)

RCSE
Royal College of Surgeons, Edinburgh

RCSI
Royal College of Surgeons, Ireland

RCT
randomized clinical trial (pharmacology and research)
root canal therapy (dentistry)
root canal treatment (dentistry)
Rorschach Content Test (psychiatry)

RCU
respiratory care unit (respiratory)

RCV
red cell volume (hematology and laboratory)

RCVS
Royal College of Veterinary Surgeons (veterinary medicine)

RD
Raynaud's disease (neurology)
reaction of degeneration (chemistry and laboratory)
registered dietitian (dietary)
renal disease (nephrology)
research and development (research)
research department (research)
resistance determinant (laboratory)
respiratory disease (respiratory)
respiratory distress (respiratory)
retinal detachment (ophthalmology)
Reye's disease (gastroenterology, neurology, and respiratory)
right deltoid [muscle] (neurology and orthopedics)
right dorsal (anatomy)
rubber dam (dentistry and otorhinolaryngology)
ruptured disc (neurology and orthopedics)

R.D.
Registered Dietitian (dietary)
right deltoid [muscle] (neurology and orthopedics)

R & D
research and development (research)

Rd
reading (education and speech and language therapy)

rd
rutherford [unit of radioactivity] (chemistry, radiation therapy, and radiology)

RDA
recommended daily allowance (dietary and pharmacology)
recommended dietary allowance (dietary and pharmacology)
right dorsoanterior [position] (obstetrics)

RdA
reading age (education and speech and language therapy)

RDC
Research Diagnostic Criteria (research)

RDDA
recommended daily dietary allowance (dietary and pharmacology)

RDE
receptor-destroying enzyme (laboratory)

R determinant
resistance determinant (laboratory)

RDH
Registered Dental Hygienist (dentistry)

R.D.H.
Registered Dental Hygienist (dentistry)

RDI
rupture-delivery interval (obstetrics)

RDMS
Registered Diagnostic Medical Sonographer (cardiovascular, obstetrics, and radiology)

R.D.M.S.
Registered Diagnostic Medical Sonographer (cardiovascular, obstetrics, and radiology)

rDNA
recombinant deoxyribonucleic acid (genetics and laboratory)

RDOD
retinal detachment, oculus dexter [right eye] (ophthalmology)

RDOS
retinal detachment, oculus sinister [left eye] (ophthalmology)

RDP
right dorsoposterior [position] (obstetrics)

RDPE
reticular degeneration of the pigment epithelium (laboratory)

RdQ
reading quotient (education and speech and language therapy)

RDRV
Rhesus diploid cell strain rabies vaccine (infectious diseases and pharmacology)

RDRV (adsorbed)
Rhesus diploid cell strain rabies vaccine (adsorbed) (infectious diseases and pharmacology)

RDS
respiratory distress syndrome (respiratory)

Rds
resistance of the airways on the oral side of the point in the airways where intraluminal pressure equals intrapleural pressure (laboratory and respiratory)

RDT
regular dialysis [hemodialysis] treatment (nephrology)
retinal damage threshold (ophthalmology)

RDVT
recurrent deep vein thrombosis (cardiovascular and orthopedics)

RDW
red cell distribution width (hematology and laboratory)
red cell size distribution width (hematology and laboratory)

RE
radium emanation (chemistry, radiation therapy, and radiology)
rectal examination (gastroenterology)
regarding [or concerning]
regional enteritis (gastroenterology)
resting energy
reticuloendothelial (hematology and laboratory)
reticuloendothelium (hematology and laboratory)
retinol equivalent (pharmacology)
right eye (ophthalmology)

R$_E$
respiratory exchange [ratio] (laboratory and respiratory)

R & E
research and education (education and research)
rest and exercise

Re
regarding [or concerning]
rhenium (chemistry)

R$_e$
Reynold's number (measurement)

re
regarding [or concerning]

REA
Radiation Emergency Area (armed forces, emergency medicine, government, and radiation medicine)
radioenzymatic assay (laboratory)
renal anastomosis (cardiovascular, nephrology, and surgery)

REACH
Reassurance to Each [to assist the families of the mentally ill] (psychiatry) {pronounced "reach"}

"reach"
{pronunciation of *REACH* [Reassurance to Each (to assist the families of the mentally ill)]} (psychiatry) {not an abbreviation}

readm
readmission (administration)

REAT
Radiological Emergency Assistance Team (armed forces, emergency medicine, government, radiation medicine, and radiology)

REB
roentgen-equivalent biological (measurement, radiation therapy, and radiology)

R-EBD-HS
recessive-epidermolysis bullosa dystrophica-Hallopeau Siemens (dermatology and genetics)

REC
reactive (laboratory)
recens [fresh]
recent

rec
recens [fresh]
recent
record
recreation
recurrent

recd
received

rec'd
received

RE CEL
reticulum cell(s) [on differential] (hematology and laboratory)

RECG
radioelectrocardiogram (cardiovascular and radiology)

Recip
recipient

Recomm
recommendation

recon
reconnaissance (armed forces) {pronounced "re-kon"}

recond
recondition (rehabilitation)
reconditioning (rehabilitation)

reconstr
reconstruction (surgery)

recryst
recrystallize (chemistry and laboratory)

RECT
rectificatus [rectified]

rect
rectal (gastroenterology and pharmacology)
rectally (gastroenterology and pharmacology)
rectificatus [rectified]
rectum (gastroenterology)
rectus [muscle] (gastroenterology and ophthalmology)

rect.
rectificatus [rectified]
rectum (gastroenterology)
rectus [muscle] (gastroenterology and ophthalmology)

recur
recurrence
recurrent

Re-D
re-evaluation deadline (rehabilitation)

redig in pulv
redigatur in pulverem [let it be reduced to powder] (pharmacology)

redig. in pulv.
redigatur in pulverem [let it be reduced to powder] (pharmacology)

RED IN PULV
redigatur in pulverem [let it be reduced to powder] (pharmacology)

red in pulv
reductus in pulverem [reduced to powder] (pharmacology)

red. in pulv.
reductus in pulverem [reduced to powder] (pharmacology)

REDNP
Regent's External Degree Nursing Program [in New York] (education and nursing)

redox
reduction oxidation (chemistry and laboratory)

REDY
ready (laboratory)

REE
rapid extinction effect (neurology)
resting energy expenditure

re-ed
re-education (rehabilitation)

Reed & C
Reed and Carnrick [pharmaceutical company] (pharmacology)

REEG
radioelectroencephalograph (neurology and radiology)

REEGT
Registered Electroencephalographic Technician (neurology)

R EEG T
Registered Electroencephalographic Technologist (neurology)

REEL
Receptive-Expressive Emergent Language Scale (speech and language therapy)

REF
referred

renal erythropoietic factor (hematology, laboratory, and nephrology)

Ref.
refused (respiratory therapy)

ref
refer
reference

REF DOC
referring doctor

ref doc
referring doctor

REFL
specimen lost by reference laboratory (laboratory)

refl
reflex (neurology)

REFMS
Recreation and Education for Multiple Sclerosis Victims (neurology and rehabilitation)

ref phys
referring physician

REFRAD
released from active duty (armed forces)

REG
Radiation Exposure Guide (measurement, radiation therapy, and radiology)
radioencephalogram (neurology and radiology)
radioencephalograph (neurology and radiology)

Reg
registered

reg
regarding
region
regular
regulation

Reg diet
regular diet (dietary)

regen
regenerate
regeneration

reg nsy
regular nursery (neonatology and pediatrics)

REG UMB
regio umbilici [umbilical region]

reg umb
regio umbilici [umbilical region]

reg. umb.
regio umbilici [umbilical region]

regurg
regurgitation (cardiovascular and gastroenterology) {pronounced "re-gurge"}

"re-gurge"
{pronunciation of *regurg* [regurgitation]} (cardiovascular and gastroenterology) {not an abbreviation}

REHAB
rehabilitation {pronounced "re-hab"}

rehab
rehabilitation {pronounced "re-hab"}

"re-hab"
{pronunciation of *REHAB* and *rehab* [rehabilitation]} {not an abbreviation}

rehabil
rehabilitation

Reid-P
Reid-Provident [pharmaceutical company] (pharmacology)

REINCH
Reinsch Test [for urine mercury and arsenic] (laboratory)

"re-kon"
{pronunciation of *recon* [reconnaissance]} (armed forces) {not an abbreviation}

REL
rate of energy loss (measurement)

Rel
religion

rel
related
relative
religion

reliq
reliquus [remainder]

REM
rapid eye movement [sleep] (neurology and psychiatry) {pronounced "rem"}
removal
roentgen equivalent man (measurement, radiation therapy, and radiology) {pronounced "rem"}

rem
removal
roentgen equivalent man (measurement, radiation therapy, and radiology) {pronounced "rem"}

"rem"
{pronunciation of *REM* [rapid eye movement (sleep)] (neurology and psychiatry) and *REM* and *rem* [roentgen equivalent man (measurement, radiation therapy, and radiology)]} {not an abbreviation}

REMAB
radiation equivalent manikin absorption (measurement, radiation therapy and radiology)

REMCAL
radiation equivalent manikin calibration (measurement, radiation therapy, and radiology)

REMP
roentgen equivalent—man period (measurement, radiation therapy, and radiology)

REMS
rapid eye movement sleep (neurology)

REN
renal (nephrology)

ren
renal (nephrology)
renovetur [renew]

ren.
renal (nephrology)
renovetur [renew]

RENAL
renal squamous cells [on urine screen] (laboratory, nephrology, and urology)

ren sem
renovetum semel [shall be renewed only once] (pharmacology)

REO
respiratory and enteric orphan [virus] (gastroenterology, laboratory, and respiratory)

REO virus
respiratory and enteric orphan virus (gastroenterology, laboratory, and respiratory)

reovirus
respiratory and enteric orphan virus (gastroenterology, laboratory, and respiratory)

REP
repair (surgery)
repeat
repetatur [let it be repeated] (pharmacology)
report
retrograde pyelogram (nephrology and radiology)
roentgen equivalent physical (measurement, radiation therapy, and radiology)

rep
repeat
repetatur [let it be repeated] (pharmacology)
report

roentgen equivalent physical (measurement, radiation therapy, and radiology)

rep.
repetatur [let it be repeated] (pharmacology)
report

repol
repolarization (cardiovascular)

req
request(ed)
required
requires

REQF
wrong test requested—floor error (laboratory)

REQL
wrong test requested—laboratory error (laboratory)

RER
renal excretion rate (laboratory, nephrology, and urology)
respiratory exchange ratio (laboratory and respiratory)
rough endoplasmic reticulum (laboratory)

RES
research
resident
reticuloendothelial system (hematology and internal medicine)

res.
research
reserve
resident

"re-sah"
{pronunciation of *RISA* [radioimmunosorbent assay]} (immunology and laboratory) {not an abbreviation}

RESC
resuscitation (cardiovascular, emergency medicine, and respiratory)

resist. ex.
resistive exercises (orthopedics and rehabilitation)

RESP
respectively
respiration(s) (respiratory)
respiratory
responsible

Resp
respiratory
response

resp
respectively
respiration(s) (respiratory)
respiratory
responsible

RESP-A
respiratory battery, acute (laboratory and respiratory)

respir
respirations (respiratory)

rest
restorative (pharmacology)

resus
resuscitation (cardiovascular and respiratory)

RET
reticulocyte (hematology and laboratory)
right esotropia (ophthalmology)

ret
retired

RETAIN
serum retained (laboratory)

retard
retarded [meaning delayed] (neurology and psychiatry) {pronounced "retard"}
{not an abbreviation} [slang term referring to a mentally retarded person]

(neurology and psychiatry) {slang}
{pronounced "re-tard"}

"re-tard"
{pronunciation of *retard* [retarded
(meaning delayed)] and also a slang
word referring to a mentally retarded
person [not an abbreviation]} (neurology and psychiatry) {not an abbrevia-
tion}

ret. cath.
retention catheter (surgery)

RETIC
reticulocyte (hematology and laboratory) {pronounced "re-tick"}

retic
reticulocyte (hematology and laboratory) {pronounced "re-tick"}

retic count
reticulocyte count (hematology and laboratory) {pronounced "re-tick-count"}

"re-tick"
{pronunciation of *RETIC* and *retic* [re-
ticulocyte]} (hematology and laboratory) {not an abbreviation}

"re-tick-count"
{pronunciation of *retic count* [reticu-
locyte count]} (hematology and laboratory) {not an abbreviation}

"re-ticks"
{pronunciation of *retics* [reticulocytes]}
(hematology and laboratory) {not an
abbreviation}

retics
reticulocytes (hematology and laboratory) {pronounced "re-ticks"}

Retro. pyelo
retrograde pyelogram (nephrology, radiology, and urology)

RETUL
reticulum cells [on differential] (hematology and laboratory)

REV
reverse
review
revolution(s) (measurement)

rev
reverse
review
revolution(s) (measurement)

reverse T$_3$
reverse tri-iodothyronine (endocrinology
and laboratory)

REVL
to be reviewed by pathologist (laboratory and pathology)

Rev of Sym
review of symptoms (medical records)

Rev of Sys
review of systems (medical records)

REW
incised wound [on autopsy] (pathology)

RF
radial fibers [of the cochlea] (otorhinolaryngology)
radiofrequency (radiology)
receptive field [of visual cortex] (neurology and ophthalmology)
Reitland-Franklin [unit] (measurement)
relative flow [rate] (measurement)
relative fluorescence (laboratory and
measurement)
releasing factor (laboratory)
renal failure (nephrology)
replicative form (genetics)
resistance factor (bacteriology and laboratory)
respiratory failure (respiratory)
reticular formation (hematology and laboratory)
rheumatic fever (cardiovascular, infectious diseases, orthopedics, and rheumatology)
rheumatoid factor (cardiovascular, infectious diseases, laboratory, orthopedics, and rheumatology)

riboflavine [also called *lactoflavin* and *vitamin B₂;* a vitamin] (dietary, laboratory, and pharmacology)
root canal, filling of (dentistry)

R_F
rate of flow [on chromatography] (laboratory and measurement)

Rf
rutherfordium (chemistry)

R_f
rate of flow [on chromatography] (laboratory and measurement)

rf
radiofrequency (electricity)

RFA
right femoral artery (cardiovascular and orthopedics)
right frontoanterior [position] (obstetrics)

R.F.A.
right frontoanterior [position] (obstetrics)

R factor
resistance factor (bacteriology and laboratory)

RFB
retained foreign body (surgery)

RFC
rosette-forming cells (laboratory)

RFL
right frontolateral [position] (obstetrics)

RFLA
rheumatoid-factor-like activity (cardiovascular, infectious diseases, laboratory, orthopedics, and rheumatology)

RFLP
restriction fragment length polymorphism (genetics and laboratory)

RFLS
rheumatoid-factor-like substance (cardiovascular, infectious diseases, laboratory, orthopedics, and rheumatology)

RFN
Registered Fever Nurse (nursing)

RFOL
results to follow (laboratory)

RFP
right frontoposterior [position] (obstetrics)

R.F.P.
right frontoposterior [position] (obstetrics)

RFPS (Glasgow)
Royal Faculty of Physicians and Surgeons of Glasgow

RFR
refraction (ophthalmology)

RFS
rapid frozen section (pathology and surgery)
renal function study (laboratory and nephrology)

RFT
right frontotransverse [position] (obstetrics)
rod-and-frame test

R.F.T.
right frontotransverse [position] (obstetrics)

RFV
right femoral vein (cardiovascular and orthopedics)

RFW
rapid-filling wave

RG
retrograde
right gluteal [muscle] (neurology and orthopedics)

R.G.
right gluteal [muscle] (neurology and orthopedics)

R-G
Radiologist, General (radiology)

Rg
Rodgers antibodies (laboratory)

RGAS
retained gastric antrum syndrome

RGC
retinal ganglial cell(s) (laboratory, neurology, and ophthalmology)

RGE
relative gas expansion (chemistry)

RGH
Riverside General Hospital (administration)

RGM
right gluteus maximus [muscle] (neurology and orthopedics)

RGN
Registered General Nurse (nursing)

RGP
retrograde pyelogram (nephrology, radiology, and urology)

RGR
relative growth rate (laboratory)

RH
radiant heat (physics)
radiological health (radiology)
reactive hyperemia (cardiovascular)
reduced haloperidol (laboratory and psychiatry)
relative humidity (climate control and weather)
releasing hormone (endocrinology and laboratory)
rheumatic (cardiovascular, infectious diseases, orthopedics, and rheumatology)
rheumatism (cardiovascular, infectious diseases, orthopedics, and rheumatology)

rheumatology (cardiovascular, infectious diseases, orthopedics, and rheumatology)
right hand (neurology and orthopedics)
right hyperphoria (ophthalmology)
room humidifier (climate control, otorhinolaryngology, and respiratory)
Royal Hospital [London] (administration)

Rh
Rhesus [referring to blood factors—Rh negative and Rh positive] (hematology and laboratory)
Rhipicephalus [a genus of cattle tick] (entomology and infectious diseases)
rhodium (chemistry)

Rh−
Rhesus negative (hematology and laboratory)

Rh+
Rhesus positive (hematology and laboratory)

^{106}Rh
radioactive rhodium (chemistry)

rh
rhonchi [râles] (respiratory)

rh.
rheumatic (cardiovascular, infectious diseases, orthopedics, and rheumatology)
rhonchi [râles] (respiratory)

r/h
roentgens per hour (measurement, radiation therapy, and radiology)

RHA
Regional Health Authority (administration and government)

RHA(T)
Regional Health Authority (Teaching) [British] (administration, education, and government)

RHB
raise head of bed (gastroenterology and respiratory)
Regional Hospital Board (administration and government)
right heart bypass [surgery] (cardiovascular)

RHBF
reactive hyperemic blood flow (cardiovascular)

RHC
resin hemoperfusion column (cardiovascular)
respirations have ceased (respiratory)
right hypochondrium (gastroenterology, orthopedics, and respiratory)

RHCC/PP
Reproductive Health Care Center/ Planned Parenthood (gynecology, obstetrics, and urology)

RHCSA
Regional Hospitals Consultants' and Specialists' Association (administration)

RHD
Radiological Health Data (radiation therapy and radiology)
relative hepatic dullness [on physical examination] (gastroenterology)
rheumatic heart disease (cardiovascular, infectious diseases, orthopedics, and rheumatology)

R.H.D.
rheumatic heart disease (cardiovascular, infectious diseases, orthopedics, and rheumatology)

RHEU
rheumatology (cardiovascular, infectious diseases, orthopedics, and rheumatology)

rheu fev
rheumatic fever (cardiovascular, infectious diseases, orthopedics, and rheumatology)

rheu ht dis
rheumatic heart disease (cardiovascular, infectious diseases, orthopedics, and rheumatology)

RHEUM
rheumatic (cardiovascular, infectious diseases, orthopedics, and rheumatology)
rheumatism (cardiovascular, infectious diseases, orthopedics, and rheumatology)

rheum
rheumatic (cardiovascular, infectious diseases, orthopedics, and rheumatology)
rheumatism (cardiovascular, infectious diseases, orthopedics, and rheumatology)

RHF
right heart failure (cardiovascular)

RHD
Radiological Health Data (radiology)

Rh factor
Rhesus factor (hematology and laboratory)

RhIg
Rhesus immune globulin (hematology, immunology, and laboratory)

Rhin
rhinologist (otorhinolaryngology)
rhinology (otorhinolaryngology)

Rhiz
Rhizobium [a bacterium] (laboratory)

RHJSC
Regional Hospital Junior Staff Committee [British] (administration and government)

RHL
right hemisphere lesion(s) (cardiovascular and neurology)

right hepatic lobe (anatomy and gastro-enterology)

RHLN
right hilar lymph node (respiratory and surgery)

RHM
roentgen per hour at one meter (measurement, radiation therapy, and radiology)

rhm
roentgen per hour at one meter (measurement, radiation therapy, and radiology)

RhMK
Rhesus monkey kidney cell(s) (laboratory)

"R-H-neg"
{pronunciation of *Rh neg.* [Rhesus factor negative]} (hematology and laboratory) {not an abbreviation}

Rh neg.
Rhesus factor negative (hematology and laboratory) {pronounced "R-H-neg"}

"R-H-null"
{pronunciation of Rh_{null} [Rhesus factor null (indicating all Rhesus factors are missing)]} (hematology and laboratory) {not an abbreviation}

Rh_{null}
Rhesus factor null [indicating all Rhesus factors are missing] (hematology and laboratory) {pronounced "R-H-null"}

$Rh_0(D)$
{not an abbreviation} [an immune human globulin] (hematology, immunology and laboratory)

rhom
rhomboid [muscle] (neurology and orthopedics) {pronounced "rhom"}

"rhom"
{pronunciation of *rhom* [rhomboid (muscle)]} (neurology and orthopedics) {not an abbreviation}

RHOV
du variant (laboratory)

"R-H-pause"
{pronunciation of *Rh pos.* [Rhesus factor positive]} (hematology and laboratory) {not an abbreviation}

Rh pos.
Rhesus factor positive (hematology and laboratory) {pronounced "R-H-pause"}

RHR
resting heart rate (cardiovascular)

R.H.R.
resting heart rate (cardiovascular)

r/hr
roentgens per hour (measurement, radiation therapy, and radiology)

RHS
right-hand side (anatomy)

RHT
right hypertropia (ophthalmology)

RHU
Registered Health Underwriter (insurance)

RHWV
CW variant (laboratory)

RI
radiation intensity (radiation therapy and radiology)
radioisotope (measurement, radiation therapy, and radiology)
Recovery, Incorporated
refractive index (ophthalmology)
regional ileitis (gastroenterology)
regular insulin (endocrinology and pharmacology)
release-inhibiting (laboratory)
remission induction (chemotherapy, oncology, pharmacology, and radiation therapy)
replicative intermediate (laboratory)

respiratory illness (respiratory)
retroactive inhibition [also called *retro-active interference*] (psychiatry)
Rhode Island [Postal Service state designation]
ribosome (genetics and laboratory)
right iliac [crest] (anatomy and orthopedics)

R/I
rule in

RIA
radioimmune assay [also called *radio-immunoassay*] (allergy, immunology, and laboratory)

RIA-DA
radioimmune assay double antibody [test; also called *radio-immunoassay double antibody*] (allergy, immunology, and laboratory)

RIAST
Reitan Indiana Aphasic Screening Test (neurology, psychiatry, and speech and language therapy)

RIC
right iliac crest (anatomy and orthopedics)
right internal carotid [artery] (cardiovascular and neurology)
Royal Institute of Chemistry (chemistry)

RICK-A
Rickettsial Battery (bacteriology and laboratory)

"rick-U"
{pronunciation of *RICU* [respiratory intensive care unit]} (respiratory) {not an abbreviation}

RICM
right intercostal margin (anatomy and cardiovascular)

RICS
right intercostal space (anatomy and cardiovascular)

RICU
respiratory intensive care unit (respiratory) {pronounced "rick-U"}

RID
radial immunodiffusion (laboratory)
reversible intravas device (urology)

RIDCSF
colloidal gold (radial immunodiffusion cerebrospinal fluid) (laboratory)

RIF
release-inhibiting factor (laboratory)
rifampicin [an antibacterial, antibiotic, and antituberculin] (infectious diseases, pharmacology, and respiratory)
rifampin [an antibacterial, antibiotic, and antituberculin] (infectious diseases, pharmacology, and respiratory)
right iliac fossa (anatomy, cardiovascular, and surgery)
right internal fixation (orthopedics)

RIFA
radio iodinated fatty acid (cardiovascular, chemistry, pharmacology, and radiology)

RIFC
rat intrinsic factor concentrate (laboratory)

RIG
rabies immune globulin (laboratory)

RIGH
rabies immune globulin, human (laboratory)

RIH
right inguinal hernia (gastroenterology and surgery)

RIHSA
radioactive iodinated human serum albumin [also called *radioiodinated human serum albumin*] (cardiovascular, chemistry, pharmacology, and radiology)

RILT
rabbit ileal loop test

RIM
radioisotope medicine (oncology, radiation therapy, and radiology)

RIMA
right internal mammary anastomosis (cardiovascular) {pronounced "rim-ah"}

"rim-ah"
{pronunciation of *RIMA* [right internal mammary anastomosis]} (cardiovascular) {not an abbreviation}

RIMR
Rockefeller Institute for Medical Research (research)

RIND
resolving ischemic neurological defect [also called *resolving ischemic neurological deficit, reversible ischemic neurological defect, reversible ischemic neurological deficit,* and *reversible ischemic neurological disorder*] (cardiovascular and neurology) {pronounced "rind"}

"rind"
{pronunciation of *RIND* [resolving ischemic neurological defect (also called *resolving ischemic neurological deficit, reversible ischemic neurological defect, reversible ischemic neurological deficit,* and *reversible ischemic neurological disorder*)]} (neurology) {not an abbreviation}

RIO
right inferior oblique [projection] (radiology)

RIOJ
recurrent intrahepatic obstructive jaundice (gastroenterology)

RIP
radioimmunoprecipitin [test] (laboratory)
rapid infusion pump (chemotherapy, oncology, and pharmacology)

RIPH
Royal Institute of Public Health

RIPHH
Royal Institute of Public Health and Hygiene

RIR
right iliac region (anatomy, orthopedics, and surgery)
right inferior rectus [muscle] (anatomy and ophthalmology)

RIRB
radio iodinated rose bengal [a dye] (laboratory and radiology)

RIS
radiology information system (radiology)

RISA
radioactive iodinated serum albumin [scan or study] (cardiovascular, chemistry, pharmacology, and radiology)
radioimmunosorbent assay (immunology and laboratory) {pronounced "re-sah"}

risa
radioactive iodinated serum albumin [scan or study] (cardiovascular, chemistry, pharmacology, and radiology)

RIST
radio immunosorbent test (allergy, immunology, and laboratory) {pronounced "wrist"}

RIT
radio iodinated triolein (chemistry, pharmacology, and radiology)
Rorschach Inkblot Test (psychiatry)

RITC
rhodamine isothiocyanate [a dye] (laboratory)

RIU
radioactive iodine uptake (endocrinology and radiology)

RIV
ramus interventricularis [of coronary arteries] (cardiovascular)
right innominate vein (cardiovascular)

RJ
radial jerk [reflex] (neurology and orthopedics)
Robert Jones [dressing] (surgery)

RK
rabbit kidney (laboratory)
radial keratoplasty (ophthalmology)
radial keratotomy (ophthalmology)
right kidney (nephrology)

RKG
radiocardiogram (cardiovascular and radiology)

RKH
Rokitansky-Kuster-Hauser [syndrome] (gynecology and obstetrics)

RKID
right kidney (urine) [sample] (laboratory and nephrology)

RKW
renal potassium wasting (nephrology)

RKY
roentgenkymography [also called *roentgen kymography*] (radiology)

RL
coarse râles [on chest auscultation] (respiratory)
Radiation Laboratory (oncology, radiation therapy, and radiology)
Record Librarian (medical records)
reduction level [of reciprocal of respiratory quotient] (respiratory)
reticular lamina (anatomy, neurology, and otorhinolaryngology)
right lateral
right leg (anatomy, neurology, and orthopedics)
right lower
right lung (anatomy and respiratory)
Ringer's lactate (pharmacology and surgery)
Royal Licence [British]
stimulus *(Reiz)* limen (neurology)

R_L
respiratory resistance (laboratory and respiratory)
total pulmonary resistance (laboratory and respiratory)

R-L
right to left

R.L.
right lateral

R/L
Ringer's lactate (pharmacology and surgery)

RL_3
many coarse râles [on chest auscultation] (respiratory)

R→L
right to left

RI
medium râles [on chest auscultation] (respiratory)

RI_2
moderate number of medium râles [on chest auscultation] (respiratory)

rl
fine râles [on chest auscultation] (respiratory)

rl_1
few fine râles [on chest auscultation] (respiratory)

RLBCD
right lower border of cardiac dullness (cardiovascular)

RLC
residual lung capacity (laboratory and respiratory)

RLD
related living donor (hematology, laboratory, nephrology, and transplant surgery)

ruptured lumbar disk (neurology and orthopedics)

RLE
right lower extremity (anatomy, neurology, and orthopedics)

R.L.E.
right lower extremity (anatomy, neurology, and orthopedics)

RLF
retained lung fluid (respiratory)
retrolental fibroplasia (neonatology, ophthalmology, and pediatrics)
right lateral femoral [injection site] (pharmacology)

RLL
right lower limb (anatomy, neurology, and orthopedics)
right lower lobe [of lung] (respiratory)

R.L.L.
right lower lobe [of lung] (respiratory)

RLM
Regional Library of Medicine (library science)

RLMD
rat liver mitochondria (and submitochondrial particles derived by) digitonin [treatment]

RLN
recurrent laryngeal nerve (otorhinolaryngology and surgery)
regional lymph node(s) (oncology and surgery)

RLND
regional lymph node dissection (oncology and surgery)

RLP
radiation-leukemia-protection (hematology, oncology, and radiation therapy)

RLQ
right lower quadrant [of abdomen] (anatomy and gastroenterology)

R.L.Q.
right lower quadrant [of abdomen] (anatomy and gastroenterology)

RLR
right lateral rectus [eye muscle] (neurology and ophthalmology)

RLS
Ringer's lactate solution (pharmacology and surgery)
{not an abbreviation} [refers to a person who stammers, having difficulty enunciating R, L, and S] (speech and language therapy)

RLSO
unit released by blood bank (hematology and laboratory)

R-L shunt
right-to-left shunt (cardiovascular)

RLT
right lateral thigh (anatomy, neurology, and orthopedics)

RM
radical mastectomy (gynecology, oncology, and surgery)
range of motion (neurology and orthopedics)
range of movement (neurology and orthopedics)
Raven's Matrices (speech and language therapy)
red marrow (hematology and laboratory)
reference material(s) (publishing)
repetitions maximum (orthopedics and rehabilitation)
respiratory movement (respiratory)
Rogosa SL medium (laboratory)

R & M
routine and microscopic (laboratory)

RM-1
Madison chromosome (genetics and laboratory)

Rm
remission (oncology)

rm
room

RMA
Registered Medical Assistant
relative medullary area [of the kidney]
(nephrology)
right mentoanterior [position] (obstetrics)

R.M.A.
right mentoanterior [position] (obstetrics)

RMAC
Regional Medical Advisory Committee
[British] (administration and govern-
ment)

RMBF
regional myocardial blood flow (cardiovascular)

RMCA
right main coronary artery (cardiovascular)
right middle cerebral artery (cardiovascular and neurology)

RMCAT
right middle cerebral artery thrombosis
(cardiovascular and neurology)

RMCL
right midclavicular line (anatomy, cardiovascular, and respiratory)

RMCT
rat mast cell technique (allergy and laboratory)

RMD
rapid movement disorder (neurology)
retromanubrial dullness [at base of skull]
(neurology and orthopedics)
right manubrial dullness [at right base of
skull] (neurology and orthopedics)

RME
right mediolateral episiotomy (obstetrics)

RMEE
right middle ear exploration (otorhinolaryngology)

RMK
Rhesus monkey kidney (laboratory)

RML
right mediolateral [episiotomy] (obstetrics)
right middle lobe [of lung] (respiratory)

R.M.L.
right middle lobe [of lung] (respiratory)

rml
right mediolateral [episiotomy] (obstetrics)

RMM
rapid micromedia method (laboratory)

RMN
Registered Mental Nurse [England and
Wales] (nursing and psychiatry)

RMO
Regional Medical Officer
Resident Medical Officer

RMP
rapidly miscible pool (laboratory)
Regional Medical Program (administration)
rifampicin [an antibacterial, antibiotic,
and antituberculin] (infectious diseases, pharmacology, and respiratory)
right mentoposterior [position] (obstetrics)

R.M.P.
right mentoposterior [position] (obstetrics)

RMPA
Royal Medico-Psychological Association
(psychology)

RMR
resting metabolic rate (laboratory)

right medial rectus [eye muscle] (neurology and ophthalmology)

RMS
rectal morphine sulfate [suppository; an analgesic] (pharmacology)
rehabilitation medicine service (rehabilitation)
respiratory muscle strength (respiratory)
root-mean-square (mathematics)
{not an abbreviation} [a brand name preparation of rectal morphine sulfate (suppository)] (pharmacology)

R.M.S.
Royal Mail Steamer (shipping)

RMSF
Rocky Mountain spotted fever (infectious diseases)

RMT
registered music therapist (rehabilitation)
relative medullary thickness [of kidney] (nephrology)
retromolar trigone (dentistry)
right mentotransverse [position] (obstetrics)

R.M.T.
right mentotransverse [position] (obstetrics)

RMV
respiratory minute volume (laboratory and respiratory)

RN
radionuclide (chemistry, laboratory, radiation therapy, and radiology)
red nucleus (hematology and laboratory)
Registered Nurse (nursing)
Royal Navy (armed forces)

R.N.
Registered Nurse (nursing)

Rn
radon (chemistry)

Rn^{222}
radioactive radon (chemistry and radiology)

RNA
radionuclide angiography (cardiovascular and radiology)
Registered Nurse Anesthetist (anesthesiology and nursing)
ribonucleic acid (genetics and laboratory)
rough, noncapsulated avirulent [referring to bacteria] (bacteriology and laboratory)

RNAase
ribonuclease (genetics and laboratory)

RNase
ribonuclease (genetics and laboratory)

RND
radical neck dissection (endocrinology, oncology, otorhinolaryngology, and surgery)
round

RNEF
resting (radio-)nuclide ejection fraction (cardiovascular and radiology)

RNIB
Royal National Institute for the Blind (ophthalmology)

RNID
Royal National Institute for the Deaf (otorhinolaryngology)

RNm
red nucleus, magnocellular [division] (hematology and laboratory)

RNMD
Registered Nurse for Mental Defectives (neurology, nursing, and psychiatry)

RNMS
Registered Nurse for Mentally Subnormal (neurology, nursing, and psychiatry)

RNMT
Registered Nuclear Medicine Technologist (radiology)

RNP
Registered Nurse Practitioner (nursing)
ribonucleoprotein [also called *ribonuclear protein*] (genetics and laboratory)

R.N.P.
Registered Nurse Practitioner (nursing)

RNP complex
ribonucleoprotein complex (genetics and laboratory)

Rnt
roentgenologist (radiology)
roentgenology (radiology)

RNV
radionuclide venography (radiology)

RO
reverse osmosis (chemistry and laboratory)
Ritter-Oleson [technique]
routine order (treatment)
rule out

R/O
rule out

r/o
rule out

ROA
right occipitoanterior [position; also called *right occiput anterior*] (obstetrics)

R.O.A.
right occipitoanterior [position; also called *right occiput anterior*] (obstetrics)

ROAD
reversible obstructive airway disease (respiratory)

ROAP
rubidazone, Oncovin [vincristine], cytosine arabinoside, and prednisone (chemotherapy, oncology, and pharmacology)

ROC
receiver operating characteristic (diagnostics)
residual organic carbon (chemistry and laboratory)

Roent
roentgenologist (radiology)
roentgenology (radiology)

roent
roentgenologist (radiology)
roentgenology (radiology)

Rogosa SL medium
Rogosa-selective *Lactobacillus* medium (laboratory)

ROH
rat ovarian hyperemia [test] (laboratory)

ROI
region of interest (radiology)

ROL
right occipitolateral [position; also called *right occiput lateral*] (obstetrics)

ROM
range of motion (neurology and orthopedics)
range of movement (neurology and orthopedics)
read only memory (computer sciences)
rupture of membranes (obstetrics)

romi
rule out myocardial infarction (cardiovascular)

ROP
Regional Occupational Program (education and rehabilitation)
retinopathy of prematurity [also called *retrolental fibroplasia*] (neonatology, ophthalmology, and pediatrics)
right occipitoposterior [position; also

called *right occiput posterior*] (obstetrics)

R.O.P.
right occipitoposterior [position; also called *right occiput posterior*] (obstetrics)

R.O.P.A.
Regional Organ Procurement Agency (cardiovascular, gastroenterology, nephrology, ophthalmology, orthopedics, and transplantation surgery)

Ror
Rorschach [test] (neurology, ophthalmology, and psychiatry)

RO & R
Rey Osterreigh and Recall [test] (psychiatry)

RoRx
radiation therapy

ROS
review of systems (medical records)

ROSC
restoration of spontaneous circulation (cardiovascular)

ROSE
rosette (laboratory)

ROT
remedial occupational therapy (rehabilitation)
right occipitotransverse [position; also called *right occiput transverse*] (obstetrics)
rotating
rotator (orthopedics)

R.O.T.
Registered Occupational Therapist (occupational therapy and rehabilitation)
right occipitotransverse [position; also called *right occiput transverse*] (obstetrics)

rot
rotate
rotating

rotation
rotator (anatomy and orthopedics)

ROUL
rouleaux [formation differential] (laboratory)

rout
routine

Roux-en-Y
{not an abbreviation} [the name of an anastomosis] (gastroenterology and surgery) {pronounced "rue-en-why"}

ROV
remotely operated vehicle (oceanography)

RP
pulse rate [index] (cardiovascular)
radial pulse (cardiovascular and orthopedics)
Raynaud's phenomenon (neurology)
reactive protein (laboratory)
refractory period (neurology and orthopedics)
Registered Pharmacist (pharmacology)
relative potency
respiratory rate (respiratory)
resting potential (neurology)
resting pressure (cardiovascular)
rest pain (neurology and orthopedics)
retinitis pigmentosa (ophthalmology)
retinitis proliferans (ophthalmology)
retrograde pyelography (nephrology, radiology, and urology)
retroperitoneal (anatomy, gastroenterology, and surgery)
ribose phosphate (laboratory)
ristocetin polymyxin [an antibiotic] (pharmacology)

R$_P$
pulmonary resistance (laboratory and respiratory)

R-P
radiologist—pediatric (pediatrics and radiology)

Reid-Provident [pharmaceutical company] (pharmacology)

R-5-P
ribose-5-phosphate (laboratory)

RPA
radial photon absorptiometry (chemistry)
resultant physiological acceleration (laboratory)
reverse passive anaphylaxis (allergy)
right pulmonary artery (cardiovascular and respiratory)

RPAC
Regional Paramedic Advisory Committee (emergency medicine)

R$_{pba}$
periosteal bone apposition rate (laboratory and orthopedics)

RPC
reticularis pontis caudalis (anatomy and neurology)

RPCF
Reiter protein complement fixation [test for syphilis] (gynecology, infectious diseases, laboratory, and urology)

RPCFT
Reiter protein complement fixation test [for syphilis] (gynecology, infectious diseases, laboratory, and urology)

RPCU
retropubic cystourethropexy (gynecology and urology)

RPD
removable partial denture (dentistry)

RPE
rating of perceived exertion (measurement)
retinal pigment epithelial (ophthalmology)
retinal pigment epithelium (ophthalmology)

RPF
relaxed pelvic floor (gynecology and urology)
renal plasma flow (cardiovascular and nephrology)

RP film
rapid processing film (radiology)

RPG
radiation protection guide (radiation therapy and radiology)
retrograde pyelogram (nephrology, radiology, and urology)

RPGG
retroplacental gamma globulin (immunology and laboratory)

RPGMEC
Regional Postgraduate Medical Educational Committee (education)

RPGN
rapidly progressive glomerulonephritis (nephrology)

RPH
Registered Pharmacist (pharmacology)
retroperitoneal hemorrhage (gastroenterology, hematology, and surgery)

RPh
Registered Pharmacist (pharmacology)

R.Ph.
Registered Pharmacist (pharmacology)

RPHA
reverse passive hemagglutination (hematology and laboratory)

RP-HPLC
reversed phase—high performance liquid chromatography (laboratory)

RPI
reticulocyte production index (hematology and laboratory)

RPICCE
round pupil intracapsular cataract extraction (ophthalmology)

RPLAD
retroperitoneal lymphoadenectomy (oncology and surgery)

RPLC
reversed-phase liquid chromatography (laboratory)

RPLND
retroperitoneal lymphadenectomy (oncology and surgery)

RPM
rapid processing mode (radiology)
Raven's Progressive Matrices (psychiatry and speech and language therapy)

rpm
revolutions per minute (measurement)

RPMI
Roswell Park Memorial Institute (administration)

RPN
renal papillary necrosis (nephrology)

RPO
right posterior oblique [view] (radiology)

R point
{not an abbreviation} [a cephalometric landmark] (neurology and radiology) {pronounced "are-point"}

RPP
rate-pressure product
retropubic prostatectomy (oncology and urology)

RPPI
role perception picture inventory (psychiatry)

RPPR
red cell precursor production rate (hematology and laboratory)

RPR
rapid plasma reagin [test for syphilis] (gynecology, infectious diseases, laboratory, obstetrics, and urology)
Reiter protein reagin (laboratory)

RPS
renal pressor substance (laboratory and nephrology)

rps
revolutions per second (measurement)

RPT
Registered Physical Therapist (physical therapy and rehabilitation)

R.P.T.
Registered Physical Therapist (physical therapy and rehabilitation)

Rpt
repeat
report (medical records)

RPTD
ruptured

RPU
retropubic urethropexy (gynecology and urology)

RPV
right pulmonary vein (cardiovascular and respiratory)

RQ
recovery quotient (rehabilitation)
respiratory quotient (respiratory)

RR
radiation reaction [cells] (laboratory, radiation therapy, and radiology)
radiation response (oncology, radiation therapy, and radiology)
recovery room (surgery)
red reflex (ophthalmology)
regular respirations (respiratory)
regular rhythm (cardiovascular)
relative response
relative risk (measurement)

renin release (laboratory)
respiratory rate (respiratory)
response rate (measurement)
risk ratio (measurement)
Riva-Rocci [sphygmomanometer] (cardiovascular)

R.R.
recovery room (surgery)

R & R
rate and rhythm [of pulse] (cardiovascular)
rest and recuperation (armed forces)

RRA
radioreceptor assay (laboratory and radiology)
Registered Record Administrator (medical records)
renal renin activity (laboratory and nephrology)

R.R.A.
Registered Record Administrator (medical records)

RRAM
repetitive and rapid alternating movements (neurology)

RRC
routine respiratory care (respiratory)
Royal Red Cross (emergency medicine and social services)

RRE
round, regular, and equal [referring to the pupils of the eyes] (ophthalmology)

RR & E
round, regular, and equal [referring to the pupils of the eyes] (ophthalmology)

RREF
resting radionuclide ejection fraction (cardiovascular and radiology)

RR-HPO
rapid recompensation–high pressure oxygen [treatment] (cardiovascular and respiratory)

RRI
{not an abbreviation} [interval between two R-waves on electrocardiograms] (cardiovascular)

RRL
Registered Record Librarian (medical records)

R.R.L.
Registered Record Librarian (medical records)

rRNA
ribosomal ribonucleic acid (genetics and laboratory)

RRND
right radical neck dissection (endocrinology, oncology, otorhinolaryngology, and surgery)

RRP
relative refractory period (neurology and orthopedics)

RRR
regular rate and rhythm (cardiovascular)
renin-release rate (laboratory)

RRRN
round, regular, and react normally [referring to the pupils of the eyes] (ophthalmology)

RRT
Registered Respiratory Therapist (respiratory)
relative retention time
resazurin reduction time (laboratory)

R.R.T.
Registered Respiratory Therapist (respiratory)

RS
rating schedule
Rauwolfia serpentina (cardiovascular, neurology, pharmacology, and psychiatry)
reading of standard

recipient's serum (hematology, laboratory, and transplant surgery)
rectal sinus (gastroenterology)
reducing substance (laboratory)
reducing sugar (laboratory)
Reed-Sternberg [cell] (laboratory and oncology)
reinforcing stimulus (neurology)
Reiter's syndrome (ophthalmology, orthopedics, and urology)
renal specialist (nephrology)
resorcinol-sulphur (dermatology and pharmacology)
respiratory syncytial [virus] (laboratory and respiratory)
response to stimulus [ratio] (neurology)
review of symptoms (medical records)
review of systems (medical records)
Reye's syndrome (gastroenterology, neurology, and pediatrics)
rheumatoid spondylitis (orthopedics and rheumatology)
rhythm strip [from electrocardiogram] (cardiovascular)
right sacrum (anatomy, neurology, and orthopedics)
right side
Ringer's solution (pharmacology and surgery)

R & S
restraints and seclusion (psychiatry)

RSA
rabbit serum albumin (laboratory)
Rehabilitation Services Administration (rehabilitation)
relative specific activity (laboratory)
relative standard accuracy (laboratory)
reticulum cell sarcoma (oncology and pathology)
right sacroanterior [position; also called *right sacrum anterior*] (obstetrics)
right subclavian artery (cardiovascular)

R.S.A.
right sacroanterior [position; also called *right sacrum anterior*] (obstetrics)

RSB
Regimental Stretcher-Bearer (armed forces)
reticulocyte standard buffer (laboratory)

right sternal border [on examination] (cardiovascular)

R.S.B.
Regimental Stretcher-Bearer (armed forces)

RSC
rested-state contraction(s) (neurology and orthopedics)
reversible sickled cell (genetics, hematology, and laboratory)
right-side colon cancer (gastroenterology and oncology)

RScA
right scapuloanterior [position] (obstetrics)

R.Sc.A.
right scapuloanterior [position] (obstetrics)

rsch
research

RSCN
Registered Sick Children's Nurse (nursing and pediatrics)

R.S.C.N.
Registered Sick Children's Nurse (nursing and pediatrics)

RScP
right scapuloposterior [position] (obstetrics)

R.Sc.P.
right scapuloposterior [position] (obstetrics)

RSCT
Rach Sentence Completion Test (psychiatry and speech and language therapy)
Rotter Sentence Completion Test (psychiatry and speech and language therapy)

RSD
reflex sympathetic dystrophy (neurology and orthopedics)
relative standard deviation (measurement)

RSDS
reflex-sympathetic dystrophy syndrome (neurology)

RSE
reverse sutured eye (ophthalmology)
right sternal edge [on examination] (cardiovascular)

RSES
Rosenberg Self-Esteem Scale (psychiatry)

RSG
Reitan Strength of Grip (psychiatry and rehabilitation)

RSH
Royal Society of Health

RSIC
Radiation Shielding Information Center (radiation therapy and radiology)

R-SICU
respiratory-surgical intensive care unit (respiratory and surgery)

RSIVP
rapid sequence intravenous pyelogram (nephrology, radiology, and urology)

RSL
right sacrolateral [position; also called *right sacrum lateral*] (obstetrics)

RSM
Royal Society of Medicine

R.S.M.
Royal Society of Medicine

RSNA
Radiological Society of North America (radiology)

R.S.N.A.
Radiological Society of North America (radiology)

RSO
Resident Surgical Officer (surgery)
right salpingo-oophorectomy (gynecology)

RSP
rhinoseptoplasty (otorhinolaryngology)
right sacroposterior [position; also called *right sacrum posterior*] (obstetrics)

R.S.P.
right sacroposterior [position; also called *right sacrum posterior*] (obstetrics)

RSPCA
Royal Society for the Prevention of Cruelty to Animals (veterinary medicine)

RSPH
Royal Society for the Promotion of Health

RSPK
recurrent spontaneous psychokinesis (parapsychology and psychiatry)

RSR
regular sinus rhythm (cardiovascular)
relative survival rate (oncology and statistics)

R.S.R.
regular sinus rhythm (cardiovascular)

rSR′
{not an abbreviation} [found on electrocardiograms] (cardiovascular) {pronounced "R-S-R-prime"}

"R-S-R-prime"
{pronunciation of *rSR′* [found on electrocardiograms {not an abbreviation}]} (cardiovascular) {not an abbreviation}

RSS
Russian spring-summer [encephalitis]
(neurology)

RSSE
Russian spring-summer encephalitis
(neurology)

RST
radiosensitivity test(ing) (laboratory)
Reagin Screen Test [for syphilis] (gynecology, infectious diseases, laboratory, and urology)
right sacrotransverse [position; also
called *right sacrum transverse*] (obstetrics)

RS-T
{not an abbreviation} [a segment on elec-
trocardiograms] (cardiovascular)

R.S.T.
right sacrotransverse [position; also
called *right sacrum transverse*] (obstetrics)

RSTL
relaxed skin tension lines (dermatology)

RSTMH
Royal Society of Tropical Medicine and
Hygiene (tropical medicine)

RSTs
Rodney Smith tubes

RST's
Rodney Smith tubes

RSV
respiratory syncytial virus (laboratory
and respiratory)
right subclavian vein (cardiovascular)
Rous sarcoma virus (laboratory, oncology, and veterinary medicine)

R-S variation
rough-smooth variation (bacteriology
and laboratory)

RSW
right-sided weakness (neurology)

RT
radiation therapy
radiologic technologist (radiology)
Radiology Technologist (radiology)
radiotherapy (radiation therapy and radiology)
radium therapy (radiation therapy)
rational therapy (psychiatry)
reaction time (laboratory and neurology)
reading test (neurology, ophthalmology,
psychiatry, and speech and language
therapy)
recreational therapy (rehabilitation)
reduction time (laboratory)
Registered Technician (American Registry of X-ray Technicians) (radiology)
Registered Technologist (radiology)
renal transplant (nephrology and transplant surgery)
resistance transfer (laboratory)
Respiratory Therapist (respiratory)
respiratory therapy (respiratory)
right
right thigh (anatomy, neurology, and orthopedics)
right triceps (anatomy, neurology, and
orthopedics)
room temperature (measurement)
running total

R$_T$
total pulmonary resistance (laboratory
and respiratory)

R.T.
Recreation Therapy (rehabilitation)
Registered Technician (radiology)

R/T
rectal temperature (measurement)
related to

Rt
right
rotundus nucleus

R/t
related to

RT$_3$
serum resin triiodothyronine [uptake]
(endocrinology and laboratory)

rT$_3$
reverse triiodothyronine (endocrinology
and laboratory)

rt
right

RTA
Radiology Telephone Access [System]
(communications and radiology)
renal tubular acidosis (laboratory and
nephrology)
road traffic accident (emergency medicine)

RTC
return to clinic
round the clock

rtc
root canal [treatment] (dentistry)

RTD
Rapid Transit District [Los Angeles]
(transportation)
retarded (neurology and psychiatry)
routine test dilution (laboratory)

Rtd
retarded (neurology and psychiatry)
retired

RTE
route

rte
route

R test
reductase test (laboratory)

RTF
replication and transfer (genetics and research)
resistance transfer factor (laboratory)
respiratory tract fluid (laboratory and
respiratory)

RtH
right-handed (neurology and orthopedics)

RTI
respiratory tract infection (respiratory)

Rti
tissue resistance (laboratory and respiratory)

RTKP
radiothermokeratoplasty (ophthalmology)

RTL
reactive to light [referring to the pupils
of the eyes] (ophthalmology)

rtl
rectal (gastroenterology)

RT LAT
right lateral

rt. lat.
right lateral

RTM
routine medical care

R$_{tmf}$
total matrix formation rate

RTN
return

R.T.(N)
Registered Technologist (Nuclear) (radiology)

rtn.
return

RT N(ARRT)
Registered Technologist in Nuclear Medicine Technology (American Registry
of Radiologic Technologists) (radiation therapy and radiology)

RT(NM)
Radiology Technologist (Nuclear Medicine) (radiology)

rTNM
retreatment tumor, nodes, and metastasis [staging of cancer] (pathology and oncology)

RTO
return to office

RTOG
Radiation Therapy Oncology Group (oncology, radiation therapy, and radiology)

R to R
Reach to Recovery (gynecology, oncology, rehabilitation, and social services)

RTPA
recombinant tissue-type plasminogen activator (cardiovascular, genetics, laboratory, pharmacology, and research)

rtPA
recombinant tissue-type plasminogen activator (cardiovascular, genetics, laboratory, pharmacology, and research)

rt-PA
recombinant tissue-type plasminogen activator (cardiovascular, genetics, laboratory, pharmacology, and research)

RTR
Recreational Therapist Registered (rehabilitation)
red blood cell turnover rate (hematology and laboratory)

R.T.(R)
Registered Technologist (Radiology) (radiology)

RT R(ARRT)
Registered Technologist in Radiography (American Registry of Radiologic Technologists) (radiation therapy and radiology)

R. Tren.
right Trendelenburg [position] (surgery)

RTRR
return to recovery room (surgery)

RTS
real time scan (radiology)

RTT
Radiation Therapy Technologist (oncology, radiation therapy, and radiology)
Respiratory Therapy Technician (respiratory)

R.T.(T)
Registered Technologist (Therapy) (oncology, radiation therapy, and radiology)

RT T(ARRT)
Registered Technologist in Radiation Therapy Technology (American Registry of Radiologic Technologists) (radiation therapy and radiology)

RT$_3$U
resin triiodothyronine uptake (endocrinology and radiology)

RTW
return to work

RTx
radiation therapy

RU
radioactive uptake (laboratory and radiology)
rat unit (gynecology and measurement)
reading of unknown
rectourethral (anatomy, gastroenterology, gynecology, and urology)
resin uptake (endocrinology and laboratory)
resistance unit (chemistry and measurement)

retrograde urogram (radiology and urology)
right upper
roentgen unit (radiation therapy and radiology)

Ru
ruthenium (chemistry)

Ru¹⁰⁶
radioactive ruthenium (chemistry and radiology)

RUA
routine urinalysis (laboratory and urology)

RUB
ruber [red]

rub
ruber [red]

RUBIDIC
rubidazone and dacarbazine [DTIC] (chemotherapy, oncology, and pharmacology)

RUE
right upper extremity (orthopedics)

"rue-en-Y"
{pronunciation of *Roux-en-Y* [an anastomosis]} (gastroenterology and surgery) {not an abbreviation}

RUG
retrograde ureterogram (radiology and urology)
retrograde urethrogram (radiology and urology)

RUI
Royal University of Ireland (education)

RUL
right upper lid (ophthalmology)
right upper lung [of lung] (respiratory)

R.U.L.
right upper lobe [of lung] (respiratory)

RUO
right upper outer [quadrant] (anatomy)

RUOQ
right upper outer quadrant (anatomy)

RUP
rat urine protein (allergy and laboratory)

rupt
rupture(d)

RUQ
right upper quadrant (anatomy)

R.U.Q.
right upper quadrant (anatomy)

RUR
resin-uptake ratio (endocrinology and laboratory)

RURTI
recurrent upper respiratory tract infection(s) (respiratory)

Rus
resistance of the airways on the alveolar side of the point in the airways where intraluminal pressure equals intrapleural pressure (laboratory and respiratory)

RUSB
right upper sternal border [on examination of heart] (cardiovascular)

RV
rat virus (laboratory)
rectovaginal [examination] (gynecology and obstetrics)
reinforcement value
residual volume (laboratory and respiratory)
respiratory volume (laboratory and respiratory)
retroversion [of uterus] (gynecology and obstetrics)
return visit
right ventricle (cardiovascular)
right ventricular (cardiovascular)

rubella vaccine (gynecology, infectious diseases, obstetrics, pediatrics, and pharmacology)

rubella virus (gynecology, infectious diseases, laboratory, obstetrics, and pediatrics)

R.V.
residual volume (laboratory and respiratory)

RVA
renal vascular resistance (cardiovascular and nephrology)

RVB
red venous blood (hematology and laboratory)

RVD
relative vertebral density (neurology, orthopedics, and radiology)

RVDV
right ventricular diastolic volume (cardiovascular)

RVE
right ventricular enlargement (cardiovascular)

RVEDP
right ventricular end-diastolic pressure (cardiovascular)

RVEDV
right ventricular end-diastolic volume (cardiovascular)

RVEF
right ventricular ejection fraction (cardiovascular)

RVESP
right ventricular end-systolic pressure (cardiovascular)

RVESV
right ventricular end-systolic volume (cardiovascular)

RVET
right ventricular ejection time (cardiovascular)

RVG
radionuclide ventriculography (cardiovascular and radiology)
right ventrogluteal (anatomy)
right visceral ganglion (neurology)

RVH
renovascular hypertension (cardiovascular and nephrology)
right ventricular hypertrophy (cardiovascular)

RVI
relative value index (measurement)

RVID
right ventricular internal dimension (cardiovascular)

RVL
right vastus lateralis [muscle] (anatomy and orthopedics)

RVLG
right ventrolateral gluteal [injection site] (pharmacology)

RVO
Regional Veterinary Officer (veterinary medicine)
relaxed vaginal outlet (gynecology and obstetrics)
retinal vein occlusion (cardiovascular and ophthalmology)
right ventricular overactivity (cardiovascular)

RVOA
right ventricular overactivity (cardiovascular)

RVOT
right ventricular outflow tract (cardiovascular)

RVP
red veterinary petrolatum (veterinary medicine)
renal venous plasma (laboratory and nephrology)

RVR
rapid ventricular response (cardiovascular)
renal vascular resistance (cardiovascular and nephrology)
resistance to venous return (cardiovascular)

RVRA
renal vein renin activity (laboratory)
renal vein renin assay (laboratory)
renal venous renin assay (cardiovascular, laboratory, and nephrology)

RV/RA
renal vein/renal activity [ratio] (cardiovascular, laboratory, and nephrology)

RVRC
renal vein renin concentration (cardiovascular, laboratory, and nephrology)

RVS
relative value scale (measurement)
relative value schedule (measurement)
relative value study (statistics)
reported visual sensation (neurology and ophthalmology)

R.V.S.
Relative Value Scale [Schedule] (measurement)

RVSW
right ventricular stroke work (cardiovascular)

RVSWI
right ventricular stroke work index (cardiovascular)

RVT
renal vein thrombosis (cardiovascular and nephrology)

R.V.T.
Registered Vascular Technologist (cardiovascular and radiology)

RV time
Russell viper time [a prothrombin test] (hematology and laboratory)

RV/TLC
residual volume to total lung capacity [ratio] (laboratory and respiratory)

RV/TLC%
residual volume to total lung capacity [ratio expressed as a percent] (laboratory and respiratory)

RVV
rubella virus vaccine (immunology, infectious diseases, and pharmacology)

RW
radiological warfare (armed forces and radiology)
ragweed (allergy)

R-W
Rideal-Walker [phenol coefficient test] (laboratory)

R wave
{not an abbreviation} [a deflection on electrocardiograms] (cardiovascular)

RWP
R-wave progression [on electrocardiograms] (cardiovascular)

RX
prescription (pharmacology)
recipe [take]
treatment

Rx
drug (pharmacology)
medication (pharmacology)
prescription [only] (pharmacology)
recipe [take]
therapy
treatment

R$_x$
drug (pharmacology)
medication (pharmacology)
prescription (pharmacology)
recipe [take]
therapy
treatment

rx
reaction (laboratory)

RXLI
recessive X-linked ichthyosis (dermatology and genetics)

RXN
reaction (laboratory)

RXT
right exotropia (ophthalmology)

RxTV
Prescription Television (communications and pharmacology)

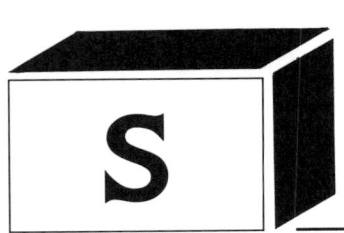

S

Σ
sigma [eighteenth letter of the Greek alphabet]
sum (mathematics)
syphilis [euphemistic abbreviation for] (gynecology, infectious diseases, laboratory, and urology)

σ
one-thousandth part of a second (measurement)
sigma [eighteenth letter of the Greek alphabet]
standard deviation (statistics)

S
entropy (physics)
mean dose per unit cumulated activity
sacral [referring to vertebrae] (neurology and orthopedics)
saline (pharmacology and surgery)
Salmonella [a bacterium] (laboratory)
same
sans (French) [*sine* (Latin), without]
saturated
saturation (laboratory)
saturation in the blood phase (laboratory and respiratory)
Schistosoma [a trematode] (laboratory)
screen-containing cassette (radiology)
second (measurement)
section
sedimentation coefficient (laboratory)
semilente [insulin] (endocrinology and pharmacology)
semis [half]
senile (neurology and psychiatry)
sensation (neurology)
sensitive (laboratory)
septum [image on transesophageal echocardiography] (cardiovascular)
serine [a supplement] (dietary and laboratory)
serum (laboratory)
siemens (measurement and physics)
signa [label, mark, sign, write] (pharmacology)

signetur [let it be written] (pharmacology)
silicate (chemistry)
sine (Latin) [sans (French), without]
single [referring to marital status]
singular
sinister [left]
sister
small
smooth [referring to bacterial colonies] (laboratory)
soft [referring to diet] (dietary and gastroenterology)
solid
soluble
solute
space
special preparations necessary for test (laboratory)
spherical
spherical lens (ophthalmology)
Spirillum [a bacterium] (laboratory)
spleen (anatomy and gastroenterology)
staff [referring to staff physician] (administration)
standard normal deviate (statistics)
Staphylococcus [a bacterium] (laboratory)
stimulus (neurology)
Streptococcus [a bacterium] (laboratory)
subcutaneous (pharmacology)
subject [of an experiment] (research)
subjective [findings]
substrate (laboratory)
suction (respiratory and surgery)
sulfur [also called *sulphur*] (chemistry and laboratory)
sum (mathematics)
supine
supravergence (ophthalmology)
surface
surgeon (surgery)
surgery

Svedberg [unit of sedimentation coefficient (10^{-13} seconds)] (laboratory)

synthesis [of deoxyribonucleic acid (DNA) in cell cycle] (genetics and laboratory)

S

surface serum glutamic-oxaloacetic transaminase [SGOT] [*Note: The abbreviation is subscripted.*] (laboratory)

S1

first heart sound [systolic] (cardiovascular)

first sacral nerve (neurology and orthopedics)

first sacral vertebra (neurology and orthopedics)

S₁

first heart sound [systolic] (cardiovascular)

first sacral nerve (neurology and orthopedics)

first sacral vertebra (neurology and orthopedics)

S2

second heart sound [diastolic] (cardiovascular)

second sacral nerve (neurology and orthopedics)

second sacral vertebra (neurology and orthopedics)

S₂

second heart sound [diastolic] (cardiovascular)

second sacral nerve (neurology and orthopedics)

second sacral vertebra (neurology and orthopedics)

S3

third heart sound [on cardiac examination; also called *summation gallop* and *ventricular gallop sound*] (cardiovascular)

third sacral nerve (neurology and orthopedics)

third sacral vertebra (neurology and orthopedics)

S₃

third heart sound [on cardiac examination; also called *summation gallop* and *ventricular gallop sound*] (cardiovascular)

S4

fourth sacral nerve (neurology and orthopedics)

fourth sacral vertebra (neurology and orthopedics)

S₄

fourth heart sound [on cardiac examination; also called *atrial gallop* and *summation gallop*] (cardiovascular)

S5

fifth sacral nerve (neurology and orthopedics)

fifth sacral vertebra (neurology and orthopedics)

s

distance

esophoria (ophthalmology)

sample standard deviation (statistics)

sans (French) [*sine* (Latin), without]

satellite [chromosomal] (genetics and laboratory)

scruple [apothecaries] (measurement and pharmacology)

second [unit of time] (measurement)

section

see

semis [half]

sensation (neurology)

sign(ed)

singular

sine (Latin) [*sans* (French), without]

sinister [left]

son

systolic (cardiovascular)

{not an abbreviation} [symbol for atomic orbital with angular momentum quantum number 0] (chemistry and physics)

s.

semis [half]

saline (pharmacology and surgery)
secundum artis legis [according to the rules of art]

Sal
Salmonella [a bacterium] (gastroenterology and laboratory)

sal
salicylate (pharmacology)
saline (pharmacology and surgery)
saliva (dentistry and otorhinolaryngology)
salt (dietary)
secundum artis legis [according to the rules of art]

SAL 12
sequential analysis of twelve chemistry constituents (laboratory)

salicyl
salicylate (pharmacology)

Salm
Salmonella [a bacterium] (gastroenterology and laboratory)

SAM
S-adenosyl-L-methionine (laboratory)
scanning acoustic microscope (laboratory)
self-administered medication (pharmacology)
sex arousal mechanism (gynecology, psychiatry, and urology)
streptozocin, Adriamycin, and methyl-CCNU [MeCCNU or semustine] (chemotherapy, oncology, and pharmacology)
sulfated acid mucopolysaccharide (laboratory)
systolic anterior motion [on two-dimensional echocardiogram] (cardiovascular)

SAMA
Student American Medical Association (education)

S.A.M.A.
Student American Medical Association (education)

SAMI
socially acceptable monitoring instrument

SAN
sinoatrial node (cardiovascular)

Sanat
sanatorium (infectious diseases and respiratory) [*Note: Do not confuse with sanitarium.* (psychiatry)]

SANC
short-arm navicular cast (orthopedics)

sang
sanguineous (laboratory)

sanit
sanitarium (psychiatry) [*Note: Do not confuse with sanatorium.* (respiratory)]
sanitary
sanitation

S-A node
sinoatrial node (cardiovascular)

SaO$_2$
arterial oxygen saturation [also called *oxygen percent saturation* (*arterial*)] (laboratory and respiratory)

SAP
serum alkaline phosphatase (gastroenterology, laboratory, and orthopedics)
serum amyloid-P (laboratory)
Staphylococcus aureus protease (laboratory)
systemic arterial pressure (cardiovascular)

SAPD
self-administration of psychotropic drugs (pharmacology and psychiatry)

sapon
saponification (chemistry and laboratory)

SAQ
short-arc quadriceps [exercises] (rehabilitation)

SAR
sexual attitude reassessment (psychiatry)
structure activity relationship (dentistry)

Sar
sulfarsphenamine [also called *sulpharsphenamine*] (chemistry and pharmacology)

SARA
System for Anesthetic and Respiratory Analysis (anesthesiology and respiratory)

sarc
sarcoma (oncology)

SAS
short-arm splint (orthopedics)
Sklar Aphasia Scale (psychiatry and speech and language therapy)
sleep apnea syndrome (neurology)
sterile aqueous suspension (pharmacology)
sulfasalazine (gastroenterology and pharmacology)
supravalvular aortic stenosis (cardiovascular)

SASE
self-addressed, stamped envelope (business)

SAT
satellite (genetics and laboratory)
saturated
saturation (laboratory and respiratory) {pronounced "sat"}
Saturday
Scholastic Achievement Test [college entrance examination] (education)
Scholastic Aptitude Test [college entrance examination] (education)
School Ability Test (education and psychiatry)
Senior Apperception Test (psychiatry)
sine acido thymonucleinico [without thymonucleic acid]

speech awareness threshold (otorhinolaryngology)
subacute thyroiditis (endocrinology)
systematized assertive therapy (psychiatry)

Sat
Saturday

sat
saturated
saturation (laboratory and respiratory) {pronounced "sat"}

"sat"
{pronunciation of *SAT* and *sat* [saturation]} (laboratory and respiratory) {not an abbreviation}

SAT-chromosome
chromosome with satellite (genetics and laboratory)

sat'd
saturated

SATL
surgical Achilles tendon lengthening (orthopedics)

satn
saturation

sat sol
saturated solution (pharmacology)

SATY
few atypical lymphocytes (laboratory)

SAU
statistical analysis unit (statistics)

SAVD
spontaneous assisted vaginal delivery (obstetrics)

SB
Scientiae Baccalaureus [Bachelor of Science] (education)
Senate Bill [followed by a numeral] (government)

S.B.
Sengstaken-Blakemore [tube] (gastroenterology)
serum bilirubin (gastroenterology and laboratory)
shortness of breath (respiratory)
sick bay (armed forces)
single breath (respiratory)
sinus bradycardia (cardiovascular)
small bowel (gastroenterology)
spina bifida (neurology)
Stanford-Binet [intelligence test] (psychiatry)
sternal border (anatomy and cardiovascular)
stillbirth (gynecology and obstetrics)
stillborn (gynecology and obstetrics)
stretcher-bearer (armed forces and emergency medicine)

S.B.
Senate Bill [followed by a numeral] (government)

Sb
stibium [antimony] (chemistry)
strabismus (ophthalmology)

SBA
sick-bay attendant (armed forces)
soy bean agglutinin (chemistry and laboratory)
stand-by assistance (rehabilitation)
{not an abbreviation} [used in measurements for orthodontistry with *S* referring to sella and *B* and *A* being reference points] (dentistry)

SBB
Specialist in Blood Bank [Technology] (hematology)

S.B.B.
Specialist Blood Banking (hematology)

SBC
standard bicarbonate (gastroenterology and pharmacology)

SBCMC
San Bernardino County Medical Center (administration)

SBD
straight bag drainage (urology)

SBE
breast self-examination (gynecology and oncology)
self breast examination (gynecology and oncology)
shortness of breath on exertion (respiratory)
subacute bacterial endocarditis (cardiovascular)

S.B.E.
subacute bacterial endocarditis (cardiovascular)

SBEP
somatosensory brain stem evoked potential(s) (neurology)

SBF
serologic-blocking factor (laboratory)
splanchnic blood flow (cardiovascular)

SBFT
small-bowel follow-through (gastroenterology and radiology)

SBG
selenite brilliant green (pharmacology)

SBGM
self blood glucose monitoring (endocrinology and laboratory)

SBH
sea blue histiocytosis (hematology)

SBH
State Board of Health (government)

S.B.H.
State Board of Health (government)

SBI
systemic bacterial infection (bacteriology and infectious diseases)

SBIS
Stanford-Binet Intelligence Scale (psychiatry)

SB-LM
Stanford-Binet Intelligent Test—Form LM (psychiatry)

SBMPL
simultaneous binaural mid plane localization test (otorhinolaryngology)

SBN
single-breath nitrogen [test] (respiratory)

SB$_{N2}$
single-breath nitrogen [test] (respiratory)

SBNS
Society of British Neurological Surgeons (neurology and neurosurgery)

SBO
small-bowel obstruction (gastroenterology and surgery)

SBOM
soybean oil meal [a protein supplement] (dietary)

SBP
scleral buckling procedure (ophthalmology)
spontaneous bacterial peritonitis (gastroenterology)
steroid-binding plasma [protein] (laboratory)
subacute bacterial peritonitis (gastroenterology)
systemic blood pressure (cardiovascular)
systolic blood pressure (cardiovascular)

SBR
strict bed rest (rehabilitation)
styrene-butadiene rubber (chemistry)

SBS
social-breakdown syndrome (psychiatry)
small-bowel syndrome (gastroenterology, radiology)

SBSRT
Spreen-Benton Sentence Repetition Test (speech and language therapy)

SBStJ
Serving Brother, Order of Saint John of Jerusalem

SBT
serum bactericidal titer(s) (laboratory)
serum bacteriological titer(s) (laboratory)
single-breath (nitrogen) test (respiratory)

SBTI
soybean trypsin inhibitor (laboratory)

SC
closure of semilunar valves (gastroenterology)
sacrococcygeal (neurology and orthopedics)
Sanitary Corps (ecology)
Schwann cell (laboratory and neurology)
sciatic [nerve] (neurology and orthopedics)
science
scientific
scilicet [namely]
sclerocorneal (ophthalmology)
scrupulus [scruple] (measurement and pharmacology)
secretory component (laboratory)
self-care (rehabilitation)
semicircular
semiclosed
service connected (armed forces)
Service Corporation
sex chromatin (genetics and laboratory)
sick call (armed forces)
sickle cell (hematology and laboratory)
sieving coefficient (laboratory)
silicone coated
single chemical (chemistry)
skin conductance (neurology)
slow component (neurology)
Snellen's chart (ophthalmology)
South Carolina [Postal Service state designation]
special care (nursing)
splenic collateral (gastroenterology)
squamous cancer (oncology)
Stepped Care

sternoclavicular (anatomy and orthopedics)
stimulus, conditioned (psychiatry)
subclavian (cardiovascular and orthopedics)
subcutaneous (pharmacology)
succinylcholine (anesthesiology, neurology, and pharmacology)
sugar coated (pharmacology)
sulfur colloid (chemistry)

S-C
sickle-cell hemoglobin C [disease] (hematology and laboratory)

Sc
scandium (chemistry)
scapula (anatomy and orthopedics)

sc
sans correction [without correction or without spectacles] (ophthalmology)
self-care (rehabilitation)
subcutaneous (pharmacology)

sc.
scilicet [certainly, evidently, of course, one may know]

SCA
selective coronary angiogram (cardiovascular and radiology)
sickle-cell anemia (hematology and laboratory)
sperm-coating antigen (laboratory)
subcutaneous abdominal [block] (anesthesiology)

S$_{Ca}$
serum calcium (laboratory)

SCAA
Skin Care Association of America (dermatology)

SCAB
streptozocin, lomustine [CCNU], Adriamycin, and bleomycin (chemotherapy, oncology, and pharmacology)

SCAN
scintiscan (radiology)
suspected child abuse and neglect (pediatrics) {pronounced "scan"}

"scan"
{pronunciation of *SCAN* [suspected child abuse and neglect]} (pediatrics) {not an abbreviation}

Scand
Scandinavian [referring to area of origin or race]

SCAT
scatula [box] (pharmacology)
School and College Ability Test (education and psychiatry)
sheep-cell agglutination test (hematology and laboratory)

scat
scatula [box] (pharmacology)

scat orig
scatula originalis [manufacturer's package and label, original package] (pharmacology)

SCB
strictly confined to bed (rehabilitation)

Sc.B
Scientiae Baccalaureus [Bachelor of Science] (education)

SCBA
self-contained breathing apparatus (oceanography and respiratory)

SCBC
small-cell bronchogenic carcinoma (oncology and respiratory)

SCC
Services for Crippled Children (pediatrics and social services)
short-course chemotherapy (chemotherapy, oncology, and pharmacology)
short-circuit current (electricity)
sickle-cell crisis (hematology)
small-cell cancer [of the lung] (oncology and respiratory)
squamous-cell carcinoma (oncology)

S.C.C.
Services for Crippled Children (pediatrics and social services)

SCCA
semiclosed circle absorber

SCCa
squamous-cell carcinoma (oncology)

SCCL
small-cell (oat cell) carcinoma of the
lung (oncology and respiratory)

SCCM
Sertoli cell culture medium (laboratory)

SCD
sequential compression device (orthopedics and surgery)
service-connected disability (armed
forces)
sickle-cell disease (hematology)
spinal cord disease (neurology)
subacute combined degeneration [of spinal cord] (neurology)
sudden cardiac death (cardiovascular)
sudden coronary death (cardiovascular)

SC (D)
sickle-cell disease (hematology)

ScD
Scientiae Doctor [Doctor of Science]
(education)

Sc.D.
Scientiae Doctor [Doctor of Science]
(education)

ScDA
scapuladextra anterior (position) [right
scapuloanterior (position)] (obstetrics)

Sc.D.A.
scapuladextra anterior (position) [right
scapuloanterior (position)] (obstetrics)

SC disease
sickle-cell disease (hematology)

ScDP
scapuladextra posterior (position)
[right scapuloposterior (position)] (obstetrics)

Sc.D.P.
scapuladextra posterior (position)
[right scapuloposterior (position)] (obstetrics)

SCE
secretory carcinoma of the endome-
trium (gynecology and oncology)
sister chromatic exchange analysis (laboratory)

SCF
Skin Cancer Foundation (dermatology
and oncology)

SCFA
short-chain fatty acid (laboratory)

SCFE
slipped capital femoral epiphysis (orthopedics)

scf/min
standard cubic feet per minute (measurement)

SCG
serum chemistry graft (laboratory)
sodium cromoglycate (pharmacology
and respiratory)

SCH
succinylcholine (anesthesiology, neurology, and pharmacology)

SCh
succinylcholine chloride (anesthesiology, neurology, and pharmacology)

SChE
serum cholinesterase [an enzyme] (laboratory)

SCHED
schedule

sched
schedule

SCHIS
schistocytes [on differential] (hematology and laboratory)

SCHIZ
schizophrenia (psychiatry) {pronounced "skizz"}

schiz
schizophrenia (psychiatry) {pronounced "skizz"}

"schrom"
{pronunciation of *SROM* [spontaneous rupture of membranes]} (obstetrics) {not an abbreviation}

SCI
Science Citation Index
Science of Creative Intelligence [transcendental meditation] (parapsychology, psychiatry, and religion)
spinal cord injury (neurology)
structured clinical interview (psychiatry)

Sci
science
scientific

SCID
severe combined immune deficiency [also called *severe combined immunodeficiency disease(s)* and *severe combined immunodeficiency disorder(s)*] (genetics and immunology)

SCIPP
sacrococcygeal to inferior pubic point (anatomy)

SCIS
spinal cord injury service (neurology and rehabilitation)

SCIV
subclavian intravenous [line] (cardiovascular and surgery)

SCJ
sclerocorneal junction (ophthalmology)
squamocolumnar junction (otorhinolaryngology)

S.C.J.
sternoclavicular joints (anatomy, orthopedics, and radiology)

SCK
serum creatine kinase (cardiovascular and laboratory)

SCL
scleroderma (dermatology and rheumatology)

ScLA
scapulolaeva (position) [left scapuloanterior (position)] (obstetrics)

Sc.L.A.
scapulolaeva (position) [left scapuloanterior (position)] (obstetrics)

SCLC
small-cell lung cancer (oncology and respiratory)

SCLE
subacute cutaneous lupus erythematosus (dermatology and rheumatology)
subcutaneous lupus erythematosus (dermatology and rheumatology)

Scler
sclerosis (cardiovascular and neurology)

ScLP
scapulolaeva posterior (position) [left scapuloposterior (position)] (obstetrics)

Sc.L.P.
scapulolaeva posterior (position) [left scapuloposterior (position)] (obstetrics)

SCLs
soft contact lenses (ophthalmology)

SCM
spondylitic caudal myelopathy (neurology and orthopedics)
State Certified Midwife (obstetrics)
sternocleidomastoid [muscle] (anatomy, orthopedics, and surgery)
streptococcal cell membrane (laboratory)

S.C.M.
Society of Computer Medicine (computer sciences)
State Certified Midwife (obstetrics)

SCMO
Senior Clerical Medical Officer (medical records)

SCN
potassium thiocyanate [also abbreviated *KSCN*] (laboratory and pharmacology)

SC$_{Na}$
sieving coefficient for sodium (laboratory)

SCND
thiocyanate (chemistry and laboratory)

SCNS
subcutaneous nerve stimulation (neurology)

S colony
smooth colony [referring to bacterial colonies] (laboratory)

SCOP
scopolamine [also called *hyoscine*] (pharmacology) {pronounced "scope"}

SCOPE
microscopic (laboratory)

"scope"
{pronunciation of *SCOP* [scopolamine; also called *hyoscine*]} (pharmacology) {not an abbreviation}

SCP
single-celled protein (laboratory)
sodium cellulose phosphate (nephrology and pharmacology)
standard care plan

scp
spherical candle power (electrical measurement)

s.c.p.
spherical candle power (electrical measurement)

SCPK
serum creatine phosphokinase (cardiovascular and laboratory)

S-CPK
serum creatine phosphokinase (cardiovascular and laboratory)

SCR
scruple (measurement and pharmacology)
silicon-controlled rectifier (electronics and laboratory)
skin conductance reading [on biofeedback] (psychiatry)
skin conductance response (psychiatry)
spondylitic caudal radioculopathy (neurology and orthopedics)

SCr
serum creatinine (laboratory and nephrology)

scr
scruple (measurement and pharmacology)

SCRAP
Simple Complex Reaction-Time Apparatus (neurology)

SCREN
screen (laboratory)

scrim
{not an abbreviation} [Slang for *speech discrimination*] (otorhinolaryngology and speech and language therapy) {pronounced "scrim"}

"scrim"
{pronunciation of *scrim* [Slang for *speech discrimination*]} (otorhinolar-

yngology and speech and language therapy) {not an abbreviation}

SCS
silicon-controlled switch (electronics)
Society of Clinical Surgery (surgery)

S.C.S.
Society of Clinical Surgery (surgery)

SCT
salmon calcitonin (endocrinology and pharmacology)
Sentence Completion Test (psychiatry)
sex chromatin test (genetics and laboratory)
sickle-cell trait (hematology and laboratory)
staphylococcal clumping test (laboratory)
sugar-coated tablet (pharmacology)

SCU
special care unit

SCUBA
self-contained underwater breathing apparatus (oceanography and respiratory) {pronounced "skoo-bah"}

scuba
self-contained underwater breathing apparatus (oceanography and respiratory) {pronounced "skoo-bah"}

SCUT
schizophrenia, chronic undifferentiated type (psychiatry)

SCV
smooth, capsulated, virulent [referring to bacteria] (laboratory)
subcutaneous vaginal [block] (anesthesiology, gynecology, and obstetrics)

SCWT
Stroop Color-Word Test (psychiatry)

SD
scleroderma (dermatology and rheumatology)
senile dementia (neurology and psychiatry)

septal defect (cardiovascular and otorhinolaryngology)
serologically defined (laboratory)
serologically determined (laboratory)
serum defect (hematology and laboratory)
shoulder disarticulation (orthopedics)
skin destruction (dermatology)
skin dose (radiation therapy and radiology)
South Dakota [Postal Service state designation]
spontaneous delivery (obstetrics)
standard deviation (statistics)
State disability (government, insurance, rehabilitation, and social services)
sterile dressing (surgery)
stone disintegration (nephrology and urology)
streptodornase (hematology and pharmacology)
sudden death (cardiovascular and respiratory)
surgical drain (surgery)
systolic discharge (cardiovascular)

S-D
sickle-cell hemoglobin D [disease] (hematology and laboratory)

S & D
stomach and duodenum (anatomy and gastroenterology)

S/D
sit and dangle (orthopedics)
systolic to diastolic (cardiovascular)

Sd
stimulus drive (psychiatry)

S^d
stimulus, discriminative (neurology)

SDA
sacrodextra anterior (position) [right sacroanterior (position)] (obstetrics)
Seventh Day Adventist [Church] (religion)
specific dynamic action [of foods] (dietary and gastroenterology)

steroid-dependent asthmatic [patient] (respiratory)

succinic dehydrogenase activity (laboratory)

S.D.A.
sacrodextra anterior (position) [right sacroanterior (position)] (obstetrics)

SD antigen
serologically defined antigen (laboratory)

SDAT
senile dementia, Alzheimer type (neurology and psychiatry)

SDC
sodium deoxycholate (laboratory)
succinyldicholine (pharmacology)

SDCL
symptom distress check list

S-D curve
strength-duration curve (pharmacology)

SDD
sterile dry dressing (surgery)

SDE
specific dynamic effect
State Department of Education (education and government)

SDF
slow death factor

SDH
serine dehydrase [a supplement] (dietary and laboratory)
sorbitol dehydrogenase [also called *L-iditol dehydrogenase*] (gastroenterology and laboratory)
spinal dorsal horn (neurosurgery)
subdural hematoma (neurology and neurosurgery)
succinate dehydrogenase [an enzyme] (laboratory)

SDHD
sudden death heart disease (cardiovascular)

SDI
standard deviation interval (statistics)
State Disability Insurance (government, insurance, rehabilitation, and social services)
Strategic Defense Initiative (armed forces)

SDL
serum digoxin level (cardiovascular and laboratory)

SDM
sensory detection method (neurology)
standard deviation of the mean (statistics)

SDMS
Society of Diagnostic Medical Sonographers (cardiovascular, obstetrics, and radiology)

SDN
sexually dimorphic nucleus (laboratory)

SDO
sudden-dosage onset (pharmacology)

SDP
sacrodextra position (position) [right sacroposterior (position)] (obstetrics)

S.D.P.
sacrodextra position (position) [right sacroposterior (position)] (obstetrics)

SDR
surgical dressing room (surgery)

SDS
same day surgery (surgery)
school dental service (dentistry and education)
Self-Rating Depression Scale (psychiatry)
sensory deprivation syndrome (neurology and psychiatry)
sexual differentiation scale (laboratory)
sodium dodecyl sulfate (pharmacology)
specific diagnosis service
State Disability Service (government, in-

surance, rehabilitation, and social services)
sudden death syndrome (cardiovascular and respiratory)

Sds
sounds

SDT
sacrodextra transversa (position) [right sacrotransverse (position)] (obstetrics)
Spache Diagnostic Test (psychiatry)
Speech Detection Threshold (otorhinolaryngology and speech and language therapy)

S.D.T.
sacrodextra transversa (position) [right sacrotransverse (position)] (obstetrics)

SDU
short double upright brace (orthopedics)
Standard Deviation Unit (statistics)

S.D.U.
Standard Deviation Unit (statistics)

SE
herself
himself
saline enema (gastroenterology and pharmacology)
sanitary engineering (ecology)
self
side effect(s)
solid extract [used as a diluent] (pharmacology)
southeast (direction)
sphenoethmoidal [suture] (otorhinolaryngology)
spherical equivalent
spin echo (radiology)
stage of exhaustion [in generalized adaptation syndrome] (psychiatry)
standard error (laboratory)
Starr-Edwards [prosthesis] (cardiovascular)

Se
selenium (chemistry)

SEA
sheep erythrocyte agglutination [test] (hematology and laboratory)
spontaneous electrical activity (neurology and physiology)
staphylococcal enterotoxin A (laboratory)
state education agency (education and government)

"sea-bahz"
{pronunciation of *CIBA's* [glutethimide (also called *Doriden*)]} (chemical dependency) {slang} {not an abbreviation}

SEA test
sheep erythrocyte agglutination test (hematology and laboratory)

SEB
staphylococcal enterotoxin B (laboratory)

SEBA
staphylococcal enterotoxin B antiserum (laboratory)

SEBM
Society for Experimental Biology and Medicine (biology and research)

S.E.B.M.
Society for Experimental Biology and Medicine (biology and research)

SEC
secundum [according to] (pharmacology)
soft elastic capsules (orthopedics)

sec
second (time measurement) {pronounced "sek"}
secondary
secretary (business)
section(s)

μsec
microsecond (measurement)

SEP
sensory evoked potential(s) (neurology)
separate
sepultus [buried]
somatosensory evoked potential(s) (neurology)
sperm entry point (laboratory, obstetrics, and urology)
systolic ejection period (cardiovascular)

separ
separately
separatum [separately]

sept
septem [seven]

SEQ. #
sequence number

seq
sequela [that which follows]
sequestration (orthopedics)
sequestrum (orthopedics)

SEQ. DEV. EX.
sequential developmental exercises (occupational therapy and rehabilitation)

seq luce
sequenti luce [the following day, the next day]

SER
service
smooth endoplasmic reticulum (laboratory)
somatosensory evoked response(s) (neurology)
systolic ejection rate (cardiovascular)

sER
smooth endoplasmic reticulum (laboratory)

Ser
serine [a supplement] (dietary and laboratory)

ser
serial
series

SER-IV
supination-external rotation type IV (four) [fracture] (orthopedics)

"serk"
{pronunciation of *Circ*, *circ*, and *circ*. [circumcision]} (neonatology, pediatrics, and urology) {not an abbreviation}

sero
serological [examination] (laboratory)

Serol
serological [examination] (laboratory)

SERs
somatosensory evoked responses (neurology)

ser sect
serial sections (laboratory and pathology)

serv
serva [keep, preserve] (pharmacology)
service(s)

SERVHEL
Service and Health [Record] (medical records)

SES
seasonal energy syndrome (psychiatry)
Society of Eye Surgeons (ophthalmology)
socioeconomic status (social services and statistics)
spatial emotional stimuli (psychiatry)

sesquih
sesquihora [an hour and a half] (time measurement)

sesunc
sesuncia [an ounce and a half] (measurement and pharmacology)

SET
systolic ejection time (cardiovascular)

sev
severe
severed

sex
sexual

s expr
sine expressione [without expressing, without pressing]

SF
sacrifice fly [in baseball] (sports medicine)
safety factor
salt-free (dietary)
scarlet fever (infectious diseases, pediatrics, and rheumatology)
science fiction (literature)
semi-Fowler's [position] (surgery)
seminal fluid (laboratory and urology)
serum fibrinogen (hematology and laboratory)
shell fragment (armed forces, radiology, and surgery)
shrapnel fragment (armed forces, radiology, and surgery)
sodium azide, fecal [medium] (laboratory)
soluble factor
sound field (otorhinolaryngology)
spinal fluid (laboratory and neurology)
sterile female (gynecology and obstetrics)
Streptococcus faecalis [a bacterium] (laboratory)
stress formula [a vitamin formula] (pharmacology)
sugar-free (dietary)
sulfation factor [also called *somatomedin* and *sulphation factor*] (laboratory)
Svedberg flotation [unit] (chemistry and laboratory)
symptom-free
synovial fluid (laboratory and orthopedics)

S.F.
salt free (dietary)

SF-6
sulfur hexafluoride [used in fluid-gas exchange] (ophthalmology)

SF$_6$
sulfur hexafluoride [used in fluid-gas exchange] (ophthalmology)

Sf
Svedberg flotation [unit] (chemistry and laboratory)

S$_f$
Svedberg flotation [unit] (chemistry and laboratory)

SFA
saturated fatty acids (cardiovascular, chemistry, dietary, and laboratory)
superficial femoral artery (cardiovascular and orthopedics)

SFC
sergeant first class (armed forces)
soluble fibrin-fibrinogen complex (hematology and laboratory)
spinal fluid count (laboratory and neurology)

SFD
short food drape (dietary and rehabilitation)
skin-film distance (radiology)

SFEMG
single-fiber electromyography (neurology)

SFFF
sedimentation field flow fractionization (hematology and laboratory)

SFGS
stratum fibrosum et griseum superficiale (neurology)

SFHb
stroma-free hemoglobin [an artificial blood] (hematology)

SFL
Sexual Freedom League (social services)

SFO
subfornical organ [also called *organum*

subfornicale] (anatomy and neurology)

SFP
screen filtration pressure (chemistry and laboratory)
simultaneous foveal perception (ophthalmology)
spinal fluid pressure (neurology)
stopped flow pressure

SFPT
standard fixation preference test (laboratory)

SFR
stroke with full recovery (neurology and rehabilitation)

SFS
serial focal seizures (neurology)
skin and fascial stapler (surgery)
split function study (laboratory)

SFT
skin-fold thickness (measurement)

SFW
shell fragment wound (armed forces and surgery)
shrapnel fragment wound (armed forces and surgery)

SG
Sachs-Georgi [test for syphilis] (gynecology, infectious diseases, laboratory, and urology)
senior grade (employment rating)
sergeant (armed forces)
serum globulin (immunology and laboratory)
serum glucose (endocrinology and laboratory)
sign(s)
skin graft (dermatology and plastic surgery)
solicitor general (law enforcement)
soluble gelatin [referring to capsules] (pharmacology)
specific gravity (laboratory and urology)
Surgeon General (government)
Swan-Ganz [catheter] (cardiovascular)

S.G.
serum glucose (endocrinology and laboratory)
specific gravity (laboratory and urology)
Swan-Ganz [catheter] (cardiovascular)

S-G
Sachs-Georgi [test for syphilis] (gynecology, infectious diseases, laboratory, and urology)

sg
specific gravity (laboratory and urology)

SGA
small for gestational age (neonatology and obstetrics)

SGAW
specific airway conductance (respiratory)

SGC
spermicide-germicide compound (gynecology and pharmacology)

SGD
straight gravity drainage (surgery)

SGE
significant glandular enlargement (endocrinology)

SGFR
single-nephron glomerular filtration rate (laboratory and nephrology)

SGIA
{not an abbreviation} [A stapling device and staples] (surgery)

s gl
sans correction [without correction] (ophthalmology)
sans glasses [without glasses] (ophthalmology)

SGM
Society for General Microbiology (laboratory and microbiology)

SGO
Surgeon General's Office (government)
surgery, gynecology, and obstetrics (gynecology, obstetrics, and surgery)

S.G.O.
Surgeon General's Office (government)
surgery, gynecology, and obstetrics (gynecology, obstetrics, and surgery)

SGOT
serum glutamic oxalo-acetic transaminase (cardiovascular, gastroenterology, and laboratory) {*Obsolete*—Now called *AST* [aspartate aminotransferase]}

SGP
serine glycerophosphatide (laboratory)
Society of General Physiologists (physiology)
soluble glycoprotein (laboratory)

S.G.P.
Society of General Physiologists (physiology)

SGPT
serum glutamic pyruvic transaminase (cardiovascular, gastroenterology, and laboratory) {*Obsolete*—Now called *ALT* [alanine aminotransferase]}

SGR
Sachs-Georgi reaction [on test for syphilis] (gynecology, infectious diseases, laboratory, and urology)
submandibular gland renin (laboratory)

S-Gt
Sachs-Georgi test [for syphilis] (gynecology, infectious diseases, laboratory, and urology)

Sgt.
sergeant (armed forces)

SG test
Sachs-Georgi test [for syphilis] (gynecology, infectious diseases, laboratory, and urology)

Sgt. Maj.
sergeant major (armed forces)

SGV
salivary gland virus (dentistry, laboratory, and otorhinolaryngology)

SH
serum hepatitis (gastroenterology, infectious diseases, and laboratory)
sex hormone (endocrinology and laboratory)
sexual harassment (psychiatry)
short
shoulder (neurology and orthopedics)
shower
sick in hospital
sinus histiocytosis (otorhinolaryngology)
social history
somatotropic (growth) hormone (endocrinology, laboratory, and pediatrics)
spontaneously hypertensive (cardiovascular)
state hospital (government)
student health (education)
sulfhydryl [also called *sulphydryl*; the univalent radical] (chemistry)
surgical history (surgery)

S.H.
state hospital (government)
student health (education)

S & H
speech and hearing (otorhinolaryngology and speech and language therapy)

S/H
suicidal/homicidal [ideation] (psychiatry)

Sh
sheep (veterinary medicine)
Shigella [a bacterium] (bacteriology and laboratory)

sh
short
shoulder (neurology and orthopedics)

SHA
superheated aerosol

SHAA
serum hepatitis–associated antigen (gastroenterology, infectious diseases, and laboratory)

SHAA-Ab
serum hepatitis–associated antigen-antibody (gastroenterology, infectious diseases, and laboratory)

SHA-Ab
serum hepatitis–associated antibody (gastroenterology, infectious diseases, and laboratory)

SHARP
School Health Additional Referral Program (education)

sharps
{not an abbreviation} [Slang for sharp surgical instruments that must be counted and accounted for during and after surgery] (surgery) {pronounced "sharpz"}

"sharpz"
{pronunciation of *sharps* [not an abbreviation (Slang for sharp surgical instruments that must be counted and accounted for during and after surgery)]} (surgery) {not an abbreviation}

SHB
subacute hepatitis with bridging (gastroenterology and infectious diseases)
sulfhemoglobin (hematology and laboratory)

SHb
sickle hemoglobin [screen] (hematology and laboratory)
sulfhemoglobin (hematology and laboratory)

SHBD
serum X-hydroxybutyrate dehydrogenase (laboratory)

SHBG
sex hormone–binding globulin (endocrinology and laboratory)

SHCO
sulfated hydrogenated castor oil (gastroenterology and pharmacology)

SHDI
supraorbital hypophysial [or hypophyseal] diabetes insipidus (endocrinology and neurology)

SHEENT
skin, hair, eyes, ears, nose and throat [or head] (dermatology, ophthalmology, and otorhinolaryngology)

SHEM
hemolyzed—unable to do test (laboratory)

SHES
School Health Education Study (education)

SHG
Sauerbruch, Herrmannsdorfer, Gerson diet [in tuberculosis] (infectious diseases and respiratory)
synthetic human gastrin (gastroenterology)

SHHD
Scottish Home and Health Department (government)

SHHP
semihorizontal heart position (cardiovascular and radiology)

SHHV
Society for Health and Human Values (social services)

Shig
Shigella [a bacterium] (bacteriology and laboratory) {pronounced "shig"}

"shig"
{pronunciation of *Shig* [*Shigella* (a bacterium)]} (bacteriology and laboratory) {not an abbreviation}

SHIS
schistocytes (hematology and laboratory)

SHLD
shoulder (neurology and orthopedics)

shld.
shoulder (neurology and orthopedics)

SHMO
Senior Hospital Medical Officer (administration)
social health maintenance organization

SHN
spontaneous hemorrhagic necrosis (hematology)
subacute hepatic necrosis (gastroenterology)

SHO
secondary hypertrophic osteoarthropathy (orthopedics)
Senior House Officer (administration)
Student Health Organization (education)

S.H.O.
Student Health Organization (education)

SHP
surgical hypoparathyroidism (endocrinology)

SHS
Sayre head sling (neurology, orthopedics, and surgery)
sheep hemolysate supernatant (laboratory)
Shipley-Hartford Scale (psychiatry and speech and language therapy)
Student Health Service (education)

SHT
simple hypocalcemic tetany (neurology and orthopedics)
subcutaneous histamine test (allergy)

SH virus
homologous serum-transmitted hepatitis virus (gastroenterology, infectious diseases, and laboratory)

SHWR
saturated hydrocarbon weathering ratio (ecology)

SHx
social history (medical records)

SI
sacroiliac (anatomy, neurology, and orthopedics)
saline injection [abortion] (obstetrics)
saturation index (measurement)
self-inflicted [injury or wound] (emergency medicine)
seriously ill
serum iron (hematology and laboratory)
sex inventory (psychiatry)
soluble insulin (endocrinology and pharmacology)
stimulation index (laboratory)
stress incontinence (gynecology and urology)
stroke index (neurology)
suicidal ideation (psychiatry)
Système Internationale d'Unités [International System of Units] (measurement)
system inventory [also called *review of systems*] (medical records)

S.I.
Système Internationale d'Unités [International System of Units] (measurement)

S & I
suction and irrigation (surgery)

Si
silicon (chemistry)

SIA
stress-induced anesthesia (neurology)
synalbumin-insulin antagonism (laboratory)

SIADH
syndrome of inappropriate antidiuretic hormone [secretion] (endocrinology and nephrology)

SIB
self-injurious behavior (emergency medicine and psychiatry)

sibs
siblings {pronounced "sibz"}

sib-ship
sibling relationship (pediatrics) {pronounced "sib-ship"}

"sib-ship"
{pronunciation of *sib-ship* [sibling relationship]} (pediatrics) {not an abbreviation}

"sibz"
{pronunciation of *sibs* [siblings]} {not an abbreviation}

sic
siccus [dry]
{not an abbreviation} [Latin word meaning *as stated, spelled in that way, thus so,* or *used in that way*] (language)

SICD
Sequenced Inventory of Communicative Development (speech and language therapy)
serum isocitric dehydrogenase (laboratory)

SICK
sickle cells (hematology and laboratory)

SICKLE
sickle cells (hematology and laboratory)

SICOR
{not an abbreviation} [A computer-assisted cardiac catheterization recording system] (cardiovascular and radiology) {pronounced "see-cor"}

SICSVA
sequential impaction cascade sieve volumetric air [sampler] (respiratory)

SICT
selective intracoronary thrombolysis (cardiovascular)

SICU
surgical intensive care unit (surgery)

SID
sudden infant death [syndrome] (neonatology, pediatrics, and respiratory)

S.I.D.
Society for Investigative Dermatology (dermatology and research)

s.i.d.
semel in die [once a day] (pharmacology)

SIDER
siderocytes [in differential] (hematology and laboratory)

SIDS
sudden infant death syndrome (neonatology, pediatrics, and respiratory) {pronounced "sidz"}

"sidz"
{pronunciation of *SIDS* [sudden infant death syndrome]} (neonatology, pediatrics, and respiratory) {not an abbreviation}

SIECUS
Sex Information and Education Council of the United States (education, gynecology, government, psychiatry, social services, and urology)

S.I.E.C.U.S.
Sex Information and Education Council of the United States (education, gynecology, government, psychiatry, social services, and urology)

SI & F
spinal instrumentation and fusion (neurology and orthopedics)

SIg
serum immune globulin (immunology and laboratory)

slg
surface immunoglobulin (immunology and laboratory)

Sig
sigmoidoscopy (gastroenterology)
signa [label, mark, write] (pharmacology) {pronounced "sig"}
signal
signature
signetur [let it be labeled, let it be written] (pharmacology) {pronounced "sig"}
significant

sig
sigmoidoscopy (gastroenterology)
signa [label, mark, write] (pharmacology) {pronounced "sig"}
signal
signature
signetur [let it be labeled, let it be written] (pharmacology) {pronounced "sig"}

"sig"
{pronunciation of *Sig* and *sig* [*signa* (label, mark, write) and *signetur* (let it be labeled, let it be written)]} (pharmacology) {not an abbreviation}

S-IgA
secretory immunoglobulin A (immunology and laboratory)

"sigh"
{pronunciation of *PSI*, *psi*, and *p.s.i.* [pounds per square inch] (measurement) and *Psy* [psychiatry]} {not an abbreviation}

"sigh-borg"
{pronunciation of *cyborg* [cybernetic organism]} (computer sciences and research) {not an abbreviation}

"sigh-call"
{pronunciation of *psychol* [psychology]} (psychiatry) {not an abbreviation}

"sigh-co"
{pronunciation of *psycho* [psychopath]} (psychiatry) {not an abbreviation}

"sigh-co-an"
{pronunciation of *psychoan* [psychoanalysis]} (psychiatry) {not an abbreviation}

"sigh-co-fizz"
{pronunciation of *psychophys* [psychophysics and psychophysiology]} (psychiatry) {not an abbreviation}

"sigh-co-ther"
{pronunciation of *psychother* [psychotherapy]} (psychiatry) {not an abbreviation}

"sigh-coz-med"
{pronunciation of *PsychosMed* [psychosomatic medicine]} (psychiatry) {not an abbreviation}

"sighk"
{pronunciation of *psych* [psychology]} (psychiatry) {not an abbreviation}

"sigh-kem"
{pronunciation of *PSYCHEM* [psychiatric chemistry]} (chemistry, pharmacology, and psychiatry) {not an abbreviation}

"sigh-path"
{pronunciation of *psy-path* [psychopath and psychopathic]} (psychiatry) {not an abbreviation}

"sigh-som"
{pronunciation of *psy-som* [psychosomatic]} (psychiatry) {not an abbreviation}

"sigh-vay-dact"
{pronunciation of *CY-VA-DACT* [cyclophosphamide, vincristine, Adriamycin, and actinomycin D] (chemotherapy, oncology, and pharmacology) {not an abbreviation}

"sigh-vay-dick"
{pronunciation of *CYVADIC* and *CY-VA-DIC* [cyclophosphamide (Cytoxan), vincristine (Oncovin), Adriamycin (doxorubicin), and dacarbazine

(DTIC)]} (chemotherapy, oncology, and pharmacology) {not an abbreviation}

sigmo
sigmoidoscopy (gastroenterology)

sigmoid
sigmoidoscopy (gastroenterology) {pronounced "sig-moid"}

"sig-moid"
{pronunciation of *sigmoid* [sigmoidoscopy]} (gastroenterology) {not an abbreviation}

sign
signature

SIG N PRO
signa nomine proprio [label with the proper name] (pharmacology)

sig n pro
signa nomine proprio [label with the proper name] (pharmacology)

sig. n. pro.
signa nomine proprio [label with the proper name] (pharmacology)

SIhPTH
serum immunoreactive human parathormone (endocrinology, immunology, and laboratory)

SIJ
sacroiliac joint (neurology and orthopedics)

SI jt
sacroiliac joint (neurology and orthopedics)

SIL
seriously ill list (administration)

SILS
Shipley Institute of Living Scale (psychiatry)

SIM
Society of Industrial Microbiology (laboratory and microbiology)

sucrase-isomaltose [deficiency; also called *disaccharide intolerance*] (gastroenterology and genetics)
sulfide, indole, motility [medium] (laboratory)

S.I.M.
Society of Industrial Microbiology (laboratory)

Simkin
simulation kinetics [analysis] (laboratory and toxicology)

simp
simple
simplex [simple]

SIMUL
simultaneously [at the same time]

simul
simultaneously [at the same time]

SIMV
synchronized intermittent mandatory ventilation (respiratory)

sine
sinusoidal (anatomy, cardiovascular, and otorhinolaryngology)

SINES
short interspaced repeated segments [of deoxyribonucleic acid] (genetics and laboratory)

SING
singular [one]
singulorum [of each] (pharmacology)

sing
singular [one]
singulorum [of each] (pharmacology)

SI NON VAL
si non valet [if it does not answer, if it is not enough, if it is not of value] (pharmacology)

SINR
Swiss Institute of Nuclear Research
(physics and research)

si n val
si non valet [if it does not answer, if it is
not enough, if it is not of value] (pharmacology)

SI OP SIT
si opus sit [if necessary] (pharmacology)

si op sit
si opus sit [if necessary] (pharmacology)

Sippy No. 1
{not an abbreviation} [a preparation of
sodium bicarbonate and calcium car-
bonate] (gastroenterology and pharmacology)

Sippy No. 2
{not an abbreviation} [a preparation of
sodium bicarbonate and magnesium
oxide] (gastroenterology and pharmacology)

sIPTH
serum immunoreactive parathyroid hormone (endocrinology, immunology,
and laboratory)

SIQ
sick in quarters (armed forces)

SIRA
Scientific Instrument Research Association [British] (manufacturing and research)

SIRS
soluble immune response suppressor
(immunology and laboratory)

SIS
sterile injectable suspension (pharmacology)

SISI
short increment sensitivity index (laboratory)

short increment sensitivity index [of
hearing] (otorhinolaryngology)

"sis-tow"
{pronunciation of *CYSTO* [cystogram
and cystoscopy] and *cysto* [cysto-
scopic examination and cystoscopy]}
(urology) {not an abbreviation}

SiSV
simian sarcoma virus (laboratory, oncology, and veterinary medicine)

SIT
serum inhibiting titer(s) (laboratory)
Slossen Intelligence Test (psychiatry)
sperm immobilization test (laboratory
and urology)

S.I. unit
Système Internationale d'Unités [Inter-
national System of Units] (measurement)

SI VIR PERM
si vires permitant [if the strength will
permit] (pharmacology)

si vir perm
si vires permitant [if the strength will
permit] (pharmacology)

SIW
self-inflicted wound (emergency medicine)

SIZE
size

SJ
Stevens-Johnson [syndrome] (dermatology, gastroenterology, ophthalmology,
orthopedics, and otorhinolaryngology)

S-J
Stevens-Johnson [syndrome] (dermatology, gastroenterology, ophthalmology,
orthopedics, and otorhinolaryngology)

SJR
Shinowara-Jones-Reinhart [unit] (laboratory)

SJS
Stevens-Johnson syndrome (dermatology, gastroenterology, ophthalmology, orthopedics, and otorhinolaryngology)

SK
senile keratosis (dermatology)
skin (dermatology)
Sloan-Kettering [combined with numbers to denote experimental compounds for treatment of cancer] (chemotherapy and oncology)
Smith Kline [Diagnostics] (laboratory and pharmacology)
solar keratosis (dermatology)
spontaneous killer [cells] (immunology and laboratory)
streptokinase (cardiovascular and pharmacology)
striae keratopathy (ophthalmology)

SK-65
{not an abbreviation} [a brand name for a preparation of propoxyphene hydrochloride] (pharmacology)

sk.
skeletal (orthopedics)
skimmed

SKA
supracondylar knee-ankle [orthosis] (orthopedics)

SKAT
Sex Knowledge and Aptitude [test] (psychiatry)

SKD
Smith Kline Diagnostics (laboratory and pharmacology)

Skel
skeletal (orthopedics)

skel
skeletal (orthopedics)

SKF
Smith, Kline, and French [manufacturer] (pharmacology)

SKI
skin (dermatology)
Sloan-Kettering Institute (administration and oncology)

"skizz"
{pronunciation of SCHIZ and schiz [schizophrenia]} (psychiatry) {not an abbreviation}

SKL
serum-killing level (pharmacology, radiation therapy, and research)

"skoo-bah"
{pronunciation of SCUBA and scuba [self-contained underwater breathing apparatus]} (oceanography and respiratory) {not an abbreviation}

SKSD
streptokinase-streptodornase [skin test for immune function] (immunology)

SK-SD
streptokinase-streptodornase [skin test for immune function] (immunology)

sk. tr.
skeletal traction (orthopedics)

sk. tx.
skeletal traction (orthopedics)

SKU
stockkeeping unit (computer science)

SKW
Sturge-Kalischer-Weber [syndrome; also called Sturge-Weber syndrome] (dermatology, genetics, and neurology)

SL
satellite-like (laboratory and pathology)
secundum legem [according to the law, according to the rules]
sensation level [of hearing] (otorhinolar-

yngology and speech and language therapy)

serious list (administration)

short-leg [cast] (orthopedics)

Sibley-Lehninger [unit] (laboratory)

Sinding Larsen [disease; also called *Larsen's disease* and *Larsen-Johansson disease*] (orthopedics)

Sjögren-Larsson [syndrome] (dermatology, genetics, neurology, and psychiatry)

slight

slit lamp (ophthalmology)

small lymphocyte(s) (hematology and laboratory)

sodium lactate [for electrolyte and fluid replacement] (pharmacology)

solidified-liquid

sound level (otorhinolaryngology and speech and language therapy)

Stein-Leventhal [syndrome] (endocrinology, gynecology, and nephrology)

streptolysin (hematology and laboratory)

Strümpell-Lorrain [disease] (genetics and neurology)

sublingual (pharmacology)

S→L

serosa to lumen (anatomy and measurement)

sl

secundum legem [according to the law, according to the rules]

sensu lato [in the broad sense]

slightly

sublingual (pharmacology)

s.l.

secundum legem [according to the rules]

sensu lato [in the broad sense]

SLA

sacrolaeva anterior (position) [left sacroanterior (position)] (obstetrics)

slide latex agglutination (laboratory)

S.L.A.

sacrolaeva anterior (position) [left sacroanterior (position)] (obstetrics)

SLA-212

cyclophosphamide, vincristine, methotrexate, daunomycin, and prednisone consolidation and maintenance (chemotherapy, oncology, and pharmacology)

SLAM

scanning laser acoustic microscope (laboratory)

SLAP

serum leucine aminopeptidase (gastroenterology, laboratory, and oncology)

SLB

short-leg brace (orthopedics)

SLC

short-leg cast (orthopedics)

SLD

serum lactate dehydrogenase (laboratory and multiple specialties)

SLDH

serum lactate dehydrogenase (laboratory and multiple specialties)

SLDS

single-level dynamic scan(ner) [radiology]

SLE

Saint Louis encephalitis (infectious diseases, laboratory, and neurology)

slit lamp examination (ophthalmology)

systemic lupus erythematosus (rheumatology)

S.L.E.

systemic lupus erythematosus (rheumatology)

"slert"

{pronunciation of *SLRT* [straight-leg-raising tenderness or test]} (neurology and orthopedics) {not an abbreviation}

SLEV

Saint Louis encephalitis virus (infectious diseases, laboratory, and neurology)

SLGXT
symptom-limited graded exercise test (cardiovascular)

SLI
splenic localization index (gastroenterology)

SLIT
little S positive (laboratory)

SLK
superior limbic keratoconjunctivitis (ophthalmology)

SLKC
superior limbic keratoconjunctivitis (ophthalmology)

SLN
superior laryngeal nerve (anatomy, endocrinology, otorhinolaryngology, and surgery)

SLO
streptolysin-O [test] (cardiovascular, laboratory, and rheumatology)

SLP
sacrolaeva posterior (position) [left sacroposterior (position)] (obstetrics)
sex-limited proteins (genetics and laboratory)

S.L.P.
sacrolaeva posterior (position) [left sacroposterior (position)] (obstetrics)

SLPP
serum lipophosphoprotein (cardiovascular and laboratory)

SLR
straight-leg raising (neurology and orthopedics)
Streptococcus lactis R [factor] (laboratory)
Streptococcus lactis, resistant (laboratory)

S.L.R.
straight-leg raising (neurology and orthopedics)

S:L ratio
sucrase to lactase ratio (laboratory)

SLR factor
folic acid (dietary, laboratory, and pharmacology)

SLRT
straight-leg-raising tenderness (neurology and orthopedics) {pronounced "slert"}
straight-leg-raising test (neurology and orthopedics) {pronounced "slert"}

SLR (t)
straight-leg-raising test (neurology and orthopedics)

SLS
segment long-spacing [collagen fibers on electrophoresis] (laboratory)
short-leg splint (orthopedics)

SLT
sacrolaeva transversa (position) [left sacrotransverse (position)] (obstetrics)
slight

S.L.T.
sacrolaeva transversa (position) [left sacrotransverse (position)] (obstetrics)

SITr
silent treatment (psychiatry)

SLWC
short-leg walking cast (orthopedics)

SM
Master of Science (education)
sadomasochism (psychiatry)
Scheuthauer-Marie [syndrome]
self-monitoring
semimembranous (anatomy)

Serratia marcescens [a bacterium] (laboratory)

sewage microparticulates (laboratory)

Sexual Myths [scale] (psychiatry)

Shigella mutant [a bacterium] (laboratory)

simple mastectomy (oncology and surgery)

skim milk (dietary)

slime mold (laboratory)

small

smoker (chemical dependency and respiratory)

smooth muscle (anatomy and neurology)

somatomedin (endocrinology, laboratory, and orthopedics)

Space Medicine (aerospace medicine)

sphingomyelin (laboratory and neurology)

stapedius muscle (neurology and otorhinolaryngology)

staphylococcus medium (laboratory)

streptomycin [an antibiotic] (pharmacology)

Strümpell-Marie [disease; also called *rheumatoid spondylitis*] (neurology, orthopedics, and rheumatology)

submandibular (anatomy)

submucosal (anatomy)

submucous (anatomy)

substitute for morphine (pharmacology)

substituted metabolites (laboratory)

suckling mice (laboratory and research)

sucrose medium (laboratory)

suction method (surgery)

superior mesenteric (cardiovascular and gastroenterology)

supramamillary (neurology)

sustained medication (pharmacology)

symptoms

synaptic membrane (anatomy, neurology, and neurosurgery)

synovial membrane (anatomy and orthopedics)

systolic mean (cardiovascular)

systolic murmur (cardiovascular)

S/M

sadism/masochism (psychiatry)

SM-1

Singh's mosquito [tissue culture medium] (laboratory)

Sm

Smith [as in *anti-Smith antibody*] (hematology and laboratory)

sm

small

SMA

sequential multiple analysis (laboratory)

Sequential Multiple Analyzer (laboratory)

simultaneous multichannel autoanalyzer (laboratory)

smooth muscle antibody (laboratory)

Society for Medical Anthropology (anthropology)

spinal muscular atrophy (neurology and orthopedics)

standard methods agar (laboratory)

superior mesenteric artery (cardiovascular, gastroenterology, and surgery)

SMA 6

{not an abbreviation} [Sequential Multiple Analyzer of serum bicarbonate, blood urea nitrogen, chloride, creatinine, potassium, and sodium] (laboratory)

SMA 12

{not an abbreviation} [Sequential Multiple Analyzer of serum albumin, alkaline phosphatase, blood urea nitrogen, calcium, cholesterol, glucose, lactate dehydrogenase, phosphorus, serum glutamic-oxaloacetic transaminase, total protein, total bilirubin, and uric acid] (laboratory)

SMA 6/60

{not an abbreviation} [Sequential Multiple Analyzer of serum bicarbonate, blood urea nitrogen, chloride, creatinine, potassium, and sodium in 60 minutes] (laboratory)

SMA 12/60

{not an abbreviation} [Sequential Multiple Analyzer of serum albumin, alkaline phosphatase, blood urea nitrogen, calcium, cholesterol, glucose, lactate dehydrogenase, phosphorus, serum glutamic-oxaloacetic transaminase, total bilirubin, total protein, and uric acid in 60 minutes] (laboratory)

SMAC
sequential multiple analyzer computerized (laboratory)

SMAC-23
{not an abbreviation} [a panel of laboratory tests] (laboratory)

SMAF
smooth muscle activating factor (laboratory)
specific macrophage arming factor (laboratory)

sm an
small animal (veterinary medicine)

SMAO
superior mesenteric artery occlusion (cardiovascular and gastroenterology)

SMAS
superficial musculoaponeurotic system [flap] (plastic surgery) {pronounced "smass"}

"smass"
{pronunciation of *SMAS* [superficial musculoaponeurotic system (flap)]} (plastic surgery) {not an abbreviation}

Smb
standard mineral base [medium] (laboratory)

SMC
Scientific Manpower Commission (business and government)
smooth-muscle cell (laboratory)
special monthly compensation (social services)
special mouth care (dentistry and otorhinolaryngology)
succinylmonocholine (pharmacology)

SM-C
somatomedin C (endocrinology, laboratory, neonatology, and pediatrics)

SMCPA
System of Multi-Cultural Pluralistic Assessment (psychiatry)

SMD
senile macular degeneration (ophthalmology)
Society of Medical-Dental Management Consultants (dentistry)
submanubrial dullness (neurology)

SMDC
sodium-*N*-methyl dithiocarbamate dihydrate [a soil sterilizing agent] (agriculture and chemistry)

SMF
streptozocin, mitomycin-C, and 5-fluorouracil (chemotherapy, oncology, and pharmacology)

SMI
Senior Medical Investigator (administration)
small volume infusion (pharmacology)
Style of Mind Inventory (psychiatry)
sustained maximal inspiration [maneuver] (respiratory)
Supplementary Medical Insurance (insurance)

S.M.I.
Senior Medical Investigator (administration)

SMJAB
State Medical Journal Advertising Bureau (publishing)

SMM
supplemental minimal medium (laboratory)

SMO
Medical Officer of Schools (education)
Senior Medical Officer (armed forces)
slip made out (laboratory)
Squadron Medical Officer (armed forces)

S.M.O.
Senior Medical Officer (armed forces)

SMo
stainless steel with molybdenum [devices] (orthopedics)

SMOH
Society of Medical Officers of Health (armed forces)
Senior Medical Officer of Health (armed forces)

SMON
subacute myelo-optical neuropathy [also called *subacute myelo-opticoneuropathy* (neurology and ophthalmology)

SMP
self-management program
slow-moving protease (laboratory)
Smith, Miller, and Patch [manufacturer] (pharmacology)
special monthly pension (finances)

SMR
senior medical resident (administration and education)
sensorimotor rhythm (neurology)
skeletal muscle relaxant (neurology, orthopedics, and pharmacology)
somnolent metabolic rate (laboratory and measurement)
standard morbidity ratio (statistics)
standard mortality rate (statistics)
standard mortality ratio (statistics)
standardized mortality ratio (statistics)
submucosal resection (otorhinolaryngology, plastic surgery, and surgery)
submucous resection (otorhinolaryngology, plastic surgery, and surgery)

SMRR
submucous resection and rhinoplasty (otorhinolaryngology, plastic surgery, and surgery)

SMS
senior medical student (education)
Socioeconomic Monitoring Survey (statistics)

S.M.S.
State Medical Society

SMSA
Standard Metropolitan Statistical Area (statistics)

SMSV
San Miguel sea lion virus (infectious diseases, laboratory, and veterinary medicine)

SMUD
smudge cell (hematology and laboratory)

SMV
submento-vertex [view] (radiology)

SMVT
sustained monomorphic ventricular tachycardia (cardiovascular)

SMWDSep
single, married, widowed, divorced, separated [marital status]

SMX
sulfamethoxazole [an antibacterial; also called *sulphamethoxazole*] (pharmacology)

SMZTMP
sulfamethoxazole and trimethoprim [antibiotics] (pharmacology)

SMZ-TMP
sulfamethoxazole and trimethoprim [antibiotics] (pharmacology)

SN
secundum naturam [according to nature]
sensory neuron (neurology, neurosurgery, and pathology)
serum neutralization (laboratory)
serum-neutralizing (laboratory)
sinus node (cardiovascular)
Staff Nurse (nursing)
Standard Nomenclature
sternal notch (anatomy)
streptonigrin (chemotherapy, oncology, and pharmacology)
Student Nurse (education and nursing)

subnormal
substantia nigra [black substance] (neurosurgery)
suprasternal notch (anatomy)

S.N.
Standard Nomenclature
Student Nurse (education and nursing)

S/N
signal-to-noise [ratio] (otorhinolaryngology)

sn
secundum naturam [according to nature]

s.n.
secundum naturam [according to nature]

SNA
Student Nurses' Association (education and nursing)
{not an abbreviation} [used in measurements for orthodontistry with *S* referring to sella, *N* referring to nasion, and *A* being a reference point] (dentistry)

S$_{Na}$
serum sodium (laboratory)

snafu
situation normal, all fouled up [also called *situation normal, all fucked up*] (slang) {pronounced "sna-fu"}

"sna-fu"
{pronunciation of *snafu* [situation normal, all fouled up, and situation normal, all fucked up]} (slang) {not an abbreviation}

SNAI
Standard Nomenclature of Athletic Injuries (orthopedics and sports medicine)

S.N.A.I.
Standard Nomenclature of Athletic Injuries (orthopedics and sports medicine)

SNAP
sensory nerve action potential (neurology) {pronounced "snap"}

"snap"
{pronunciation of *SNAP* [sensory nerve action potential]} (neurology) {not an abbreviation}

SNB
scalene node biopsy (pathology and surgery)
Silverman needle biopsy (pathology and surgery)
{not an abbreviation} [used in measurements for orthodontistry with *S* referring to sella, *N* referring to nasion, and *B* being a reference point] (dentistry)

SNCV
sensory nerve conduction velocity (neurology)

SND
sinus node dysfunction (cardiovascular)

SNDO
Standard Nomenclature of Diseases and Operations

S.N.D.O.
Standard Nomenclature of Diseases and Operations

SNE
spatial nonemotional stimuli (psychiatry)
subacute necrotizing encephalomyelopathy (neurology)

SNEF
skilled nursing extended (care) facility (administration and nursing)

SNF
skilled nursing facility (administration and nursing) {pronounced "sniff"}

SNGFR
single nephron glomerular filtration rate (laboratory and nephrology)

SNHL
sensorineural hearing loss (otorhinolaryngology)

"sniff"
{pronunciation of *SNF* [skilled nursing facility]} (administration and nursing) {not an abbreviation}

SNIVT
Society of Non-Invasive Vascular Technology (cardiovascular)

SNM
Society of Nuclear Medicine (radiology)
sulfanilamide [an antibacterial] (pharmacology)

S.N.M.
Society of Nuclear Medicine (nuclear medicine and radiology)

SNMA
Student National Medical Association (education)

SNMT
Society of Nuclear Medical Technologists (nuclear medicine and radiology)

SNM-TS
Society of Nuclear Medicine—Technology Section (nuclear medicine and radiology)

SNOP
Standard Nomenclature of Pathology (College of American Pathologists) (pathology)
Systematized Nomenclature of Pathology (pathology)

S.N.O.P.
Systematized Nomenclature of Pathology (pathology)

SNP
School Nurse Practitioner (education and nursing)

sodium nitroprusside (cardiovascular, pharmacology, and surgery)

SNR
signal-to-noise ratio (otorhinolaryngology)

snRNA
small nuclear ribonucleic acid (genetics and laboratory)

SNS
Senior Nursing Sister [British] (nursing)
Society of Neurological Surgeons (neurosurgery)
sympathetic nervous system (neurology and psychiatry)

S.N.S.
Society of Neurological Surgeons (neurosurgery)

SNT
sinuses, nose, and throat (otorhinolaryngology)

SNV
spleen necrosis virus (gastroenterology and laboratory)

SO
salpingo-oophorectomy (gynecology)
second opinion
sex offender (law enforcement and psychiatry)
south
spheno-occipital [synchondrosis] (otorhinolaryngology)
standing orders
superior oblique [muscle] (ophthalmology)
supraoptic [nucleus] (ophthalmology)

S & O
salpingo-oophorectomy (gynecology)

S-O
salpingo-oophorectomy (gynecology)

S/O
significant other

SO$_2$
arterial oxygen saturation (laboratory and respiratory)
sulfur dioxide (chemistry)

So
south

so
south

SOA
supraorbital artery (cardiovascular and ophthalmology)
swelling of ankle(s) (cardiovascular, obstetrics, orthopedics, and respiratory)

SOAA
signed out against advice (administration)

SOA-MCA
superficial occipital artery to middle cerebral artery [anastomosis and bypass procedure] (cardiovascular and neurology)

SOAP
subjective data, objective data, assessment, and plan(s) (medical records)
subjective, objective, assessment, and plan(s) (medical records)

S.O.A.P.
subjective data, objective data, assessment, and plan(s) (medical records)
subjective, objective, assessment, and plan(s) (medical records)

SOB
see order blank (laboratory)
shortness of breath (respiratory)
short of breath (respiratory)
son of a bitch [slang]
suboccipitobregmatic [sutures] (neurosurgery)

S.O.B.
shortness of breath (respiratory)

SOC
sequential-type oral contraceptive (endocrinology, gynecology, obstetrics, and pharmacology)

S & OC
signed and on chart [referring to permit] (medical records and surgery)

SoC
state of consciousness (neurology and psychiatry)

soc
social

SocSec
Social Security (government and social services)

SOD
superoxide dismutase [also called *orgotein*; an anti-inflammatory and antirheumatic] (orthopedics, pharmacology, and rheumatology)
surgical officer of the day (administration and surgery)

Sod
sodomy (gynecology, pediatrics, psychiatry, and urology)

sod
sodium (chemistry, dietary, laboratory, and pharmacology)

sod acid phos
sodium acid phosphatase [also called *sodium biphosphate*] (pharmacology)

sod. bicarb.
sodium bicarbonate [also called *baking soda* and *bicarbonate of soda*] (pharmacology) {pronounced "sowed-bi-carb"}

SOL
solution (pharmacology)
space-occupying lesion (neurology, neurosurgery, and radiology)

sol
soluble
solutio [a solution] (pharmacology)
solution (pharmacology)

---

solidif
solidification

SOLN
solution (pharmacology)

soln
solution (pharmacology)

SOLV
solve [dissolve] (pharmacology)
solvent (chemistry)

solv
solve [dissolve] (pharmacology)
solvent (chemistry)

SOM
secretory otitis media (otorhinolaryngology)
serous otitis media (otorhinolaryngology)
somatotropin [also called *growth hormone*] (endocrinology and pediatrics)
somnolent [metabolic test] (laboratory)
sulformethoxine [also called *sulfadoxine, sulforthomidine,* and *sulphormethoxine*; an antibacterial] (pharmacology)

SOMA
Student Osteopathic Medical Association (education and osteopathic medicine) {pronounced "so-mah"}

"so-mah"
{pronunciation of *SOMA* [Student Osteopathic Medical Association]} (education and osteopathic medicine) {not an abbreviation}

somat
somatic [pertaining to the body or the body wall] (anatomy)

SOMI
skull occipital mandibular immobilization [orthosis] (dentistry and otorhinolaryngology)
sterno-occipital mandibular immobilization (dentistry and otorhinolaryngology)

SOMOS
Society of Military Orthopedic Surgeons (armed forces and orthopedics)

S.O.M.O.S.
Society of Military Orthopedic Surgeons (armed forces and orthopedics)

SONK
spontaneous osteonecrosis of the knee (orthopedics)

sono
sonogram (obstetrics and radiology) {pronounced "so-no"}
sonography (obstetrics and radiology) {pronounced "so-no"}

"so-no"
{pronunciation of *sono* [sonogram and sonography]} (obstetrics and radiology) {not an abbreviation}

SONP
solid organs not palpable [on examination]

SOP
standard operating procedure (administration and surgery)

s op s
si opus sit [if it is necessary, if necessary] (pharmacology)

s. op. s.
si opus sit [if it is necessary, if necessary] (pharmacology)

S OP SIT
si opus sit [if it is necessary, if necessary] (pharmacology)

s op sit
si opus sit [if it is necessary, if necessary] (pharmacology)

S-O-R
stimulus-organism-response (neurology)

sor
short open reading [frame] (genetics and laboratory)

Sorb
sorbitol (endocrinology, nephrology, and pharmacology)

SORT
Slosson Oral Reading Test (psychiatry)

SOS
si opus sit [if it is necessary, if necessary] (pharmacology)
speed of sound (physics)
supplemental oxygen system (respiratory)
{not an abbreviation} [The international code signal of extreme distress—an urgent appeal for help.]

S.O.S.
si opus sit [if it is necessary, if necessary] (pharmacology)

sos
si opus sit [if it is necessary, if necessary] (pharmacology)

s.o.s.
si opus sit [if it is necessary, if necessary] (pharmacology)

SOSSUS
Study of Surgical Services in the United States (surgery)

SOT
same old thing
stream of thought (psychiatry)

SOTT
synthetic medium old tuberculin trichloracetic acid precipitated (laboratory, pharmacology, and respiratory)

"sowed-bi-carb"
{pronunciation of *sod. bicarb.* [sodium bicarbonate]} (pharmacology) {not an abbreviation}

SP
sacrum posterior [position] (obstetrics)

sacrum to pubis (anatomy, measurement, and surgery)
Schwangerschaftsprotein
sequential pulse
shunt procedure (surgery)
skin potential (neurology)
species (laboratory)
speech pathology (speech and language therapy)
sphingomyelin (laboratory and neurology)
spine (anatomy, neurology, and orthopedics)
spiritus [spirit] (pharmacology)
standard practice (administration)
standard procedure (administration)
staphylococcal protein A (laboratory)
status post
steady potential (neurology)
stool preservative [Hajna] (gastroenterology and laboratory)
subliminal perception (psychiatry)
substance P [a peptide] (gastroenterology, laboratory, and neurology)
suicide precautions (psychiatry)
summating potential
suprapubic (anatomy and urology)
symphysis pubis (anatomy and orthopedics)
systolic pressure (cardiovascular)

S/P
status post

2-S P
{not an abbreviation} [a transport medium utilized for mycoplasma isolation] (laboratory)

Sp
speech (speech and language therapy)
spine (anatomy, neurology, and orthopedics)
Spirillum [a bacterium] (laboratory)
summation potential

sp
space
species (laboratory)
specific
spinal (neurology and orthopedics)

spiritus [spirit] (pharmacology)

s/p
status post

SPA
salt-poor albumin [*Obsolete;* now called
  albumin human] (gastroenterology,
  nephrology, and pharmacology)
stimulation-produced analgesia (neurology)
suprapubic aspiration (urology)

SPAD
subcutaneous peritoneal access device
  (nephrology and surgery)

SPAG
small-particle aerosol generator

SPAI
steroid protein activity index (laboratory)

SPAM
scanning photo-acoustic microscopy
  (laboratory)

Span
Spanish [referring to language or national origin]
spansule (pharmacology)

SPBI
serum protein bound iodine (endocrinology and laboratory)

SPBT
suprapubic bladder tap (urology)

SPC
salicyamide, phenacetin, and caffeine
  (pharmacology)
standard platelet count (hematology and
  laboratory)

SPCA
serum prothrombin conversion accelerator (factor VII) [also called *proconvertin*] (hematology and laboratory)
Society for the Prevention of Cruelty to
  Animals (research and veterinary
  medicine)

sp cd
spinal cord (neurology, neurosurgery,
  and orthopedics)

SPD
sociopathic personality disorder (psychiatry)

SPE
serum protein electrolytes (laboratory)
serum protein electrophoresis (laboratory)
superficial punctate erosions (ophthalmology)

SPEC
specimen (laboratory, pathology, and
  surgery)

Spec
specimen (laboratory, pathology, and
  surgery)

spec
special
specialist
specific
specification {pronounced "speck"}
specimen (laboratory, pathology, and
  surgery)
speculum (obstetrics and surgery) {pro-
  nounced "speck"}

spec diet
special diet (dietary)

Spec Ed
special education (education)

spec grav
specific gravity (laboratory and urology)

specif
specification

"speck"
{pronunciation of *spec* [specification and
  speculum (obstetrics and surgery)]}
  {not an abbreviation}

SPECT
single photon emission computer tomography (radiology) {pronounced "spekt"}

"spekt"
{pronunciation of *SPECT* [single photon emission computer tomography]} (radiology) {not an abbreviation}

Spencer-M
Spencer-Mead [company] (pharmacology)

SPEP
serum protein electrophoresis (laboratory) {pronounced "es-pep" or "S-pep"}

"S-pep"
{pronunciation of *SPEP* [serum protein electrophoresis]} (laboratory) {not an abbreviation}

S period
the period of deoxyribonucleic acid (DNA) synthesis in the mitotic cycle (chemistry, genetics, and laboratory)

SPF
skin protection factor [rating system used in sun tan protection products] (pharmacology)
specific pathogen free (laboratory)
spectrophotofluorometer (laboratory)
split products of fibrin (hematology and laboratory)

SPFI
solid-phase fluorescent immunoassay (laboratory and oncology)

sp fl
spinal fluid (laboratory and neurology)

sp. fl.
spinal fluid (laboratory and neurology)

SPFT
Sixteen Personality Factors Test (psychiatry)

SPG
sphenopalatine ganglion (neurology and orthopedics)

Sp.G.
specific gravity (laboratory and urology)

sp g
specific gravity (laboratory and urology)

SP GR
specific gravity (laboratory and urology)

sp gr
specific gravity (laboratory and urology)

sp. gr.
specific gravity (laboratory and urology)

SP GRV
specific gravity (laboratory and urology)

SPH
secondary pulmonary hemosiderosis (hematology and respiratory)
severely and profoundly handicapped (neurology, orthopedics, and rehabilitation)
spherical
spherical [lens] (ophthalmology)

Sph
sphingomyelin (laboratory and neurology)

sph
spherical
spherical [lens] (ophthalmology)

SPHE
Society of Public Health Educators (education and public health)
spherocytes (hematology and laboratory)

SPHER
spherocytes (hematology and laboratory)

sp ht
specific heat (chemistry and laboratory)

SPI
serum precipitable iodine (endocrinology, hematology, and laboratory)
Stuttering Prediction Instruction (speech and language therapy)

sp indet
species indeterminata [species indeterminate] (laboratory)

sp inquir
species inquirendae [species of doubtful status] (laboratory)

SPIR
spiral
spiritual (religion)
spiritus [spirit] (pharmacology)

spir
spiral
spiritual (religion)
spiritus [spirit] (pharmacology)

spiss
spissus [dried] (pharmacology)

SPK
spinnbarkeit [referring to cervical mucosa] (gynecology, laboratory, and obstetrics)
superficial punctate keratitis (ophthalmology)

SPL
skin potential level (neurology)
sound pressure level (otorhinolaryngology)
spontaneous lesion (dermatology)

"splat"
{pronunciation of *SPLATT* [split anterior tibial transfer]} (orthopedics) {not an abbreviation}

SPLATT
split anterior tibial transfer (orthopedics) {pronounced "splat"}

SPLATT TALTFR
split anterior tibial transfer, tendo Achillis lengthening, and toe flexor release (orthopedics)

SPM
suspended particulate matter (laboratory)

SpM
spiriformis medialis [nucleus]

SPMA
spinal progressive muscle atrophy (neurology and orthopedics)

SPMB
strong partial maternal behavior (psychiatry)

SPMI
status post myocardial infarction (cardiovascular)

SPN
solitary pulmonary nodule (radiology and respiratory)
Student Practical Nurse (education and nursing)
sympathetic preganglionic neuron (laboratory, neurology, neurosurgery, and pathology)

sp n
species novum [new species] (laboratory)

sp nov
species novum [new species] (laboratory)

SPO
status postoperative (surgery)

spon
spontaneous

SPONT
spontaneous [delivery] (obstetrics)

spont
spontaneous [delivery] (obstetrics)

spont. Ab.
spontaneous abortion (gynecology and obstetrics)

SPOOL
simultaneous peripheral operation on-line (computer sciences) {pronounced "spool"}

"spool"
{pronunciation of *SPOOL* [simultaneous peripheral operation on-line (computer sciences)]} {not an abbreviation}

SPORO
sporotrichosis [a fungal infection] (dermatology and multiple systems)

SPP
Sexuality Preference Profile (psychiatry)
suprapubic prostatectomy (oncology, surgery, and urology)

spp
species [plural form of the singular *species*] (laboratory)

Sp Path
speech pathology (speech and language therapy)

SPPS
stable plasma protein solution (laboratory)

SPR
serial probe recognition
Society for Pediatric Radiology (pediatrics and radiology)
Society for Pediatric Research (pediatrics and research)
Society for Psychical Research (parapsychology)

SPRIA
solid phase radioimmunoassay (laboratory)

SPRM
spermatozoa (laboratory and urology)

SPROM
spontaneous premature rupture of membranes (obstetrics)
spontaneous rupture of membranes (obstetrics)

SPROM NIL
spontaneous rupture of membranes, not in labor (obstetrics)

SPRU
Science Policy Research Unit [University of Sweden] (research)

SPS
Society of Pelvic Surgeons (gynecology, obstetrics, surgery, and urology)
sodium polyanetholesulfonate (hematology, obstetrics, and pharmacology)
sodium polyethylene sulfonate [an antibiotic] (pharmacology)
sulfadiazine [agar] (laboratory)
sulfite polymyxin [agar] (laboratory)
sulfite polymyxin sulfadiazine [agar] (laboratory)
Symond's Picture Story (psychiatry)

SPS agar
sulfite polymyxin sulfadiazine agar (laboratory)

SPT
skin prick test (allergy and immunology)
spiritus [spirit] (pharmacology)

spt
spiritus [spirit] (pharmacology)

SP TAP
spinal tap (neurology and neurosurgery)

SPTI
systolic pressure time index (cardiovascular)

SP tube
suprapubic tube (urology)

S-P tube
suprapubic tube (urology)

SPTURP
status post transurethral resection of the prostate (oncology and urology)

SPU
short procedure unit (surgery)

Society of Pediatric Urology (pediatrics
and urology)

SPUT
sputum (laboratory and respiratory)

SPV
Shope papilloma virus (laboratory and
oncology)

SPVR
systemic peripheral vascular resistance
(cardiovascular)

SQ
Sick Quarters [British] (armed forces)
social quotient (psychiatry)
subcutaneous [injection] (pharmacology)

sq
square (measurement)
subcutaneous [injection] (pharmacology)

Sq CCa
squamous-cell carcinoma (oncology and
pathology)

sq cell ca
squamous-cell carcinoma (oncology and
pathology)

sq cm
square centimeter (measurement)

sq. cm.
square centimeter (measurement)

sq m
square meter (measurement)

sq. m.
square meter (measurement)

sq mm
square millimeter (measurement)

sq. mm.
square millimeter (measurement)

sqq
sequentia [and following]

SQ3R
survey, question, read, review, recite
(psychiatry)

SQU
squamous (laboratory)

SQUAM
squamous (laboratory)

SQUID
superconducting quantum interference
device (physics)

SR
sarcoplasmic reticulum (laboratory)
screen (laboratory)
secretion rate (laboratory)
sedimentation rate (hematology and laboratory)
seizure resistant (neurology)
senior
Senior Registrar
sensitivity response (allergy)
sensitization response (allergy)
service record (armed forces)
sex ratio (statistics)
side rails (rehabilitation)
sigma reaction
sinus rhythm (cardiovascular)
skin resistance (neurology)
soluble, repository [referring to penicil-
lin] (pharmacology)
spontaneous discharge rate (measurement)
stage of resistance [referring to general
adaptation syndrome] (psychiatry)
stimulus-response (neurology and psychiatry)
stomach rumble (gastroenterology)
stretch reflex (neurology and orthopedics)
strong reactive (laboratory)
sulfonamide resistant (laboratory)
superficial reflex (neurology)
superior rectus [muscle] (ophthalmology)
surgical removal (surgery)
sustained release (pharmacology)
suture removal (surgery)
system(s) review (medical records)

systemic resistance (cardiovascular)
systems research (research)

S.R.
sedimentation rate (hematology and laboratory)

S/R
suture removal (surgery)

sr
steradian (measurement)

SRAN
surgical resident's admission note (education and medical records)

SRaw
specific resistance, airway [also called *specific airway resistance*] (respiratory)

SRBC
sheep red blood cells (laboratory)
sickle red blood cells (hematology and laboratory)

SRBOW
spontaneous rupture of bag of water(s) (obstetrics)

SRC
sedimented red cell(s) (hematology and laboratory)
sheep red cells (laboratory)
social rehabilitation center (psychiatry)

SR cells
sensitization response cells [referring to vaginal smears] (gynecology, laboratory, and pathology)

SRD
Society for the Relief of Distress (social services)
Society for the Right to Die (social services)
soluble, repository, plus dihydrostreptomycin [referring to penicillin] (pharmacology)

SRF
skin reactive factor (laboratory)
skin respiratory factor

somatotropin-releasing factor (endocrinology and laboratory)
split renal function (laboratory and nephrology)
subretinal fluid (ophthalmology)

SRF-A
slow releasing factor of anaphylaxis (laboratory)

SRFS
split renal function study (laboratory and nephrology)

SRH
single radical hemolysis (hematology)
somatotropin-releasing hormone (endocrinology and laboratory)
spontaneously resolving hyperthyroidism (endocrinology)

SRHL
Southwestern Radiological Health Laboratory (radiology)

SRI
severe renal insufficiency (nephrology)

SRIF
somatotropin-releasing inhibiting factor (endocrinology and laboratory)

SRM
standard reference materials (publishing)
superior rectus muscle (ophthalmology)

S.R.M.
Standard Reference Material (publishing)

SRMD
stress-related mucosal damage

SRN
State Registered Nurse [England and Wales] (nursing)
Student Registered Nurse (education and nursing)
subretinal neovascularization (ophthalmology)

S.R.N.
State Registered Nurse [England and Wales] (nursing)
Student Registered Nurse (education and nursing)

SRNA
soluble ribonucleic acid (genetics and laboratory)

sRNA
soluble ribonucleic acid (genetics and laboratory)

SR/NE
sinus rhythm, no ectopy (cardiovascular)

SRNS
steroid-responsive nephrotic syndrome (nephrology)

SROM
spontaneous rupture of membrane(s) (obstetrics) {pronounced "S-rom"}

"S-rom"
{pronunciation of *SROM* [spontaneous rupture of membrane(s)]} (obstetrics) {not an abbreviation}

SRP
State Registered Physiotherapist (physical therapy)
Society for Radiological Protection (nuclear science, radiation therapy, and radiology)

SRPM
Standard Raven's Progressive Matrix (psychiatry)

SRR
slow rotation room

SR-RSV
Schmidt-Ruppin strain Rous sarcoma virus (laboratory and oncology)

SRS
Silver-Russell syndrome (genetics and neonatology)
slow-reacting substance (laboratory)
Social and Rehabilitation Service [of the Department of Health and Human Services] (government, rehabilitation, and social services)

S.R.S.
Social and Rehabilitation Service [of the Department of Health and Human Services] (government, rehabilitation, and social services)

SRSA
slow-reacting substance of anaphylaxis (laboratory)

SRS-A
slow-reacting substance of anaphylaxis (laboratory)

SRS-RSV
Schmidt-Ruppin strain Rous sarcoma virus (laboratory and oncology)

SRT
science, research, technology (research)
sedimentation rate test (hematology and laboratory)
simple reaction time (measurement)
sinus node recovery time (cardiovascular)
smoke removal tube [used in laser therapy] (gynecology and surgery)
social relations test (psychiatry)
speech reception test (otorhinolaryngology and speech and language therapy)
speech reception threshold (otorhinolaryngology and speech and language therapy)
Stroke Rehabilitation Technician (cardiovascular, neurology, and rehabilitation)
sustained-release theophylline (pharmacology and respiratory)

S.R.T.
Stroke Rehabilitation Technician (cardiovascular, neurology, and rehabilitation)

SRU
side rails up (nursing and rehabilitation)

S-R variation
smooth-rough variation (laboratory)

SS
saline soak (pharmacology)
saline solution (pharmacology)
saliva sample (laboratory and otorhinolaryngology)
Salmonella and *Shigella* [agar; also
  called *Shigella and Salmonella
  (agar)*] (laboratory)
salt substitute (dietary)
Sanarelli-Shwartzman [reaction]
saturated solution (pharmacology)
schizophrenia spectrum (psychiatry)
seizure sensitive (neurology)
semis [one-half]
serum sickness (hematology)
seizure sensitive (neurology)
Shigella sonnei [a bacterium] (bacteriology and laboratory)
short stay
siblings
sickle cell [anemia] (hematology and
  laboratory)
side-to-side [anastomosis] (cardiovascular and surgery)
signs and symptoms
single-stranded [deoxyribonucleic acid
  (DNA)] (genetics and laboratory)
Sjögren's syndrome (immunology)
skull series (neurology and radiology)
slip sent (laboratory)
slow (wave) sleep (neurology)
soap solution (pharmacology)
soap suds [enema] (gastroenterology and
  pharmacology)
Social Security (government and social
  services)
social service (social services)
sodium salicylate [an analgesic, antipy-
  retic, and antirheumatic] (pharmacology)
somatostatin (endocrinology and laboratory)
sparingly soluble
special senses (neurology, ophthalmology, and otorhinolaryngology)
special services (administration, armed
  forces, and government)
stable sarcoidosis (multiple specialties)
staccato syndrome (otorhinolaryngology
  and speech and language therapy)

standard score (psychiatry and statistics)
statistically significant (statistics)
steady state [also called *dynamic equi-
  librium*] (biology)
sterile solution (pharmacology)
steroid sulfurylation (pharmacology)
Strachan-Scott [syndrome] (neurology,
  ophthalmology, and orthopedics)
subaortic stenosis (cardiovascular)
subscapularis [muscle] (orthopedics)
subsegmental (respiratory)
subsequent sibling
substernal (anatomy and cardiovascular)
suction socket
sum of squares (mathematics)
supersaturated (chemistry and pharmacology)
surging sine (mathematics)
symmetrical strength (neurology and orthopedics)
systemic sclerosis [also called *scleroderma*] (rheumatology)

S & S
Salmonella and *Shigella* [bacteria] (laboratory)
signs and symptoms
support and stimulation (rehabilitation)

S/S
signs and symptoms

S-S
sickle cell [anemia] (hematology and
  laboratory)

SS#
Social Security number [followed by nu-
  merals] (government and social services)

ss
saturated solution (pharmacology)
semis [one-half]
sensu stricto [in the strict sense]

$\overline{ss}$
sans [without]
semi- [a prefix meaning one-half] {not an
  abbreviation}

semis [one-half]
semisse [a half]
semissem [one-half]

SSA
salicylsalicylic acid [former name of *salsalate*] (orthopedics, pharmacology, and rheumatology)
skin-sensitizing antibody (allergy and laboratory)
Social Security Administration (government and social services)
Smith surface antigen (laboratory)
sulfosalicylic acid [test] (laboratory)

SS-A
Sjögren's syndrome antigen A (immunology and laboratory)

S.S.A.
Social Security Administration (government and social services)

SS-Ab
Sjögren's syndrome antibody (immunology and laboratory)

SS agar
Salmonella-Shigella agar (laboratory)

SS-B
Sjögren's syndrome antigen B (immunology and laboratory)

SSBR
see separate bacteriology report (bacteriology and laboratory)

SSCA
single shoulder contrast arthrography (orthopedics and radiology)

SSCQT
Selective Service College Qualifying Test (armed forces and education)

SSC
stainless steel crown (dentistry)

SSCr
stainless steel crown (dentistry)

SSCT
Sacks Sentence Completion Test (psychiatry)

SSD
silver sulfadiazine [an anti-infective used in burn therapy] (dermatology and emergency medicine)
Social Security disability (government and social services)
source-skin distance [source-to-skin distance] (radiation therapy and radiology)
source-to-skin distance [source-skin distance] (radiation therapy and radiology)
sudden sniffing death
sum of square deviations (mathematics)

SS (D)
sickle cell (disease) (hematology)

SSDI
Social Security disability income (government and social services)

SSE
saline solution enema (gastroenterology and pharmacology)
skin self-examination (dermatology)
soap suds enema (gastroenterology and pharmacology)
systemic side effects (pharmacology)

SSEC
Solar System Exploration Committee (aerospace)

S.S. enema
soap suds enema (gastroenterology and pharmacology)

SSEP
somatosensory evoked potential (neurology)

SSEP's
somatosensory evoked potentials (neurology)

SSFP
steady-state free precession [magnetic resonance imaging] (radiology)

SSI
Social Security income (government and social services)
Stuttering Severity Index (speech and language therapy)
subshock insulin (endocrinology and pharmacology)
Supplemental Security Income (government and social services)
Synthetic Sentence Identification (speech and language therapy)
System Sign Inventory

S.S.I.
Supplemental Security Income (government and social services)

SSIDS
sibling(s) of sudden infant death syndrome [victim(s)] (neonatology and pediatrics)

SSI/SSP
Supplemental Security Income/State Supplemental Payment (government and social services)

SSKI
saturated solution of potassium iodide (endocrinology, pharmacology, and respiratory)
{not an abbreviation} [a trade name for a preparation of saturated solution of potassium iodide] (endocrinology, pharmacology, and respiratory)

SSM
sesquiterpenoid stress metabolites (laboratory)
subsynaptic membrane (laboratory, neurosurgery, and pathology)
superficial spreading melanoma (dermatology, oncology, and pathology)

SSN
severely subnormal (laboratory)

SSO
Society of Surgical Oncology (oncology and surgery)

SSOP
Second Surgical Opinion Program (surgery)

SSP
Sanarelli-Shwartzman phenomenon (research)
State Supplemental Payment (government and social services)
subacute sclerosing panencephalitis (neurology)
supersensitivity perception (neurology)

SSPE
subacute sclerosing panencephalitis (neurology)

SSPL
saturation sound pressure level (otorhinolaryngology)

SSS
scaled skin syndrome (dermatology)
sick sinus syndrome (cardiovascular)
specific soluble substance [polysaccharide hapten] (laboratory)
sterile saline soak (pharmacology)
stratum super stratum [layer upon layer]
strong soap solution (pharmacology)

sss
stratum super stratum [layer upon layer]

s.s.s.
stratum super stratum [layer upon layer]

SSSS
staphylococcal scalded skin syndrome (dermatology)

SSStJ
Serving Sister, Order of Saint John of Jerusalem (nursing)

s str
sensu stricto [in the strict sense]

s. str.
sensu stricto [in the strict sense]

SSU
self-service unit
sterile supply unit

SSV
simian sarcoma virus (laboratory, oncology, and pathology)
sub signo veneni [under a poison label] (pharmacology)

ssv
sub signo veneni [under a poison label] (pharmacology)

s.s.v.
sub signo veneni [under a poison label] (pharmacology)

SSW
staggered spondiac word test (speech and language therapy)

SSX
sulfisoxazole [an anti-infective sulfa] (pharmacology)

ST
esotropia [usually written with an *l* (left) or an *r* (right)] (ophthalmology)
sedimentation time (hematology and laboratory)
sinus tachycardia (cardiovascular)
skin test (allergy and immunology)
slight trace (laboratory)
speech therapist (speech and language therapy)
speech therapy (speech and language therapy)
speech threshold (speech and language therapy)
sphincter tone (gastroenterology and urology)
split thickness [skin graft] (dermatology and plastic surgery)
standardized test (psychiatry)
station (neurology, obstetrics, and orthopedics)
sternothyroid (anatomy)
stet [let it stand] (pharmacology)
stimulus (neurology)
straight

stress testing (cardiovascular)
subtalar (orthopedics)
subtotal
superior turbinate (otorhinolaryngology)
surface tension (chemistry)
Surgical Technologist (surgery)
survival time (oncology)
{not an abbreviation} [a segment of electrocardiograms] (cardiovascular)

S-T
sickle-cell thalassemia (hematology)

S.T.
stress test (cardiovascular)

S.T. 37.
hexylresorcinol [an antiseptic] (pharmacology)

St
slight
stoke (chemistry and measurement)
stomach (gastroenterology)
subtype (laboratory)

st
stage (laboratory, pathology, and oncology)
stent [let them stand] (pharmacology)
stet [let it stand] (pharmacology)
stomach (gastroenterology)
stool (gastroenterology)

st.
stage [of disease]
stent [let them stand] (pharmacology)
stet [let it stand] (pharmacology)
straight

STA
serum thrombotic accelerator (hematology and laboratory)
superficial temporal artery (cardiovascular and neurosurgery)

sta
station (neurology, obstetrics, and orthopedics)

stab
{not an abbreviation} [*stab cell* is also known as *band cell, band form, nonsegmented polymorphonuclear leukocyte,* and *staff cell*] (hematology and laboratory) {pronounced "stab"}

"stab"
{pronunciation of *stab* [stab (cell)]} (hematology and laboratory) {not an abbreviation}

stabs
{not an abbreviation} [*stab cells* are also known as *band cells, band forms, nonsegmented polymorphonuclear leukocytes,* and *staff cells*] (hematology and laboratory) {pronounced "stabz"}

"stabz"
{pronunciation of *stabs* [stab cells]} (hematology and laboratory) {not an abbreviation}

"staff"
{pronunciation of *STAPH* and *Staph* [*Staphylococcus*] and *staph* [*staphylococcus*]} (bacteriology and laboratory) {not an abbreviation}

STAG
split thickness autogenous graft (dermatology and plastic surgery)

STAINP
stain pattern (laboratory)

"stair-E-oh"
{pronunciation of *Stereo* [stereophonic (sound system)]} (electronics) {not an abbreviation}

STA-MCA
superior temporal artery to middle cerebral artery [anastomosis and bypass procedure] (cardiovascular and neurosurgery)

standard
standardization {pronounced "standard"}
standardized {pronounced "stan-dard"}

"stan-dard"
{pronunciation of *standard* [standardization and standardized]} {not an abbreviation}

StanPsych
Standard Psychiatric [nomenclature] (psychiatry)

STAPH
Staphylococcus [a bacterium] (bacteriology and laboratory) {pronounced "staff"}

Staph
Staphylococcus [a bacterium] (bacteriology and laboratory) {pronounced "staff"}

staph
staphylococcus [a bacterium] (bacteriology and laboratory) {pronounced "staff"}

Staph epi
Staphylococcus epidermidis [a bacterium] (bacteriology and laboratory)

STAT
statim [at once, immediately] {pronounced "stat"}

stat
statim [at once, immediately] {pronounced "stat"}
statistic {pronounced "stat"}
{not an abbreviation} [German unit of radiation emanation] (radiation therapy and radiology)

"stat"
{pronunciation of *stat* [*statim* (at once, immediately) or statistics]} {not an abbreviation}

stats
statistics {pronounced "statz"}

"statz"
{pronunciation of *stats* [statistics]} {not an abbreviation}

STB
stillborn (obstetrics)

Stb
stillborn (obstetrics)

ST BY
stand by [anesthesia] (anesthesiology)

STC
soft tissue calcification (dermatology and radiology)

STD
saturated
sexually transmitted disease(s) (gynecology, infectious diseases, and urology)
skin test dose (radiation therapy and radiology)
skin to tumor distance (radiation therapy and radiology)
sodium tetradecyl sulfate (cardiovascular, gastroenterology, and pharmacology)
standard test dose (pharmacology and radiation therapy)

std
standard
standardized

std.
saturated
standard

STD TF
standard tube feeding (dietary and gastroenterology)

2-step
Master "2-step" exercise test (cardiovascular)

Stereo
stereogram (radiology)
stereophonic [sound system] (electronics) {pronounced "stair-E-oh"}

STET
submaximal treadmill exercise test (cardiovascular)

stet
{not an abbreviation} [Latin word meaning let it stand] (pharmacology)

STF
special tube feeding (dietary and gastroenterology)

STFA
step-father

STG
short-term goal (occupational and physical therapy and rehabilitation)
split thickness graft (dermatology and plastic surgery)

STH
soft tissue hematoma (hematology and surgery)
somatotropin (growth) hormone (endocrinology and laboratory)

STI
serum trypsin inhibitor (laboratory)
systolic time interval (cardiovascular)

STIA
Scientific, Technological, and International Affairs

stillat
stillatim [by drops, in small quantities] (pharmacology)

stillat.
stillatim [by drops, in small quantities] (pharmacology)

still B.
stillborn (obstetrics)

stillb
stillborn (obstetrics)
stillbirth (obstetrics)

stim
stimulation (neurology) {pronounced "stim"}

"stim"
{pronunciation of *stim* [stimulation]} (neurology) {not an abbreviation}

stimn
stimulation (neurology)

STIP
basophilic stippling (laboratory)

STJ
subtalar joint (orthopedics)

STK
streptokinase [a thrombolytic] (cardiovascular and pharmacology)

STL
swelling, tenderness, limitation [of movement] (orthopedics)

STl
esotropia, left (ophthalmology)

STM
scanning tunneling microscope (laboratory)
short-term memory (neurology)
streptomycin [an antibiotic and antituberculin] (infectious diseases, pharmacology, and respiratory)

STMO
step-mother

STN
subthalamic nucleus (neurology)

sTNM
surgical-evaluative staging of cancer [Classification of malignant tumors with *T* referring to the size of the tumor, *N* referring to the clinical status of the nodes, and *M* referring to metastases.] (oncology, pathology, and surgery)

STNR
symmetrical tonic neck reflex (neurology)

STOM
stomatocytes (hematology and laboratory)

STORCH
syphilis, toxoplasmosis, other agents, rubella, cytomegalovirus, and herpes [maternal infections] (laboratory, neonatology, obstetrics, and pediatrics)

STP
2,5-dimethoxy-4-methylamphetamine [an illicit hallucinogenic drug; also called *methyldimethoxy-amphetamine* and *DOM*] (chemical dependency, law enforcement, and pharmacology) {slang}
scientifically treated petroleum (chemistry)
sodium thiopental [also called *thiopental sodium*; a general anesthetic] (anesthesiology and pharmacology)
standard (normal) temperature and pulse
standard temperature and pressure

STPD
standard temperature and pressure, dry [temperature zero degrees centigrade, pressure 760 millimeters of mercury, and dry (zero water vapor] (laboratory and respiratory)

St. Quo
status quo

STR
special treatment room
streptococcus [a bacterium] (bacteriology and laboratory)

STr
esotropia, right (ophthalmology)

Strep
Streptococcus [a bacterium] (bacteriology and laboratory) {pronounced "strep"}

strep
streptococcus [a bacterium] (bacteriology and laboratory) {pronounced "strep"}
streptomycin [an antibacterial and antituberculin] (infectious diseases, phar-

macology, and respiratory) {pro-
nounced "strep"}

"strep"
{pronunciation of *Strep* [*Streptococcus*
(bacteriology and laboratory)] and
strep [*streptococcus* (bacteriology
and laboratory) and streptomycin (infectious diseases, pharmacology, and
respiratory)]} {not an abbreviation}

strept
streptococcus [a bacterium] (bacteriology and laboratory)

Str pyogenes
Streptococcus pyogenes [a bacterium]
(bacteriology and laboratory)

struct
structural

Str viridans
Streptococcus viridans [a bacterium]
(bacteriology and laboratory)

STRW
straw [colored] (laboratory)

STS
serological test for syphilis (gynecology,
infectious diseases, laboratory, and
urology)
Society of Thoracic Surgeons (cardiovascular, respiratory, surgery, and
thoracic surgery)
soft-tissue swelling (radiology)
standard test for syphilis (gynecology,
infectious diseases, laboratory, and
urology)
subtrapezial space (orthopedics, radiology)
suprasonic transport (aviation)

STSA
Southern Thoracic Surgical Association
(thoracic surgery)

ST segment
{not an abbreviation} [a segment on elec-
trocardiograms] (cardiovascular)

STSG
split thickness skin graft (plastic surgery)

STS-QN
serological test for syphilis—quantita-
tion (gynecology, infectious diseases,
laboratory, and urology)

STT
scaphotrapeziotrapezoid [joint] (orthopedics)
sensitization test (allergy and immunology)
serial thrombin time (hematology and
laboratory)
standard triple therapy [for hyperten-
sion] (cardiovascular and pharmacology)

ST & T
ST segment and T-waves [found on elec-
trocardiograms] (cardiovascular)

STT joint
scaphotrapeziotrapezoid [joint] (orthopedics)

STU
shock trauma unit (emergency medicine)
skin test unit (allergy and immunology)

STV
soft-tissue view (radiology)

STVA
subtotal villose atrophy (laboratory and
pathology)

STYCAR
Screening Tests for Young Children and
Retardates (genetics, neurology, pedi-
atrics, and psychiatry)

S.T.Y.C.A.R.
Screening Tests for Young Children and
Retardates (genetics, neurology, pedi-
atrics, and psychiatry)

STZ
streptozocin [also called *Zanosar*] (chemotherapy, oncology, and pharmacology)

SU
salicyluric acid (laboratory)
sensation unit (neurology)
sensory urgency (neurology)
sigma unit(s)
Somogyi unit(s) (laboratory)
strontium unit (chemistry, measurement, and radiation therapy)
sulfonamide [an antibiotic] (pharmacology)
sumat [let him take, let the person take] (pharmacology)
surgery

S & U
supine and upright

su
sumat [let him take, let the person take] (pharmacology)

su.
sumat [let him take, let the person take] (pharmacology)

SUA
sedative urinary antibiotic (neurology, pharmacology, and urology)
serum uric acid (laboratory)
single umbilical artery (neonatology and obstetrics)

SUB
Skene's, urethral, and Bartholin's [glands] (anatomy and gynecology)

sub
submarine (armed forces and oceanography)

subac
subacute

"sub-cong"
{pronunciation of *subconj* [subconjunctival]} (ophthalmology) {not an abbreviation}

subconj
subconjunctival (ophthalmology) {pronounced "sub-cong"}

subcrep
subcreptitant (orthopedics and respiratory)

subcu
subcutaneous [injection] (pharmacology) {pronounced "sub-Q"}
subcutaneous [tissue] (surgery)
subcuticular (dermatology and surgery) {pronounced "sub-Q"}

subcut
subcutaneous
subcutaneously

sub fin coct
sub finem coctionis [towards the end of boiling] (pharmacology)

sub fin. coct.
sub finem coctionis [towards the end of boiling] (pharmacology)

subling
sublingual (dentistry, otorhinolaryngology, and pharmacology)

submand
submandibular (dentistry and otorhinolaryngology)

Sub-Q
subcutaneous [injection] (pharmacology) {pronounced "sub-Q"} [*Note: This is a dangerous abbreviation.*]
subcuticular (dermatology and surgery) {pronounced "sub-Q"} [*Note: This is an dangerous abbreviation.*]

"sub-Q"
{pronunciation of *subcu, subq, Sub-Q,* and *sub-q* [subcutaneous (injection) (pharmacology) and subcuticular (dermatology and surgery)]} {not an abbreviation}

799

subq
subcutaneous [injection] (pharmacology) {pronounced "sub-Q"} [*Note: This is a dangerous abbrevation.*]
subcutaneous [tissue] (surgery)
subcuticular (dermatology and surgery) {pronounced "sub-Q"} [*Note: This is a dangerous abbreviation.*]

sub-q
subcutaneous [injection] (pharmacology) {pronounced "sub-Q"} [*Note: This is a dangerous abbreviation.*]
subcuticular (dermatology and surgery) {pronounced "sub-Q"} [*Note: This is a dangerous abbreviation.*]

subsp
subspecies (laboratory)

substd
substandard

suc
succus [juice] (pharmacology)

suc.
succus [juice] (pharmacology)

Succ
succinate (laboratory)

SUD
skin unit dose (radiation therapy and radiology)
sudden unexpected death
sudden unexplained death

SUDS
single unit diagnostic system [experimental acquired immunodeficiency syndrome (AIDS) testing device] (immunology, infectious diseases, and laboratory) {pronounced "sudz"}
subjective units of distress [on biofeedback] (psychiatry)

"sudz"
{pronunciation of *SUDS* [single unit diagnostic system]} (immunology, infectious diseases, and laboratory) {not an abbreviation}

"sue-per"
{pronunciation of *super* [superintendent]} {not an abbreviation}

SUF
sequential ultrafiltration (laboratory and nephrology)

suf
sufficient

SUID
sudden unexplained infant death (neonatology and pediatrics)

SUIH
State University of Iowa Hospitals (administration)

SULF
sulfur (chemistry, multiple specialties, and pharmacology)

sulf
sulfate (chemistry, laboratory, and pharmacology)

SULFHB
sulfhemoglobin [also called *sulfmethemoglobin*] (gastroenterology, hematology, laboratory, and pathology)

SULF-PRIM
sulfamethoxazole and trimethoprim [antibacterials] (immunology, pharmacology, and urology)

sulph
sulphate [also called *sulfate*] (chemistry, laboratory, and pharmacology)

sulpha
sulphonamide [also called *sulfonamide*] [an antibacterial] (pharmacology)

SUM
sumantur [let it be taken] (pharmacology)
sumat [let him take, let the person take] (pharmacology)
sume [take] (pharmacology)

sumendum [to be taken] (pharmacology)

sum
sumantur [let it be taken] (pharmacology)
sumat [let him take, let the person take] (pharmacology)
sume [take] (pharmacology)
sumendum [to be taken] (pharmacology)

sum.
sumantur [let it be taken] (pharmacology)
sumat [let him take, let the person take] (pharmacology)
sume [take] (pharmacology)
sumendum [to be taken] (pharmacology)

sum tal
sumat talem [let the person take one like this, take one like this] (pharmacology)

sum. tal.
sumat talem [let the person take one like this, take one like this] (pharmacology)

SUN
Standard Units and Nomenclature (measurement)
serum urea nitrogen [also called *blood urea nitrogen*] (laboratory, nephrology, and urology)

SUP
superficial
superior
supervised (rehabilitation)
supination (neurology and orthopedics)
supinator (neurology and orthopedics)

sup
superior
supination (neurology and orthopedics)
supine
supra [above, superior]

super
superintendent {pronounced "sue-per"}

Supp
suppository (pharmacology)

supp
suppository (pharmacology)

suppl
supplement
supplementary

suppos
suppository (pharmacology)

supra cit
supra citato [cited above]

supt
superintendent

SUR
surgical (surgery)
surgery

"surf" test
surfactant test [of amnionic fluid] (laboratory, neonatology, and obstetrics) {slang} {pronounced "surf-test"}

"surf-test"
{pronunciation of *"surf" test* [surfactant test (of amnionic fluid)]} (laboratory, neonatology, and obstetrics) {not an abbreviation}

SURG
surgeon (surgery) {pronounced "surge"}
surgery {pronounced "surge"}
surgical (surgery) {pronounced "surge"}

Surg
surgeon (surgery) {pronounced "surge"}
surgery {pronounced "surge"}
surgical (surgery) {pronounced "surge"}

surg
surgeon (surgery) {pronounced "surge"}
surgery {pronounced "surge"}
surgical (surgery) {pronounced "surge"}

"surge"
{pronunciation of *SURG, Surg,* and *surg*

[surgeon, surgery, and surgical]} (surgery) {not an abbreviation}

SUS
suppressor sensitive (laboratory)
stained urinary sediment (laboratory and urology)

susp
suspension (pharmacology)

SUUD
sudden, unexpected, unexplained death

SUV
sociated unilamellar vesicles (anatomy)

SUX
succinylcholine (anesthesiology, gastroenterology, neurology, orthopedics, pharmacology, and respiratory)

SV
sarcoma virus (laboratory and oncology)
satellite virus (laboratory)
scalp vein (cardiovascular and neurosurgery)
severe
sigmoid volvulus (gastroenterology and surgery)
simian virus (laboratory)
single ventricle (cardiovascular)
sinus venosus (anatomy, cardiovascular, neonatology, and pediatrics)
snake venom (chemistry, laboratory, and pharmacology)
spiritus vini [alcoholic spirit]
spoken voice (otorhinolaryngology and speech and language therapy)
stimulus valve
stock volume
stroke volume (cardiovascular)
subclavian vein (cardiovascular)
supraventricular (cardiovascular)
supravital (laboratory)

S/V
surface to volume [ratio] (measurement)

S.V.
supraventricular (cardiovascular)

SV 40
simian virus 40 (laboratory)

Sv
Sievert [unit] (radiation therapy and radiology)

sv
single vibrations
spiritus vini [alcoholic spirit]

s.v.
spiritus vini [alcoholic spirit]

SVAS
supravalvular aortic stenosis (cardiovascular)

SVBPG
saphenous vein bypass graft (cardiovascular)

SVC
slow vital capacity (respiratory)
superior vena cava (cardiovascular)

SVCG
spatial vectorcardiogram (cardiovascular)

SVCO
superior vena cava obstruction (cardiovascular)

SVCP
Special Virus Cancer Program (oncology and research)

SVC-RPA
superior vena cava to right pulmonary artery [shunt] (cardiovascular)

SVCS
superior vena cava syndrome (cardiovascular)

SVD
spontaneous vaginal delivery (obstetrics)
spontaneous vertex delivery (obstetrics)

SVE
sterile vaginal examination (obstetrics)

SVG
saphenous vein graft (cardiovascular)

SVI
stroke volume index (cardiovascular)

SVM
syncytiovascular membrane (cardiovascular)

SVN
small volume nebulizer (pharmacology)

SVPB
supraventricular premature beat (cardiovascular)

SVPT
supraventricular paroxysmal tachycardia (cardiovascular)

SVR
spiritus vini rectificatus [rectified spirit of alcohol, rectified spirit of wine]
supraventricular rhythm (cardiovascular)
systemic vascular resistance (cardiovascular)

svr
spiritus vini rectificatus [rectified spirit of alcohol, rectified spirit of wine]

s.v.r.
spiritus vini rectificatus [rectified spirit of alcohol, rectified spirit of wine]

SVRI
systemic vascular resistance index (cardiovascular)

SVS
Society for Vascular Surgery (cardiovascular)

SVT
spiritus vini tenuis [proof spirit]
supraventricular tachyarrhythmia (cardiovascular)
supraventricular tachycardia (cardiovascular)

svt
spiritus vini tenuis [proof spirit]

s.v.t.
spiritus vini tenuis [proof spirit]

SW
Schwartz-Watson [test; also called *Watson-Schwartz (test)*] (dermatology, gastroenterology, genetics, hematology, and neurology)
seriously wounded (emergency medicine)
slow wave [on electroencephalogram] (neurology)
social worker (social services)
southwest
spiral wound (emergency medicine)
stab wound (emergency medicine)
sterile water (pharmacology)
stroke work (cardiovascular)
water fraction of serum (laboratory)

S.W.
social worker (social services)

Sw
swine (veterinary medicine)

SWA
seriously wounded in action (armed forces)

S-wave
{not an abbreviation} [found on electrocardiograms] (cardiovascular)

SWD
short-wave diathermy (physical therapy)

SWE
slow-wave encephalography (neurology)

SWFI
sterile water for injection (pharmacology)

SWI
sterile water for injection (pharmacology)
stroke work index (cardiovascular)

SWIM
sperm-washing insemination method

(obstetrics and urology) {pronounced "swim"}

"swim"
{pronunciation of *SWIM* [sperm-washing insemination method]} (obstetrics and urology) {not an abbreviation}

SWOG
Southwest Oncology Group [protocols] (chemotherapy, oncology, and pharmacology)

SWR
sperm Wassermann reaction (laboratory and urology)

SWS
slow-wave sleep (neurology)
Social Work Service (social services)
Sturge-Weber syndrome (cardiovascular, dermatology, genetics, and neurology)
student ward secretary (clerical, education, and nursing)

SWT
stab wound of the throat (emergency medicine and otorhinolaryngology)

SWU
septic workup (laboratory)

SX
surgeries

Sx
signs
surgery
symptoms

S$_x$
signs
symptoms

sx
suction (surgery)

SXT
sulfamethoxazole [an antibacterial] (pharmacology)

SY
symmetrical

symmetry
symptoms

SYC
small, yellow, constipated [stool] (gastroenterology)

SYM
symmetrical
symptom(s)

sym
symmetrical
symptom(s)

symb
symbol
symbolic

SYMP
symptom(s)

symp
symptom(s)

sympath
sympathetic

sympt
symptom(s)

SYN
synthetic

syn
synonym
synovial (orthopedics)

synd
syndrome

syn fl
synovial fluid (laboratory and orthopedics)

syn. fl.
synovial fluid (laboratory and orthopedics)

synth
synthetic

syph
syphilis (gynecology, infectious diseases, laboratory, and urology)
syphilologist (gynecology, infectious diseases, and urology)
syphilology (gynecology, infectious diseases, and urology)

syr
syrup (pharmacology)
syrupus [syrup] (pharmacology)

sys
system
systemic

syst
systemic
systolic (cardiovascular)

syst m
systolic murmur (cardiovascular)

SZ
schizophrenia (psychiatry)
schizophrenic (psychiatry)
seizure (neurology)
streptozocin (chemotherapy, oncology, and pharmacology)
suction (surgery)

Sz
schizophrenia (psychiatry)
schizophrenic (psychiatry)
seizure (neurology)
skin impedance (neurology)

SZN
streptozocin (chemotherapy, oncology, and pharmacology)

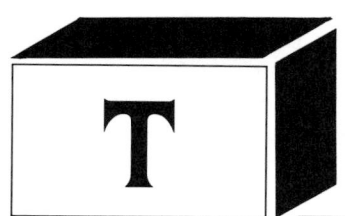

T

_τ_
tau [nineteenth letter of the Greek alphabet]
{not an abbreviation} [symbol for lifetime of pharmaceuticals and radioactive isotopes] (chemistry, pharmacology, physics, and radiology)

_τ½_
{not an abbreviation} [symbol for halflife time of pharmaceuticals and radioactive isotopes] (chemistry, pharmacology, physics, and radiology)

_θ_
theta [eighth letter of the Greek alphabet]

T
absolute temperature (physics)
intraocular tension (ophthalmology)
period [of time] (measurement)
tablespoon (measurement)
Taenia [a genus of tapeworm] (gastroenterology and laboratory)
tamoxifen (chemotherapy, oncology, and pharmacology)
tau [nineteenth letter of the Greek alphabet]
temperature (measurement)
temporary
tension [intraocular] (ophthalmology)
tera- {not an abbreviation} [prefix for 10^{12}] (measurement)
tetra- {not an abbreviation} [prefix meaning four]
term
tetracycline [an antibiotic] (pharmacology)
thoracic (cardiovascular, orthopedics, radiology, and respiratory)
thorax (cardiovascular, orthopedics, radiology, and respiratory)
threonine [an amino acid] (endocrinology and laboratory)
thrill (cardiovascular)
thymidine (genetics and laboratory)

thymine (endocrinology and laboratory)
thymus-derived [lymphocyte] (hematology, immunology, and laboratory)
thyroid (endocrinology, laboratory, and pharmacology)
tidal gas [respiration] (laboratory and respiratory)
time
topical (pharmacology)
torque (dentistry)
total
toxicity (pharmacology)
trace
transition point
transmittance [symbol used in spectrophotometry] (laboratory)
transverse
Treponema [a bacterium] (laboratory)
Trichophyton [a fungus] (dermatology and laboratory)
tritium (chemistry)
Trypanosoma [a parasite] (laboratory)
tumor (oncology and pathology)
T-wave [found on electrocardiograms] {not an abbreviation} (cardiovascular)
type

T.
Taenia [a genus of tapeworm] (gastroenterology and laboratory)
tesla (measurement and physics)
Treponema [a bacterium] (laboratory)
Trichomonas [a parasite] (gastroenterology, gynecology, laboratory, and urology)
Trichophyton [a fungus] (dermatology and laboratory)
Trypanosoma [a parasite] (laboratory)

T#
temperature (measurement)

T°
temperature (measurement)

T+
increased tension [intraocular; followed by a numeral indicating stage of increase] (ophthalmology)

T−
decreased tension [intraocular; followed by a numeral indicating stage of decrease] (ophthalmology)

T.
tesla (measurement and physics)

T½
{not an abbreviation} [symbol for one-half lifetime of radioactive isotope] (chemistry and physics)

T½
{not an abbreviation} [symbol for one-half lifetime of pharmaceuticals and radioactive isotopes] (chemistry, pharmacology, physics, and radiology)

T1
first thoracic nerve (neurology and orthopedics)
first thoracic vertebra (neurology, orthopedics, and radiology)
longitudinal relaxation time constant [used as "T1 weighted" on magnetic resonance imaging (MRI) scans; also called *spin-lattice relaxation time constant*] (radiology)

T₁
first thoracic nerve (neurology and orthopedics)
first thoracic vertebra (neurology, orthopedics, and radiology)
longitudinal relaxation time constant [used as "T₁ weighted" on magnetic resonance imaging (MRI) scans; also called *spin-lattice relaxation time constant*] (radiology)
tricuspid first sound (cardiovascular)

T+1
{not an abbreviation} [symbol indicating stage of increased intraocular tension] (ophthalmology)

T-1
{not an abbreviation} [symbol indicating stage of decreased intraocular tension] (ophthalmology)

T2
second thoracic nerve (neurology and orthopedics)
second thoracic vertebra (neurology, orthopedics, and radiology)
transverse relaxation time constant [used as "T2 weighted" on magnetic resonance imaging (MRI) scans; also called *spin-spin relaxation time constant*] (radiology)

T₂
second thoracic nerve (neurology and orthopedics)
second thoracic vertebra (neurology, orthopedics, and radiology)
transverse relaxation time constant [used as "T₂ weighted" on magnetic resonance imaging (MRI) scans; also called *spin-spin relaxation time constant*] (radiology)

T+2
{not an abbreviation} [symbol indicating stage of increased intraocular tension] (ophthalmology)

T-2
T-2 protocol [a four-cycle chemotherapy regimen including dactinomycin, doxorubicin (Adriamycin), vincristine (Oncovin), cyclophosphamide (Cytoxan), and radiation therapy] (chemotherapy, oncology, pharmacology, and radiation therapy)
{not an abbreviation} [symbol indicating stage of decreased intraocular tension] (ophthalmology)

T3
third thoracic nerve (neurology and orthopedics)
third thoracic vertebra (neurology, orthopedics, and radiology)
tri-iodothyronine (endocrinology and laboratory)

T₃
third thoracic nerve (neurology and orthopedics)
third thoracic vertebra (neurology, orthopedics, and radiology)
tri-iodothyronine (endocrinology and laboratory)

T-3
tri-iodothyronine (endocrinology and laboratory)

T4
fourth thoracic nerve (neurology and orthopedics)
fourth thoracic vertebra (neurology, orthopedics, and radiology)
thyroxine [also called *levothyroxine (L-thyroxine)* and *tetraiodothyronine*] (endocrinology, laboratory, and pharmacology)

T₄
fourth thoracic nerve (neurology and orthopedics)
fourth thoracic vertebra (neurology, orthopedics, and radiology)
thyroxine [also called *levothyroxine (L-thyroxine)* and *tetraiodothyronine*] (endocrinology, laboratory, and pharmacology)

T-4
T-4 cell [also called *helper/inducer thymus-derived cell*] (hematology, immunology, and laboratory)
thyroxine [also called *levothyroxine (L-thyroxine)* and *tetraiodothyronine*] ´ (endocrinology, laboratory, and pharmacology)

T5
fifth thoracic nerve (neurology and orthopedics)
fifth thoracic vertebra (neurology, orthopedics, and radiology)

T₅
fifth thoracic nerve (neurology and orthopedics)
fifth thoracic vertebra (neurology, orthopedics, and radiology)

T6
sixth thoracic nerve (neurology and orthopedics)
sixth thoracic vertebra (neurology, orthopedics, and radiology)

T₆
sixth thoracic nerve (neurology and orthopedics)
sixth thoracic vertebra (neurology, orthopedics, and radiology)

T7
seventh thoracic nerve (neurology and orthopedics)
seventh thoracic vertebra (neurology, orthopedics, and radiology)

T₇
seventh thoracic nerve (neurology and orthopedics)
seventh thoracic vertebra (neurology, orthopedics, and radiology)

T8
eighth thoracic nerve (neurology and orthopedics)
eighth thoracic vertebra (neurology, orthopedics, and radiology)

T₈
eighth thoracic nerve (neurology and orthopedics)
eighth thoracic vertebra (neurology, orthopedics, and radiology)

T-8
T-8 suppressor cell [also called *cytotoxic cell* and *suppressor cell*] (hematology, immunology, and laboratory)

T9
ninth thoracic nerve (neurology and orthopedics)
ninth thoracic vertebra (neurology, orthopedics, and radiology)

T₉
ninth thoracic nerve (neurology and orthopedics)

ninth thoracic vertebra (neurology, orthopedics, and radiology)

T10
tenth thoracic nerve (neurology and orthopedics)
tenth thoracic vertebra (neurology, orthopedics, and radiology)

T₁₀
tenth thoracic nerve (neurology and orthopedics)
tenth thoracic vertebra (neurology, orthopedics, and radiology)

T11
eleventh thoracic nerve (neurology and orthopedics)
eleventh thoracic vertebra (neurology, orthopedics, and radiology)

T₁₁
eleventh thoracic nerve (neurology and orthopedics)
eleventh thoracic vertebra (neurology, orthopedics, and radiology)

T12
twelfth thoracic nerve (neurology and orthopedics)
twelfth thoracic vertebra (neurology, orthopedics, and radiology)

T₁₂
twelfth thoracic nerve (neurology and orthopedics)
twelfth thoracic vertebra (neurology, orthopedics, and radiology)

T-1824
Evans blue [dye] (cardiovascular, hematology, and radiology)

t
teaspoon (measurement)
temporal (cardiovascular and neurology)
ter [three times]
terminal
tertiary
test of significance (laboratory)
time
translocation (genetics and laboratory)

t.
temporal (cardiovascular and neurology)
ter [three times]
terminal
tertiary
test of significance (laboratory)
translocation (genetics and laboratory)

t.
temporal

t½
{not an abbreviation} [symbol for one-half lifetime of pharmaceuticals and radioactive isotopes] (chemistry, pharmacology, physics, and radiology)

t½
{not an abbreviation} [symbol for one-half lifetime of pharmaceuticals and radioactive isotopes] (chemistry, pharmacology, physics, and radiology)

TA
tannic acid (laboratory and urology)
Teaching Assistant (education)
temperature, axillary [also called *axillary temperature*] (measurement)
tendo Achilis [reflex] (neurology and orthopedics)
tension applanation (ophthalmology)
Test of Articulation (Goldman Fristoe) (speech and language therapy)
therapeutic abortion (obstetrics)
thermophilic *Actinomyces* [a bacterium] (laboratory)
thoracoabdominal [stapler] (surgery)
thyroid autoantibody (endocrinology and laboratory)
titratable acid (laboratory)
total alkaloids (laboratory)
toxin-antitoxin (pharmacology)
traffic accident (emergency medicine)
Transactional Analysis (psychiatry)
transaldolase (laboratory)
transplantation antigen (laboratory and transplant surgery)
tricuspid atresia (cardiovascular)
true anomaly
truncus arteriosus (cardiovascular)
tryptophane acid [reaction] (laboratory)

tryptose agar (laboratory)
tube agglutination (laboratory)
tuberculin, alkaline [also called *alkaline tuberculin*] (infectious diseases, pharmacology, and respiratory)
tumor-associated (oncology)

TA.

tuberculin, alkaline [also called *alkaline tuberculin*] (infectious diseases, pharmacology, and respiratory)

T.A.

toxin-antitoxin (pharmacology)

T(A)

temperature, axillary (measurement)

T & A

tonsillectomy and adenoidectomy (otorhinolaryngology)
tonsillitis and adenoiditis (otorhinolaryngology)
tonsils and adenoids (otorhinolaryngology)

TA₄

tetraiodothyroacetic acid (laboratory)

Ta

atrial T-wave [found on electrocardiograms] (cardiovascular)
intraocular pressure applanation (ophthalmology)
tantalum [used in prostheses and wire sutures] (chemistry, orthopedics, and surgery)
tonometry applanation (ophthalmology)

TAA

thoracic aortic aneurysm (cardiovascular)
total ankle arthroplasty (orthopedics)
transverse aortic arch (cardiovascular)
triamcinolone acetonide (dentistry, dermatology, otorhinolaryngology, orthopedics, and pharmacology)
tumor-associated antibody(ies) (laboratory and oncology)
tumor-associated antigen(s) (laboratory and oncology)

TAAF

thromboplastic activity of amnionic

fluid (laboratory, neonatology, and obstetrics)

TAB

tablet (pharmacology)
therapeutic abortion (obstetrics) {pronounced "tab"}
triple antibiotic [bacitracin, neomycin, and polymyxin] (pharmacology) [*Note: This is considered a dangerous abbreviation.*]
typhoid, paratyphoid A, and paratyphoid B [vaccine] (infectious diseases and pharmacology) {pronounced "tab"}

Tab

tabella [tablet] (pharmacology) {pronounced "tab"}
tablet (pharmacology) {pronounced "tab"}

tab

tabella [tablet] (pharmacology) {pronounced "tab"}
tablet (pharmacology) {pronounced "tab"}

tab.

tabella [tablet] (pharmacology) {pronounced "tab"}
tablet (pharmacology) {pronounced "tab"}

"tab"

{pronunciation of *TAB* (therapeutic abortion [obstetrics] and typhoid, paratyphoid A, and paratyphoid B (vaccine) [infectious diseases and pharmacology]) and *Tab, tab,* and *tab.* (*tabella*, tablet [pharmacology])]} {not an abbreviation}

TABC

total aerobic bacteria count (laboratory)
typhoid-paratyphoid A, B, and C [vaccine] (infectious diseases and pharmacology)

tabs
tablets (pharmacology) {pronounced "tabz"}

Tab-Strap
{not an abbreviation} [a knee immobilizer] (orthopedics)

TABT
combined typhoid, paratyphoid A, and paratyphoid B, and tetanus toxoid [vaccine] (infectious diseases and pharmacology)

TABTD
combined typhoid, paratyphoid A, and paratyphoid B, tetanus toxoid, and diphtheria toxoid [vaccine] (infectious diseases and pharmacology)

TAB vaccine
typhoid, paratyphoid A, and paratyphoid B vaccine (infectious diseases and pharmacology) {pronounced "tab-vak-seen"}

"tab-vak-seen"
{pronunciation of *TAB vaccine* [typhoid, paratyphoid A, and paratyphoid B vaccine]} (infectious diseases and pharmacology) {not an abbreviation}

"tabz"
{pronunciation of *tabs* [tablets]} (pharmacology) {not an abbreviation}

TAC
terminal atrial contraction (cardiovascular)
triamcinolone cream (dermatology and pharmacology) {pronounced "tack"}

TACE
tripara-anisylchloroethylene {pronounced "tace"}
{not an abbreviation} [trademark for preparation of *chlorotrianisene* used for estrogen therapy] (chemotherapy, gynecology, oncology, and pharmacology) {pronounced "tace"}

"tace"
{pronunciation of *TACE* [*tripara-anisylchloroethylene* and a trademark preparation of *chlorotrianisene* used for estrogen therapy {not an abbreviation} (chemotherapy, gynecology, oncology, and pharmacology)] and *T'ASE* [tryptophane synthetase (laboratory)]} {not an abbreviation}

tach
tachycardia (cardiovascular) {pronounced "tack"}

tacho-
{not an abbreviation} [prefix indicating relationship to speed] {pronounced "tack-oh"}

tachy
tachycardia (cardiovascular) {pronounced "tack-E"}

tachy-
{not an abbreviation} [prefix indicating rapid or swift] {pronounced "tack-E"}

"tack"
{pronunciation of *TAC* [triamcinolone cream] (dermatology and pharmacology)] and *tach* [tachycardia] (cardiovascular)]} {not an abbreviation}

"tack-E"
{pronunciation of *tachy* [tachycardia (cardiovascular)] and *tachy-* [prefix indicating rapid or shift {not an abbreviation}] {not an abbreviation}

TACL
Test for Auditory Comprehension of Language (speech and language therapy)

"tack-oh"
{pronunciation of *tacho-* [prefix indicating relationship to speed {not an abbreviation}]} {not an abbreviation}

TAD
thioguanine, cytosine arabinoside, and daunomycin (chemotherapy, oncology, and pharmacology)
thoracic asphyxiant dystrophy (neurol-

ogy, otorhinolaryngology, and respiratory)

transverse abdominal diameter (measurement)

TADAC
therapeutic abortion, dilation, aspiration, curettage (obstetrics)

TAE
transcatheter arterial embolization (cardiovascular)

taenia-
{not an abbreviation} [prefix meaning a flat band or tapeworm] {pronounced "tea-knee-ah"}

TAF
tissue angiogenesis factor (laboratory)
toxoid-antitoxin floccules (laboratory)
trypsin-aldehyde-fuchsin (laboratory)
Tuberculin Albumose-frei [also called *albumose-free tuberculin*] (infectious diseases, pharmacology, and respiratory)
tumor-angiogenesis factor (laboratory, oncology, and pathology)

TAG
thymine, adenine, guanine (laboratory)

TAH
total abdominal hysterectomy (gynecology)
total artificial heart (cardiovascular)
transabdominal hysterectomy (gynecology)

TAH-BSO
total abdominal hysterectomy and bilateral salpingo-oophorectomy (gynecology)

TAL
talis [of such, such a one]
tendo Achillis lengthening [also called *Achilles tendon lengthening*] (orthopedics)
thymic alymphoplasia (immunology)

Tal.
talis [of such, such a one]

tal
talis [of such, such a one]

tal.
talis [of such, such a one]

T-ALL
T-cell acute lymphoblastic leukemia (hematology and oncology)

TALTFR
teno [or tendo] Achillis lengthening and toe flexor release (orthopedics and podiatry)

TALWIN
Talwin [an analgesic] (pharmacology)

TAM
tamoxifen (chemotherapy, oncology, and pharmacology)
thermoacidurans agar modified (laboratory)
toxoid-antitoxin mixture [for diphtheria immunization] (infectious diseases and pharmacology)

T.A.M.
toxoid-antitoxoid mixture [for diphtheria immunization] (infectious diseases and pharmacology)

TAME
toluene-sulfo-trypsin arginine methyl ester [also called *p-toluenesulfonyl-L-arginine methylester* and *tosylarginine methylester*] (laboratory)

TAMe
toluene-sulfo-trypsin arginine methyl ester [also called *p-toluenesulfonyl-L-arginine methylester* and *tosylarginine methylester*] (laboratory)

T.-A. mixture
toxin-antitoxin mixture [for diphtheria immunization] (infectious diseases and pharmacology)

TAMIS
Telemetric Automated Microbial Identification System (laboratory)

TAN
total ammonia nitrogen (laboratory)

tan
tangent

tan.
tangent

TANI
total axial [lymph] node irradiation (oncology and radiation therapy)

TANS
Territorial Army Nursing Service (armed forces and nursing)

TAO
thromboangiitis obliterans (cardiovascular)
triacetyloleandomycin [an antibiotic] (pharmacology)
troleandomycin [an antibacterial] (pharmacology)
{not an abbreviation} [trademark for preparation of troleandomycin; an antibiotic] (pharmacology)

TAPVC
total anomalous pulmonary venous connection (cardiovascular and respiratory)

TAPVD
total anomalous pulmonary venous drainage (cardiovascular and respiratory)

TAPVR
total anomalous pulmonary venous return (cardiovascular and respiratory)

TAR
thrombocytopenia with absent radius [or radii] (hematology and laboratory)
total ankle replacement (orthopedics)
Treatment Authorization Request [for Medi-Cal] (insurance) {pronounced "tar"}

"tar"
{pronunciation of TAR [Treatment Authorization Request (for Medi-Cal)]} (insurance) {not an abbreviation}

TARA
total articular replacement arthroplasty (orthopedics) {pronounced "tar-ah"}

"tar-ah"
{pronunciation of TARA [total articular replacement arthroplasty]} (orthopedics) {not an abbreviation}

TARGET
target cell (hematology and laboratory)

tarso-
{not an abbreviation} [prefix indicating relationship to the edge of the eyelid (ophthalmology) or to the instep of the foot (orthopedics and podiatry)] {pronounced "tar-so"}

"tarso"
{pronunciation of tarso- [prefix indicating relationship to the edge of the eyelid (ophthalmology) or to the instep of the foot (orthopedics and podiatry) {not an abbreviation}]} {not an abbreviation}

TART
tart cell (hematology and laboratory)

TAS
Therapeutic Activities Specialist (physical therapy)

T'ASE
tryptophane synthetase (laboratory) {pronounced "tace"}

TA stapler
thoracoabdominal stapler (surgery)

TAT
tetanus antitoxin (infectious diseases and pharmacology)
thematic apperception test (psychiatry)

thromboplastin activation time (hematology and laboratory)
till all taken (pharmacology)
total antitryptic activity (laboratory)
toxin-antitoxin (pharmacology)
turnaround time (laboratory)
tyrosine aminotransferase (laboratory)

T.A.T.
toxin-antitoxin (pharmacology)

TATST
tetanus antitoxin skin test (infectious diseases and pharmacology)

tauto-
{not an abbreviation} [prefix meaning the same] {pronounced "taw-toe"}

"taw-toe"
{pronunciation of *tauto-* [prefix meaning the same {not an abbreviation}]} {not an abbreviation}

TB
Mycobacterium tuberculosis [a bacterium] (infectious diseases, laboratory, and respiratory)
terminal bronchiole (respiratory)
thromboxane B (hematology and laboratory)
thymol blue (laboratory)
toluidine blue (laboratory)
total base (laboratory)
total body
tracheal bronchiolar [region] (respiratory)
tracheobronchitis (respiratory)
trapezoid body (neurology)
tubercle bacillus (infectious diseases, laboratory, and respiratory)
tuberculin (infectious diseases, pharmacology, and respiratory)
tuberculosis (infectious diseases, laboratory, and respiratory)

T-B
Thomas-Binetti [test] (laboratory, oncology, and pathology)

Tb
terbium (chemistry)
tubercle bacillus (infectious diseases, laboratory, and respiratory)

tuberculosis (infectious diseases, laboratory, and respiratory)

T.b.
tubercle bacillus (infectious diseases, laboratory, and respiratory)
tuberculosis (infectious diseases, laboratory, and respiratory)

TBA
tertiary butyl acetate (chemistry)
testosterone-binding affinity (endocrinology and laboratory)
thiobarbituric acid (pharmacology)
thyroxine-binding albumin (endocrinology and laboratory)
to be absorbed (pharmacology)
to be added
to be admitted
to be announced
tubercle bacillus (infectious diseases, laboratory, and respiratory)
tuberculosis (infectious diseases, laboratory, and respiratory)

T banding
telomere banding (genetics and laboratory)
terminal banding (genetics and laboratory)

TBB
transbronchial biopsy (pathology and respiratory)

TBBM
total body bone mineral (laboratory)

TBC
thyroxine-binding coagulin (endocrinology and laboratory)
tuberculosis (infectious diseases, laboratory, and respiratory)

Tbc
tuberculosis (infectious diseases, laboratory, and respiratory)

Tbc.
tuberculosis (infectious diseases, laboratory, and respiratory)

tbc
tuberculosis (infectious diseases, laboratory, and respiratory)

tbc.
tuberculosis (infectious diseases, laboratory, and respiratory)

TB charcoal agar
{not an abbreviation} (laboratory and respiratory)

TBD
total body density

TBE
tick-born(e) encephalitis (neurology)
tuberculin bacillary emulsion (infectious diseases, pharmacology, and respiratory)
tuberculin bacillen emulsion (infectious diseases, pharmacology, and respiratory)

T.B.E.
bacillen emulsion tuberculin (infectious diseases, pharmacology, and respiratory)

TBF
total body fat (laboratory)

TBG
testosterone-binding globulin (endocrinology and laboratory)
thyroglobulin (endocrinology, laboratory, and pharmacology)
thyroid-binding globulin (endocrinology and laboratory)
thyroxine-binding globulin [also called T_4-binding globulin] (endocrinology and laboratory)

TBG cap
thyroxine-binding capacity of thyroxine-binding globulin assays (endocrinology and laboratory)

TBGP
total blood granulocyte pool (hematology and laboratory)

TBH
total body hematocrit (hematology and laboratory)

TBI
thyrobinding index (endocrinology and laboratory)
thyroxine-binding index (endocrinology and laboratory)
tooth brushing instruction (dentistry and rehabilitation)
total body irradiation (radiation therapy)
traumatic brain injury (emergency medicine, neurology, and rehabilitation)

TBII
thyroid-stimulating hormone (TSH) binding inhibitory immunoglobulin (endocrinology and laboratory)

T. BIL
total bilirubin (gastroenterology and laboratory)

T. Bili
total bilirubin (gastroenterology and laboratory) {pronounced "tea-bill-E"}

T bili
total bilirubin (gastroenterology and laboratory) {pronounced "tea-bill-E"}

TBK
total body potassium (laboratory)

tbl
tablespoon (measurement)

TBLB
transbronchial lung brush (laboratory, oncology, pathology, and respiratory)

TBLC
term birth, living child (obstetrics)

TBLI
term birth, living infant (obstetrics)

TBM
tuberculous meningitis (infectious diseases and neurology)
tubular basement membrane (anatomy and laboratory)
tubule basement membrane (anatomy and laboratory)

TBN
bacillus emulsion (infectious diseases, pharmacology, and respiratory)

TBNA
treated but not admitted (emergency medicine)

TBP
bithionol [a bacteriostatic] (pharmacology)
testosterone-binding protein (endocrinology and laboratory)
thyroxine-binding protein (endocrinology and laboratory)
tributyl phosphate (chemistry, genetics, and laboratory)
tuberculous peritonitis (gastroenterology and infectious diseases)

TBPA
thyroxine-binding prealbumin [also called *T$_4$-binding protein*] (endocrinology and laboratory)

TBR
total bed rest
total bilirubin (gastroenterology and laboratory)

TB-RD
tuberculosis-respiratory disease (infectious diseases and respiratory)

TBS
total body solute
tribromosalicylanilide [a bacteriostatic; also called *tribromsalan*] (pharmacology)
triethanolamine-buffered saline (pharmacology)

tbs
tablespoon (measurement)

TBSA
total body surface area (measurement)
total burn surface area (measurement)

Tbsp
tablespoon (measurement)

tbsp
tablespoon (measurement)

tbsp.
tablespoon (measurement)

TBT
tolbutamine test (endocrinology and laboratory)
tracheobronchial toilet (respiratory)

TBTNR
Toronto Biculture Test of Nonverbal Reasoning (speech and language therapy)

TBV
total blood volume (hematology and laboratory)
transluminal balloon valvuloplasty (cardiovascular)

TB-Vis
isoniazid [an antibacterial] (infectious diseases, pharmacology, and respiratory)

TBVp
total blood volume predicted from body surface (hematology and laboratory)

TBW
total body water (measurement)
total body weight (measurement)

TBX
total body irradiation [also called *whole body irradiation*] (radiation therapy)

TBX$_2$
thromboxane B$_2$ (hematology and laboratory)

TBZ
{not an abbreviation} [brand name for *thiabendazole;* an antihelmintic] (veterinary medicine)

TC
taurocholate [also called *cholytaurine* and *taurocholic acid*] (laboratory)
temperature compensation
tetracycline [an antibiotic] (pharmacology)
thermal conductivity (physics)
thoracic cage (anatomy, cardiovascular, and respiratory)
throat culture (laboratory and otorhinolaryngology)
thyrocalcitonin [also called *calcitonin*] (laboratory, orthopedics, and pharmacology)
tissue culture (laboratory)
to contain
total capacity
total cholesterol (cardiovascular and laboratory)
total colonoscopy (gastroenterology)
traffic collision (emergency medicine)
transcobalamin (hematology and laboratory)
transcutaneous
treatment completed
tropocollagen (genetics and laboratory)
true conjugate (ophthalmology)
tuberculin, contagious (infectious diseases, pharmacology, and respiratory)
tubocurarine (anesthesiology, neurology, and surgery)
type and crossmatch [for blood transfusion] (hematology and surgery)

T.C.
traffic collision (emergency medicine)
tuberculin contagious (infectious diseases, laboratory, and respiratory)

T & C
turn and cough (respiratory)
type and cross (blood bank, hematology, and laboratory)
type and crossmatch (blood bank, hematology, and laboratory)

T/C
to consider

T₄(C)

$T_4(C)$
serum thyroxine [measured by column chromatographic technique] (endocrinology and laboratory)

Tc
generation time (laboratory and research)
technetium (chemistry and radiology)

⁹⁹ᵐTc

^{99m}Tc
technetium 99m [a radioactive technetium] (chemistry and radiology)

TCA
terminal cancer (oncology)
terminal carcinoma (oncology)
transluminal coronary angioplasty (cardiovascular, radiology)
tricalcium aluminate
tricarboxylic acid [cycle] (laboratory)
trichloroacetate [a herbicide] (chemistry)
trichloroacetic acid (dermatology, laboratory, and pharmacology)
tricuspid atresia (cardiovascular)
tricyclic antidepressant (pharmacology and psychiatry)

TCABG
triple coronary artery bypass graft (cardiovascular)

TCAD
tricyclic antidepressant (pharmacology and psychiatry)

TCAP
trimethyl-cetyl-ammonium pentachlorphenate [a fungicide] (pharmacology)

T-CAP
Baker's Antifol, cyclophosphamide, Adriamycin, and cisplatin (chemotherapy, oncology, and pharmacology)

TCAT
transmission computer-assisted tomography

TCB
total cardiopulmonary bypass (cardiovascular)
tumor cell burden (laboratory, oncology,
and pathology)

TCBS
thiosulfate citrate bile salts sucrose
[agar] (laboratory)

TCBS agar
thiosulfate citrate bile salts sucrose agar
(laboratory)

TCC
thromboplastic cell component (hematology and laboratory)
transitional-cell carcinoma (laboratory,
oncology, and pathology)
trichlorocarbanilide (laboratory)

TCCB
transitional-cell carcinoma of bladder
(oncology and urology)

TC CO$_2$
transcutaneous carbon dioxide [monitor]
(laboratory and respiratory)

Tc^{99} colloid
technetium isotope (chemistry and radiology)

Tc$_{99}$ colloid
technetium isotope (chemistry and radiology)

TCD
tissue culture dose (laboratory)

TCD$_{50}$
median tissue culture dose (laboratory)

TCDB
turn, cough, and deep breath(e) (respiratory)

T,C,DB
turn, cough, and deep breath(e) (respiratory)

T.C. & D.B.
turn, cough, and deep breath(e) (respiratory)

TCDC
taurochenodeoxycholate [also called
chenodeoxycholytaurine] (gastroenterology and laboratory)

TCDD
2,3,6,7-tetrachlorodibenzo-p-dioxin
(chemistry)
2,3,7,8-tetrachlorodibenzo-p-dioxin [a
herbicide; also called tetra-
chlorodibenzodioxin] (chemistry)

TC detector
thermal conductivity detector (physics)

TCE
tetrachloro-diphenyl-ethane [an insecti-
cide] (chemistry)
tetrachloroethylene [a solvent] (chemistry)
trichloroethanol [an anesthetic and hyp-
notic] (pharmacology)

T cell
thymus-dependent lymphocyte [also
called T-lymphocyte] (hematology, immunology, and laboratory)

T-4
T-4 cell [also called helper/inducer thymus-derived cell] (hematology, immunology, and laboratory)

T-8 cell
T-8 suppressor cell [also called cytotoxic
cell and suppressor cell] (hematology,
immunology, and laboratory)

TCES
transcutaneous cranial electrical stimulation (neurology)

TCESOM
trichlorethylene-extracted soybean-oil
meal [a supplement] (dietary)

TCF
total coronary flow (cardiovascular)

TCGF
thymus cell growth factor [also called in-

terleukin 2] (chemotherapy, oncology, and pharmacology)

TCH
total circulating hemoglobin (hematology and laboratory)
turn, cough, and hyperventilate (respiratory)

Tchg
teaching (education)

TcHIDA
technetium hepatoiminodiacetic acid [scan] (radiology)

T^{c}H$_2$O
free water reabsorption

Tchr
teacher (education)

TCI
to come in [to hospital]
transient cerebral ischemia (neurology)

TCID
tissue culture infective dose (laboratory)

TCID$_{50}$
median tissue culture infective dose (laboratory)

TCIE
transient cerebral ischemic episode (neurology)

T-CLL
T-cell chronic lymphatic leukemia (hematology, laboratory, and pathology)

TCM
tissue culture medium (laboratory)
transcutaneous monitor (laboratory and respiratory)

Tc^{99m}
technetium medronate [scan] (radiology)

TCMH
tumor-direct cell-mediated hypersensitivity (laboratory and oncology)

TCMZ
trichlormethiazide [a diuretic] (cardiovascular and pharmacology)

TCN
tetracycline [an antibiotic] (pharmacology)

TCNS
transcutaneous nerve stimulator (neurology and orthopedics)

T-COAP
vincristine, prednisone, cytosine arabinoside, cyclophosphamide, and 6-thioguanine (chemotherapy, oncology, and pharmacology)

TCOM
transcutaneous oxygen monitor (laboratory and respiratory)

TCP
therapeutic continuous penicillin [an antibiotic] (pharmacology)
trichlorophenol [an antiseptic and disinfectant] (pharmacology)
tricresyl phosphate [an antiesterase] (pharmacology)

^{99m}Tc-PIPIDA scan
technetium pertechnetate/N-paraisopropylacetanilide-iminodiacetic acid scan (radiology)

TCPM
{not an abbreviation} [a pneumatic tourniquet system] (orthopedics)

TC pO$_2$
transcutaneous partial pressure of oxygen [monitor] (laboratory and respiratory)

TCR
thalamocortical relay (neurology)

tcRNA
translation control ribonucleic acid (genetics and laboratory)

TCS
tripanel, convoluted, Y-strap [knee immobilizer] (orthopedics)

TCSA
tetrachlorosalicylanilide

TCT
thrombin-clotting time (hematology and laboratory)

thyrocalcitonin [also called *calcitonin*] (laboratory, orthopedics, and pharmacology)

turbid creamy layer on top (laboratory)

TcT
tympanostomy with tube placement (otorhinolaryngology)

TCu
copper T [an intrauterine contraceptive device] (gynecology and pharmacology)

TCV
thoracic cage volume (cardiovascular and respiratory)

TCVA
thromboembolic cerebrovascular accident (cardiovascular and neurology)

TD
Takayasu's disease (cardiovascular and neurology)

tardive dyskinesia (neurology)

temporary disability

terminal device

tetanus and diphtheria [toxoids] (infectious diseases, pediatrics, and pharmacology)

therapy discontinued

thermal dilution

thoracic duct (anatomy and otorhinolaryngology)

three times a day (pharmacology)

threshold dose (radiation therapy)

threshold of discomfort (neurology)

thymus-dependent [cells] (hematology, immunology, and laboratory)

tidal [volume] (laboratory and respiratory)

time disintegration (radiation therapy)

timed disintegration (radiation therapy)

to deliver

tone decay (otorhinolaryngology)

torsion dystonia [also called *dystonia musculorum deformans*] (genetics and neurology)

total disability

total dose [of radiation] (radiation therapy and radiology)

totally disabled

touchdown (sports medicine)

toxic dose (pharmacology and radiation therapy)

transdermal

transverse diameter (measurement)

traveler's diarrhea (gastroenterology)

treating distance (radiation therapy)

treatment discontinued

tuberoinfundibular dopaminergic (neurology)

tumor dose (radiation therapy)

typhoid-dysentery (gastroenterology and infectious diseases)

T₄(D)
serum thyroxine [measured by displacement analysis] (endocrinology and laboratory)

TD₅₀
median toxic dose (pharmacology and radiation therapy)

Td
tetanus-diphtheria [toxoid] (infectious diseases and pharmacology)

td
ter die [three times daily] (pharmacology)

t.d.
ter die [three times daily] (pharmacology)

TDA
thyroid-stimulating hormone displacing antibody (endocrinology and laboratory)

TDC
taurodeoxycholate (gastroenterology
and laboratory)
total dietary calories (dietary)

TDD
Telecommunication Device for the Deaf
(electronics and otorhinolaryngology)
tetradecadiene (chemistry)
thoracic duct drainage (otorhinolaryngology)
Tuberculous Diseases Diploma (education, infectious diseases, and respiratory)

TDDA
tetradecadiene acetate (chemistry)

TDE
tetrachlorodiphenylethane [an insecti-
cide] (chemistry)
total daily energy [requirement] (dietary)
total digestible energy (dietary)

TDEC
test no longer offered (laboratory)

TDF
thoracic duct fistula (otorhinolaryngology)
thoracic duct flow (otorhinolaryngology)
tumor dose fractionation (oncology and
radiation therapy)

TDI
Therapy Dogs International (ophthalmology, rehabilitation, social services,
and veterinary medicine)
toluene diisocyanate [also called *toluene
2,4-diisocyanate*] (chemistry)
total dose infusion (pharmacology)

TDK
tardive dyskinesia (neurology)

TDL
thoracic duct lymph (otorhinolaryngology)
thoracic duct lymphocyte(s) (laboratory)
thymus-dependent lymphocyte(s) (hematology, immunology, and laboratory)

TDM
therapeutic drug monitoring (pharmacology)

TDN
total digestible nutrients (dietary)

T-DNA
transferred deoxyribonucleic acid (genetics and laboratory)

TDP
thoracic duct pressure (otorhinolaryngology)
thymidine diphosphate (genetics and
laboratory)

TdP
torsade de pointes [found on electrocardiograms; French meaning *fringe of
pointed tips*] (cardiovascular)

TdR
thymidine (genetics and laboratory)

TdR-³H
tritiated thymidine (genetics and laboratory)

TDS
ter die sumendum [to be taken three
times a day] (pharmacology)
temperature, depth, salinity (laboratory)
temperature-determined sex (laboratory)

tds
ter die sumendum [to be taken three
times a day] (pharmacology)

t.d.s.
ter die sumendum [to be taken three
times a day] (pharmacology)

TDT
tentative drainage tomorrow (surgery)
terminal deoxynucleotidyl transferase
(laboratory)
terminal deoxytransferase (laboratory)
thermal death time (laboratory)
tone decay test (otorhinolaryngology)

TdT
terminal deoxytransferase (laboratory)

Tdt
terminal deoxytransferase (laboratory)

TDTA
Templin Darley Test of Articulation (speech and language therapy)

TDWB
touch-down weight-bearing (orthopedics and rehabilitation)

TDZ
thymus-dependent zone [of lymph node] (immunology and laboratory)

TE
Teacher of Electrotherapy (education and physical therapy)
tennis elbow (orthopedics and sports medicine)
test ear (otorhinolaryngology)
tetanus (cardiovascular, infectious diseases laboratory, and pharmacology)
tetracycline [an antibiotic] (pharmacology)
threshold energy
thromboembolism (cardiovascular and hematology)
thymus epithelial [cell] (immunology and laboratory)
thyrotoxic exophthalmos (endocrinology and ophthalmology)
time echo
time estimation
tissue-equivalent
tonsillectomy (otorhinolaryngology)
tonsils excised (otorhinolaryngology)
tooth extracted (dentistry)
total estrogen [excretion] (endocrinology, gynecology, laboratory, and obstetrics)
totally embedded
toxoplasma encephalitis (neurology)
trace elements (chemistry)
tracheoesophageal (otorhinolaryngology and gastroenterology)
treadmill exercise (cardiovascular)
trial and error

T & E
trial and error

Te
tellurium (chemistry)
tetanus (cardiovascular, infectious diseases, laboratory, and pharmacology)

T-e
erythrocyte tri-iodothyronine (endocrinology and laboratory)

TEA
tetraethylammonium (cardiovascular and pharmacology)
thromboendarterectomy (cardiovascular) {pronounced "tea"}
total elbow arthroplasty (orthopedics) {pronounced "tea"}
total endarterectomy (cardiovascular) {pronounced "tea"}

"tea"
{pronunciation of *TEA* [thromboendarterectomy (cardiovascular), total elbow arthroplasty (orthopedics), and total endarterectomy (cardiovascular)]} {not an abbreviation}

TEAB
tetraethylammonium bromide (cardiovascular and pharmacology)

"tea-bill-E"
{pronunciation of *T. Bili* and *T bili* [total bilirubin]} (gastroenterology and laboratory) {not an abbreviation}

TEAC
tetraethylammonium chloride (cardiovascular and pharmacology)

"tea-knee-ah"
{pronunciation of *taenia-* and *tenia-* [prefixes meaning a flat band or tapeworm {not abbreviations}]} {not an abbreviation}

"tea-lenz"
{pronunciation of *T-lens* [therapeutic contact lens]} (ophthalmology) {not an abbreviation}

"tea-max"
{pronunciation of *T-MAX* [temperature maximum]} (measurement) {not an abbreviation}

"tea-no"
{pronunciation of *teno-* [prefix indicating relationship to a tendon {not an abbreviation}]} (neurology and orthopedics) {not an abbreviation}

"tea-peed"
{pronunciation of *TP'd* [toilet papered (a practical joke)]} {not an abbreviation}

TEAR
tear drop (laboratory and ophthalmology)

"tear-ah"
{pronunciation of *tera-* [prefix for 10^{12} {not an abbreviation}]} (measurement) {not an abbreviation}

"tear-ah-toe"
{pronunciation of *terato-* [prefix indicating relationship to a monster {not an abbreviation}]} {not an abbreviation}

"tea-re"
{pronunciation of *tere* [a word meaning *rub* {not an abbreviation}]} (cardiovascular and respiratory) {not an abbreviation}

"tea-sect"
{pronunciation of *T sect* [cross section or transverse section]} {not an abbreviation}

"tea-set"
{pronunciation of *T-set* [tracheostomy set]} (emergency medicine, respiratory, and surgery)

TEB
tris-ethylenediaminetetra-acetate borate (laboratory and pharmacology)

TeBG
testosterone-binding globulin (endocrinology and laboratory)
testosterone-estradiol-binding globulin (endocrinology and laboratory)

TEC
total eosinophil count (hematology and laboratory)
transient erythroblastopenia of childhood (hematology, laboratory, and pediatrics)

T & EC
Trauma and Emergency Center (emergency medicine)

TECA
technetium albumin study (radiology)

tech
technical
technician {pronounced "tek"}
technology {pronounced "tek"}

TED
Tasks of Emotional Development (psychiatry)
threshold erythema dose (radiation therapy)
thromboembolic disease (cardiovascular)

T.E.D.
threshold erythema dose (radiation therapy)

TED hose
thromboembolic disease hose (cardiovascular)

TEDS
thromboembolic disease stockings (cardiovascular) {pronounced "tedz"}
{not an abbreviation} [brand name for thromboembolic disease stockings] (cardiovascular) {pronounced "tedz"}

TED stockings
antiembolism stockings [acronym for *thromboembolic disease*] (cardiovascular)

"tedz"
{pronunciation of *TEDS* [thromboembolic disease stockings and brand name for thromboembolic disease

stockings {not an abbreviation}]} (cardiovascular) {not an abbreviation}

TEE
transesophageal echocardiography (cardiovascular)
tyrosine ethyl ester (endocrinology and laboratory)

TEF
tetralogy of Fallot (cardiovascular, neonatology, and pediatrics)
tracheoesophageal fistula (gastroenterology, otorhinolaryngology, respiratory, and surgery)
transmission electron microscopy (laboratory)
trunk extension-flexion [unit] (rehabilitation)

TE (F)
tracheoesophageal (fistula) (gastroenterology, otorhinolaryngology, and respiratory)

TEG
thromboelastogram [of blood] (cardiovascular, hematology, and laboratory)

TEIB
triethyleneiminobenzoquinone (chemistry)

"tek"
{pronunciation of *tech* [technician and technology]} {not an abbreviation}

TEL
tetraethyl lead (chemistry)

tele
telemetry (cardiovascular) {pronounced "tell-E"}
telephone (communications) {pronounced "tell-E"}
television (communications) {pronounced "tell-E"}

tele-
{not an abbreviation} [prefix indicating relation to the end or operating at a distance or far away] {pronounced "tell-E"}

"tell-E"
{pronunciation of *tele* [telemetry (cardiovascular) and telephone and television (communications)] and *tele-* [prefix indicating relation to the end or operating at a distance or far away {not an abbreviation}]} {not an abbreviation}

"tell-oh"
{pronunciation of *telo-* [prefix indicating relationship to an end {not an abbreviation}]} {not an abbreviation}

telo-
{not an abbreviation} [prefix indicating relationship to an end] {pronounced "tell-oh"}

TEM
transmission electron microscope (laboratory)
triethylenemelamine (chemotherapy, oncology, and pharmacology)

Temp
temperature (measurement) {pronounced "temp"}

temp
temperature (measurement) {pronounced "temp"}
temporal
temporary {pronounced "temp"}

"temp"
{pronunciation of *Temp* [temperature (measurement)] and *temp* [temperature (measurement) and temporary]} {not an abbreviation}

temp dext
tempori dextro [to the right temple]

temp. dext.
tempori dextro [to the right temple]

temp sinist
tempori sinistro [to the left temple]

825

temp. sinist.
tempori sinistro [to the left temple]

TEN
total enteral nutrition (dietary and gastroenterology)
total excreted nitrogen (laboratory)
total excretory nitrogen (laboratory)
toxic epidermal necrolysis (dermatology)

TENAC
tenaculum (surgery) {pronounced "ten-ack"}

tenac.
tenaculum (surgery) {pronounced "ten-ack"}

"ten-ack"
{pronunciation of *TENAC* and *tenac.* [tenaculum]} (surgery) {not an abbreviation}

tendo
{not an abbreviation} [Latin word meaning *tendon*] (neurology and orthopedics)

tenia-
{not an abbreviation} [prefix meaning a flat band or tapeworm] {pronounced "tea-knee-ah"}

teno-
{not an abbreviation} [prefix indicating relationship to a tendon] (neurology and orthopedics) {pronounced "teano" or "ten-oh"}

"ten-oh"
{pronunciation of *teno-* [prefix indicating relationship to a tendon {not an abbreviation}]} (neurology and orthopedics) {not an abbreviation}

tenonto-
{not an abbreviation} [prefix indicating relationship to a tendon] (neurology and orthopedics) {pronounced "ten-on-to"}

"ten-on-to"
{pronunciation of *tenonto-* [prefix indi-

cating relationship to a tendon {not an abbreviation}]} (neurology and orthopedics) {not an abbreviation}

TENS
transcutaneous electrical nerve stimulation (neurology and physical therapy) {pronounced "tenz"}
transcutaneous electrical nerve stimulator (neurology and physical therapy) {pronounced "tenz"}

T.E.N.S.
transcutaneous electrical nerve stimulation (neurology and physical therapy) {pronounced "tenz"}
transcutaneous electrical nerve stimulator (neurology and physical therapy) {pronounced "tenz"}

"tenz"
{pronunciation of *TENS* and *T.E.N.S.* [transcutaneous electrical nerve stimulation and transcutaneous electrical nerve stimulator]} (neurology and physical therapy) {not an abbreviation}

TEP
thromboendophlebectomy (cardiovascular)

TEPA
triethylenephosphoramide (chemotherapy, oncology, and pharmacology)

TEPP
tetraethylpyrophosphate [an insecticide] (chemistry)

TEQU
test equivocal, possible low titer (laboratory)

TER
three times (pharmacology)
threefold
total endoplasmic reticulum (laboratory)
transcapillary escape rate
transcapillary escape route

ter
tere [rub] (cardiovascular and respiratory)
tertiary
three times (pharmacology)
threefold

ter-
{not an abbreviation} [prefix meaning three or three-fold] {pronounced "ter"}

"ter"
{pronunciation of *ter-* [prefix meaning three or three-fold {not an abbreviation}]} {not an abbreviation}

tera-
{not an abbreviation} [prefix for 10^{12}] (measurement) {pronounced "tear-ah"}

terato-
{not an abbreviation} [prefix indicating relationship to a monster] {pronounced "tear-ah-toe"}

tere
{not an abbreviation} [a word meaning *rub*] (cardiovascular and respiratory) {pronounced "tea-re"}

Terleu
tertiary leucine (endocrinology and laboratory) {pronounced "tur-lu"}

term
terminal

ter sim
tere simul [rub together]

ter. sim.
tere simul [rub together]

tert.
tertiary

TES
transcutaneous electrical stimulation (neurology and physical therapy)
transmural electrical stimulation (cardiovascular)
Treatment Emergent Symptoms

trimethylaminoethanesulfonic acid (chemistry)

TESPA
triethylenethiophosphoramide [also called *Thiotepa, thiotepa,* and *thiophosphoramide*] (chemotherapy, oncology, and pharmacology) {pronounced "tess-pah"}

"tess-pah"
{pronunciation of *TESPA* [triethylenethiophosphoramide (also called *Thiotepa, thiotepa,* and *thiophosphoramide*)]} (chemotherapy, oncology, and pharmacology) {not an abbreviation}

TESTOS
testosterone (endocrinology, laboratory, pharmacology, and urology)

TET
Teacher of Electrotherapy (physical therapy)
tetralogy of Fallot (cardiovascular, neonatology, and pediatrics) {pronounced "tet"}
treadmill exercise test (cardiovascular)

tet
tetanus (cardiovascular, infectious diseases, laboratory, and pharmacology)
tetralogy of Fallot (cardiovascular and pediatrics) {pronounced "tet"}

"tet"
{pronunciation of *TET* and *tet* [tetralogy of Fallot]} (cardiovascular, neonatology, and pediatrics) {not an abbreviation}

TETA
test-estrin time(d) action (chemotherapy, oncology, and pharmacology)

TETCYC
tetracycline [an antibiotic] (pharmacology)

TETD
tetraethylthiuram disulfide [also called *disulfiram*] (chemical dependency and pharmacology)

tetra-
{not an abbreviation} [prefix meaning *four*] {pronounced "tet-rah"}

TETRAC
tetraiodothyroacetic acid (endocrinology and laboratory)

"tet-rah"
{pronunciation of *tetra-* [prefix meaning four {not an abbreviation}]} {not an abbreviation}

"tet" spell
{not an abbreviation} [slang for *spell typical of tetralogy of Fallot*] (cardiovascular and pediatrics) {pronounced "tet-spell"}

"tet-spell"
{pronunciation of *"tet" spell* [slang for *spell typical of tetralogy of Fallot* {not an abbreviation}]} (cardiovascular and pediatrics) {not an abbreviation}

tet. tox.
tetanus toxoid (infectious diseases and pharmacology)

TEV
talipes equinovarus (orthopedics and podiatry)

TeV
tera-electron-volt [equals 10^{12} volts] (measurement and physics)

TF
tactile fremitus (respiratory)
temperature factor
tetralogy of Fallot (cardiovascular, neonatology, and pediatrics)
thymidine factor (genetics and laboratory)
thymol flocculation (laboratory)
tissue-damaging factor (laboratory)
to follow
total flow

tracheal fistula (otorhinolaryngology and respiratory)
transfer factor (allergy, immunology, laboratory, and pharmacology)
transferrin [also called *siderophilin*] (hematology and laboratory)
tube feeding (dietary and gastroenterology)
tuberculin filtrate (infectious diseases and laboratory)
tubular fluid (laboratory)
tuning fork (otorhinolaryngology)

T.F.
to follow
tuberculin filtrate (infectious diseases and laboratory)

Tf
transferrin [also called *siderophilin*] (hematology and laboratory)

TFA
total fatty acids (laboratory)

TFB
trifascicular block (cardiovascular)

TFC
transferrin, common form [also called *siderophilin*] (hematology and laboratory)

TFE
polytetrafluoroethylene (chemistry)
Teflon [trademark for preparations of polytef (polytetrafluoroethylene)] (chemistry)
tetrafluoroethylene (chemistry)

TFEV
timed forced expiratory volume (laboratory and respiratory)

Tf-Fe
transferrin-bound iron (hematology and laboratory)

T fibers
{not an abbreviation} [a type of nerve

fiber] (anatomy, laboratory, and neurology)

TFL
tensor fascia lata (anatomy and orthopedics)

Tfm
testicular feminization syndrome (endocrinology and urology)

TFN
total fecal nitrogen (gastroenterology and laboratory)

TFNS
Territorial Force Nursing Service (nursing)

TF/P
tubular fluid-to-plasma [ratio] (laboratory)
tubule fluid-to-plasma [ratio] (laboratory)

(TF/P)In
tubule fluid-to-plasma inulin ratio (laboratory)

TFR
total fertility rate (statistics analysis)

T fracture
{not an abbreviation} (orthopedics)

TFS
testicular feminization syndrome (endocrinology and urology)

TFT
thyroid function test(s) (endocrinology and laboratory)
tight fingertip [dilation of cervix] (obstetrics)
transfer factor test (allergy, immunology, laboratory, and pharmacology)
trifluorothymidine [also called *trifluridine*] (genetics and laboratory)

TFT's
thyroid function tests (endocrinology and laboratory)

TG
tendon graft (orthopedics)
testosterone glucuronide (endocrinology and laboratory)
tetraglycine (laboratory)
thioglycolate broth (laboratory)
thioguanine (chemotherapy, oncology, and pharmacology)
thromboglobulin (laboratory)
thyroglobulin (endocrinology and laboratory)
toxic goiter (endocrinology)
triglyceride(s) (cardiovascular and laboratory)

ΔTG
delta triglyceride increments (cardiovascular and laboratory)

6TG
6-thioguanine (chemotherapy, oncology, and pharmacology)

6-TG
6-thioguanine (chemotherapy, oncology, and pharmacology)

Tg
generation time (measurement)
type genus (laboratory)

TGA
taurocholate gelatin agar (laboratory)
total glycoalkaloids (laboratory and pharmacology)
transient global amnesia (neurology and psychiatry)
transposition of the great arteries (cardiovascular, neonatology, and pediatrics)
tumor glycoprotein assay (laboratory and oncology)

TGAR
total graft area rejected (dermatology and plastic surgery)

TGC
time gain compensation (radiology)

TGE
transmissible gastroenteritis [virus of swine] (gastroenterology, veterinary medicine, and virology)
tryptone glucose extract [broth or agar] (laboratory)

T.G.E.
transmissible gastroenteritis [virus of swine] (gastroenterology, veterinary medicine, and virology)

TGF
transformin growth factor (endocrinology and laboratory)

TGFA
triglyceride fatty acid (laboratory)

TGG
turkey gamma globulin (immunology and laboratory)

TGIF
thank God, it's Friday {slang}
thank goodness, it's Friday {slang}

TGL
triglyceride (cardiovascular and laboratory)
triglyceride lipase (cardiovascular and laboratory)

T globulin
{not an abbreviation} (immunology and laboratory)

TGR
tenderness, guarding, rigidity [on abdominal examination]
thioguanosine (chemotherapy, oncology, and pharmacology)

6-TGR
thioguanine riboside (chemotherapy, oncology, and pharmacology)

T group
training group [a sensitivity group] (psychiatry)

T-group
training group [a sensitivity group] (psychiatry)

TGS
tincture of green soap (pharmacology)

TGT
thromboplastin generation test (hematology and laboratory)
thromboplastin generation time (hematology and laboratory)

TGV
thoracic gas volume (respiratory)
transposition of the great vessels (cardiovascular, neonatology, and pediatrics)

TGY
tryptone glucose yeast (agar) [also called *tryptophane peptone glucose yeast (agar)*] (laboratory)

TH
tetrahydrocortisol (endocrinology and laboratory)
T-helper [cell] (immunology, infectious diseases, laboratory, and oncology)
theophylline (pharmacology and respiratory)
thoracic (cardiovascular, neurology, orthopedics, and respiratory)
thrill (cardiovascular)
thyrohyoid (anatomy, endocrinology, and surgery)
thyroid hormone [also called *thyroxine*] (endocrinology, laboratory, and pharmacology)
total hysterectomy (gynecology)

Th
thenar (anatomy, neurology, and orthopedics)
thoracic (cardiovascular, neurology, orthopedics, and respiratory)
thorax (cardiovascular, neurology, orthopedics, and respiratory)
thorium (chemistry, gastroenterology, and radiology)

th.
thoracic (cardiovascular and respiratory)

THA
tetrahydroaminoacridine [an experimental drug] (neurology and pharmacology)
total hip arthroplasty (orthopedics)
total hydroxyapatite (dentistry, laboratory, and orthopedics)
transient hemispheric attack (cardiovascular and neurology)

ThA
thoracic aorta (cardiovascular)

Thal.
thalassemia (hematology)

THAM
2-amino-2-(hydroxymethyl)-1,3-propanediol
trihydroxymethylaminomethane [an alkalinizer; also called *tris(hydroxymethyl)aminomethane* and *tromethamine*] (pharmacology)
{not an abbreviation} [brand name for *tromethamine*; an alkalinizer] (pharmacology)

THAN
transient hyperammonemia of newborn (neonatology)

"than-ah-to"
{pronunciation of *thanato-* [prefix indicating relationship to death {not an abbreviation}]} {not an abbreviation}

thanato-
{not an abbreviation} [prefix indicating relationship to death] {pronounced "than-ah-to"}

THC
tetrahydrocannabinol [derived from marijuana; an illicit drug used experimentally in cancer research as an antiemetic (dronabinol)] (chemical dependency, chemotherapy, oncology, and pharmacology)
tetrahydrocortisol (endocrinology and laboratory)
thiocarbanidin [an antibacterial] (pharmacology)
transhepatic cholangiogram (gastroenterology and radiology)

TH-CULT
throat culture (laboratory and otorhinolaryngology)

THDOC
tetrahydrodeoxycorticosterone (endocrinology and laboratory)

THE
tetrahydrone E [also called *tetrahydrocortisone*] (endocrinology and laboratory)
tonic hind-limb extension (veterinary medicine)
transhepatic embolization (cardiovascular, gastroenterology, and hematology)

THELEP
Chemotherapy of Leprosy Program [of the World Health Organization] (chemotherapy, infectious diseases, and pharmacology)

T-helper
{not an abbreviation} [refers to the *T-helper cell*] (immunology, laboratory, and oncology)

theo
theophylline (pharmacology and respiratory)

theor
theoretical

theo toxicity
theophylline toxicity (laboratory, pharmacology, and respiratory)

THER
therapeutic
therapeutic [range] (laboratory)
therapy
thermometer (measurement)

ther
therapeutic
therapy
thermometer (measurement)

THERAP
therapeutic

therap.
therapeutic

Ther Ex
therapeutic exercise (physical therapy)

ther ex
therapeutic exercise (physical therapy)

therm
{not an abbreviation} [a unit of heat]
(measurement)

therm-
{not an abbreviation} [prefix indicating
relationship to heat] {pronounced
"therm"}

"therm"
{pronunciation of *therm-* [prefix indicating relationship to heat {not an abbre-
viation}]} {not an abbreviation}

thermo-
{not an abbreviation} [prefix indicating
relationship to heat] {pronounced
"ther-moe"}

"ther-moe"
{pronunciation of *thermo-* [prefix indicating relationship to heat {not an ab-
breviation}]} {not an abbreviation}

THF
tetrahydrocortisol (endocrinology and
laboratory)
tetrahydro F [also called *tetrahydrocortisone*] (endocrinology and laboratory)
tetrahydrofluorenone [an amebicide and
fungistatic] (pharmacology)
tetrahydrofolate (laboratory)
tetrahydrofolic acid (laboratory)
tetrahydrofuran [a solvent] (chemistry)
thymic humoral factor (hematology, laboratory, and research)

THFA
tetrahydrofolic acid (laboratory)
tetrahydrofurfuryl alcohol [a solvent]
(chemistry)

THI
transient hypogammaglobinemia of in-
fancy (immunology and pediatrics)
trihydroxyindole (laboratory)

THIA
thiamylal [an anesthetic] (anesthesiology
and pharmacology)

"thigh-me-ah"
{pronunciation of *-thymia* [suffix indicating a condition of the mind {not an
abbreviation}]} (neurology and psychiatry) {not an abbreviation}

"thigh-moe"
{pronunciation of *thymo-* [1. prefix indicating relationship to the thymus
gland (endocrinology) {not an abbrevi-
ation}; 2. prefix indicating relationship
to the emotions or the soul (psychiatry) {not an abbreviation}]} {not an ab-
breviation}

"thigh-oh"
{pronunciation of *thio-* [prefix indicating
the presence of sulfa {not an abbrevia-
tion}]} {not an abbreviation}

"thigh-oh-tea"
{pronunciation of *Thio-T* [triethyl-
enethiophosphoramide (also called
thiotepa and *thiophosphoramide*)]}
(chemotherapy, oncology, and pharmacology)

"thigh-oh-teh-pah"
{pronunciation of *Thio-TEPA, Thiotepa,*
and *thiotepa* [triethylenethiophos-
phoramide (also called thiophosphoramide)]} (chemotherapy, oncology,
and pharmacology) {not an abbrevia-
tion}

"thigh-re-oh"
{pronunciation of *thyreo-* [prefix indicating relationship to the thyroid gland
{not an abbreviation}]} (endocrinology) {not an abbreviation}

"thigh-row"
{pronunciation of *thyro-* [prefix indicating relationship to the thyroid gland {not an abbreviation}]} (endocrinology) {not an abbreviation}

THIO
thiopental sodium [an anesthetic] (anesthesiology, pharmacology, and surgery)

thio-
{not an abbreviation} [prefix indicating the presence of sulfa] {pronounced "thigh-oh"}

Thio-T
triethylenethiophosphoramide [also called *Thiotepa, thiotepa* and *thiophosphoramide*] (chemotherapy, oncology, and pharmacology) {pronounced "thigh-oh-tea"}

Thio-TEPA
{not an abbreviation} [triethylenethiophosphoramide (also called *thiotepa* and *thiophosphoramide*)] (chemotherapy, oncology, and pharmacology) {pronounced "thigh-oh-teh-pah"}

Thiotepa
{not an abbreviation} [triethylenethiophosphoramide (also called *thiotepa* and *thiophosphoramide*)] (chemotherapy, oncology, and pharmacology) {pronounced "thigh-oh-teh-pah"}

thiotepa
{not an abbreviation} [triethylenethiophosphoramide (also called *Thiotepa* and *thiophosphoramide*)] (chemotherapy, oncology, and pharmacology) {pronounced "thigh-oh-teh-pah"}

THIQ
tetrahydraisoquinolon (chemical dependency and laboratory)

THM
total heme mass (hematology and laboratory)

THO
titrated water (laboratory)

tritium-labeled water (laboratory)

TH₂O
titrated water (laboratory)

ThO₂
thorium dioxide (chemistry, gastroenterology, and radiology)

THOR
thoracentesis [fluid] (cardiovascular, laboratory, and respiratory)

Thor
thoracic (cardiovascular, neurology, orthopedics, respiratory)
thorax (cardiovascular, neurology, orthopedics, respiratory)

thoraco-
{not an abbreviation} [prefix indicating relationship to the chest] (cardiovascular and respiratory) {pronounced "thor-ah-co"}

"thor-ah-co"
{pronunciation of *thoraco-* [prefix indicating relationship to the chest {not an abbreviation}]} (cardiovascular and respiratory) {not an abbreviation}

THP
total hydroxyproline (endocrinology, hematology, laboratory, and orthopedics)
trihexphenidyl hydrochloride [an anticholinergic] (neurology and pharmacology)

THPA
tetrahydropteric acid

THR
target heart rate (cardiovascular and sports medicine)
total hip replacement (orthopedics)

T.H.R.
target heart rate (cardiovascular and
   sports medicine)

Thr
threonine (genetics and laboratory)

THR-CT
thrombin control (hematology and laboratory)

THRF
thyrotropic hormone-releasing factor
   (endocrinology and laboratory)

"thrickz"
{pronunciation of -*thrix* [suffix meaning
   hair {not an abbreviation}]} {not an
   abbreviation}

-thrix
{not an abbreviation} [suffix meaning
   hair] {pronounced "thrickz"}

Throm
thrombosis (cardiovascular and hematology)

THROMB
thrombin time tritium (hematology and
   laboratory)

Thromb
thrombosis (cardiovascular and hematology)

thromb.
thrombosis (cardiovascular and hematology)

thrombo
thrombophlebitis (cardiovascular and
   hematology) {pronounced "throm-
   bow"}

thrombo-
{not an abbreviation} [prefix indicating
   relationship to a clot or thrombus]
   (cardiovascular and hematology) {pro-
   nounced "throm-bow"}

"throm-bow"
{pronunciation of *thrombo* [throm-
   bophlebitis] and thrombo- [prefix indi-

cating relationship to a clot or thrombus {not an abbreviation}]}
   (cardiovascular and hematology) {not
   an abbreviation}

thru
{not an abbreviation} [a variant of
   through]

THS
tetrahydro-compound S [also called *tet-
   rahydro-11-deoxycortisol*] (endocrinology, laboratory, and neurology)
Times Health Supplement (publishing)

THSC
totipotent hematopoietic stem cell (hematology and laboratory)

THT
Teacher of Hydrotherapy (education
   and physical therapy)

-thymia
{not an abbreviation} [suffix indicating a
   condition of the mind] (neurology and
   psychiatry) {pronounced "thigh-me-
   ah"}

thymo-
{not an abbreviation} [1. prefix indicating relationship to the thymus gland
   (endocrinology); 2. prefix indicating
   relationship to the emotions or the
   soul (psychiatry)] {pronounced "thigh-
   moe"}

Thymol turb
thymol turbidity [test; obsolete test of
   hepatic function] (gastroenterology
   and laboratory)

thyreo-
{not an abbreviation} [prefix indicating
   relationship to the thyroid gland] (endocrinology) {pronounced {thigh-re-
   oh"}

thyro-
{not an abbreviation} [prefix indicating
   relationship to the thyroid gland] (en-

docrinology) {pronounced "thigh-row"}

THYROID PERCHL WO
thyroid uptake with perchlorate washout (endocrinology, oncology, radiation therapy, and radiology)

THYROID RE-RX
thyroid retreatment (endocrinology, oncology, radiation therapy, and radiology)

THYROID RX MEDS
thyroid therapy medications (endocrinology, pharmacology, and radiology)

THYROID RX 10 mCi
thyroid therapy, 10 millicuries (endocrinology, oncology, radiation therapy, and radiology)

THYROID S ONLY
thyroid scan only (endocrinology, oncology, radiation therapy, and radiology)

THYROID STIM
thyroid stimulation (endocrinology, oncology, radiation therapy, and radiology)

THYROID SUPP
thyroid suppression (endocrinology, oncology, radiation therapy, and radiology)

THYROID U.
thyroid uptake (endocrinology, oncology, radiation therapy, and radiology)

THYROID U & S
thyroid uptake and scan (endocrinology, oncology, radiation therapy, and radiology)

THz
terahertz (measurement)

TI
terminal ileum (gastroenterology)
Texas Instruments (manufacturer)
thalassemia intermedia (hematology)
thoracic index (cardiovascular, measurement, radiology, and respiratory)

thymus-independent [cells] (hematology, immunology, and laboratory)
time interval
tissue-impacted (laboratory and pathology)
tissue invasiveness (laboratory and pathology)
transverse inlet [diameter between ischia] (obstetrics and radiology)
tricuspid incompetence (cardiovascular)
tricuspid insufficiency (cardiovascular)
tumor-inducing (laboratory)

T₄I
total serum thyroxine iodine [also called *tri-iodothyronine*] (endocrinology and laboratory)

Ti
titanium (chemistry and orthopedics)

TIA
transient ischemic attack (cardiovascular and neurology)

T.I.A.
transient ischemic attack (cardiovascular and neurology)

TIA-IR
transient ischemic attack—incomplete recovery (cardiovascular, neurology, and rehabilitation)

TIAs
transient ischemic attacks (cardiovascular and neurology)

TIA's
transient ischemic attacks (cardiovascular and neurology)

Tib
tibia (anatomy and orthopedics) {pronounced "tib"}

tib
tibia (anatomy and orthopedics) {pronounced "tib"}
tibialis [muscle] (anatomy and orthopedics) {pronounced "tib"}

"tib"
{pronunciation of *Tib* [tibia] and *tib*
  [tibia and tibialis (muscle)]} (anatomy
  and orthopedics) {not an abbreviation}

TIBC
total iron-binding capacity (hematology
  and laboratory)

T.I.B.C.
total iron-binding capacity (hematology
  and laboratory)

Tib.-Fib.
tibia-fibula (anatomy and orthopedics)
  {pronounced "tib-fib"}
tibial-fibular (anatomy and orthopedics)
  {pronounced "tib-fib"}

"tib-fib"
{pronunciation of *Tib.-Fib.* [tibia-fibula
  and tibial-fibular]} (anatomy and orthopedics) {not an abbreviation}

TIC
trypsin-inhibitory capacity (laboratory)

tic
diverticulum (gastroenterology) {pro-
  nounced "tick"}

"tick"
{pronunciation of *tic* [*diverticulum*]}
  (gastroenterology) {not an abbrevia-
  tion}

TID
ter in die [three times daily] (pharmacology)
titrated initial dose (pharmacology)

T.I.D.
ter in die [three times daily] (pharmacology)

tid
ter in die [three times daily] (pharmacology)

t.i.d.
ter in die [three times daily] (pharmacology)

TIE
transient ischemic episode (cardiovascular and neurology)

"tie-co"
{pronunciation of *Tyco* [slang for *Tylenol
  with Codeine* (acetaminophen with
  codeine)]} (pharmacology) {not an ab-
  breviation}

"tie-co-num-ber-four"
{pronunciation of *TYCO #4* [Tylenol No.
  4 (acetaminophen with 60 milligrams
  of codeine)]} (pharmacology) {not an
  abbreviation}

"tie-co-num-ber-one"
{pronunciation of *TYCO #1* [Tylenol No.
  1 (acetaminophen with 7.5 milligrams
  of codeine)]} (pharmacology) {not an
  abbreviation}

"tie-co-num-ber-three"
{pronunciation of *TYCO #3* [Tylenol No.
  3 (acetaminophen with 30 milligrams
  of codeine)]} (pharmacology) {not an
  abbreviation}

"tie-co-num-ber-two"
{pronunciation of *TYCO #2* [Tylenol No.
  2 (acetaminophen with 15 milligrams
  of codeine)]} (pharmacology) {not an
  abbreviation}

"tie-row"
{pronunciation of *tyro-* [prefix indicating
  relationship to cheese {not an abbrevi-
  ation}]} {not an abbreviation}

TIF
tumor-inducing factor (laboratory and
  oncology)

"tif-low"
{pronunciation of *typhlo-* [1. prefix indicating relationship to the cecum {not
  an abbreviation} (gastroenterology); 2.
  prefix indicating relationship to blindness {not an abbreviation} (ophthalmology)]} {not an abbreviation}

TIG
tetanus immune globulin (immunology, infectious diseases, laboratory, and neurology)

TIg
tetanus immune globulin (immunology, infectious diseases, laboratory, and neurology)

TIGAN
Tigan [brand name for a preparation of *trimethobenzamide hydrochloride;* an anticholinergic] (pharmacology)

TIM
transthoracic intracardiac monitoring (cardiovascular)

TIMC
tumor-induced cytatocity (laboratory and oncology)

TIME
time urine (laboratory and urology)

TIN
ter in nocte [three times nightly] (pharmacology)
tubulointerstitial nephropathy (nephrology)

T.I.N.
ter in nocte [three times nightly] (pharmacology)

tin
ter in nocte [three times nightly] (pharmacology)

t.i.n.
ter in nocte [three times nightly] (pharmacology)

tinc
tinctura [tincture] (pharmacology)
tincture (pharmacology)

TINCT
tinctura [tincture] (pharmacology)
tincture (pharmacology)

tinct
tinctura [tincture] (pharmacology)

tincture (pharmacology)

TIP
Threshold by Identification of Pictures
translation-inhibiting protein (laboratory)
tumor-inhibiting principle (laboratory)

TIRR
Texas Institute of Rehabilitation and Research (rehabilitation and research)

TIS
tetracycline-induced steatosis [also called *tetracycline-induced fatty liver*] (gastroenterology, laboratory, and pathology)
trypsin-insoluble segment (laboratory)
tumor in situ (laboratory, oncology, and pathology)

TIT
Treponema immobilization test (laboratory)
tri-iodothyronine (endocrinology and laboratory)

TITER
titer (laboratory)

TIU
trypsin-inhibiting unit (laboratory)

TIUV
total intrauterine volume (gynecology and obstetrics)

TIVC
thoracic inferior vena cava (cardiovascular)

+tive
positive

TIW
[*Note: This is considered a dangerous abbreviation.*]
three times a week (pharmacology)
twice a week (pharmacology)

tiw
[*Note: This is considered a dangerous abbreviation.*]
three times a week (pharmacology)
twice a week (pharmacology)

t.i.w.
[*Note: this is considered a dangerous abbreviation.*]
three times a week (pharmacology)
twice a week (pharmacology)

TJ
tendon jerk (neurology and orthopedics)
terajoule (measurement)
triceps jerk (neurology and orthopedics)
Troell-Junet [syndrome] (genetics, endocrinology, and orthopedics)

TJB
time-sharing job block (computer science)

TJN
twin jet nebulizer (pharmacology and respiratory)

TJR
total joint replacement (orthopedics)

TK
thymidine kinase [deficient] (genetics and laboratory)
tokodynamometer (obstetrics)
transketolase (laboratory)

TKA
total knee arthroplasty (orthopedics)
transketolase activity (laboratory)

TKD
thymidine kinase deficiency (genetics and laboratory)
tokodynamometer (obstetrics)

TKG
tokodynagraph (obstetrics)

TKLI
tachykinin-like immunoreactivity (laboratory)

TKNO
to keep needle open (pharmacology)

TKP
thermokeratoplasty (ophthalmology)

TKO
technical knockout (sports medicine)
to keep open [referring to vein for administration of intravenous fluids] (pharmacology)

TKR
total knee replacement (orthopedics)

TL
team leader
temporal lobe (anatomy and neurology)
terminal limen
thymic lymphoma (oncology and pathology)
thymic-derived lymphocyte (hematology, immunology, and laboratory)
thymus leukemia [antigen] (hematology, laboratory, and oncology)
thymus lymphoma (neurology and oncology)
time lapse
time-limited
total lipids (cardiovascular and laboratory)
trial leave (psychiatry)
tubal ligation (gynecology)

T-L
thymus-dependent lymphocyte (hematology, immunology, and laboratory)

Tl
thallium (cardiovascular, chemistry, and radiology)

Tl-201
thallium-201 [a radioactive isotope] (cardiovascular, chemistry, and radiology)

TLA
translumbar aortogram (cardiovascular and radiology)
transluminal angioplasty (cardiovascular)

TLAA

T-lymphocyte-associated antigen (hematology, immunology, laboratory, and oncology)

TLC

maximum recoil pressure (laboratory and respiratory)
tender loving care
thin-layer chromatography (laboratory)
total light chain concentration (immunology and laboratory)
total lung capacity (laboratory and respiratory)
total lung compliance (respiratory)
total lymphocyte count (hematology and laboratory)

T.L.C.

tender loving care
total lung capacity (laboratory and respiratory)

^{201}TlCl

thallium chloride [a radioactive isotope] (cardiovascular, chemistry, and radiology)

TLD

thermoluminescent dosimeter [also called *thermal luminescent dosimeter*] (radiology)
thermoluminescent dosimetry [also called *thermal luminescent dosimetry*] (radiology)
thoracic lymph duct (anatomy and otorhinolaryngology)
tumor lethal dose (oncology and radiation therapy)

T/LD$_{100}$

minimum dose causing malformation or death of 100 percent of fetuses (radiation therapy)

TLE

temporal lobe epilepsy (neurology)
thin-layer electrophoresis (laboratory)
total lipid extract (laboratory)

T-lens

therapeutic contact lens (ophthalmology) {pronounced "tea-lenz"}

TLI

thymidine labelling index (laboratory)
total lymphoid irradiation (radiation therapy)

TLQ

total living quotient

TLS

testing the limits for sex (psychiatry)
thoracolumbosacral [drain] (surgery)

TLV

threshold limit value
total lung volume (laboratory and respiratory)

TLX

trophoblast/lymphocyte cross-reactive antigens (laboratory)

T-lymphocyte

thymus-dependent lymphocyte [also called *T-cell*] (immunology and laboratory)

TM

temporomandibular [joint; also called *temporal mandibular (joint)*] (dentistry, orthopedics, and otorhinolaryngology)
thalassemia major (hematology)
Thayer-Martin [medium] (laboratory)
time-motion technique (radiology)
tobramycin [an antibiotic] (pharmacology)
trabecular meshwork
trademark (government and manufacturing)
transcendental meditation (psychiatry and religion)
transitional mucosa (anatomy and laboratory)
transmediastinal (cardiovascular and respiratory)
transmetatarsal (orthopedics and podiatry)
transport mechanism (laboratory)
transport medium (laboratory)
transport messenger (laboratory)
Tropical Medicine

tympanic membrane (otorhinolaryngology)

T-M
Thayer-Martin [medium] (laboratory)

T & M
Trichomonas and *Monilia* [cultures] (gynecology and laboratory)

Tm
maximal renal tubular excretory capacity [also called *maximal tubular excretory capacity of kidney*] (laboratory, nephrology, and urology)
transport maximum (laboratory)
transport mechanism (laboratory)

T$_m$
maximum tubular excretory capacity of the kidneys (laboratory, nephrology, and urology)

TMA
tetramethylammonium [a toxin] (laboratory and oceanography)
thyroid microsomal antibody (endocrinology and laboratory)
transmetatarsal amputation (orthopedics and podiatry)
trimethyloxyamphetamine [a hallucinogen] (chemical dependency, pharmacology, and psychiatry)
trimethoxyphenyl aminopropane [a hallucinogen] (pharmacology and psychiatry)
trimethylamine (chemistry and laboratory)

TMAS
Taylor Manifest Anxiety Scale (psychiatry)

T-MAX
temperature maximum (measurement) {pronounced "tea-max"}

T$_{max}$
time of maximum concentration (laboratory)

TMB
transient monocular blindness (neurology and ophthalmology)

TMC
Terramycin capsules [an antibiotic] (pharmacology)
transmural colitis (gastroenterology)
triamcinolone [an anti-inflammatory] (pharmacology)

TMCA
trimethylcolchicinic acid (chemotherapy, oncology, and pharmacology)

TME
Teacher of Medical Electricity (education and physical therapy)
total metabolizable energy (dietary)

TMET
treadmill exercise test (cardiovascular)

TMF
transformed mink fibroblast [cell line] (laboratory)

TMG
maximum tubular reabsorption rate for glucose [of kidney] (laboratory and nephrology)
3,3-tetramethyleneglutaric acid (laboratory)

TM$_G$
maximum tubular reabsorption rate for glucose [of kidney] (laboratory and nephrology)

TmG
maximum tubular reabsorption rate for glucose [of kidney] (laboratory and nephrology)

Tm$_G$
maximum tubular reabsorption rate for glucose [of kidney] (laboratory and nephrology)

TMI
threatened myocardial infarction (cardiovascular)
Three Mile Island [site of nuclear reactor accident] (oncology, radiation diseases, and radiology)
transmural infarction (cardiovascular)

TMIC
Toxic Materials Information Center (toxicology)

TMIF
tumor-cell migratory inhibition factor (laboratory)

TMIS
Technical Medical Information System

TMJ
temporomandibular joint (dentistry, orthopedics, and otorhinolaryngology)

T.M.J.
temporomandibular joint (dentistry, orthopedics, and otorhinolaryngology)

TM joint
temporomandibular joint (dentistry, orthopedics, and otorhinolaryngology)

TMJS
temporomandibular joint syndrome (dentistry, orthopedics, and otorhinolaryngology)

TML
tetramethyl lead (chemistry)

TMMG
Teacher of Massage and Medical Gymnastics (education, physical therapy, and sports medicine)

T-MOP
methotrexate, 6-thioguanine, vincristine, and prednisone (chemotherapy, oncology, and pharmacology)

TMP
thallium myocardial perfusion [test] (cardiovascular)
thymidine monophosphate [also called *thymidine-5'-phosphate*] (genetics and laboratory)
thymine ribonucleoside-5'-phosphate (genetics and laboratory)
transmembrane potential(s) (laboratory)
transmembrane pressure (laboratory)
trimethoprim [an antibacterial] (pharmacology)

Tm$_{PAH}$
maximum tubular excretory capacity for *para*-aminohippuric acid [of kidney] (laboratory and nephrology)

T$_{mPAH}$
maximum tubular excretory capacity for *para*-aminohippuric acid [of kidney] (laboratory and nephrology)

TMPD
tetramethylparaphenylinediamine (chemistry and laboratory)

TMP/SMX
trimethoprim-sulfamethoxazole [antibacterials] (pharmacology and urology)

TMP/SMZ
trimethoprim-sulfamethoxazole [antibacterials] (pharmacology and urology)

TMR
topical magnetic resonance (radiology)
trainable mentally retarded (genetics, pediatrics, and rehabilitation)

TMS
thallium myocardial scintigraphy (cardiovascular and radiology)
trimethoprim and sulfamethoxazole [antibacterials] (pharmacology and urology)
trimethylsilane (chemistry)
trimethylsilyl (chemistry and laboratory)

TMST
treadmill stress test [also called *treadmill stress study*] (cardiovascular)

TMT
tarsometatarsal [joint] (orthopedics and podiatry)
Trail Making Test (psychiatry)

TMTC
too many to count (laboratory)

TMTD
tetramethylthiuram disulfide [also called *thiram*; an antifungal] (dermatology and pharmacology)

TMV
tobacco mosaic virus (agriculture)

TMX
tamoxifen (chemotherapy, oncology, and pharmacology)

TN
team nursing (nursing)
temperature normal
Tennessee [Postal Service state designation]
total negatives
true negative (laboratory)

Tn
intraocular tension (ophthalmology)
normal intraocular pressure (ophthalmology)
normal intraocular tension (ophthalmology)

TNAS
Tuberculosis Nursing Advisory Service (infectious diseases, nursing, and respiratory)

TNB
Tru-Cut needle biopsy (oncology, pathology, and surgery)

TNC
turbid, no creamy layer (laboratory)

TND
term normal delivery (gynecology and obstetrics)

TNF
tumor necrosis factor (laboratory)

TNG
nitroglycerin (cardiovascular and pharmacology)
tongue (dentistry and otorhinolaryngology)
trinitroglycerin [also abbreviated *TNT*] (armed forces and chemistry)

Tng
training

TNI
total nodal irradiation (oncology and radiation therapy)

TNM
tumor node (lymph) metastasis (laboratory, oncology, and pathology)
tumor, node, and metastasis [criteria for staging] (laboratory, oncology, and pathology)
{not an abbreviation} [a cancer-staging classification system, with T referring to the primary tumor size, N to the clinical status of regional lymph node metastasis, and M to the remote metastasis; letters followed by numbers to indicate staging (T1N1M1, $T_1N_1M_1$, or T1-N1-M1) using the numerals 0, 1, 2, and 3] (laboratory, oncology, and pathology)

TNR
tonic neck reflex (neurology)
true negative rate

TNS
transcutaneous nerve stimulation (neurology)
tumor necrosis serum (laboratory)

T.N.S.
transcutaneous nerve stimulation (neurology)

TNT
trinitrotoluene [also called *2,4,6-trinitrotoluene*] (armed forces and chemistry)

T.N.T.
trinitrotoluene (armed forces and chemistry)

TNTC
too numerous to count (laboratory)

TNT test
{not an abbreviation} [urine test for trinitrotoluene] (laboratory)

TNV
tobacco necrosis virus (agriculture and
laboratory)

TO
no evidence of primary tumor (oncology
and pathology)
old tuberculin [also called *original tuberculin*] (infectious diseases, pharmacology, and respiratory)
target organ (radiology)
telephone order (nursing)
temperature, oral (measurement)
tinctura opii [tincture of opium] (pharmacology)
tincture of opium (pharmacology)
tracheo-oesophageal [British spelling]
(gastroenterology, otorhinolaryngology, and respiratory)
tuberculin ober [supernatant portion]
(infectious diseases, laboratory, pharmacology, and respiratory)
tubo-ovarian (gynecology and obstetrics)
turnover [number]

T(O)
oral temperature (measurement)

T.O.
original tuberculin (infectious diseases,
laboratory, pharmacology, and respiratory)
telephone order (nursing)

T/O
telephone order (nursing)

to
tinctura opii [tincture of opium] (pharmacology)
tincture of opium (pharmacology)

t.o.
tinctura opii [tincture of opium] (pharmacology)
tincture of opium (pharmacology)

TOA
time of arrival (transportation)
tubo-ovarian abscess (gynecology and
obstetrics)

TOAP
thioguanine, Oncovin [vincristine], cytosine arabinoside [cytarabine], and
prednisone (chemotherapy, oncology,
and pharmacology)

"to-berk"
{pronunciation of *TUBERC* and *tuberc*
[tuberculosis]] (infectious diseases
and respiratory) {not an abbreviation}

TOBP
tobramycin, peak [an antibiotic] (laboratory)

TOBT
tobramycin, trough [an antibiotic] (laboratory)

TOC
test of cure
total organic compound (chemistry)
tubo-ovarian complex (anatomy, gynecology, and obstetrics)

toco-
{not an abbreviation} [prefix indicating
relationship to childbirth or labor]
(obstetrics) {pronounced "toe-co"}

TOCP
tri-*o*-cresyl phosphate [also called *trior-
thocresyl phosphate*] (chemistry)
tail-on detector (radiology)

T.O.D.
titanium optimized design [plate] (orthopedics)

TOE
Epidermatophyton [a fungus] (dermatology and laboratory)
theory of everything [meaning all theo-
ries fit the universe] (physics)
tracheo-oesophageal [British spelling]
(gastroenterology, otorhinolaryngology, and respiratory)

"toe-co"
{pronunciation of *toco-* and *toko-* [pre-
fixes indicating relationship to child-

birth or labor {not abbreviations}]}
(obstetrics) {not an abbreviation}

"toe-me"
{pronunciation of -*tomy* [suffix indicating the operation of cutting or incision {not an abbreviation}]} (surgery)
{not an abbreviation}

"toe-moe"
{pronunciation of *TOMO* and *Tomo* [to-
mogram and tomography (radiology)]
and *tomo*- [prefix indicating relationship to a cutting or to a designated
layer (pathology, radiology, and surgery) {not an abbreviation}]} {not an
abbreviation}

"toe-no"
{pronunciation of *tono*- [prefix indicating relationship to tension or tone {not
an abbreviation}]} {not an abbrevia-
tion}

"toe-poe"
{pronunciation of *topo*- [prefix meaning
place {not an abbreviation}]} {not an
abbreviation}

TOF
tetralogy of Fallot (cardiovascular, neonatology, and pediatrics)
tracheo-esophageal fistula (gastroenterology, otorhinolaryngology, and respiratory)

T of A
transposition of the aorta (cardiovascular, neonatology, and pediatrics)

TOFRAN
Tofranil [an antidepressant; also called
imipramine hydrochloride] (pharmacology and psychiatry)

TOGV
transposition of the great vessels (cardiovascular, neonatology, and pediatrics)

toko-
{not an abbreviation} [prefix indicating
relationship to childbirth or labor]
(obstetrics) {pronounced "toe-co"}

TOL
trial of labor (obstetrics)

tol
tolerated

-tome
{not an abbreviation} [a suffix indicating
an instrument for cutting or a seg-
ment] (surgery) {pronounced "tome"}

"tome"
{pronunciation of -*tome* [a suffix indicating an instrument for cutting or a segment {not an abbreviation}]} (surgery)
{not an abbreviation}

TOMO
tomogram (radiology) {pronounced
"toe-moe"}
tomography (radiology) {pronounced
"toe-moe"}

Tomo
tomogram (radiology) {pronounced
"toe-moe"}
tomography (radiology) {pronounced
"toe-moe"}

tomo-
{not an abbreviation} [prefix indicating
relationship to a cutting or to a designated layer] (pathology, radiology,
and surgery) {pronounced "toe-moe"}

-tomy
{not an abbreviation} [suffix indicating
the operation of cutting or incision]
(surgery) {pronounced "toe-me"}

tono-
{not an abbreviation} [prefix indicating
relationship to tension or tone] {pro-
nounced "toe-no"}

TONOC
tonight

tonoc.
tonight

TOP

termination of pregnancy (gynecology and obstetrics)
transovarial passage (entomology)

top

topically (dermatology and pharmacology)

topo-

{not an abbreviation} [prefix meaning *place*] {pronounced "toe-poe"}

TOPS

Take Pounds Off Sensibly [a weight-reduction program] (dietary) {pronounced "topz"}

TOPV

trivalent oral poliovirus vaccine (infectious diseases, neurology, and pharmacology)

"topz"

{pronunciation of TOPS [*Take Pounds Off Sensibly* (a weight reduction program)]} (dietary) {not an abbreviation}

TORCH

toxoplasmosis, other viruses (hepatitis, syphilis, herpes zoster), rubella, cytomegalovirus, and herpes virus [titer] (infectious diseases, laboratory, neonatology, and pediatrics) {pronounced "torch"}
toxoplasmosis, rubella, cytomegalovirus, and herpes simplex [titer] (infectious diseases, laboratory, neonatology, and pediatrics) {pronounced "torch"} [*Note: Derived from the letters in each word as to-r-c-h.*]
toxoplasmosis, rubella, cytomegalovirus, and infectious and congenital herpes [titer] (infectious diseases, laboratory, neonatology, and pediatrics) {pronounced "torch"} [*Note: Derived from the letters in each word as to-r-c-h.*]

T.O.R.C.H.

toxoplasmosis, other viruses (hepatitis, syphilis, herpes zoster), rubella, cytomegalovirus, and herpes virus [titer] (infectious diseases, laboratory, neo-

natology, and pediatrics) {pronounced "torch"}
toxoplasmosis, rubella, cytomegalovirus, and herpes simplex [titer] (infectious diseases, laboratory, neonatology, and pediatrics) {pronounced "torch"} [*Note: Derived from the letters in each word as to-r-c-h.*]
toxoplasmosis, rubella, cytomegalovirus infectious, and congenital herpes [titer] (infectious diseases, laboratory, neonatology, and pediatrics) {pronounced "torch"} [*Note: Derived from the letters in each word as to-r-c-h.*]

"torch"

{pronunciation of TORCH and T.O.R.C.H. [toxoplasmosis, other viruses (hepatitis, syphilis, herpes zoster), rubella, cytomegalovirus, and herpes virus (titer) and toxoplasmosis, rubella, cytomegalovirus, and herpes simplex (titer) and toxoplasmosis, rubella, cytomegalovirus infectious, and congenital herpes (titer)]} (infectious diseases, laboratory, neonatology, and pediatrics) {not an abbreviation}

TORCHS

toxoplasmosis, other viruses (hepatitis, herpes zoster), rubella, cytomegalovirus, herpes virus, and syphilis [titer] (infectious diseases, laboratory, neonatology, and pediatrics) {pronounced "torchs"}

"torchs"

{pronunciation of TORCHS [toxoplasmosis, other viruses (hepatitis, herpes zoster), rubella, cytomegalovirus, herpes virus, and syphilis (titer)]} (infectious diseases, laboratory, neonatology, and pediatrics) {not an abbreviation}

"torch-tie-tur"

{pronunciation of TORCH titer [toxoplasma, other viruses, rubella, cytomegalovirus, and herpes virus titer and toxoplasmosis, rubella, cytomegalovirus, and herpes simplex titer and toxoplasmosis, rubella, cytomegalovirus infectious, and congenital herpes titer]} (infectious diseases, laboratory, neonatology, and pediatrics) {not an abbreviation}

TORCH titer
toxoplasma, other viruses, rubella, cytomegalovirus, and herpes virus titer (infectious diseases, laboratory, neonatology, and pediatrics) {pronounced "torch-tie-tur"}
toxoplasmosis, rubella, cytomegalovirus, and herpes simplex titer (infectious diseases, laboratory, neonatology, and pediatrics) {pronounced "torch-tie-tur"}
toxoplasmosis, rubella, cytomegalovirus infectious, and congenital herpes titer (infectious diseases, laboratory, neonatology, and pediatrics) {pronounced "torch-tie-tur"}

TORP
total ossicular chain replacement prosthesis (otorhinolaryngology) {pronounced "torp"}
total ossicular replacement prosthesis (otorhinolaryngology) {pronounced "torp"}

"torp"
{pronunciation of *TORP* [total ossicular chain replacement prosthesis and total ossicular replacement prosthesis]} (otorhinolaryngology) {not an abbreviation}

torr
{not an abbreviation} (measurement)

TOS
thoracic outlet syndrome (neurology and orthopedics)

TOT
tincture of time [slang meaning *with the passage of time*]

total lymph ct
total lymphocyte count (hematology and laboratory)

TOT PROT
total protein (laboratory)

tot. prot.
total protein (laboratory)

TOWER
testing, orientation, work, evaluation, rehabilitation (rehabilitation) {pronounced "tow-er"}

"tow-er"
{pronunciation of *TOWER* [testing, orientation, work, evaluation, rehabilitation]} (rehabilitation) {not an abbreviation}

TOX
toxic {pronounced "tox"}
toxicity {pronounced "tox"}

tox
toxic {pronounced "tox"}
toxicity {pronounced "tox"}

"tox"
{pronunciation of *TOX* and *tox* [toxic and toxicity]} {not an abbreviation}

"tox-ah-co"
{pronunciation of *toxico-* [prefix meaning poisonous or indicating relationship to poison {not an abbreviation}]} {not an abbreviation}

TOXGR
toxic granulation—differential (laboratory)

TOXI
toxic granulation (laboratory)

toxico-
{not an abbreviation} [prefix meaning poisonous or indicating relationship to poison] {pronounced "tox-ah-co"}

TOXO
toxoplasmosis (laboratory) {pronounced "tox-oh"}

Toxo
toxoplasmosis (laboratory) {pronounced
  "tox-oh"}

toxo-
{not an abbreviation} [prefix indicating
  relationship to a poison or toxin] {pro-
  nounced "tox-oh"}

"tox-oh"
{pronunciation of *TOXO* and *Toxo* [toxo-
  plasmosis (laboratory)] and *toxo-* [pre-
  fix meaning poisonous or indicating
  relationship to poison {not an abbrevi-
  ation}]} {not an abbreviation}

TP
temperature and pressure
temporoparietal (anatomy, neurology,
  and radiology)
terminal phalanx (orthopedics and podiatry)
testosterone propionate (endocrinology,
  gynecology, oncology, pharmacology,
  and urology)
threshold potential (neurology)
thrombocytopenic purpura (hematology)
thymic polypeptide (endocrinology and
  laboratory)
thymidine phosphorylase (genetics and
  laboratory)
thymus protein (endocrinology and laboratory)
Todd's paralysis (neurology)
toilet paper
total positives (laboratory)
total protein (laboratory)
transforming principle (bacteriology and
  laboratory)
transverse process (neurology, neurosurgery, and orthopedics)
Treponema pallidum [the bacterium
  causing syphilis] (gynecology, infectious diseases, laboratory, and urology)
trigger point (neurology and orthopedics)
triphosphate (laboratory)
true positive (laboratory)
tryptophan [an amino acid] (dietary, laboratory, and pharmacology)
tube precipitin (laboratory)
tuberculin precipitation (laboratory)

T.P.
total protein (laboratory)

T+P
temperature and pulse

tp
mean transit time (radiology)
time-to-peak tension

TPA
tannic acid, polyphosphomolybdic acid,
  amido acid [staining technique] (laboratory)
12-*o*-tetradecanoyl phorbol-13-acetate
  (chemistry)
tissue-type plasminogen activator (cardiovascular, hematology, and laboratory)
tissue polypeptide antigen (laboratory)
total parenteral alimentation (dietary
  and gastroenterology)
Treponema pallidum agglutination (gynecology, infectious diseases, laboratory, and urology)
tumor polypeptide antigen (laboratory
  and oncology)

tPA
tissue-type plasminogen activator (acti-
  vase) [protocol for use in myocardial
  infarction patients] (cardiovascular,
  hematology, and pharmacology)

TPB
tryptone phosphate broth (laboratory)

TPBF
total pulmonary blood flow (cardiovascular and respiratory)

TPBS
three-phase radionuclide bone scanning
  (radiology)

TPC
thromboplastic plasma component (hematology and laboratory)
total patient care (nursing)
Treponema pallidum complement [fixa-

tion test for syphilis] (gynecology, infectious diseases, laboratory, and urology)

TPCF
Treponema pallidum complement fixation [test for syphilis] (gynecology, infectious diseases, laboratory, and urology)

TPCF test
Treponema pallidum complement fixation test [for syphilis] (gynecology, infectious diseases, laboratory, and urology)

TPCK
L-(1-tosylamido-2-phenyl) ethyl chloromethyl ketone (chemistry)

TPCP
Treponema pallidum cryolysis complement fixation [test for syphilis] (gynecology, infectious diseases, laboratory, and urology)

TPCV
total packed cell volume (hematology)

TPD
thiamine propyl disulfide [prosultiamine] (laboratory)
tropical pancreatic diabetes (endocrinology)
tumor-producing dose (pharmacology)

TP'd
toilet-papered [a practical joke] {pronounced "tea-peed"}

TPE
therapeutic plasma exchange (hematology)
total protective environment (immunology and infectious diseases)

TPEY
tellurite polymyxin egg yolk [agar] (laboratory)

TPF
thymus permeability factor (laboratory)

TPG
transmembrane potential gradient
transplacental gradient (obstetrics)
tryptophan peptone glucose [broth] (laboratory)

TPGY
trypticose-peptone-glucose-yeast extract-trypsin [medium] (laboratory)

TPH
thromboembolic pulmonary hypertension (cardiovascular and respiratory)
transplacental hemorrhage (obstetrics)

TPHA
treponemal hemagglutination [test for syphilis] (gynecology, infectious diseases, laboratory, and urology)

TPI
treponemal immobilization [test for syphilis] (gynecology, infectious diseases, laboratory, and urology)
Treponema pallidum immobilization [test for syphilis] (gynecology, infectious diseases, laboratory, and urology)
triose phosphate isomerase (laboratory)

TPIA
Treponema pallidum immobilization (immune) adherence [test for syphilis] (gynecology, infectious diseases, laboratory, and urology)

TPL-6
titanium proximal loading—6-inch stem [total hip system] (orthopedics)

TPM
temporary pacemaker (cardiovascular)
total passive motion (orthopedics and rehabilitation)
triphenylmethane (chemistry and laboratory)

TPN
thalamic projection neuron(s) (laboratory and neurology)

total parenteral nutrition (dietary and gastroenterology)

triphosphopyridine nucleotide [also called *nicotinamide-adenine-dinucleotide phosphate*] (genetics and laboratory)

TPN²
triphosphopyridine nucleotide [also called *nicotinamide-adenine-dinucleotide phosphate*] (genetics and laboratory)

TPNH
triphosphopyridine nucleotide, reduced form [also called *nicotinamide adenine dinucleotide phosphate, reduced*] (genetics and laboratory)

TPN line
total parenteral nutrition line (dietary and gastroenterology)

TPO
thyroid peroxidase (laboratory)
tryptophan peroxidase (laboratory)

TPP
thiamine pyrophosphate [a vitamin; also called *diphosphothiamine*] (dietary, laboratory, and pharmacology)

TP & P
time, place, and person (neurology)

TPPN
total peripheral parenteral nutrition (dietary and gastroenterology)

TPR
temperature (measurement)
temperature, pulse, and respiration (measurement)
testosterone production rate (endocrinology, laboratory, and urology)
total peripheral resistance (cardiovascular)
total pulmonary resistance (cardiovascular and respiratory)
true positive rate (laboratory)

T.P.R.
temperature, pulse, and respiration (measurement)

TPRI
total peripheral resistance index (cardiovascular)

TPS
trypsin (gastroenterology and laboratory)
tumor polysaccharide substance (laboratory and oncology)

TPST
true positive stress test

TPT
tetraphenyl tetrazolium [a stain] (laboratory)
time-to-peak tension
total protein tuberculin (infectious diseases, laboratory, pharmacology, and respiratory)
typhoid-paratyphoid [vaccine] (infectious diseases and pharmacology)

TPTHS
total parathyroid hormone secretion [rate] (endocrinology and laboratory)

TPTX
thyroid-parathyroidectomized (endocrinology and surgery)
thyroid-parathyroidectomy (endocrinology and surgery)

T-PTX
thyroid-parathyroidectomized (endocrinology and surgery)
thyroid-parathyroidectomy [also called *thyroparathyroidectomy*] (endocrinology and surgery)

TPTZ
tripyridyltriazine [a reagent] (chemistry)

TPUR
transperineal urethral resection (surgery and urology)

TPVR
total peripheral vascular resistance (cardiovascular)

total pulmonary vascular resistance (cardiovascular and respiratory)

TQ
tourniquet (emergency medicine and surgery)

Tq.
tourniquet (emergency medicine and surgery)

TR
teaching and research (education and research)
temperature, rectal (measurement)
tetrazolium reduction (laboratory)
therapeutic radiology (radiation therapy and radiology)
time recovery (radiology)
time release(d) (pharmacology)
tincture (pharmacology)
total resistance (cardiovascular)
total response (pharmacology)
trace (laboratory)
tricuspid regurgitation (cardiovascular)
tuberculin R [also called *new tuberculin*] (infectious diseases, laboratory, pharmacology, and respiratory)
tuberculin residue (infectious diseases, laboratory, pharmacology, and respiratory)
tuberculin rest (infectious diseases, laboratory, pharmacology, and respiratory)
tubular reabsorption (laboratory)
turbidity reducing (laboratory)

T.R.
tuberculin residue (infectious diseases, laboratory, pharmacology, and respiratory)

T(R)
rectal temperature (measurement)

TR-28
{not an abbreviation} [a hip prosthesis] (orthopedics)

Tr
tincture (pharmacology)
trace (laboratory)
treatment
tremor (neurology)

Tr.
tincture (pharmacology)
trace (laboratory)

tr
tincture (pharmacology)
trace (laboratory)
traction (orthopedics)
treatment
tremor (neurology)

TRA
therapeutic recreation associate (rehabilitation)
total renin activity (laboratory)
transaldolase [an enzyme] (laboratory)

Trach
trachea(l) (otorhinolaryngology and respiratory) {pronounced "trayk"}
tracheostomy (otorhinolaryngology and respiratory) {pronounced "trayk"}
tracheotomy (otorhinolaryngology and respiratory) {pronounced "trayk"}

trach
trachea(l) (otorhinolaryngology and respiratory) {pronounced "trayk"}
tracheostomy (otorhinolaryngology and respiratory) {pronounced "trayk"}
tracheotomy (otorhinolaryngology and respiratory) {pronounced "trayk"}

trachelo-
{not an abbreviation} [prefix indicating relationship to the neck or to a neck-like structure] {pronounced "tray-key-low"}

tracheo-
{not an abbreviation} [prefix indicating relationship to the trachea] (otorhinolaryngology and respiratory) {pronounced "tray-key-oh"}

"track"
{pronunciation of *tract.* [traction]} (orthopedics) {not an abbreviation}

tract.
traction (orthopedics) {pronounced "track"}

train
training (education)

TRAM
transverse rectus abdominis myocutaneous [breast reconstruction] (gynecology, plastic surgery, and surgery)
Treatment Rating Assessment Matrix
Treatment Response Assessment Method

TRAN NOT DONE
transfusion not done (hematology)

"trank"
{pronunciation of *tranq* [*tranquilize(r)*]} (neurology, pharmacology, and psychiatry) {not an abbreviation}

tranq
tranquilize(r) (neurology, pharmacology, and psychiatry) {pronounced "trank"}

trans
transaction {pronounced "tranz"}
transfer {pronounced "tranz"}
transverse {pronounced "tranz"}
{not an abbreviation} [1. a word in organic chemistry meaning having certain atoms or radicals on opposite sides; 2. a word in genetics meaning having one or two mutant genes of a pseudoallele on each homologous chromosome] {pronounced "tranz"}

trans-
{not an abbreviation} [prefix meaning *across, beyond,* or *through*] {pronounced "tranz"}

trans D
transverse diameter (measurement) {pronounced "tranz-dee"}

transm
transmission

transpl
transplant (surgery)
transplantation (surgery)

trans sect
transverse section {pronounced "tranz-sect"}

transsex
transsexual (endocrinology, gynecology, psychiatry, surgery, and urology) {pronounced "tranz-sex"}

"tranz"
{pronunciation of *trans* [transaction, transfer, and transverse], trans [1. a word in organic chemistry meaning having certain atoms or radicals on opposite sides; 2. a word in genetics meaning having one or two mutant genes of a pseudoallele on each homologous chromosome {not an abbreviation}], and *trans-* [prefix meaning *across, beyond,* or *through* {not an abbreviation}]} {not an abbreviation}

"tranz-dee"
{pronunciation of *trans D* [*transverse diameter*]} (measurement) {not an abbreviation}

"tranz-sect"
{pronunciation of *trans sect* [*transverse section*]} {not an abbreviation}

"tranz-sex"
{pronunciation of *transsex* [transsexual]} (endocrinology, gynecology, psychiatry, surgery, and urology) {not an abbreviation}

TRAP
thioguanine, rubidomycin, ara-C, and prednisone (chemotherapy, oncology, and pharmacology) {pronounced "trap"}

trap
trapezius [muscle] (neurology and orthopedics) {pronounced "trap"}

"trap"
{pronunciation of *TRAP* [thioguanine, rubidomycin, ara-C, and prednisone (chemotherapy, oncology, and phar-

macology)] and *trap* [trapezius (muscle) (neurology and orthopedics)]} {not an abbreviation}

trau
trauma
traumatic

traumato-
{not an abbreviation} [prefix indicating relationship to trauma or to an injury or wound] {pronounced "trau-mat-oh"}

"trau-mat-oh"
{pronunciation of traumato- [prefix indicating relationship to trauma or to an injury or wound {not an abbreviation}]} {not an abbreviation}

"trayk"
{pronunciation of *Trach* and *trach* [trachea(l), tracheostomy, and tracheotomy]} (otorhinolaryngology and respiratory) {not an abbreviation}

"tray-key-low"
{pronunciation of *trachelo-* [prefix indicating relationship to the neck or to a neck-like structure {not an abbreviation}]} {not an abbreviation}

"tray-key-oh"
{pronunciation of *tracheo-* [prefix indicating relationship to the trachea {not an abbreviation}]} (otorhinolaryngology and respiratory) {not an abbreviation}

TRBF
total renal blood flow (cardiovascular and nephrology)

TRC
tanned red cell(s) [antibody titer] (endocrinology and laboratory)
therapeutic referral center
therapeutic residential center
total renin concentration (laboratory)
total ridge count

TRCH
tanned-red-cell hemagglutination (endocrinology and laboratory)

TRCHI
tanned-red-cell hemagglutination (endocrinology and laboratory)

TRCV
total red cell volume (laboratory)

TRD
traction retinal detachment (ophthalmology)

TRE
true radiation emission (radiation therapy and radiology)

TREA
triethanolamine

treat
treatment {pronounced "treat"}

"treat"
{pronunciation of *treat* [*treatment*]} {not an abbreviation}

T₁ relaxation time

T_1 **relaxation time**
longitudinal relaxation time constant [on magnetic resonance imaging (MRI) scans; also called *spin-lattice relaxation time constant*] (radiology)

T_2 **relaxation time**
transverse relaxation time constant [on magnetic resonance imaging (MRI) scans; also called *spin-spin relaxation time constant*] (radiology)

Tren
Trendelenburg [position] (surgery)

Trep
Treponema [a bacterium] (laboratory)

TRF
T-cell replacing factor (immunology, laboratory, and oncology)
thymus-dependent cell-replacing factor (hematology, immunology, and laboratory)
thyroid-stimulating-hormone releasing factor (endocrinology and laboratory)

thyrotropin-releasing factor (endocrinology and laboratory)

trf
transfer

TRFC
total rosette-forming cell (laboratory)

trg
training (education)

TRGI
triglycerides incalculable (laboratory)

TRH
thyrotropin-releasing hormone (endocrinology and laboratory)

TRI
tetrazolium-reduction inhibition (laboratory)
Thyroid Research Institute (endocrinology and research)
total response index (psychiatry)
trichloroethylene [a solvent] (chemistry)
tubuloreticular inclusion

tri-
{not an abbreviation} [prefix meaning *three* or *thrice*] {pronounced "tri"}

"tri"
{pronunciation of *tri-* [prefix meaning *three* or *thrice* {not an abbreviation}]} {not an abbreviation}

T₃RIA
triiodothyronine radioimmunoassay (endocrinology and laboratory)

T₃(RIA)
serum triiodothyronine radioimmunoassay (endocrinology and laboratory)

T₄RIA
thyroxine radioisotope assay (endocrinology and laboratory)

T₄(RIA)
serum thyroxine radioisotope assay (endocrinology and laboratory)

TRIAC
tri-iodothyroacetic acid (endocrinology and laboratory)

Triac.
tri-iodothyroacetic acid (endocrinology and laboratory)

TRIC
trachoma-inclusion conjunctivitis (ophthalmology) {pronounced "trick"}
trichloroethylene [a solvent] (chemistry) {pronounced "trike"}
Trichomonas [a parasite] (laboratory) {pronounced "trick"}

triCB
trichlorobiphenyl (chemistry)

TRICH
trichinosis (gastroenterology and laboratory)
Trichomonas [a parasite] (laboratory) {pronounced "trick"}

Trich
Trichomonas [a parasite] (laboratory) {pronounced "trick"}

tricho-
{not an abbreviation} [prefix indicating relationship to hair] {pronounced "trick-oh"}

Trich V
Trichomonas vaginitis [a parasite] (gynecology, laboratory, obstetrics, and urology) {pronounced "trick-vee"}

"trick"
{pronunciation of *TRIC* [trachoma-inclusion conjunctivitis (ophthalmology) and *Trichomonas* (laboratory)] and *TRICH* and *Trich* [*Trichomonas* (laboratory)]} {not an abbreviation}

"trick-oh"
{pronunciation of *tricho-* [prefix indicating relationship to hair {not an abbreviation}]} {not an abbreviation}

"trick-vee"
{pronunciation of *Trich V* [*Trichomonas vaginitis*]} (gynecology, laboratory, obstetrics, and urology)

Trid.
triduum [three days]

trid
triduum [three days]

trid.
triduum [three days]

"tri-en"
{pronunciation of *-triene* [chemical suffix indicating the presence of three double bands {not an abbreviation}]} (chemistry) {not an abbreviation}

-triene
{not an abbreviation} [chemical suffix indicating the presence of three double bands] (chemistry) {pronounced "tri-en"}

TRIG
triglycerides (cardiovascular and laboratory)

Trig.
triglycerides (cardiovascular and laboratory)

"trike"
{pronunciation of *TRIC* [trichloroethylene (a solvent)]} (chemistry) {not an abbreviation}

TRIMIS
Tri-Service Medical Information Service

triple A
abdominal aortic aneurysm (cardiovascular)
Automobile Association of America (insurance)

"trip-see"
{pronunciation of *-tripsy* [suffix indicating a surgical procedure involving intentionally crushing a structure {not an abbreviation}]} (surgery) {not an abbreviation}

-tripsy
{not an abbreviation} [suffix indicating a surgical procedure involving intentionally crushing a structure] (surgery) {pronounced "trip-see"}

TRIS
tris(hydroxymethyl)aminomethane [also called *trometamol*; an alkalizer] (pharmacology)

TRIT
tri-iodothyronine (endocrinology and laboratory)
tritura [triturate] (pharmacology)

Trit.
tritura [triturate] (pharmacology)

trit.
tritura [triturate] (pharmacology)

TRK
transketolase [an enzyme] (laboratory)

TRMC
tetramethylrhodaminoisothiocyanate (laboratory)

TRML
terminal

TRM-SMX
trimethoprim-sulfamethoxazole [antibacterials] (pharmacology and urology)

tRNA
transfer ribonucleic acid (genetics and laboratory)

TROCH
troche [lozenge, *trochiscus*] (pharmacology) {pronounced "trouch"}
trochiscus [lozenge, troche] (pharmacology) {pronounced "trouch"}

troch
troche [lozenge, *trochiscus*] (pharmacology) {pronounced "trouch"}

trochiscus [lozenge, troche] (pharmacology) {pronounced "trouch"}

troch.
troche [lozenge, *trochiscus*] (pharmacology) {pronounced "trouch"}
trochiscus [lozenge, troche] (pharmacology) {pronounced "trouch"}

"tro-fee"
{pronunciation of -*trophy* [suffix indicating food or nutrition {not an abbreviation}]} {not an abbreviation}

"tro-fik"
{pronunciation of -*trophic* [suffix indicating relationship to nutrition {not an abbreviation}]} {not an abbreviation}

"tro-fin"
{pronunciation of -*trophin* [1. suffix indicating relationship to nutrition {not an abbreviation}; 2. suffix meaning having an affinity for the thing indicated by the root word {not an abbreviation}]} {not an abbreviation}

"tro-foe"
{pronunciation of *tropho-* [prefix indicating relationship to food or nourishment {not an abbreviation}]} {not an abbreviation}

-trophic
{not an abbreviation} [suffix indicating relationship to nutrition] {pronounced "tro-fik"}

-trophin
{not an abbreviation} [1. suffix indicating relationship to nutrition; 2. suffix meaning having an affinity for the thing indicated by the root word] {pronounced "tro-fin"}

tropho-
{not an abbreviation} [prefix indicating relationship to food or nourishment] {pronounced "tro-foe"}

-trophy
{not an abbreviation} [suffix indicating food or nutrition] {pronounced "tro-fee"}

-tropin
{not an abbreviation} [suffix meaning having an affinity for the thing indicated by the root word] {pronounced "tro-pin"}

"tro-pin"
{pronunciation of -*tropin* [suffix meaning having an affinity for the thing indicated by the root word {not an abbreviation}]} {not an abbreviation}

Trop Med
tropical medicine

"trouch"
{pronunciation of *troch* and *troch.* [lozenge, troche, and *trochiscus*]} (pharmacology) {not an abbreviation}

TRP
total refraction period (neurology and orthopedics)
total refractory period (neurology and orthopedics)
trichorhinophalangeal [syndrome]
tubular reabsorption of phosphate (laboratory)

Trp
tryptophan (dietary, laboratory, and pharmacology)

TRPA
tryptophan-rich prealbumin (laboratory)

TRPC
triple phosphate (laboratory)

TRPS
trichorhinophalangeal syndrome

TRPT
theoretical renal phosphorus threshold (laboratory and nephrology)

TRS
total reducing sugars (laboratory)

TRSV
tobacco ringspot virus (agriculture and laboratory)

TRT
thermoradiotherapy (radiation therapy)
treatment

trt
treatment

TRU
turbidity reducing unit (laboratory)

T3RU
triiodothyronine resin uptake [value] (endocrinology and laboratory)

T$_3$RU
triiodothyronine resin uptake [test] (endocrinology and laboratory)

TR unit
turbidity reducing unit (laboratory)

TRX
transsexual (gynecology, psychiatry, surgery, and urology)

Try
tryptophan (dietary, laboratory, and pharmacology)

Try.
tryptophan (dietary, laboratory, and pharmacology)

TRYPSN
trypsin [an enzyme] (gastroenterology and laboratory)

TS
technical school (education)
temperature-sensitive (chemistry, laboratory, and pharmacology)
temporal stem (anatomy and neurology)
Teratology Society (embryology, genetics, and pathology)
terminal [or greater] sensation (neurology)
test solution (laboratory)
thoracic surgery (cardiovascular, respiratory, surgery, and thoracic surgery)

total solids (gastroenterology)
Tourette syndrome [also called *Gilles de la Tourette's syndrome*] (neurology)
toxic substance (chemistry)
training school (education)
transsexual (gynecology, endocrinology, psychiatry, surgery, and urology)
transverse section
transverse tubular system
tricuspid stenosis (cardiovascular)
triple strength (pharmacology)
tropical sprue (gastroenterology)
trypticase soy [plate] (laboratory)
T-suppressor [cell] (immunology, laboratory, and oncology)
tuberous sclerosis
tubular [tracheal] sound (respiratory)
tumor-specific (laboratory and oncology)
Turner syndrome
type-specific [antibodies] (laboratory)

T$_s$
tension, Schiøtz' (ophthalmology)

T.S.
test solution (laboratory)

T/S
thyroid : serum [radioiodide ratio] (endocrinology and laboratory)

Ts
intraocular pressure-Schiøtz (ophthalmology)

TSA
technical surgical assistance (surgery)
Test of Syntactic Abilities (speech and language therapy)
tissue-specific antigens (laboratory)
toluene sulfonic acid [test] (laboratory)
total shoulder arthroplasty (orthopedics)
toxic shock antigen (laboratory)
trypticase soy agar (laboratory)
tumor-specific antibody (laboratory and oncology)
tumor-specific antigen (laboratory and oncology)
type-specific antibody (laboratory)

T₄SA
thyroxine-specific activity (endocrinology and laboratory)

Tsa
{not an abbreviation} [a virus mutant] (laboratory)

TSAb
thyroid-stimulating antibody (endocrinology and laboratory)

TSAP
toxic shock-associated protein (laboratory)

TSAR
{not an abbreviation} [trademark for tape surrounded Appli-rulers]

TSAS
total severity assessment score

TSB
trypticase soy broth (laboratory)
typtone soy broth (laboratory)

TSBB
transtracheal selective bronchial brushing (respiratory)

TSC
technetium sulfur colloid (radiology)
thiosemicarbazide [a reagent] (laboratory)
tryptose-sulfite cyclosterone [agar] (laboratory)

TSD
target skin distance (radiation therapy)
Tay-Sachs disease (genetics, neurology, and ophthalmology)
theory of signal detectability
transfer summary dictated [followed by date] (medical records)

TSE
testicular self-examination (oncology and urology)
total skin examination (dermatology)
trisodium edetate (pharmacology)

TSEB
total skin electron beam

T sect
transverse section [also called *cross section*] {pronounced "tea-sect"}

T-set
tracheostomy set (emergency medicine, otorhinolaryngology, respiratory, and surgery) {pronounced "tea-set"}

TSF
thrombopoietic stimulating factor (hematology and laboratory)
tissue-coding factor (laboratory and pathology)
triceps skin fold [thickness] (measurement)

TSG
tumor-specific glycoprotein (laboratory and oncology)

TSH
thyroid-stimulating hormone [also called *serum thyrotropin* and *thyrotropic hormone*] (endocrinology and laboratory)

T-shaped
T-shaped fracture (orthopedics)

TSH-RF
thyroid-stimulating hormone-releasing factor [also called *thyrotropin releasing factor*] (endocrinology and laboratory)

TSH-RH
thyroid-stimulating hormone-releasing hormone (endocrinology and laboratory)

TSI
thyroid-stimulating immunoglobulin (endocrinology, immunology, and laboratory)
triple sugar [lactose, glucose, sucrose], iron [agar] (laboratory)

TSIA
triple sugar [lactose, glucose, sucrose], iron agar (laboratory)

TSI agar
triple sugar [lactose, glucose, sucrose], iron agar (laboratory)

TSM
type-specific M [protein] (bacteriology and laboratory)

TSN
tryptophan peptone sulfide neomycin [agar] (laboratory)

TSP
teaspoon (measurement)
total serum protein (laboratory)
trisodium phosphate

tsp
teaspoon (measurement)

TSPA
triethylenethiophosphoramide [also called *Thiotepa, thiotepa,* and *thiophosphoramide*] (chemotherapy, oncology, and pharmacology)

TSPAP
total serum prostatic acid phosphatase (laboratory, oncology, and urology)

T-spine
thoracic spine (neurology, orthopedics, and radiology)

T/spine
thoracic spine (neurology, orthopedics, and radiology)

TSPP
technetium stannous pyrophosphate [rectilinear bone scan] (oncology, orthopedics, and radiology)

TSR
testosterone sterilized [female] rate (research)
thyroid-to-serum ratio (endocrinology and laboratory)
total shoulder replacement (orthopedics)

TSS
toxic shock syndrome (gynecology and obstetrics)

transverse spinal sclerosis (orthopedics)
tropical splenomegaly syndrome (gastroenterology)

TSSA
tumor-specific cell surface antigen (laboratory and oncology)

TSSE
toxic shock syndrome exoprotein (laboratory)

TSST
toxic shock syndrome toxin (laboratory)

TSSU
theater sterile supply unit (surgery)

TST
titmus stereocuity test
treadmill stress test(ing) (cardiovascular)
tumor skin test (laboratory and oncology)

TSTA
tumor-specific tissue antigen (laboratory and oncology)
tumor-specific transplantation antigen (laboratory and oncology)

TSU
triple sugar [lactose, glucose, sucrose] urea [agar] (laboratory)

T-suppressor
T-suppressor cell (hematology, immunology, and laboratory)

TSY
trypticase soy yeast (laboratory)

TT
tablet triturate (pharmacology)
tendon transfer (orthopedics)
tetanus toxin (infectious diseases and laboratory)
tetanus toxoid (infectious diseases and pharmacology)
tetrathionate [broth] (laboratory)
tetrazol (laboratory)

thrombin time (hematology and laboratory)

thymol turbidity [obsolete test of hepatic function] (gastroenterology and laboratory)

tibial torsion (orthopedics)

tibial tubercle (anatomy and orthopedics)

tilt table (orthopedics and surgery)

Token Test (speech and language therapy)

tooth, treatment of (dentistry)

total thyroxine (endocrinology and laboratory)

total time

transient tachypnea (respiratory)

transit time [of blood through heart and lungs] (cardiovascular and respiratory)

transthoracic (cardiovascular, gastroenterology, and respiratory)

transtracheal (otorhinolaryngology and respiratory)

tuberculin tested [milk] (infectious diseases and laboratory)

twitch tension (neurology)

T.T.

tablet triturate (pharmacology)

tetanus toxoid (infectious diseases and pharmacology)

T & T

time and temperature (measurement)

touch and tone (neurology)

tympanostomy with tube placement (otorhinolaryngology)

T/T

trace of/trace of [referring to findings of traces of different substances on tests] (laboratory)

TT4

total thyroxine (endocrinology and laboratory)

TTA

total toe arthroplasty (orthopedics)

transtracheal aspiration (otorhinolaryngology and respiratory)

TTC

triphenyltetrazolium chloride [also called *red tetrazolium*] (chemistry and laboratory)

TTD

tissue tolerance dose (radiation therapy)

TTG

tellurite, taurocholate, and gelatin (laboratory)

TTGA

tellurite-taurocholate-gelatin agar (laboratory)

TTH

thyrotropic hormone [also called *thyroid-stimulating hormone*] (endocrinology and laboratory)

tritiated thymidine (pharmacology)

TTI

tension-time index [also called *time-tension index*] (neurology)

TTIB

tension-time index per beat (neurology)

TTL

Training and Test Lung [simulator] (respiratory)

transistor-transistor logic (computer science and electronics)

TTN

transient tachypnea of the newborn (neonatology, pediatrics, and respiratory)

TTNB

transient tachypnea of the newborn (neonatology, pediatrics, and respiratory)

TTO

to take out

TTP

thrombotic thrombocytopenic purpura (hematology)

thymidine triphosphate (genetics and laboratory)

time-to-peak [tension] (neurology)
total triose phosphate (laboratory)

TTPA
triethylene thiophosphoramide [also called thiotepa] (chemotherapy, oncology, and pharmacology)

TTS
temporary threshold shift
through the skin
transdermal therapeutic system (pharmacology)

TTT
tolbutamide tolerance test (endocrinology and laboratory)

TTTT
test tube turbidity test (laboratory)

T-tube
{not an abbreviation} [a self-retaining drainage tube] (surgery)

TTVP
temporary transvenous pacemaker (cardiovascular)

TTX
tetrodotoxin (laboratory)

TTY
teletypewriter [for hearing and speech impaired persons] (otorhinolaryngology and hearing and speech therapy)

TU
thiouracil (chemotherapy, oncology, and pharmacology)
Todd unit(s) (measurement)
toxic unit (measurement and research)
transmission unit
tuberculin unit (infectious diseases, measurement, pharmacology, and respiratory)
turbidity unit (laboratory and measurement)

T.U.
toxic unit (measurement and research)
tuberculin unit (infectious diseases, measurement, pharmacology, and respiratory)

T$_3$U
tri-iodothyronine resin uptake [test] (endocrinology and laboratory)

TUB
tubouterine [junction] (gynecology and obstetrics) {pronounced "tub"}

"tub"
{pronunciation of *TUB* [tubouterine (junction)]} (gynecology and obstetrics) {not an abbreviation}

TUBERC
tuberculosis (infectious diseases and respiratory) {pronounced "to-berk"}

tuberc
tuberculosis (infectious diseases and respiratory) {pronounced "to-berk"}

TUD
total urethral discharge (gynecology and urology)

TUG
total urinary gonadotropin (endocrinology, laboratory, and urology)

TUIP
transurethral incision of the prostate (urology)

TULAR
tularemia [an infectious, plague-like disease] (infectious diseases, veterinary medicine, and multiple specialties)

T$_3$UP
tri-iodothyronine uptake (endocrinology and radiology)

TUR
transurethral resection [of bladder tumor or of prostate] (urology)

T.U.R.
transurethral resection [of bladder tumor or of prostate] (urology)

T₃UR
triiodothyronine uptake radio (endocrinology and laboratory)

TURB
transurethral resection of the bladder (urology)
turbid(ity) (laboratory)

turb
turbid(ity) (laboratory)
turbinate (anatomy and otorhinolaryngology)

TURBN
transurethral resection of bladder neck (urology)

TURBT
transurethral resection of bladder tumor (urology)

"tur-lu"
{pronunciation of *Terleu* [tertiary leucine]} (endocrinology and laboratory) {not an abbreviation}

TURP
transurethral resection of prostate (urology) {pronounced "turp"}

T.U.R.P.
transurethral resection of prostate (urology) {pronounced "turp"}

turp
turpentine (chemistry) {pronounced "turp"}

"turp"
{pronunciation of *TURP* and *T.U.R.P.* [transurethral resection of prostate (urology)] and *turp* [turpentine (chemistry)]} {not an abbreviation}

TURV
transurethral resection of valves (urology)

TUS
tussis [cough] (otorhinolaryngology and respiratory)

tus
tussis [cough] (otorhinolaryngology and respiratory)

TV
talipes varus (orthopedics)
television (communications)
tetrazolium violet (laboratory)
tidal volume (laboratory and respiratory)
total volume (measurement)
transvenous
transvestite (psychiatry)
trial visit (psychiatry and rehabilitation)
Trichomonas vaginalis [a parasite] (gynecology, laboratory, and obstetrics)
Trichomonas vaginitis [a parasitic infection] (gynecology, laboratory, obstetrics, and urology)
tricuspid valve [apparatus] (cardiovascular)
truncal vagotomy (gastroenterology and surgery)
tuberculin volutin (infectious diseases, laboratory, and respiratory)

T.V.
tidal volume (laboratory and respiratory)

TVC
timed vital capacity (respiratory)
total viable cells (laboratory)
total vital capacity (respiratory)
total volume capacity (measurement)
transvaginal cone (gynecology)
triple-voiding cystogram (radiology and urology)
true vocal cord(s) (otorhinolaryngology and respiratory)

TVD
transmissible virus dementia (neurology and psychiatry)
triple-vessel disease (cardiovascular)

TVDALV
triple-vessel disease with abnormal left
ventricle (cardiovascular)

TVF
tactile vocal fremitus (otorhinolaryngology and speech and language therapy)

TVH
total vaginal hysterectomy (gynecology)
transvaginal hysterectomy (gynecology)
turkey virus hepatitis

TVI
temperature-viscosity index (laboratory)

TVL
tenth value layer [referring to radiation]
(physics, radiation therapy, and radiology)

TVP
transvenous pacemaker (cardiovascular)
transvesical prostatectomy (urology)
tricuspid valve prolapse (cardiovascular)

TYP-H
typhoid H (infectious diseases)

TVR
total vascular resistance (cardiovascular)
tricuspid valve replacement (cardiovascular)

TVT
tunica vaginalis testis (anatomy and
urology)

TVU
total volume urine [in twenty-four hours]
(nephrology and urology)

TVV
transmissible venereal virus gynecology,
infectious diseases (laboratory, and
urology)

TW
tapwater (dietary and pharmacology)
test weight (measurement)
total body water (measurement)

TW3
That Was the Week that Was [television
program] (communications)

TWA
time weighted average (measurement)

T-wave
{not an abbreviation} [found on electro-
cardiograms] (cardiovascular)

TWD
total white and differential count (hematology and laboratory)

TWE
tapwater enema (gastroenterology and
pharmacology)

T1 weighted
longitudinal relaxation time constant
[used as "T1 weighted" on magnetic
resonance imaging (MRI) scans; also
called *spin-lattice relaxation time
constant*] (radiology)

T_1 weighted
longitudinal relaxation time constant
[used as "T_1 weighted" on magnetic
resonance imaging (MRI) scans; also
called *spin-lattice relaxation time
constant*] (radiology)

T2 weighted
transverse relaxation time constant
[used as "T2 weighted" on magnetic
resonance imaging (MRI) scans; also
called *spin-spin relaxation time constant*] (radiology)

T_2 weighted
transverse relaxation time constant
[used as "T_2 weighted" on magnetic
resonance imaging (MRI) scans; also
called *spin-spin relaxation time constant*] (radiology)

TWETC
tapwater enema till clear (gastroenterology and pharmacology)

TWL
transepidermal water loss (internal medicine)

TWSb/6
antimony sodium dimercaptosuccinate [also called *stibocaptate*] (pharmacology)

TWWD
tapwater wet dressing (surgery)

TX
Texas [Postal Service state designation]
thromboxane (hematology and laboratory)
traction (orthopedics)
transplant (surgery and transplantation surgery)
transplantation (surgery and transplantation surgery)
treatment
{not an abbreviation} [symbol for a contagious tuberculin derivative] (infectious diseases, laboratory, pharmacology, and respiratory)

T & X
type and crossmatch (hematology and laboratory)

Tx
therapy
traction (neurology and orthopedics)
transfuse (hematology)
transplant (surgery and transplantation surgery)
treatment

TxA
thromboxane A (hematology and laboratory)

TxA$_2$
thromboxane A$_2$ (hematology and laboratory)

TxB$_2$
thromboxane B$_2$ (hematology and laboratory)

TY
type (laboratory)

typhoid (infectious diseases and laboratory)

Ty
thyroxine (endocrinology, laboratory, and pharmacology)
type (laboratory)

ty.
type (laboratory)
typhoid (infectious diseases and laboratory)

Tyco
{not an abbreviation} [slang for *Tylenol with Codeine*] (pharmacology) {pronounced "tie-co"}

TYCO #1
Tylenol No. 1 [acetaminophen with 7.5 milligrams of codeine] (pharmacology) {pronounced "tie-co-num-ber-one"}

TYCO #2
Tylenol No. 2 [acetaminophen with 15 milligrams of codeine] (pharmacology) {pronounced "tie-co-num-ber-two"}

TYCO #3
Tylenol No. 3 [acetaminophen with 30 milligrams of codeine] (pharmacology) {pronounced "tie-co-num-ber-three"}

TYCO #4
Tylenol No. 4 [acetaminophen with 60 milligrams of codeine] (pharmacology) {pronounced "tie-co-num-ber-four"}

Tyl
Tylenol (pharmacology)
tyloma [also called a *callus*] (orthopedics and podiatry)

Tymp
tympanicity [referring to auscultation of the chest] (cardiovascular and respiratory)

tymp
tympanostomy (otorhinolaryngology)

tymp memb
tympanic membrane (otorhinolaryngology)

tymp & tubes
tympanostomy with tube placement (otorhinolaryngology)

typ
typical

typhlo-
{not an abbreviation} [1. prefix indicating relationship to the cecum (gastroenterology); 2. prefix indicating relationship to blindness (ophthalmology)] {pronounced "tif-low"}

Tyr
tyrosine (endocrinology, laboratory, and pharmacology)

TyRIA
thyroid radioisotope assay (endocrinology and radiology)

tyro-
{not an abbreviation} [prefix indicating relationship to cheese] {pronounced "tie-row"}

TZ
tuberculin zymboplastiche (infectious diseases, laboratory, pharmacology, and respiratory)

Tz
tuberculin zymboplastiche (infectious diseases, laboratory, pharmacology, and respiratory)

Tzn
total estrogens after zinc and hydrochloric acid [Zn-HCl] treatment (laboratory)

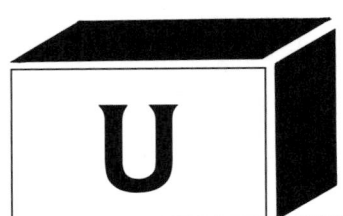

U

U
International Unit [of enzyme activity] (laboratory and measurement)
ultralente insulin (endocrinology and pharmacology)
unerupted (dentistry)
unit (measurement)
unknown
upper
uracil (chemotherapy, laboratory, oncology, and pharmacology)
uranium (chemistry)
uridine (laboratory)
urine (laboratory and urology)
urologist (urology)
urology
utendus [to be used] (pharmacology)
U-wave [on electrocardiogram] (cardiovascular)

U.
unit (measurement)

"U"
unit (measurement)

U/
at the umbilicus (obstetrics)

μU
micro- [prefix for 10^{-6}] (measurement)
microunit (measurement)

U/1
one finger breadth below the umbilicus (measurement and obstetrics)

1/U
one finger breadth above the umbilicus (measurement and obstetrics)

U/3
upper third [referring to long bones] (orthopedics and radiology)

235U
radioactive uranium (chemistry)

U-8344
{not an abbreviation} (chemotherapy, oncology, and pharmacology)

u
micron (measurement)
unit (measurement)

u.
unit (measurement)

UA
ultra-audible (otorhinolaryngology)
umbilical artery (cardiovascular and neonatology)
unaggregated (laboratory)
unauthorized absence (armed forces)
uncertain about
unstable angina (cardiovascular)
uric acid (laboratory, orthopedics, and rheumatology)
urinalysis [also called *urine analysis*] (laboratory and urology)
urinary basement membrane antigen(s) (laboratory and urology)
uterine aspiration (gynecology and obstetrics)

U/A
urinalysis (laboratory and urology)

ua
umbilical artery (cardiovascular and neonatology)
usque ad [as far as, up to]

u.a.
usque ad [as far as, up to]

UAC
umbilical artery catheter (cardiovascular and neonatology) {pronounced "U-ak"}
uric acid (laboratory, orthopedics, and rheumatology)

UA/C
uric acid to creatinine [ratio] (laboratory, orthopedics, and rheumatology)

UA/C ratio
uric acid to creatinine ratio (laboratory, orthopedics, and rheumatology)

UAD
upper-airway disease (respiratory)

UAE
unilateral absence of excretion (nephrology)

UAI
uterine activity interval (obstetrics)

"U-ak"
{pronunciation of *UAC* (umbilical artery catheter)} (cardiovascular and neonatology) {not an abbreviation}

UAL
umbilical artery line (cardiovascular and neonatology)

UAN
uric acid nitrogen (laboratory)

UAO
upper-airway obstruction (otorhinolaryngology and respiratory)

UAT
up as tolerated (rehabilitation)

UAVC
univentricular atrioventricular connection (cardiovascular)

UB
ultimobranchial [body] (anatomy, endocrinology, and laboratory)

UBA
undenatured bacterial antigen (laboratory)

UBBC
unsaturated vitamin cyanocobalamin [B$_{12}$] binding capacity (hematology and laboratory)

UBC
University of British Columbia (education)

UBC brace
University of British Columbia brace (orthopedics)

UBF
unknown black female (emergency medicine)
uterine blood flow (cardiovascular, gynecology, and obstetrics)

UBG
ultimobranchial glands (anatomy, endocrinology, and laboratory)
urobilinogen (gastroenterology and laboratory)

UBI
ultraviolet blood irradiation (hematology, laboratory, and radiation therapy)

UBL
undifferentiated B-cell lymphoma (laboratory and oncology)

UBM
unknown black male (emergency medicine)

UBO
unidentified bright object (radiology)

UBP
ureteral back pressure (nephrology and urology)

UC
ulcerative colitis (gastroenterology)
ultracentrifugal (laboratory)
unchanged
unclassifiable (laboratory)
unit clerk (administration)
University of California (education)
unsatisfactory condition
urea clearance (laboratory and nephrology)

urethral catheterization (gynecology and urology)
urinary catheter (gynecology and urology)
urine culture (laboratory and urology)
uterine contraction(s) (obstetrics)

U.C.
uterine contraction(s) (obstetrics)

U/C
urine culture (gynecology, laboratory, and urology)

U & C
urethral and cervical [cultures] (gynecology, laboratory, obstetrics, and urology)
usual and customary

U$_{Ca}$V
urinary calcium excretion (laboratory)

UCB
University of California, Berkeley (education)

UCBR
unconjugated bilirubin (gastroenterology and laboratory)

UCC
urgent care center (emergency medicine)

UCD
University of California, Davis (education)
urine-collection device (laboratory and urology)
usual childhood diseases (pediatrics)

UCDMC
University of California, Davis, Medical Center (administration, education, and research)

UCF
University of Central Florida (education)

UCG
ultrasonic cardiogram (cardiovascular and radiology)

urinary chorionic gonadotropin [pregnancy test] (endocrinology, gynecology, obstetrics, and laboratory)

UCHD
usual childhood diseases (pediatrics)

UCHI
usual childhood illnesses (pediatrics)

UCI
University of California, Irvine (education)
urinary catheter in (urology)
usual childhood illnesses

UCIMC
University of California, Irvine, Medical Center (administration, education, and research)

UCL
uncomfortable loudness [sound level] (otorhinolaryngology)
urea clearance [test] (laboratory and nephrology)

UCLA
University of California, Los Angeles (education)

UCO
urinary catheter out (gynecology and urology)

UCP
urinary coproporphyrin (laboratory and multiple specialties)
urinary C-peptide (endocrinology and laboratory)

U.C.P.
United Cerebral Palsy (genetics and neurology)

UCPT
urinary coproporphyrin test (dermatology, gastroenterology, genetics, hematology, laboratory, neurology, and psychiatry)

UCR
unconditioned response (neurology and psychiatry)
University of California, Riverside (education)
usual, customary, and reasonable

UCS
unconditioned stimulus (neurology and psychiatry)
unconscious (emergency medicine and neurology)

Ucs
unconscious (emergency medicine and neurology)

ucs
unconscious (emergency medicine and neurology)

UCSB
University of California, Santa Barbara (education)

UCSC
University of California, Santa Cruz (education)

UCSD
University of California, San Diego (education)

UCSF
University of California, San Francisco (education)

UCTD
unclassified connective tissue disease (internal medicine)

UCV
uncontrolled variable

UCX
urine culture (laboratory and urology)

UD
ud dictum [as directed] (pharmacology)
ulcerative dermatitis (dermatology)
ulnar deviation (orthopedics)
under direct vision
unit dose package (pharmacology)

urethral discharge (gynecology and urology)
uridine diphosphate (laboratory)
uroporphyrinogen decarboxylase (dermatology, gastroenterology, genetics, hematology, laboratory, neurology, and psychiatry)

ud
ud dictum [as directed] (pharmacology)

u.d.
ud dictum [as directed] (pharmacology)

UDA
under direct vision

UDC
undeveloped countries [now called *third world countries*] (economics and government)
usual diseases of childhood (pediatrics)

UDCA
ursodeoxycholic acid [used to dissolve gallstones] (gastroenterology and pharmacology)

UDE
undetermined etiology

UDP
uridine diphosphate (laboratory)

UDPG
uridine diphosphate glucose [also called *uridine diphosphoglucose*] (laboratory)

UDPGA
uridine diphosphoglucuronic acid [also called *uridine diphosphate glucuronic acid*] (laboratory)

UPDgal
uridine diphosphogalactose [also called *uridine diphosphate galactose*] (laboratory)

UDP-galactose
uridine diphosphogalactose [also called

uridine diphosphate galactose] (laboratory)

UDPglu

uridine diphosphoglucose [also called *uridine diphosphate glucose*] (laboratory)

UDP-glucose

uridine diphosphoglucose [also called *uridine diphosphate glucose*] (laboratory)

UDP-glucuronate

uridine diphosphoglucuronate (laboratory)

UDPGT

uridine diphosphoglucuronyl transferase (laboratory)

UDRP

uridine diribose phosphate (laboratory)

UDS

ultra-Doppler sonography (radiology and multiple specialties)

unscheduled deoxynucleic acid synthesis (laboratory)

UE

uncertain etiology upper esophagus (gastroenterology)

upper extremity (neurology and orthopedics)

urinary energy (urology)

U/E

upper extremity (neurology and orthopedics)

UEM

universal electron microscope (laboratory)

UEMC

unidentified endosteal marrow cell (hematology and laboratory)

UES

upper esophageal sphincter (anatomy and gastroenterology)

u/ext

upper extremity (neurology and orthopedics)

UF

ultrafiltrable (laboratory)

ultrafiltration [volume] (laboratory and measurement)

ultrafine (laboratory)

umbrella filter (cardiovascular and hematology)

universal feeder

unknown factor

UFA

unesterified fatty acids [also called *free fatty acids* and *nonesterified fatty acids*] (laboratory)

UFO

unflagged order (laboratory)

unidentified flying object (aerospace science and parapsychology)

unidentified foreign object (radiology and surgery)

UFR

ultrafiltration rate (laboratory)

UG

urogenital (gynecology and urology)

ug

microgram (measurement)

UGA

under general anesthesia (surgery)

UGDP

University Group Diabetes Program (endocrinology and research)

UGF

unidentified growth factor (endocrinology and laboratory)

UGH

uveitis, glaucoma, and hyphema [syndrome] (ophthalmology) {pronounced "ugh"}

UGH

uveitis, glaucoma, and hyphema plus vitreous hemorrhage [syndrome] (ophthalmology)

"ugh"

{pronunciation of *UGH* [uveitis, glaucoma, and hyphema (syndrome)]} (ophthalmology) {not an abbreviation}

UGI

upper gastrointestinal (gastroenterology)

U.G.I.

upper gastrointestinal (gastroenterology)

UGIS

upper gastrointestinal series (gastroenterology and radiology)

UGS

urogenital sinus (gynecology and urology)

UH

upper half

U24H

twenty-four-hour urine (laboratory and urology)

UHBI

upper hemibody irradiation (oncology and radiation therapy)

UHD

unstable hemoglobin disease (hematology)

UHDDS

Uniform Hospital Discharge Data Set (administration)

UHF

ultrahigh frequency (physics)

UHL

universal hypertrichosis lanuginosa (endocrinology, genetics, and oncology)

UHR

underlying heart rhythm (cardiovascular)

UHSC

university health services clinic

UHT

ultrahigh temperature

UI

ureteral-intestinal (gastroenterology and urology)

uroporphyrin isomerase (dermatology, gastroenterology, genetics, hematology, laboratory, neurology, and psychiatry)

U/I

unidentified

UIBC

unsaturated iron-binding capacity (hematology and laboratory)

UICC

Union International Contra le Cancrum [International Union Against Cancer] (oncology)

UID

uno in die [once daily] (pharmacology) [*Note: This is considered a dangerous abbreviation.*]

UIF

undegraded insulin factor (endocrinology and laboratory)

UIH

University of Iowa Hospitals (administration, education, and research)

UIMC

International Union of Railway Medical Services (administration, insurance, and transportation)

UIP

usual interstitial pneumonia (respiratory)

usual interstitial pneumonitis (respiratory)

UIQ
upper inner quadrant (anatomy)

UJT
unijunction transistor (electronics and physics)

UK
United Kingdom (government)
unknown
urokinase [also called *plasminogen activator*] (cardiovascular, hematology, laboratory, and pharmacology)

UKAEA
United Kingdom Atomic Energy Authority (government and physics)

"U-knee"
{pronunciation of *uni-* [prefix meaning one {not an abbreviation}]} {not an abbreviation}

"U-knee-lat"
{pronunciation of *unilat* [*unilateral*]} {not an abbreviation}

U$_K$V
potassium-excretion rate (laboratory, multiple specialties, and nephrology)

UL
undifferentiated lymphoma (oncology and pathology)
upper lobe (anatomy and respiratory)

U & L
upper and lower

U/L
upper and lower

U/l
units per liter (measurement)

ULBW
ultralow birth weight (neonatology)

ule-
{not an abbreviation} [1. prefix indicating relationship to a cicatrix or scar;

2. prefix indicating relationship to the gingivae (dentistry and otorhinolaryngology)] {pronounced "U-lee"}

"U-lee"
{pronunciation of *ule-* [1. prefix indicating relationship to a cicatrix or scar {not an abbreviation}; 2. prefix indicating relationship to the gingivae (dentistry and otorhinolaryngology) {not an abbreviation}]} {not an abbreviation}

ULL
uncomfortable loudness level (otorhinolaryngology)

ULN
upper limits of normal (laboratory)

ULO
{not an abbreviation} [trademark for a preparation of *chlophedianol hydrochloride;* a cough suppressant] (otorhinolaryngology, pharmacology, and respiratory)

ulo-
{not an abbreviation} [1. prefix indicating relationship to a cicatrix or scar; 2. prefix indicating relationship to the gingivae (dentistry and otorhinolaryngology)] {pronounced "U-low"}

"U-low"
{pronunciation of *ulo-* [1. prefix indicating relationship to a cicatrix or scar {not an abbreviation}; 2. prefix indicating relationship to the gingivae (dentistry and otorhinolaryngology) {not an abbreviation}]} {not an abbreviation}

ULQ
upper left quadrant [of abdomen] (anatomy and gastroenterology)

ULT
ultrahigh temperature [for pasteurization] (chemistry)

ult
ultimately
ultimus [last, ultimately]

ult.
ultimately
ultimus [last, ultimately]

ult praes
ultimum praescriptus [last prescribed]
(pharmacology)

ult. praes.
ultimum praescriptus [last prescribed]
(pharmacology)

ultra-
{not an abbreviation} [prefix indicating
beyond or excess] {pronounced "ul-
trah"}

"ul-trah"
{pronunciation of *ultra-* [prefix indicating beyond or excess {not an abbrevi-
ation}]} {not an abbreviation}

UM
unmarried
upper motor [neuron] (neurology)
uracil mustard (chemotherapy, oncology, and pharmacology)

um
micron (measurement)

Umax
maximum solute concentration (chemistry, laboratory, and pharmacology)
maximum urinary osmolality (laboratory
and urology)

Umax.
maximum urinary osmolality (laboratory
and urology)

UMB
umbilical (neonatology)
umbilicus (anatomy and neonatology)

umb
umbilical (neonatology)
umbilicus (anatomy and neonatology)

Umb. + #F
umbilicus plus number of finger
breadths [height of fundus (including
a numeral)] (obstetrics)

umbo
{not an abbreviation} [a word meaning a
round projection] {pronounced "um-
bow"}

"um-bow"
{pronunciation of *umbo* [a word meaning a round projection {not an abbre-
viation}]} {not an abbreviation}

umb ven
umbilical vein (cardiovascular and neonatology)

U$_{Mg}$V
magnesium excretion (cardiovascular,
laboratory, and neurology)

UMMC
University of Michigan Medical Center
(administration, education, and research)

UMN
upper motor neuron (neurology)

U.M.N.
upper motor neuron (neurology)

UMNB
upper motor neurogenic bladder (neurology and urology)

UMNL
upper motor neuron lesion (neurology)

UMP
uridine-5'-phosphate [also called *uridine
monophosphate* and *uridylic acid*]
(laboratory)

UMS
urethral manipulation syndrome (urology)

UMT
Units of Medical Time [British] (measurement)

UN
ulnar nerve (anatomy, neurology, and orthopedics)
unilateral neglect (neurology and rehabilitation)
United Nations (government)
urea nitrogen (laboratory, nephrology, and urology)
urinary nitrogen (laboratory, nephrology, and urology)

UNA
urinary nitrogen appearance (laboratory, nephrology, and urology)

UNa
urine sodium (laboratory and nephrology)

U$_{Na}$
urinary concentration of sodium (laboratory and nephrology)

"U-nah-cef"
{pronunciation of *Unicef* [*United Nations International Children's Emergency Fund*]} {not an abbreviation}

U$_{Na}$V
sodium excretion (laboratory and nephrology)
sodium excretion [rate] (laboratory and nephrology)
urine sodium (laboratory and nephrology)

uncomp
uncompensated

uncond
unconditioned

uncond ref
unconditioned reflex (neurology)

UNCOR
uncorrected

UnCS
uncorrected stimulus (neurology)

unct
unctus [smeared] (pharmacology)

unct.
unctus [smeared] (pharmacology)

undet ori
undetermined origin

Unesco
United Nations Education, Scientific, and Cultural Organization (government) {pronounced "U-nez-co"}

"U-nez-co"
{pronunciation of *Unesco* [*United Nations Education, Scientific, and Cultural Organization*]} (government) {not an abbreviation}

UNG
unguentum [ointment] (pharmacology)

Ung
unguentum [ointment] (pharmacology)

ung
unguentum [ointment] (pharmacology)

ung.
unguentum [ointment] (pharmacology)

U$_{NH4}$+
urinary ammonium (gastroenterology, laboratory, and nephrology)

uni-
{not an abbreviation} [prefix meaning one] {pronounced "U-knee"}

Unicef
United Nations International Children's Emergency Fund (government) {pronounced "U-nah-cef"}

UNID
unidentified (laboratory)

unil
unilateral

unilat
unilateral {pronounced "U-knee-lat"}

Univ
university (education)

univ
universal

UNK
unknown
unofficial

Unk
unknown

unk
unknown

UNKN
unknown

unkn
unknown

UNRRA
United Nations Relief and Rehabilitation
  Administration (government)

UnS
unconditioned stimulus (neurology and
  psychiatry)

uns
unsatisfactory
unsymmetrical

unsat
unsaturated (laboratory)

unsym
unsymmetrical

UO
ureteral orifice (urology)
urinary output (urology)

U/O
under observation

UOA
United Ostomy Association (gastroenterology, nephrology, respiratory, and
  urology)

UOQ
upper outer quadrant (anatomy)

Uosm
urinary osmolality (laboratory and urology)

UOZ
upper outer zone [also called *upper
  outer quadrant*] (anatomy)

UP
under proof
upright posture (orthopedics)
ureteropelvic (anatomy, nephrology,
  and urology)
urine-plasma [ratio] (laboratory and
  urology)
uroporphyrin (dermatology, gastroenterology, genetics, hematology, laboratory, neurology, and psychiatry)
uteropelvic (gynecology)

U/P
urine-plasma [ratio] (laboratory and
  urology)

UPA
unpressurized aerosol [therapy] (pharmacology and respiratory)

up ad lib
up *ad libitum* [ambulatory, patient may
  walk] {pronounced "up-ad-lib"}

"up-ad-lib"
{pronunciation of *up ad lib* [up *ad libitum* (ambulatory, patient may walk)]}
{not an abbreviation}

UPEP
urine protein electrophoresis (laboratory) {pronounced "U-pep" or "you-
  pep"}

"U-pep"
{pronunciation of *UPEP* [urine protein electrophoresis]} (laboratory) {not an abbreviation}

UPF
universal proximal femur [prosthesis] (orthopedics)

UPG
uroporphyrinogen (dermatology, gastroenterology, genetics, hematology, laboratory, neurology, and psychiatry)

UPI
uteroplacental insufficiency (obstetrics)
uteroplacental ischemia (obstetrics)

UPJ
ureteropelvic junction (anatomy, nephrology, and urology)
uteropelvic junction (anatomy and gynecology)

UP (J)
ureteropelvic (junction) (anatomy, nephrology, and urology)

UPL
unusual position of limbs

UPOR
usual place of residence

UPP
universal proximal femoral prosthesis (orthopedics)
urethral pressure profile (urology)
uvulopalatopharyngoplasty (otorhinolaryngology)
uvulopalatoplasty (otorhinolaryngology)

UPPP
uvulopalatopharyngoplasty (otorhinolaryngology)

U/P ratio
urine-to-plasma concentration ratio (laboratory)

UPS
ultraviolet photoelectron (spectroscopy laboratory)

uninterruptable power source (computer science and electricity)
United Parcel Service (business)
United States Pharmacopoeia (pharmacology)
uterine progesterone system (gynecology and laboratory)

Upsher-S
Upsher-Smith [company] (pharmacology)

UPT
urine pregnancy test (gynecology, laboratory, and obstetrics)

U$_p$V
phosphate excretion rate (laboratory)

UQ
ubiquinone [also called *coenzyme Q*] (laboratory)
upper quadrant [of abdomen] (anatomy and gastroenterology)

UR
unconditioned reflex (neurology and psychiatry)
unconditioned response (neurology and psychiatry)
unsatisfactory report
upper respiratory (respiratory)
urinal (urology)
urine (urology)
urology
utilization review (medical records)

Ur
urine (laboratory and urology)

ur.
urine (laboratory and urology)

ur-
{not an abbreviation} [prefix indicating relationship to the urinary tract, urination, or urine] (urology) {pronounced "ur"}

"ur"
{pronunciation of *ur*- [prefix indicating relationship to the urinary tract, uri-

nation, or urine {not an abbreviation}]}
(urology) {not an abbreviation}

URA
uracil (chemotherapy, laboratory, oncology, and pharmacology)

"U-rah-nis-ko"
{pronunciation of *uranisco-* [prefix indicating relationship to the palate {not an abbreviation}]} (dentistry and otorhinolaryngology) {not an abbreviation}

ur anal
urine analysis [also called *urinalysis*] (laboratory and urology)

uranisco-
{not an abbreviation} [prefix indicating relationship to the palate] (dentistry and otorhinolaryngology) {pronounced "U-rah-nis-ko"}

urano-
{not an abbreviation} [1. prefix indicating relationship to the palate (dentistry and otorhinolaryngology);
2. prefix indicating relationship to heaven or the sky] {pronounced "U-ran-oh"}

"U-ran-oh"
{pronunciation of *urano-* [1. prefix indicating relationship to the palate {not an abbreviation} (dentistry and otorhinolaryngology); 2. prefix indicating relationship to heaven or the sky {not an abbreviation}]} {not an abbreviation}

URC
upper rib cage (anatomy, cardiovascular, orthopedics, and respiratory)
utilization review committee (medical records)

URC A
uric acid (laboratory, orthopedics, and rheumatology)

URC SP
uric acid—urine spot [test] (laboratory, orthopedics, and rheumatology)

URD
upper respiratory disease (respiratory)

UREA
urea nitrogen (laboratory, nephrology, and urology)

urea-
{not an abbreviation} [prefix indicating relationship to urea] (laboratory, nephrology, and urology) {pronounced "U-re-ah"}

"U-re-ah"
{pronunciation of *urea-* [prefix indicating relationship to urea (laboratory, nephrology, and urology) {not an abbreviation}] and *-uria* [suffix indicating a characteristic or component of the urine as indicated by the root word {not an abbreviation} (urology)]} {not an abbreviation}

UREA-S
urea nitrogen—urine spot [test] (laboratory, nephrology, and urology)

URED
unable to read (laboratory)

"U-re-no"
{pronunciation of *urino-* [prefix indicating relationship to urine {not an abbreviation}]} (urology) {not an abbreviation}

ureo-
{not an abbreviation} [prefix indicating relationship to urea] (laboratory, nephrology, and urology) {pronounced "U-re-oh"}

"U-re-oh"
{pronunciation of *ureo-* [prefix indicating relationship to urea (laboratory, nephrology, and urology) {not an abbreviation}]} {not an abbreviation}

uretero-
{not an abbreviation} [prefix indicating

relationship to the ureter] (urology)
{pronounced "U-re-ter-oh"}

"U-re-ter-oh"
{pronunciation of *uretero-* [prefix indicating relationship to the ureter {not
an abbreviation}]} (urology) {not an
abbreviation}

ureth
urethra(l) (anatomy, gynecology, and
urology)

urethro-
{not an abbreviation} [prefix indicating
relationship to the urethra] (anatomy,
gynecology, and urology) {pronounced
"U-re-thro"}

"U-re-thro"
{pronunciation of *urethro-* [prefix indi-
·cating relationship to the urethra {not
an abbreviation}]} (anatomy, gynecology, and urology) {not an abbrevia-
tion}

URF
relaxin (gynecology, laboratory, obstetrics, and pharmacology)
uterine-relaxing factor (gynecology, laboratory, and obstetrics)

UR-FST
urine—fasting (laboratory and urology)

urg
urgent

UR#HR
urine—number of hours/glucose tolerance [*The symbol is replaced with
the correct numeral.*] (endocrinology
and laboratory)

URI
upper respiratory infection (respiratory)
upper-respiratory-tract infection (respiratory)

U.R.I.
upper respiratory infection (respiratory)
upper-respiratory-tract infection (respiratory)

-uria
{not an abbreviation} [suffix indicating a
characteristic or component of the
urine as indicated by the root word]
(urology) {pronounced "U-re-ah"}

URIN
random urine (laboratory and urology)

urino-
{not an abbreviation} [prefix indicating
relationship to urine] (urology) {pro-
nounced "U-re-no"}

url
unrelated

UR & M
urinalysis—routine and microscopic
(laboratory and urology)

URO
urology
uroporphyrin (dermatology, gastroenterology, genetics, hematology, laboratory, neurology, and psychiatry)

uro-
{not an abbreviation} [prefix indicating
relationship to the urinary tract, urination, or urine] (nephrology and
urology) {pronounced "U-row"}

UROBIL
urobilinogen (dermatology, gastroenterology, genetics, hematology, laboratory, neurology, and psychiatry)

uro-gen
urogenital (gynecology and urology)

URO-2H
urobilinogen—2 hour (gastroenterology
and laboratory)

urol
urological (urology)
urologist (urology)
urology

urono-
{not an abbreviation} [prefix indicating relationship to the urinary tract, urination, or urine] (nephrology and urology) {pronounced "U-ron-oh"}

"U-ron-oh"
{pronunciation of *urono-* [prefix indicating relationship to the urinary tract, urination, or urine {not an abbreviation}]} (nephrology and urology) {not an abbreviation}

"U-row"
{pronunciation of *uro-* [prefix indicating relationship to the urinary tract, urination, or urine {not an abbreviation}]} (nephrology and urology) {not an abbreviation}

URQ
upper right quadrant [of abdomen] (anatomy and gastroenterology)

URS
ultrasonic renal scanning (nephrology and radiology)

URT
upper respiratory tract (respiratory)

URTI
upper-respiratory-tract infection (respiratory)

UR-TIM
urine—time (laboratory and urology)

URVD
unilateral renovascular disease (cardiovascular and nephrology)

UR VOL
urine volume (urology)

US
ultrasonic (cardiovascular, obstetrics, and radiology)
ultrasonography (cardiovascular, obstetrics, and radiology)
ultrasound (cardiovascular, obstetrics, and radiology)
unconditioned stimulus (neurology and psychiatry)
unit secretary (administration)
United States [of America] (government)
unknown significance (laboratory)
urinary space (urology)

U/S
ultrasound (cardiovascular, obstetrics, and radiology)

USA
unit services assistant (administration)
United States Army (armed forces)
United States of America (government)

USAF
United States Air Force (armed forces)

USAFH
United States Air Force Hospital (armed forces)

USAFRHL
United States Air Force Radiological Health Laboratory (armed forces, radiation therapy, and radiology)

USAH
United States Army Hospital (armed forces)

USAHC
United States Army Health Clinic (armed forces)

USAHS
United States Army Hospital Ship (armed forces)

USAMEDS
United States Army Medical Service (armed forces)

USAN
United States Adopted Names [Council] (pharmacology) {pronounced "U-san"}

"U-san"
{pronunciation of *USAN* [United States Adopted Names (Council)]} (pharmacology) {not an abbreviation}

USASI
United States of America Standards Institute {obsolete} [formerly American Standards Association (ASA); now American National Standards Institute (ANSI)] (government and measurement)

USB
United States Biochemical [Corporation] (chemistry)
upper sternal border (anatomy, cardiovascular, and respiratory)

USBS
United States Bureau of Standards (government and measurement)

USBuStand
United States Bureau of Standards (government and measurement)

USC
University of Southern California (education)

USCG
United States Coast Guard (armed forces)

USD
United States Dispensary (government)

USCI
United States Catheter Instrument (cardiovascular, manufacturing, and surgery)

USDA
United States Department of Agriculture (agriculture and government)

USDHHS
United States Department of Health and Human Service (government and social services)

USDT
United States Department of Transportation (government and transportation)

USG
ultrasonograph (cardiovascular, obstetrics, and radiology)

USHL
United States Hygienic Laboratory (laboratory)

USHMAC
United States Health Manpower Advisory Council (business and government)

USI
urinary stress incontinence (gynecology and urology)

USMC
United States Marine Corps (armed forces)

USMG
United States Medical Graduate (education)

USMH
United States Marine Hospital (armed forces)

USN
ultrasonic nebulizer (pharmacology and respiratory)
United States Navy (armed forces)

U.S.N.
ultrasonic nebulizer (pharmacology and respiratory)

USNH
United States Naval Hospital (armed forces)

USO
unilateral salpingo-oophorectomy (gynecology)
United Service Organizations (social services)

USP
United States Pharmacopeia (pharmacology)

U.S.P.
United States Pharmacopeia (pharmacology)

USPE
unsatisfactory specimen (laboratory)

USPHS
United States Public Health Service (government and public health)

USPS
United States Postal Service (government)

U.S.P. unit
{not an abbreviation} [used by the United States Pharmacopeia to express potency of a drug] (pharmacology)

USR
unheated serum reagin [test] (laboratory)

USS
ultrasound scanning (cardiovascular, obstetrics, and radiology)
United States Ship [precedes name of ship] (armed forces)

ust
ustus [burnt]

ust.
ustus [burnt]

USV
USV Pharmaceutical Corporation (pharmacology)

USVB
United States Veterans Bureau (armed forces and government)

USVH
United States Veterans Hospital (administration, armed forces, and government)

USVMD
urine specimen volume measuring device (laboratory and urology)

USVMS
urine sample volume measuring system (laboratory and urology)

UT
untested (laboratory)
untreated
urinary tract (gynecology, nephrology, and urology)
Utah [Postal Service state designation]
uterus (anatomy, gynecology, and obstetrics)

U$_{TA}$
urinary titratable acidity (laboratory)

UTBG
unbound testosterone-binding globulin (endocrinology and laboratory)
unbound thyroxine-binding globulin (endocrinology and laboratory)

UTD
up-to-date

UT DICT
ut dictum [as directed] (pharmacology)

ut dict
ut dictum [as directed] (pharmacology)

ut dict.
ut dictum [as directed] (pharmacology)

UTEND
utendus [to be used] (pharmacology)

utend
utendus [to be used] (pharmacology)

utend.
utendus [to be used] (pharmacology)

utend mor sol
utendus more solito [to be used in the usual manner] (pharmacology)

utend. mor. sol.
utendus more solito [to be used in the usual manner] (pharmacology)

utero-
{not an abbreviation} [prefix indicating relationship to the uterus] (gynecol-

ogy and obstetrics) {pronounced "U-ter-oh"}

"U-ter-oh"
{pronunciation of *utero-* [prefix indicating relationship to the uterus {not an abbreviation}]} (gynecology and obstetrics) {not an abbreviation}

UTF
usual throat flora (laboratory and otorhinolaryngology)

UTI
urinary tract infection(s) (nephrology and urology)

U.T.I.
urinary tract infection(s) (nephrology and urology)

UTI's
urinary tract infections (nephrology and urology)

UTLD
Utah Test of Language Development (speech and language therapy)

UTO
upper tibial osteotomy (orthopedics)

UTP
uridine triphosphate (laboratory)

UTZ
ultrasound (cardiovascular, obstetrics, and radiology)

UU
urine urobilin (gastroenterology and laboratory)
urine urobilinogen (gastroenterology and laboratory)

uU
micro- [prefix for 10^{-6}] (measurement)

UUN
urinary urea nitrogen (laboratory and nephrology)
urine urea nitrogen (laboratory and nephrology)

UUP
urine uroporphyrin (dermatology, gastroenterology, genetics, hematology, laboratory, neurology, and psychiatry)

U urea
urinary concentration of urea (laboratory and nephrology)

UV
ultrafine
ultraviolet [light] (dermatology, orthopedics, and physical therapy)
umbilical vein (anatomy, cardiovascular, and neonatology)
ureterovesical (urology)
urethrovesical (urology)
urinary volume (measurement and urology)

U.V.
ultraviolet [light] (dermatology, orthopedics, and physical therapy)

U$_v$
Uppsala virus [also called *U virus*] (laboratory)

uv
umbilical vein (anatomy, cardiovascular, and neonatology)

UVA
ultraviolet light, long wave [also called *ultraviolet A light*] (dermatology, orthopedics, and physical therapy)
ureterovesical angle (gynecology and urology)
urethrovesical angle (gynecology and urology)

UVB
ultraviolet light, midrange sunbeam spectrum [also called *ultraviolet B light*] (dermatology, orthopedics, and physical therapy)

UVC
umbilical vein catheter (cardiovascular and neonatology)

UVI
ultraviolet irradiation (dermatology, orthopedics, and physical therapy)

UVJ
ureterovesical junction (urology)
urethrovesical junction (urology)

UVL
ultraviolet light (dermatology, orthopedics, and physical therapy)

UVP
ultraviolet photometry (dermatology, orthopedics, and physical therapy)

UV/P
{not an abbreviation} [formula for clearance of a substance or ratio with *U* referring to the concentration of solute in urine, *V* referring to the quantity of urine excreted in a given unit of time, and *P* the concentration of the substance in plasma] (laboratory)

UVR
ultraviolet radiation (dermatology, orthopedics, and physical therapy)

U-wave
{not an abbreviation} [found on electrocardiograms] (cardiovascular)

UWF
unknown white female (emergency medicine)

UWM
unknown white male (emergency medicine)
University of Wisconsin, Milwaukee (education)

ux
uxor [wife]

ux.
uxor [wife]

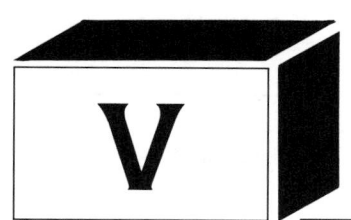

V

V
chest (respiratory)
coefficient of variation
dead space (respiratory and surgery)
five [Roman numeral]
gas volume [in gas phase] (laboratory and respiratory)
gas volume per unit time (laboratory and respiratory)
minute volume (laboratory)
tidal volume-mechanical (respiratory)
vaccinated (immunology, infectious diseases, pediatrics, and pharmacology)
vagina (anatomy, gynecology, and obstetrics)
valine [an amino acid] (endocrinology and laboratory)
valve (cardiovascular)
vanadium (chemistry and pharmacology)
variation
varnish (dentistry)
vector
vein (cardiovascular)
velocity
ventilation (respiratory)
ventral
ventricular (cardiovascular)
verbal
verbalization (speech and language therapy)
verbalize(s) (speech and language therapy)
vertex (obstetrics)
very
Vibrio [a bacterium] (bacteriology and laboratory)
vide [see]
viel [coarse]
violet
virgin
virulence
virus (laboratory)
vision (ophthalmology)
visit
visitor
visual acuity (ophthalmology)

voice (otorhinolaryngology and speech and language therapy)
volt (measurement)
voltage (electricity)
volume (measurement)
vomiting (gastroenterology)
{not an abbreviation} [unipolar chest lead on electrocardiogram] (cardiovascular)

V.
Vibrio [a bacterium] (bacteriology and laboratory)
vision (ophthalmology)
visual acuity (ophthalmology)

μV
microvolt (measurement)

μv
microvolt (measurement)

V₁
fifth cranial nerve, ophthalmic division (neurology and ophthalmology)
{not an abbreviation} [placement position of a precordial lead on fourth intercostal space at right sternal border for an electrocardiogram] (cardiovascular)

V₂
fifth cranial nerve, maxillary division (neurology and otorhinolaryngology)
{not an abbreviation} [placement position of a precordial lead at fourth intercostal space at left sternal border for an electrocardiogram] (cardiovascular)

V₃
fifth cranial nerve, mandibular division (neurology and otorhinolaryngology)
{not an abbreviation} [placement position of a precordial lead equidistant

between V_2 and V_4 for an electrocardiogram] (cardiovascular)

V₄
{not an abbreviation} [placement position of a precordial lead at fifth intercostal space in left midclavicular line for an electrocardiogram] (cardiovascular)

V₅
{not an abbreviation} [placement position of a precordial lead at anterior axillary line for an electrocardiogram] (cardiovascular)

V₆
{not an abbreviation} [placement position of a precordial lead at midaxillary line for an electrocardiogram] (cardiovascular)

V
mixed venous blood (laboratory and respiratory)
vel [or]
venous in the blood phase (laboratory and respiratory)
versus
very
vide [see]
vitamin (dietary, laboratory, and pharmacology)
volt (measurement)
von [of (German; used in names of people and places)]

v
(Note: The v is subscripted.)
venous blood (cardiovascular and laboratory)

v.
specific volume (measurement)
vein (cardiovascular)
velocity
vena [vein] (cardiovascular)
versus
very
vide [see]
virus (laboratory)
vitamin (dietary, laboratory, and pharmacology)
volt (measurement)

V̄
mixed venous in the blood phase (laboratory and respiratory)

V̇
flow [gas volume/unit time] (laboratory and respiratory)

v-
{not an abbreviation} [prefix referring to vicinal isomer] (chemistry)

v-:
vicinal isomer (chemistry)

VA
vacuum aspiration (respiratory)
valproic acid (neurology and pharmacology)
venoarterial (cardiovascular)
ventriculoatrial (cardiovascular)
vertebral artery (cardiovascular, neurology, and orthopedics)
Veterans Administration (armed forces and government)
viral antigen (laboratory)
Virginia [Postal Service state designation]
visual acuity (ophthalmology)
visual aid (ophthalmology)
volt-ampere (measurement)

V.A.
visual acuity (ophthalmology)

V$_A$
alveolar gas volume (laboratory and respiratory)
alveolar ventilation per minute (laboratory and respiratory)

V.A.
Veterans Administration (armed forces and government)

Va
alveolar ventilation (respiratory)
visual acuity (ophthalmology)
volt-ampere (measurement)

V$_a$
alveolar ventilation (respiratory)

va
variety
volt-ampere (measurement)

VAB
vinblastine, actinomycin D, and bleomycin (chemotherapy, oncology, and pharmacology)

VAB-II
vinblastine, actinomycin D, bleomycin, and cisplatin (chemotherapy, oncology, and pharmacology)

VAB-III
vinblastine, actinomycin D, bleomycin, cisplatin, cycylophosphamide, and chlorambucil (chemotherapy, oncology, and pharmacology)

VAB-III modified
vinblastine, actinomycin D, bleomycin, cisplatin, and cycylophosphamide (chemotherapy, oncology, and pharmacology)

VAB-IV
vinblastine, actinomycin D, bleomycin, cisplatin, cyclophosphamide, chlorambucil, and Adriamycin (chemotherapy, oncology, and pharmacology)

VAB-V
vinblastine, actinomycin D, bleomycin, cisplatin, and cyclophosphamide (chemotherapy, oncology, and pharmacology)

VAC
ventriculoarterial connections (cardiovascular)
ventriculoatrial conduction (cardiovascular)
vincristine, actinomycin D [dactinomycin], and cyclophosphamide [Cytoxan] (chemotherapy, oncology, and pharmacology) {pronounced "vak"}
vincristine, Adriamycin [doxorubicin], and cyclophosphamide [Cytoxan] (chemotherapy, oncology, and pharmacology) {pronounced "vak"}

virus capsid antigen (laboratory)

VAC Pulse
vincristine [Oncovin], actinomycin D [dactinomycin], and cyclophosphamide [Cytoxan] (chemotherapy, oncology, and pharmacology) {pronounced "vak-pulse"}

VAC Standard
vincristine [Oncovin], actinomycin D [dactinomycin], and cyclophosphamide [Cytoxan] (chemotherapy, oncology, and pharmacology) {pronounced "vak-stan-dard"}

vac
vacuum

vac.
vaccine (immunology, infectious diseases, pediatrics, and pharmacology)
vacuum

VACAR
vincristine, Adriamycin, cyclophosphamide, and actinomycin D (chemotherapy, oncology, and pharmacology)

vacc
vaccination (immunology, infectious diseases, pediatrics, and pharmacology)

"vack-ter-el"
{pronunciation of *VACTERL* [vertebral, anal, cardiac, tracheoesophageal, renal, and limb (defects) and vertebral or vascular defects, anorectal malformation (imperforate anus), cardiac anomaly, tracheoesophageal fistula, renal anomaly, and limb anomaly (syndrome)]} (cardiovascular, gastroenterology, genetics, nephrology, neonatology, orthopedics, and pediatrics) {not an abbreviation}

VACTERL
vertebral, anal, cardiac, tracheoesophageal, renal, and limb [defects] (cardiovascular, gastroenterology, genetics, nephrology, neonatology, orthopedics,

and pediatrics) {pronounced "vack-ter-el"}

vertebral or vascular defects, anorectal malformation (imperforate anus), cardiac anomaly, tracheoesophageal fistula, renal anomaly, and limb anomaly [syndrome] (cardiovascular, gastroenterology, genetics, nephrology, neonatology, orthopedics, and pediatrics) {pronounced "vack-ter-el"}

VAD
vascular access device (cardiovascular and nephrology)
venous access device (cardiovascular and nephrology)
ventricular assist device (cardiovascular)
vitamin A deficiency (ophthalmology)
Voluntary Aid Detachment

VAd
Veterans Administration (armed forces and government)

VADA
vincristine, Adriamycin, cyclophosphamide, and actinomycin D (chemotherapy, oncology, and pharmacology)

VADRC
vincristine, Adriamycin, and cyclophosphamide (chemotherapy, oncology, and pharmacology)

V$_A$eff
effective alveolar ventilation (laboratory and respiratory)

VAFAC
vincristine, Adriamycin, 5-fluorouracil, methotrexate, and cyclophosphamide (chemotherapy, oncology, and pharmacology)

VAG
vagina(l) (anatomy, gynecology, and obstetrics)

Vag
vagina(l) (anatomy, gynecology, and obstetrics)

vag
vagina(l) (anatomy, gynecology, and obstetrics)
vaginitis (gynecology and obstetrics)

VAG HYST
vaginal hysterectomy (gynecology)

vagino-
{not an abbreviation} [prefix indicating relationship to the vagina] (gynecology and obstetrics) {pronounced "vah-gin-oh"}

VAH
Veterans Administration Hospital (administration, armed forces, and government)
virilizing adrenal hyperplasia [also called *adrenogenital syndrome*] (endocrinology, genetics, gynecology, and urology)

"vah-gin-oh"
{pronunciation of *vagino-* [prefix indicating relationship to the vagina {not an abbreviation}]} (gynecology and obstetrics) {not an abbreviation}

VAHS
virus-associated hemophagocytic syndrome (hematology)

VAIN
vaginal intraepithelial neoplasia (gynecology and oncology)

"vak"
{pronunciation of *VAC* [vincristine (Oncovin), actinomycin D (dactinomycin), and cyclophosphamide (Cytoxan) and vincristine (Oncovin), Adriamycin (doxorubicin), and cyclophosphamide (Cytoxan) {not an abbreviation}]} (chemotherapy, oncology, and pharmacology) {not an abbreviation}

"vak-pulse"
{pronunciation of *VAC Pulse* [vincristine (Oncovin), actinomycin D (dactino-

mycin), and cyclophosphamide (Cytoxan)]} (chemotherapy, oncology, and pharmacology) {not an abbreviation}

"vak-stan-dard"
{pronunciation of *VAC Standard* [vincristine (Oncovin), actinomycin D (dactinomycin), and cyclophosphamide (Cytoxan) {not an abbreviation}]} (chemotherapy, oncology, and pharmacology) {not an abbreviation}

VAKT
visual, association, kinaesthetic, tactile [referring to reading] (speech and language therapy)

VAL
valine [an amino acid] (endocrinology and laboratory)

Val
valine [an amino acid] (endocrinology and laboratory)
Valium [a tranquilizer] (chemical dependency, neurology, and pharmacology) {pronounced "val"}

"val"
{pronunciation of *Val* [Valium (a tranquilizer]} (chemical dependency, neurology, and pharmacology) {not an abbreviation}

VALE
visual acuity, left eye (ophthalmology)

Vals
Valium [a tranquilizer] {slang} (chemical dependency, neurology, and pharmacology) {pronounced "valz"}

"valz"
{pronunciation of *Vals* [Valium (a tranquilizer)]} (chemical dependency, neurology, and pharmacology) {not an abbreviation}

VAM
VP-16 [etoposide], Adriamycin, and methotrexate (chemotherapy, oncology, and pharmacology)

VAMC
Veterans Administration Medical Center (armed forces and government)

VAMP
vincristine, actinomycin, methotrexate, and prednisone (chemotherapy, oncology, and pharmacology) {pronounced "vamp"}
vincristine, methotrexate [Amethopterine], 6-mercaptopurine, and prednisone (chemotherapy, oncology, and pharmacology) {pronounced "vamp"}

"vamp"
{pronunciation of *VAMP* [vincristine, actinomycin, methotrexate, and prednisone or vincristine, methotrexate (Amethopterine), 6-mercaptopurine, and prednisone]} (chemotherapy, oncology, and pharmacology) {not an abbreviation}

VAP
variant angina pectoris (cardiovascular)
vincristine, Adriamycin, and prednisone (chemotherapy, oncology, and pharmacology)
vincristine, Adriamycin, and procarbazine (chemotherapy, oncology, and pharmacology)

VAP-II
vinblastine, actinomycin D, and cisplatin (chemotherapy, oncology, and pharmacology)

VA/Q
ventilation-perfusion [ratio] (radiology and respiratory)

V_A/Q_C ratio
ventilation-perfusion ratio (radiology and respiratory)

VAR
variant
variation

var
variable

variation
variety

var.
variant
variation
variety

"var-ah-co"
{pronunciation of *varico-* [prefix indicating relationship to a varix (cardiovascular) or meaning swollen and twisted {not an abbreviation}]} {not an abbreviation}

VARE
visual acuity, right eye (ophthalmology)

varico-
{not an abbreviation} [prefix indicating relationship to a varix (cardiovascular) or meaning swollen and twisted] {pronounced "var-ah-co"}

VAS
vascular (cardiovascular)
vesicle attachment site (anatomy)
visual analogue scale (ophthalmology)

vas
vas deferens (urology)

vas.
vasectomy (urology)

VASC
vascular (cardiovascular)
Verbal-Auditory Screen for Children (otorhinolaryngology and pediatrics)
Visual-Auditory Screen Test for Children (ophthalmology, otorhinolaryngology, and pediatrics)

vasc
vascular (cardiovascular)

vasio-Para
Veterans Administration Seating Interface Orthosis for Paraplegics (neurology, orthopedics, and rehabilitation)

vaso-
{not an abbreviation} [prefix indicating

relationship to a duct or a vessel] (cardiovascular) {pronounced "vay-zoe"}

VAS RAD
vascular radiology (cardiovascular and radiology)

vas vit
vas vitreum [a glass vessel]

vas. vit.
vas vitreum [a glass vessel]

VAT
variable antigen type (laboratory)
ventricular activation time (cardiovascular)
vincristine, cytosine arabinoside, 6-thioguanine, and daunomycin (chemotherapy, oncology, and pharmacology)
visual action time (ophthalmology)
visual apperception test (ophthalmology)
voice-activated transcription [machine] (business)
voice-activated typewriter (business)

VATER
vertebral defects, imperforate anus, tracheoesophageal fistula, and radial and renal dysplasia [syndrome] (gastroenterology, genetics, nephrology, neurology, orthopedics, otorhinolaryngology, and pediatrics) {pronounced "vay-ter"}
vertebral and/or vascular defects, anorectal malformation, tracheoesophageal fistula, and radial, ray, or renal anomaly [syndrome] (gastroenterology, genetics, nephrology, neurology, orthopedics, otorhinolaryngology, and pediatrics) {pronounced "vay-ter"}

VATERL
vertebral defects, imperforate anus, tracheoesophageal fistula, radial and renal dysplasia, and limb anomalies [syndrome] (gastroenterology, genetics, nephrology, neurology, orthopedics, and pediatrics) {pronounced "vay-ter-el"}

VATH
vinblastine, Adriamycin, ThioTEPA, and halotensin (chemotherapy, oncology, and pharmacology)

VAV
VP-16 [etoposide], Adriamycin, and vincristine (chemotherapy, oncology, and pharmacology)

"vay-ter"
{pronunciation of *VATER* [vertebral defects, imperforate anus, tracheoesophageal fistula, and radial and renal dysplasia (syndrome) and vertebral and/or vascular defects, anorectal malformation, tracheoesophageal fistula, and radial, ray, or renal anomaly (syndrome)]} (gastroenterology, genetics, nephrology, neurology, orthopedics, otorhinolaryngology, and pediatrics) {not an abbreviation}

"vay-ter-el"
{pronunciation of *VATERL* [vertebral defects, imperforate anus, tracheoesophageal fistula, radial and renal dysplasia, and limb anomalies [syndrome]] } (gastroenterology, genetics, nephrology, neurology, orthopedics, and pediatrics) {not an abbreviation}

"vay-zoe"
{pronunciation of *vaso-* [prefix indicating relationship to a duct or a vessel {not an abbreviation}]} (cardiovascular) {not an abbreviation}

VB
van Buren [catheter] (surgery)
ventrobasal [complex of thalamus] (anatomy and neurology)
vertebral body (anatomy, orthopedics, and radiology)
viable birth (obstetrics)
vinblastine (chemotherapy, oncology, and pharmacology)

V-B1
vitamin B_1 [also called *thiamine*] (pharmacology)

V-B6
vitamin B_6 [also called *pyridoxine*] (pharmacology)

V-B12
vitamin B_{12} [also called *cyanocobalamine*] (pharmacology)

VBA
V. B. Anderson Company [oxygen equipment] (pharmacology and respiratory)

VBAC
vaginal birth after cesarean [section] (obstetrics) {pronounced "vee-back"}

VBAP
vincristine, 1,3-bis(2-chloroethyl)-1-nitrososurea [BCNU or carmustine], Adriamycin, and prednisone (chemotherapy, oncology, and pharmacology)

VBC
vincristine, bleomycin, and cisplatin (chemotherapy, oncology, and pharmacology)

VBD
vinblastine, bleomycin, and cisplatin (chemotherapy, oncology, and pharmacology)

VBG
vertical banded gastroplasty (gastroenterology and surgery)

VBI
vertebral basilar insufficiency [also called *vertebrobasilar insufficiency*] (cardiovascular and neurology)

VBL
vinblastine (chemotherapy, oncology, and pharmacology)

VBOS
veronal-buffered oxalated saline [barbital] (anesthesiology, neurology, and pharmacology)

VBMCP
vincristine, 1,3-bis(2-chloroethyl)-1-nitrososurea [BCNU or carmustine], L-phenylalanine mustard, cyclophosphamide, and prednisone (chemotherapy, oncology, and pharmacology)

VBP
vinblastine, bleomycin, and cisplatin [Platinol] (chemotherapy, oncology, and pharmacology)

VBS
vacation bible school (education and religion)
veronal-buffered saline [medium] (laboratory)
vertebral basilar [artery] system [also called *vertebrobasilar (artery) system*] (cardiovascular and neurology)

VBS:FBS
veronal-buffered saline—fetal bovine serum (laboratory)

VBT
vertebral body tenderness (neurology and orthopedics)

VC
acuity of color vision (ophthalmology)
color vision (ophthalmology)
vasoconstriction (cardiovascular)
vasoconstrictor (cardiovascular and pharmacology)
vena cava (cardiovascular)
venereal case (gynecology, infectious diseases, and urology)
ventilatory capacity (respiratory)
ventral column (anatomy)
Veterinary Corps (veterinary medicine)
videocassette
Viet Cong (armed forces and government)
vincristine (chemotherapy, oncology, and pharmacology)
vinyl chloride (chemistry)
visual capacity (ophthalmology)
visual cortex (ophthalmology)
vital capacity (laboratory and respiratory)
vitamin capsule (pharmacology)
vocal cord(s) (otorhinolaryngology)

V.C.
vital capacity (respiratory)

V/C
ventilation-to-circulation [ratio] (cardiovascular and respiratory)

V_c
pulmonary capillary blood volume (cardiovascular and respiratory)

VCA
vancomycin, colistin, and anisomycin [inhibitor] (laboratory and pharmacology)
viral capsid antibody (laboratory)
viral capsid antigen (laboratory)

VCAP
vincristine, cyclophosphamide, Adriamycin, and prednisone (chemotherapy, oncology, and pharmacology)

VCAP-I
VP-16 [etoposide], cyclophosphamide, Adriamycin, and cisplatin (chemotherapy, oncology, and pharmacology)

VDC
vibrational circular dichroism

VCE
vagina, ectocervix, and endocervix (gynecology and obstetrics)

VCC
vasoconstrictor center (cardiovascular)

V_{CE}
velocity of contractile element

VCF
vincristine, 5-fluorouracil, and cyclophosphamide (chemotherapy, oncology, and pharmacology)

V_{CF}
velocity of circumferential shortening

VCG
vectorcardiogram (cardiovascular)

VCI
volatile corrosion inhibitor (chemistry)

V-Cillin
{not an abbreviation} [brand name for *penicillin V*] (pharmacology) {pronounced "vee-sill-en"}

VCMP
vincristine, melphalan, cyclophosphamide, and prednisone (chemotherapy, oncology, and pharmacology)

VCN
vancomycin hydrochloride, colistimethate sodium, nystatin [medium] (laboratory)

V_{CO}
carbon monoxide [endogenous production] (respiratory)

VCO_2
carbon dioxide production (respiratory)

V_{CO_2}
carbon dioxide output (laboratory and respiratory)

V_{CO_2}
carbon dioxide production per minute (laboratory and respiratory)

VCP
Veterinary Creolin-Pearson [an antiseptic and parasiticide] (chemistry, pharmacology, and veterinary medicine)
vincristine, cyclophosphamide, and prednisone (chemotherapy, oncology, and pharmacology)
Virus Cancer Program (oncology and research)

VCP-1
VP-16 [etoposide], cyclophosphamide, and cisplatin (chemotherapy, oncology, and pharmacology)

VCR
vincristine sulfate [also called *leurocristine*] (chemotherapy, oncology, and pharmacology)

V-C ratio
ventilation-circulation ratio (cardiovascular and respiratory)

VCS
vasoconstrictor substance (cardiovascular, laboratory, and pharmacology)
Vocabulary Comprehension Scale (speech and language therapy)

VCT
venous clotting time (hematology and laboratory)

VCU
videocystourethrography (radiology and urology)
voiding cystourethrogram (radiology and urology)

VCUG
vesicoureterogram (radiology and urology)
voiding cystourethrogram (radiology and urology)

VD
vapor density (chemistry)
vascular disease (cardiovascular)
vasodilation (cardiovascular)
vasodilator (cardiovascular and pharmacology)
venereal disease (gynecology, infectious diseases, and urology)
ventricular dilator (cardiovascular and pharmacology)
vertical deviation
viral diarrhea (gastroenterology and infectious diseases)
virus diarrhea (gastroenterology and infectious diseases)
voided (urology)
volume of distribution

V.D.
venereal disease (gynecology, infectious diseases, and urology)

V_D
physiologic dead-space volume (respiratory)

ventilation per minute of the physiological dead-space [wasted ventilation] (respiratory)

Vd
void (urology)
volume dead air space (respiratory)

V$_d$
apparent volume of distribution [also called *V area*] (respiratory)

vd
double vibrations [referring to cycles]
void (urology)

VDA
venous digital angiogram (cardiovascular and radiology)
visual discriminatory acuity (ophthalmology)

V$_D$A
alveolar dead-space volume (respiratory)
ventilation of the alveolar dead-space (respiratory)

VDAC
vaginal delivery after cesarean section (obstetrics) {pronounced "vee-dack"}

V$_D$an
ventilation per minute of the anatomic dead-space (respiratory)
volume of the anatomic dead-space (respiratory)

VDBR
volume of distribution of bilirubin (gastroenterology and laboratory)

VDC
vasodilator center (cardiovascular)

VDEL
Venereal Disease Experimental Laboratory (gynecology, infectious diseases, research, and urology)

VDEM
vasodepressor material (cardiovascular, laboratory, and pharmacology)

VDF
ventricular diastolic fragmentation (cardiovascular)

VDG
venereal disease—gonorrhea (gynecology, infectious diseases, and urology)
voiding (urology)

V.D.G.
venereal disease—gonorrhea (gynecology, infectious diseases, and urology)

Vdg
voiding (urology)

vdg.
voiding (urology)

VDH
valvular disease of the heart (cardiovascular)

V.D.H.
valvular disease of the heart (cardiovascular)

VDL
vasodepressor lipid (cardiovascular and laboratory)
visual detection level

VDM
vasodepressor material (cardiovascular, laboratory, and pharmacology)

V$_{DM}$
volume of mechanical dead space (respiratory)

VDP
vincristine, daunomycin [daunorubicin], and prednisone (chemotherapy, oncology, and pharmacology)

VDR
venous diameter ratio (cardiovascular)

V$_D$rb
rebreathing ventilation (respiratory)

rebreathing volume [of any external respiratory apparatus] (respiratory)

VDRL

Venereal Disease Research Laboratory (gynecology, infectious diseases, research, and urology)

{not an abbreviation} [The VDRL test is produced by the Venereal Disease Research Laboratory.] (gynecology, infectious diseases, laboratory, and urology)

VDRL antigen

{not an abbreviation} [an alcohol solution used to produce standard reactivity] (gynecology, infectious diseases, laboratory, and urology)

VDRL test

{not an abbreviation} [The VDRL test is produced by the Venereal Disease Research Laboratory.] (gynecology, infectious diseases, laboratory, and urology)

VDRR

vitamin D–resistant rickets (orthopedics)

VDRS

Verdun Depression Rating Scale (psychiatry)

VDRT

Venereal Disease Reference Test [of Harris] (gynecology, infectious diseases, laboratory, and urology)

VDS

vasodilator substance (cardiovascular, laboratory, and pharmacology)
venereal disease—syphilis (gynecology, infectious diseases, and urology)
vindesine (chemotherapy, oncology, and pharmacology)

V.D.S.

venereal disease—syphilis (gynecology, infectious diseases, and urology)

VDT

video display terminal (computer sciences)

visual display terminal (computer sciences)

VDV

ventricular end-diastolic volume (cardiovascular)

V_DV_T

physiologic dead space in percent of tidal volume (respiratory)

VE

minute ventilation (respiratory)
vaginal examination (gynecology and obstetrics)
venous emptying (cardiovascular)
ventilation (respiratory)
ventricular extrasystole (cardiovascular)
vertex (obstetrics)
vesicular exanthema (dermatology)
viral encephalitis (neurology)
visual efficiency (ophthalmology)
volume ejection (cardiovascular)
voluntary effort

V.E.

vaginal examination (gynecology and obstetrics)

V_E

airflow per unit of time (respiratory)
environmental variance
respiratory minute volume (respiratory)
volume of expired gas (respiratory)

V & E

Vinethene and ether (anesthesiology and pharmacology)

VEA

ventricular ectopic activity (cardiovascular)
viral envelope antigen(s) (laboratory)

VEB

ventricular ectopic beat(s) (cardiovascular)

VECG

vector electrocardiogram (cardiovascular)

VECP
visually evoked cortical potential(s)
(neurology)

VED
ventricular ectopic depolarization (cardiovascular)
vitral exhaustion and depression

VEE
vagina, ectocervix, and endocervix (gynecology and obstetrics)
Venezuelan equine encephalitis (infectious diseases and neurology)
Venezuelan equine encephalomyelitis (infectious diseases and neurology)

"vee-back"
{pronunciation of *VBAC* [vaginal birth after cesarean (section)]} (obstetrics) {not an abbreviation}

"vee-dack"
{pronunciation of *VDAC* [vaginal delivery after cesarean section]} (obstetrics) {not an abbreviation}

"vee-fib"
{pronunciation of *V Fib, V. Fib., V fib,* and *Vfib* [ventricular fibrillation]} (cardiovascular) {not an abbreviation}

"vee-no"
{pronunciation of *veno-* [prefix indicating relationship to a vein {not an abbreviation}]} (cardiovascular) {not an abbreviation}

"veer-ooh"
{pronunciation of *veru* [verumontanum]} (anatomy and urology) {not an abbreviation}

"vee-sill-en"
{pronunciation of *V-Cillin* [brand name for penicillin V]} (pharmacology) {not an abbreviation}

"vee-tack"
{pronunciation of *V-TACH, V tach,* and *v. tach.* [ventricular tachycardia]} (cardiovascular) {not an abbreviation}

"vee-vah"
{pronunciation of *vivi-* [prefix meaning alive or indicating relationship to life {not an abbreviation}]} {not an abbreviation}

VEE virus
Venezuelan equine encephalomyelitis virus (infectious diseases and neurology)

VEF
ventricular ejection fraction (cardiovascular)

"veg-gee"
{pronunciation of *veggie* [vegetable]} (dietary) {not an abbreviation}

veggie
vegetable (dietary) {pronounced "veg-gee"}

V$_{EH}$
extrahepatic distribution (gastroenterology)

vehic
vehicle
vehiculum [vehicle]

vehic.
vehicle
vehiculum [vehicle]

V$_{EH}^{(+)}$
extrahepatic tri-iodthyronine distribution volume, timed (gastroenterology and radiology)

vel
velocity

vel.
velocity

veloc
velocity

veloc.
velocity

VEM
vasoexcitor material (cardiovascular, laboratory, and pharmacology)

V$_{Emax}$
maximum flow per unit of time (respiratory)

V$_{Emax}$
maximum flow per unit of time (respiratory)

VEMP
vincristine, cyclophosphamide [Endoxan], 6-mercaptopurine, and prednisone (chemotherapy, oncology, and pharmacology)

veno-
{not an abbreviation} [prefix indicating relationship to a vein] (cardiovascular) {pronounced "vee-no"}

VENT
ventricular (cardiovascular and neurology)

Vent
ventricle (cardiovascular and neurology)

vent
ventilation (respiratory)
ventilator (respiratory)
ventral
ventricular (cardiovascular and neurology)

vent.
ventral
ventricular (cardiovascular and neurology)

vent fib
ventricular fibrillation (cardiovascular)

vent. fib.
ventricular fibrillation (cardiovascular)

"ven-tree"
{pronunciation of *ventri-* [prefix indicating relationship to the belly or to the anterior or front aspect of the body {not an abbreviation}]} {not an abbreviation}

ventri-
{not an abbreviation} [prefix indicating relationship to the belly or to the anterior or front aspect of the body] {pronounced "ven-tree"}

ventric
ventricle (cardiovascular and neurology)
ventricular (cardiovascular and neurology)

"ven-trick-U-low"
{pronunciation of *ventriculo-* [prefix indicating relationship to a ventricle of the brain or the heart {not an abbreviation}]} (cardiovascular and neurology) {not an abbreviation}

ventriculo-
{not an abbreviation} [prefix indicating relationship to a ventricle of the brain or the heart] (cardiovascular and neurology) {pronounced "ven-trick-U-low"}

ventro-
{not an abbreviation} [prefix indicating relationship to the belly or to the anterior or front aspect of the body] {pronounced "ven-tro"}

"ven-tro"
{pronunciation of *ventro-* [prefix indicating relationship to the belly or to the anterior or front aspect of the body {not an abbreviation}]} {not an abbreviation}

VEP
ventricular escape rhythm (cardiovascular)
visual evoked potential(s) (neurology)

VER
visual evoked response(s) (neurology)

Vert
vertebra(l) (neurology and orthopedics)

vert
vertebra(l) (neurology and orthopedics)
vertical

vert.
vertebra(l) (neurology and orthopedics)
vertical

"ver-tee-bro"
{pronunciation of *vertebro-* [prefix indicating relationship to a vertebra or to the vertebral column {not an abbreviation}]} (neurology and orthopedics) {not an abbreviation}

vertebro-
{not an abbreviation} [prefix indicating relationship to a vertebra or to the vertebral column] (neurology and orthopedics) {pronounced "ver-tee-bro"}

veru
verumontanum (anatomy and urology) {pronounced "veer-ooh"}

VES
vesica [bladder] (urology)
vessel (cardiovascular)

ves
vesica [bladder] (urology)
vesicular [referring to breath sounds] (respiratory)

ves.
vesica [bladder] (urology)
vesicular [referring to breath sounds] (respiratory)

"ves-ah-co"
{pronunciation of *vesico-* [prefix indicating relationship to the bladder (urology) or to a blister (dermatology) {not an abbreviation}]} {not an abbreviation}

VESIC
vesicula [a blister, *vesicatorium*] (dermatology)
vesicatorium [a blister, *vesicula*] (dermatology)

vesic
vesicula [a blister, *vesicatorium*] (dermatology)
vesicatorium [a blister, *vesicula*] (dermatology)

vesic.
vesicula [a blister, *vesicatorium*] (dermatology)
vesicatorium [a blister, *vesicula*] (dermatology)

vesico-
{not an abbreviation} [prefix indicating relationship to the bladder (urology) or to a blister (dermatology)] {pronounced "ves-ah-co"}

vesp
vesper [evening]

vesp.
vesper [evening]

ves ur
vesica urinaria [urinary bladder] (urology)

ves. ur.
vesica urinaria [urinary bladder] (urology)

VESV
vesicular exanthema of swine virus (dermatology and veterinary medicine)

VET
vestigial testis (endocrinology, research, and urology)
vestigial testis [rat] (endocrinology, research, urology, and veterinary medicine)
veteran (armed forces) {pronounced "vet"}
veterinary (veterinary medicine) {pronounced "vet"}

Vet
veteran (armed forces) {pronounced "vet"}
veterinary (veterinary medicine) {pronounced "vet"}

vet
veterinary (veterinary medicine) {pronounced "vet"}

v et
vide etiam [see also]

v. et.
vide etiam [see also]

"vet"
{pronunciation of *VET* and *Vet* [veteran (armed forces) and veterinary (veterinary medicine)] and *vet* [veterinary] (veterinary medicine)]} {not an abbreviation}

VetAdmin
Veterans Administration (armed forces and government)

Vet Med
veterinary medicine {pronounced "vet-med"}

"vet-med"
{pronunciation of *Vet Med* [veterinary medicine]} {not an abbreviation}

VetSci
veterinary science (veterinary medicine) {pronounced "vet-sigh"}

"vet-sigh"
{pronunciation of *VetSci* [veterinary science]} (veterinary medicine) {not an abbreviation}

VF
ventricular fibrillation (cardiovascular)
ventricular fluid (cardiovascular and neurology)
vision field (ophthalmology)
visual field (ophthalmology)
vocal fremitus (respiratory)
{not an abbreviation} [position of left leg electrode for electrocardiogram] (cardiovascular)

V.F.
visual field (ophthalmology)
vocal fremitus (respiratory)

Vf
visual field (ophthalmology)

Vf.
ventricular fibrillation (cardiovascular)

V.f.
field of vision (ophthalmology)

V factor
verbal comprehension factor (psychiatry and speech and language therapy)

VFAM
vincristine, 5-fluorouracil, Adriamycin, and mitomycin C (chemotherapy, oncology, and pharmacology)

VFDF
very fast death factor

V Fib
ventricular fibrillation (cardiovascular) {pronounced "vee-fib"}

V. Fib.
ventricular fibrillation (cardiovascular) {pronounced "vee-fib"}

Vfib
ventricular fibrillation (cardiovascular) {pronounced "vee-fib"}

V fib
ventricular fibrillation (cardiovascular) {pronounced "vee-fib"}

VFIT
visual field(s) intact (ophthalmology)

VFL
ventricular filling pressure (cardiovascular)
ventricular flutter (cardiovascular)

VFP
ventricular fluid pressure (cardiovascular and neurology)
vitreous fluorophotometry (ophthalmology)

VFT
ventricualr fibrillation threshold (cardiovascular)
Verbal Fluency Test (speech and language therapy)

VG
vein graft (cardiovascular)
ventricular gallop (cardiovascular)
ventrogluteal (anatomy and orthopedics)
very good

V$_G$
genetic variance (genetics and laboratory)

VGH
Vancouver General Hospital [Canada]
(administration)
very good health
veterinary general hospital (veterinary
medicine)

VH
vaginal hysterectomy (gynecology)
venous hematocrit (hematology and laboratory)
ventricular hypertrophy (cardiovascular)
Veterans Hospital (armed forces and
government)
viral hepatitis (gastroenterology and infectious diseases)
visually handicapped (ophthalmology
and rehabilitation)
vitreous hemorrhage (ophthalmology)

V$_H$
hepatic distribution volume (gastroenterology)

V.H.
ventricular hypertrophy (cardiovascular)

VHD
valvular heart disease (cardiovascular)
ventricular heart disease (cardiovascular)
viral hematodepressive disease (hematology and virology)

VHDL
very high-density lipoprotein (cardiovascular and laboratory)

VHF
very high frequency
visual half-field (ophthalmology)

VHP
viral hepatitis panel (hematology and
laboratory)

V. Hyst.
vaginal hysterectomy (gynecology)

VI
six [Roman numeral]
vaginal irrigation (gynecology and obstetrics)
variable interval [reinforcement]
vastus intermedius [muscle] (anatomy
and orthopedics)
Virgin Islands [Postal Service designa-
tion]
virgo intacta (gynecology)
virulence
viscosity index (laboratory)
visual impairment (ophthalmology)
visual inspection
volume index (laboratory)

V$_I$
inspired volume per minute (respiratory)

Vi
virginium (chemistry)
virulence
virulent

VIA
virus-inactivating agent (laboratory)
virus-infection–associated antigen (laboratory)

via
{not an abbreviation} [by way of]

VIB
vibration

vocational interest blank (psychiatry and rehabilitation)

vib
vibration

VIBS
vocabulary, information, block design, similarities (psychiatry)

VIC
vasoinhibitory center (cardiovascular)
vehicle for initial crawling (physical therapy and rehabilitation)

vic
vices [times]

vic.
vices [times]

VID
vaginal intraepithelial dysplasia (gynecology, oncology, and pathology)
videodensitometry (laboratory)

vid
vide [see]

vid.
vide [see]

VIF
virus-induced interferon (chemotherapy, immunology, oncology, pharmacology, and research)

VIG
vaccinia immune globulin (immunology and laboratory)

VIg
vaccinia immune globulin (immunology and laboratory)

vig
vigorous

VII
seven [Roman numeral]

VIII
eight [Roman numeral]

VIII_VWF
von Willebrand's factor VIII (hematology and laboratory)

VIII-vwf
von Willebrand's factor VIII (hematology and laboratory)

VIM
video intensification microscopy (laboratory)

VIN
vaginal intraepithelial neoplasia (gynecology, oncology, and pathology)
vinbarbital [a hypnotic and sedative] (neurology and pharmacology)
vinum [wine]
vulvular intraepithelial neoplasia (gynecology, oncology, and pathology)

vin
vinum [wine]

vin.
vinum [wine]

VIP
vasoactive intestinal polypeptide [also called *vasoactive intestinal peptide*] (endocrinology and laboratory)
vasoinhibitory peptide (laboratory)
venous impedance plethysmography (cardiovascular)
very important patient {pronounced "vip"}
very important person {pronounced "vip"}
Vital Initial of Pregnancy [in vitro fertilization] (obstetrics)
voluntarily interrupted pregnancy (obstetrics)
voluntary interruption of pregnancy (obstetrics)

"vip"
{pronunciation of *VIP* [very important patient and very important person]} {not an abbreviation}

VIQ
Verbal Intelligence Quotient

VIR
virology

vir
viridus [green]
virulent

vir.
viridus [green]
virulent

VIR AC
viral antibody, acute (laboratory)

VIS
vaginal irrigation smear (gynecology, laboratory, and obstetrics)
visible
visual information storage

vis
vision (ophthalmology)
visiting
visitor

VISC
vitreous infusion suction cutter (ophthalmology)

visc
visceral
viscosity (laboratory)
viscous (laboratory)

viscero-
{not an abbreviation} [prefix indicating relationship to the organs (viscera) of the body] {pronounced "vis-er-oh"}

"vis-er-oh"
{pronunciation of *viscero-* [prefix indicating relationship to the organs (viscera) of the body {not an abbreviation}]} {not an abbreviation}

VISTAR
Vistaril [a central nervous system depressant; also called *hydroxyzine*] (anesthesiology, neurology, and pharmacology)

VIT
venom immunotherapy (emergency medicine, immunology, and pharmacology)
vital
vitamin (dietary, laboratory, and pharmacology)
vitellus [yolk] (dietary, laboratory, and pharmacology)

Vit
vitamin [followed by the letter(s) indicating which vitamin] (dietary, laboratory, and pharmacology)

vit
vital
vitamin [followed by the letter(s) indicating which vitamin] (dietary, laboratory, and pharmacology)

vit.
vitamin [followed by the letter(s) indicating which vitamin] (dietary, laboratory, and pharmacology)
vitellus [yolk] (dietary, laboratory, and pharmacology)

VitA
vitamin A [used to indicate either *dehydroretinol (vitamin A₂)* or *retinol (vitamin A₁)*] (dietary, laboratory, and pharmacology)

Vit A
vitamin A [used to indicate either *dehydroretinol (vitamin A₂)* or *retinol (vitamin A₁)*] (dietary, laboratory, and pharmacology)

VitA₁
vitamin A₁ [also called *retinol*] (dietary, laboratory, and pharmacology)

Vit A₁
vitamin A₁ [also called *retinol*] (dietary, laboratory, and pharmacology)

VitA₂
vitamin A₂ [also called *dehydroretinal*]

(dietary, laboratory, and pharmacology)

Vit A$_2$
vitamin A$_2$ [also called *dehydroretinal*] (dietary, laboratory, and pharmacology)

vitals
vital signs [on physical examination]

VitB
vitamin B [a member of the vitamin B complex] (dietary, laboratory, and pharmacology)

Vit B
vitamin B [a member of the vitamin B complex] (dietary, laboratory, and pharmacology)

VitB$_1$
vitamin B$_1$ [also called *thiamine*] (dietary, laboratory, and pharmacology)

Vit B$_1$
vitamin B$_1$ [also called *thiamine*] (dietary, laboratory, and pharmacology)

VitB$_2$
vitamin B$_2$ [also called *riboflavin*] (dietary, laboratory, and pharmacology)

Vit B$_2$
vitamin B$_2$ [also called *riboflavin*] (dietary, laboratory, and pharmacology)

VitB$_3$
vitamin B$_3$ [also called *niacin* and *nicotinamide*] (dietary, laboratory, and pharmacology)

Vit B$_3$
vitamin B$_3$ [also called *niacin* and *nicotinamide*] (dietary, laboratory, and pharmacology)

VitB$_5$
vitamin B$_5$ [also called *calcium pantothenate* and *pantothenic acid*] (dietary, laboratory, and pharmacology)

Vit B$_5$
vitamin B$_5$ [also called *calcium panto-

thenate and *pantothenic acid*] (dietary, laboratory, and pharmacology)

VitB$_6$
vitamin B$_6$ [water-soluble substances including pyridoxine, pyridoxal, and pyridoxamine] (dietary, laboratory, and pharmacology)

Vit B$_6$
vitamin B$_6$ [water-soluble substances including pyridoxine, pyridoxal, and pyridoxamine] (dietary, laboratory, and pharmacology)

VitB$_{12}$
vitamin B$_{12}$ [also called *cobalamin* and *cyanocobalamin*] (dietary, laboratory, and pharmacology)

Vit B$_{12}$
vitamin B$_{12}$ [also called *cobalamin* and *cyanocobalamin*] (dietary, laboratory, and pharmacology)

VitB$_{12b}$
vitamin B$_{12b}$ [also called *hydroxycobalamin*] (dietary, laboratory, and pharmacology)

Vit B$_{12b}$
vitamin B$_{12b}$ [also called *hydroxycobalamin*] (dietary, laboratory, and pharmacology)

VitB$_c$
vitamin B$_c$ [also called *folic acid*] (dietary, laboratory, and pharmacology)

Vit B$_c$
vitamin B$_c$ [also called *folic acid*] (dietary, laboratory, and pharmacology)

VitB$_c$ conjugate
vitamin B$_c$ [also called *folic acid*] (dietary, laboratory, and pharmacology)

Vit B$_c$ conjugate
vitamin B$_c$ [also called *folic acid*] (dietary, laboratory, and pharmacology)

VitB complex
vitamin B complex (dietary, laboratory, and pharmacology)

Vit B complex
vitamin B complex (dietary, laboratory, and pharmacology)

VITC
vitamin C [also called *ascorbic acid*] (dietary, laboratory, and pharmacology)

VitC
vitamin C [also called *ascorbic acid*] (dietary, laboratory, and pharmacology)

Vit C
vitamin C [also called *ascorbic acid*] (dietary, laboratory, and pharmacology)

VIT CAP
vital capacity (respiratory)

vit cap
vitamin capsule (dietary, laboratory, and pharmacology)

vit. cap.
vital capacity (respiratory)

VitD
vitamin D [also called *calciferol;* collective name for several fat-soluble compounds including cholecalciferol (vitamin D_3) and ergocalciferol (vitamin D_2)] (dietary, laboratory, and pharmacology)

Vit D
vitamin D [also called *calciferol;* collective name for several fat-soluble compounds including cholecalciferol (vitamin D_3) and ergocalciferol (vitamin D_2)] (dietary, laboratory, and pharmacology)

VitD$_2$
vitamin D_2 [also called *ergocalciferol*] (dietary, laboratory, and pharmacology)

Vit D$_2$
vitamin D_2 [also called *ergocalciferol*] (dietary, laboratory, and pharmacology)

VitD$_3$
vitamin D_3 [also called *cholecalciferol* and *natural vitamin D*] (dietary, laboratory, and pharmacology)

Vit D$_3$
vitamin D_3 [also called *cholecalciferol* and *natural vitamin D*] (dietary, laboratory, and pharmacology)

VitE
vitamin E [also called *alpha-tocopherol*] (dietary, laboratory, and pharmacology)

Vit E
vitamin E [also called *alpha-tocopherol*] (dietary, laboratory, and pharmacology)

vitel
vitellus [yolk]

VitG
vitamin G [also called *riboflavin*] (dietary, laboratory, and pharmacology)

Vit G
vitamin G [also called *riboflavin*] (dietary, laboratory, and pharmacology)

VitH
vitamin H [also called *biotin*] (dietary, laboratory, and pharmacology)

Vit H
vitamin H [also called *biotin*] (dietary, laboratory, and pharmacology)

VitK
vitamin K [a group of fat-soluble vitamins that promote clotting of the blood] (dietary, hematology, laboratory, and pharmacology)

Vit K
vitamin K [a group of fat-soluble vitamins that promote clotting of the blood] (dietary, hematology, laboratory, and pharmacology)

VitK$_1$
vitamin K$_1$ [also called *phytonadione*] (dietary, hematology, laboratory, and pharmacology)

Vit K$_1$
vitamin K$_1$ [also called *phytonadione*] (dietary, hematology, laboratory, and pharmacology)

VitK$_2$
vitamin K$_2$ [also called *menaquinone*] (dietary, hematology, laboratory, and pharmacology)

Vit K$_2$
vitamin K$_2$ [also called *menaquinone*] (dietary, hematology, laboratory, and pharmacology)

VitK$_3$
vitamin K$_3$ [also called *menadione*] (dietary, hematology, laboratory, and pharmacology)

Vit K$_3$
vitamin K$_3$ [also called *menadione*] (dietary, hematology, laboratory, and pharmacology)

VitL
vitamin L [a factor necessary for lactation in rats] (dietary, laboratory, pharmacology, and veterinary medicine)

Vit L
vitamin L [a factor necessary for lactation in rats] (dietary, laboratory, pharmacology, and veterinary medicine)

VitL$_1$
vitamin L$_1$ [a factor necessary for lactation in rats and found in beef-liver extract] (dietary, laboratory, pharmacology, and veterinary medicine)

Vit L$_1$
vitamin L$_1$ [a factor necessary for lactation in rats and found in beef-liver extract] (dietary, laboratory, pharmacology, and veterinary medicine)

VitL$_2$
vitamin L$_2$ [a factor necessary for lactation in rats and found in yeast] (dietary, laboratory, pharmacology, and veterinary medicine)

Vit L$_2$
vitamin L$_2$ [a factor necessary for lactation in rats and found in yeast] (dietary, laboratory, pharmacology, and veterinary medicine)

VitM
vitamin M [also called *folic acid*] (dietary, laboratory, and pharmacology)

Vit M
vitamin M [also called *folic acid*] (dietary, laboratory, and pharmacology)

vit ov sol
vitello ovi solutus [dissolved in yolk of egg]

VitPP
vitamin PP [also called *nicotinamide* and *nicotinic acid*] (dietary, laboratory, and pharmacology)

Vit PP
vitamin PP [also called *nicotinamide* and *nicotinic acid*] (dietary, laboratory, and pharmacology)

vitr
vitreous (ophthalmology)
vitreum [glass]

vitr.
vitreous (ophthalmology)
vitreum [glass]

vits.
vitamins (dietary, laboratory, and pharmacology) {pronounced "vitz"}

VitU
vitamin U [also called *antiulcer vitamin* and *cabagin vitamin*] (dietary, laboratory, and pharmacology)

Vit U
vitamin U [also called *antiulcer vitamin* and *cabagin vitamin*] (dietary, laboratory, and pharmacology)

Vit V
vitamin V [also called *Valium*] {slang} (chemical dependency and pharmacology)

"vitz"
{pronunciation of *vits.* [vitamins]} (dietary, laboratory, and pharmacology) {not an abbreviation}

vivi-
{not an abbreviation} [prefix meaning alive or indicating relationship to life] {pronounced "vee-vah"}

VIX
nine [Roman numeral]

viz
videlicet [namely]

viz.
videlicet [namely]

VJ
Vogel : Johnson [agar] (laboratory)

VKC
vernal keratoconjunctivitis (ophthalmology)

VKH
Vogt-Koyanagi-Harada [syndrome] (ophthalmology)

VL
{not an abbreviation} [placement of left arm electrode for electrocardiogram] (cardiovascular)
ventralis lateralis [nucleus] (neurology)
vision, left (ophthalmology)

V$_L$
actual volume of the lung (respiratory)

expired volume per minute (respiratory)

VLB
vincaleucoblastine [also called vinblastine] (chemotherapy, oncology, and pharmacology)

VLBR
very low birth rate (statistics)

VLBW
very low birth weight (neonatology)

VLD
very low density (laboratory)

VLDL
very-low-density lipoprotein (cardiovascular, dietary, endocrinology, and laboratory)

VLDLP
very-low-density lipoprotein (cardiovascular, dietary, endocrinology, and laboratory)

VLDS
Verbal Language Development Scale (speech and language therapy)

VLH
ventrolateral nucleus of the hypothalamus (neurology)

VLM
visceral larval migrans [also called *larva migrans, visceral*] (gastroenterology, hematology, laboratory, and respiratory)

VLP
vincristine, L-asparaginase, and prednisone (chemotherapy, oncology, and pharmacology)
virus-like particle (laboratory)

VLSI
very-large-scale integration (computer sciences)

VM
vasomotor (cardiovascular, neurology, orthopedics, and otorhinolaryngology)
ventricular muscle (cardiovascular)
vestibular membrane (otorhinolaryngology)
viomycin [an antibiotic] (pharmacology)
viral myocarditis (cardiovascular)
voltmeter (electricity)

VM-26
{not an abbreviation} [also called *teniposide*] (chemotherapy, oncology, and pharmacology)

Vm
viomycin [an antibiotic] (pharmacology)

VMA
vanillylmandelic acid [also called *vanilmandelic acid*] (laboratory)

V-Mask
Venturi mask (respiratory)

V$_{max}$
maximum velocity (measurement)

VmaxX
forced expiratory flow related to total lung capacity or the actual volume of the lung at which the measurement is made [Example: Vmax75% = instantaneous forced expiratory flow when the lung is at 75% of its total lung capacity] (respiratory)

VMC
vasomotor center (cardiovascular, neurology, orthopedics, and otorhinolaryngology)
VP-16 [etoposide], methotrexate, and citrovorum factor (chemotherapy, oncology, and pharmacology)

VMCG
vector magnetocardiogram (cardiovascular)

VMCP
vincristine, melphalan, cyclophosphamide, and prednisone (chemotherapy, oncology, and pharmacology)

VMD
Veterinariae Medicinae Doctor [Doctor of Veterinary Medicine] (education and veterinary medicine)

VMH
ventromedial hypothalamic [neurons and nuclei] (neurology)

VMN
ventromedial nucleus (neurology)

VMO
vastus medialis oblique [muscle] (orthopedics)

VMR
vasomotor rhinitis (otorhinolaryngology)

VMSC
Vineland Measurement of Social Competence (speech and language therapy)

VMV
vincristine, methotrexate, and VP-16 [etoposide] (chemotherapy, oncology, and pharmacology)

VN
Vietnam (government)
Vietnamese [national origin]
virus neutralization (laboratory)
Visiting Nurse (nursing)
Vocational Nurse (nursing)
vomeronasal (otorhinolaryngology)

VNA
Visiting Nurse Association (nursing)

V.N.A.
Visiting Nurse Association (nursing)

VNE
verbal nonemotional stimuli (psychiatry)

VNO
vomeronasal organ (otorhinolaryngology)

VNS
villonodular synovitis (orthopedics and rheumatology)
Visiting Nurse Service (nursing)

VO
verbal order (nursing)

V.O.
verbal order (nursing)

V/O
verbal order (nursing)

VO₂
volume oxygen consumption (respiratory)

V$_{O2}$
oxygen consumption per minute (respiratory)
oxygen uptake (respiratory)
volume oxygen consumption (respiratory)

voc
vocational (rehabilitation)

VOCA
Voice Output Communication Aid (otorhinolaryngology and speech and language therapy)
VP-16 [etoposide], vincristine, cyclophosphamide, and Adriamycin (chemotherapy, oncology, and pharmacology)

VOCAB
vincristine, VP-16 [etoposide], cyclophosphamide, Adriamycin, and cisplatin (chemotherapy, oncology, and pharmacology)

vocab
vocabulary (speech and language therapy) {pronounced "voe-cab"}

VOCAP
vincristine, VP-16 [etoposide], cyclophosphamide, Adriamycin, and cisplatin (chemotherapy, oncology, and pharmacology)

VOCTOR
void on call to operating room

VOD
venous occlusive disease [also called *venocclusive disease*] (cardiovascular)
visio oculus dextra [vision, right eye; also called *visio oculus dexter*] (ophthalmology)

V.O.D.
visio oculus dextra [vision, right eye; also called *visio oculus dexter*] (ophthalmology)

"voe-cab"
{pronunciation of *vocab* [vocabulary]} (speech and language therapy) {not an abbreviation}

VOL
volume (measurement)
voluntary

Vol
volume (measurement)

vol
volar
volatile (chemistry)
volitilis [volatile] (chemistry)
volume (measurement)
volumetric (measurement)
voluntary
volunteer
volvendus [to be rolled]

vol%
volume percent (measurement)

vol adm
voluntary admission (psychiatry)

volt
volatile (chemistry)
volatize (chemistry)
{not an abbreviation} (electricity and measurement)

vol/vol
volume ratio [volume per volume] (laboratory and pharmacology)

VOM
vinyl chloride monomer (chemistry)
volt-ohm-milliammeter (electricity and measurement)
vomited (gastroenterology)

VON
Victorian Order of Nurses [Canada] (nursing)

VOP
Viral Oncology Program (oncology, research, and virology)

VOR
vestibulo-ocular reflex [also called *vestibular ocular reflex*] (neurology and ophthalmology)

VOS
visio oculus sinister [vision, left eye] (ophthalmology)
vitello ovi solutus [dissolved in yolk of egg] (pharmacology)

vos
vitello ovi solutus [dissolved in yolk of egg] (pharmacology)

v.o.s.
vitello ovi solutus [dissolved in yolk of egg] (pharmacology)

VOU
visio oculus uterque [vision, each eye] (ophthalmology)

voxel
volume element (communications, computer science, and electronics) {pronounced "vox-el"}

"vox-el"
{pronunciation of *voxel* [volume element]} (communications, computer science, and electronics) {not an abbreviation}

VP
vapor pressure (measurement)

variegate porphyria (dermatology, gastroenterology, genetics, and neurology)
vasopressin (cardiovascular, endocrinology, nephrology, neurology, and pharmacology)
venipuncture (cardiovascular and laboratory)
venous pressure (cardiovascular)
ventricular-peritoneal [also called *ventriculoperitoneal*] (neurology and surgery)
ventricular premature [beat] (cardiovascular)
vincristine [Oncovin] and prednisone (chemotherapy, oncology, and pharmacology)
viral protein (laboratory)
Voges-Proskauer [reaction or test] (laboratory)
volume pressure (measurement)
vulnerable period

V$_P$
plasma volume (laboratory)

V-P
ventricular-peritoneal [also called *ventriculoperitoneal*] (neurology and surgery)

V & P
vagotomy and pyloroplasty (gastroenterology and surgery)
ventilation and perfusion [scan] (radiology and respiratory)

VP-16
{not an abbreviation} [also called *etoposide* and *VePesid*] (chemotherapy, oncology, and pharmacology)

VPA
valproic acid (neurology and pharmacology)

VPB
ventricular premature beat (cardiovascular)

VPC
vapor-phase chromatography (laboratory)
ventricular premature contraction (cardiovascular)
volume-packed cells (hematology)
volume percent (measurement)

VPCMF
vincristine, prednisone, cyclophosphamide, methotrexate, and 5-fluorouracil (chemotherapy, oncology, and pharmacology)

VPD
ventricular premature depolarization (cardiovascular)

VPD's
ventricular premature depolarizations (cardiovascular)

VPI
velopharyngeal insufficiency (otorhinolaryngology)

VPL
ventral posterolateral [nucleus; also called *ventroposterolateral nucleus*] (neurology and neurosurgery)

VP-L-Asparaginase
vincristine [Oncovin], prednisone, and L-asparaginase (chemotherapy, oncology, and pharmacology)

VPO
vapor pressure osmometry (laboratory)

VPP
viral porcine pneumonia (infectious diseases, respiratory, and veterinary medicine)

V-P ratio
ventilation-perfusion ratio (radiology and respiratory)

VPRC
volume of packed red cells (hematology)

VPS
valvular pulmonic stenosis (cardiovascular and respiratory)

ventriculoperitoneal shunt (neurology and neurosurgery)

vps
vibrations per second (measurement)

V P shunt
ventriculoperitoneal shunt (neurology and neurosurgery)

VQ
ventilation coefficient (respiratory)

V/Q
ventilation-perfusion [lung scan using xenon (Xe^{133})] (radiology and respiratory)

V/Q ratio
ventilation-perfusion ratio (radiology and respiratory)

VR
valve replacement (cardiovascular)
variable rate [reinforcement]
variable rate
vascular resistance (cardiovascular)
venous reflux (cardiovascular)
venous return (cardiovascular)
ventilation rate (respiratory)
ventilation ratio (respiratory)
ventral root (neurology and orthopedics)
ventricular rhythm (cardiovascular)
verbal reprimand (psychiatry)
vision, right eye (ophthalmology)
vital reaction [on autopsy] (pathology)
vital records (medical records)
vocal resonance (otorhinolaryngology and speech and language therapy)
vocational rehabilitation (rehabilitation)
{not an abbreviation} [position of right arm electrode for electrocardiogram] (cardiovascular)

V.R.
vocal resonance (otorhinolaryngology and speech and language therapy)

V3R
{not an abbreviation} [placement posi-

tion of a precordial lead equidistant
between right sternal border (at the
fourth intercostal space) and right
midclavicular line (at the fifth intercostal space) for an electrocardio-
gram] (cardiovascular)

Vr
relaxation volume (measurement)
ventral root [of a spinal nerve] (neurology and orthopedics)

vr
ventral root [of a spinal nerve] (neurology and orthopedics)

VRA
Vocational Rehabilitation Administration (administration and rehabilitation)

V.R.A.
Vocational Rehabilitation Administration (administration and rehabilitation)

VRBC
red blood cell volume (hematology and
laboratory)

VR CON
viral antibody, convalescent (laboratory)

VR & E
vocational rehabilitation and education
(education and rehabilitation)

VRI
viral respiratory infection (respiratory)

VRL
Virus Reference Laboratory (laboratory
and virology)

VRNA
viral ribonucleic acid (laboratory)

VRP
very reliable product [used on prescrip-
tions] (pharmacology)

VRV
ventricular residual volume (cardiovascular)

VS
vaccination scar (dermatology)
vagal stimulation
venisection [also called *phlebotomy*]
(laboratory)
ventricular septum (cardiovascular)
verbal scale [of intelligence quotient]
(psychiatry)
versus [against]
vesicular sound [on auscultation of
chest] (respiratory)
vesicular stomatitis (veterinary medicine)
Veterinary Surgeon (veterinary medicine)
villonodular synovitis (orthopedics and
rheumatology)
visual storage
vital sign(s) [on physical examination]
voids (urology)
volatile solids (chemistry)
volumetric solution
voluntary sterilization (gynecology, obstetrics, and urology)
without glasses (ophthalmology)

V.S.
vital sign(s) [on physical examination]
volumetric solution

V/S
vital sign(s) [on physical examination]

Vs
venaesectio [venesection; also called
phlebotomy and *venisection*] (laboratory)

Vs.
venaesectio [venesection; also called
phlebotomy and *venisection*] (laboratory)

vs
single vibration [cycles]
versus [against]
vibration seconds (measurement)

vide supra [see above]
voids (urology)

vs.
versus [against]

v.s.
vide supra [see above]

VSA
variant-specific surface antigen (laboratory)

VsB
venaesectio brachii [bleeding in the arm]

VSD
ventricular septal defect [also called *ventriculoseptal defect*] (cardiovascular, neonatology, and pediatrics)
virtual safe dose (pharmacology and radiation therapy)

V.S.D.
ventricular septal defect [also called *ventriculoseptal defect*] (cardiovascular, neonatology, and pediatrics)

VSFP
venous stop-flow pressure (cardiovascular)

VSG
variant surface glycoprotein (laboratory)

VSL
very serious list (administration)

VSM
vascular smooth muscle (anatomy)

VSMS
Vineland Social Maturity Scale (psychiatry)

vsn
vision (ophthalmology)

VSOK
vital signs normal [on physical examination]
vital signs okay [on physical examination]

VSPFT
Vitalor screening pulmonary function test (respiratory)

VSR
venous stasis retinopathy (ophthalmology)

VSS
vital signs stable [on physical examination]

VSULA
vaccination scar, upper left arm (dermatology)

VSV
vesicular stomatitis virus (veterinary medicine)

VSW
ventricular stroke work (cardiovascular and neurology)

VT
tetrazolium violet [a stain] (laboratory)
tidal volume (respiratory)
vacuum tuberculin (infectious diseases, pharmacology, and respiratory)
vasotocin (chemistry)
venous thrombosis (cardiovascular)
ventricular tachycardia (cardiovascular)
Vermont [Postal Service state designation]

V_T
tidal volume (respiratory)
tissue volume (laboratory)

V.T.
vacuum tuberculin (infectious diseases, pharmacology, and respiratory)

V & T
volume and tension [of pulse] (cardiovascular)

Vt
tidal volume (respiratory)

V$_t$
tidal volume (respiratory)

V$_T$A
alveolar tidal volume (laboratory and respiratory)

V-TACH
ventricular tachycardia (cardiovascular) {pronounced "vee-tack"}

V tach
ventricular tachycardia (cardiovascular) {pronounced "vee-tack"}

v. tach.
ventricular tachycardia (cardiovascular) {pronounced "vee-tack"}

VTE
venous thromboembolism (cardiovascular and hematology)
vicarious trial and error (psychiatry)

V-test
Voluter test (radiology)

VTG
volume thoracic gas (respiratory)

VTI
volume thickness index (measurement)

VTM
mechanical tidal volume (respiratory)

VTOL
vertical takeoff and landing [aircraft] (armed forces and transportation)

VTR
video tape recorder (communications and electronics)

VTSRS
Verdun Target Symptom Rating Scale

VTVM
vacuum tube voltmeter (electricity)

VTX
vertex (obstetrics)

Vtx
vertex (obstetrics)

VU
varicose ulcer (cardiovascular and dermatology)
very urgent

vulvo-
{not an abbreviation} [prefix indicating relationship to the vulva] (gynecology and obstetrics) {pronounced "vul-voh"}

"vul-voh"
{pronunciation of *vulvo-* [prefix indicating relationship to the vulva {not an abbreviation}]} (gynecology and obstetrics) {not an abbreviation}

VUR
vesicoureteric reflex [also called *vesicoureteral reflex*] (urology)

VV
varicose veins (cardiovascular)
veins (cardiovascular)
venae [veins] (cardiovascular)
venovenous (cardiovascular)
vesicovaginal (Ob/Gyn, radiology)
viper venom (emergency medicine, laboratory, and pharmacology)
vulva and vagina (gynecology and obstetrics)

V & V
vulva and vagina (gynecology and obstetrics)

V/V
volume-to-volume [ratio] (laboratory and pharmacology)

v/v
volume of solute per volume of solution (laboratory and pharmacology)

vv
veins (cardiovascular)
venae [veins] (cardiovascular)
verses
vice versa [the other way around]

vv.
veins (cardiovascular)
venae [veins] (cardiovascular)

v/v
percent volume [of solute] in volume [of solvent] (laboratory)

VVFR
vesicovaginal fistula repair (gynecology and urology)

V/VI
grade five on a scale of six basis (measurement)

VVOR
visual-vestibulo-ocular reflex (ophthalmology)

VW
vessel wall (cardiovascular)
von Willebrand [disease and factor] (hematology and laboratory)

V.W.
vessel wall (cardiovascular)

V wave
vertex sharp transient [on electroencephalogram] (neurology)

v-wave
{not an abbreviation} [an early diastolic wave found on electrocardiograms] (cardiovascular)

VWD
von Willebrand's disease (hematology)

VWF
von Willebrand factor (hematology and laboratory)

vWF
von Willebrand factor (hematology and laboratory)

VWM
ventricular wall motion (cardiovascular)

Vx
vertex (obstetrics)

Vx.
vertex (obstetrics)

V-Y
{not an abbreviation} [V-Y procedure; shape of incision] (dermatology, plastic surgery, and surgery)

V-Y flap
{not an abbreviation} [shape of incision] (dermatology, plastic surgery, and surgery)

V-Y plasty
{not an abbreviation} [V-Y plasty of bladder neck; shape of incision] (urology)

VZ
varicella zoster (dermatology, infectious diseases, and pediatrics)

V-Z
varicella-zoster (dermatology, infectious diseases, and pediatrics)
varicella-zoster [antibody] (dermatology, infectious diseases, laboratory, and pediatrics)

VZIG
varicella zoster immune globulin (dermatology, infectious diseases, laboratory, pediatrics, and pharmacology)

VZIg
varicella zoster immune globulin (dermatology, infectious diseases, laboratory, pediatrics, and pharmacology)

VZV
varicella zoster virus (dermatology, infectious diseases, laboratory, and pediatrics)

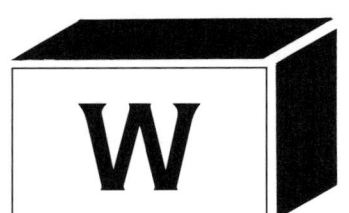

ω
omega [twenty-fourth letter of the Greek
   alphabet]

Ω
ohm (measurement)

W
mechanical work of breathing (laboratory and respiratory)
tryptophan [an amino acid] (dietary, laboratory, and pharmacology)
water
watt (measurement)
Weber [test] (otorhinolaryngology)
week
wehnelt [unit of roentgen ray hardness]
   (measurement and radiology)
weight (measurement)
wenig [fine]
west
white
whole [response]
widow(er)
widowed
width (measurement)
wife
with
wolframium [also called *tungsten*]
   (chemistry)
word fluency (psychiatry and speech
   and language therapy)
work

W.
wehnelt [unit of roentgen ray hardness]
   (measurement and radiology)

W+
weakly positive (laboratory)

*μ***W**
microwatt (measurement)

W ♀
white female

W ♂
white male

w
watt (measurement)
week
white
widowed
wife
with

w.
watt (measurement)
week
wife
with

w/
with

*μ***w**
microwatt (measurement)

WA
Washington [Postal Service state desig-
   nation]
when awake
when taken (pharmacology)
while awake
Woman's Auxiliary

W/A
while awake

WAB
Western Aphasia Battery (speech and
   language therapy)

WABT
Western Aphasia Battery Test (speech
   and language therapy)

WAC
Women's Army Corps (armed forces)

WACH
wedge adjustable cushioned heel [shoe] (orthopedics and podiatry) {pronounced "watch"}

WAIS
Wechsler Adult Intelligence Scale (psychiatry) {pronounced WAYSS}

WAIS-R
Wechsler's Adult Intelligence Scale-Revised (psychiatry) {pronounced WAYSS}

WAK
wearable artificial kidney (nephrology)

WAP
wandering atrial pacemaker (cardiovascular)
white Anglo-Saxon protestant [nationality or race and religion]

WAPT
Weidels Auditory Processing Test (speech and language therapy)

WARDS
Welfare of Animals Used for Research in Drugs and Therapy (research and veterinary medicine)

WARF
warfarin (cardiovascular, hematology, and pharmacology) {pronounced "warf"}

"warf"
{pronunciation of WARF [warfarin]} (cardiovascular, hematology, and pharmacology) {not an abbreviation}

Warren-T
Warren-Teed [manufacturer] (pharmacology)

WAS
Wiskott-Aldrich syndrome (dermatology, genetics, hematology, and otorhinolaryngology)
World Association for Sexology (psychiatry)

WASAMA
Woman's Auxiliary to the Student American Medical Association (education)

WASP
white, Anglo-Saxon, protestant (nationality or race and religion)
World Association of Societies of Pathology (pathology)

WASS
Wasserman [test for syphilis] (gynecology, infectious diseases, laboratory, and urology) {pronounced "waz"}

Wass
Wasserman [test for syphilis] (gynecology, infectious diseases, laboratory, and urology) {pronounced "waz"}

"watch"
{pronunciation of WACH [wedge adjustable cushioned heel [shoe]} (orthopedics and podiatry) {not an abbreviation}

"waz"
{pronunciation of WASS and Wass [Wasserman (test for syphilis)]} (gynecology, infectious diseases, laboratory, and urology) {not an abbreviation}

WB
washable base
water bottle
Wechsler-Bellevue [scale] (psychiatry)
weight-bearing (orthopedics and podiatry)
well baby (neonatology and pediatrics)
wet-bulb
whole blood (hematology)
whole body
Willowbrook [virus] (laboratory)
Wilson Blair [agar] (laboratory)

W.B.
whole blood (hematology)

Wb
weber [unit of magnetic flux] (chemistry, measurement, and physics)

WBA
whole body activity

WBAPTT
whole blood activated partial thromboplastin time (hematology and laboratory)

WBAT
weight-bearing as tolerated (orthopedics and podiatry)

WBC
weight-bearing with crutches (orthopedics and podiatry)
whole blood cell count (hematology and laboratory)
white blood cell(s) (hematology and laboratory)
white blood (cell) count (hematology and laboratory)
white blood corpuscles (hematology and laboratory)

W.B.C.
white blood (cell) count (hematology and laboratory)

wbc
white blood cell(s) (hematology and laboratory)

w.b.c.
white blood cell(s) (hematology and laboratory)

WBCC
white blood cell count (hematology and laboratory)

WBC/hpf
white blood cells per high powered field (hematology and laboratory)

wbc/hpf
white blood cells per high powered field (hematology and laboratory)

WBCT
whole blood clotting time (hematology and laboratory)

WBE
whole body extract (laboratory)

WBF
whole body folate (laboratory)

WBH
whole blood hematocrit (hematology and laboratory)
whole body hyperthermia (emergency medicine)

WB-I
Wechsler-Bellevue I [Test] (psychiatry)

W.B.I.
will be in

WB-II
Wechsler-Bellevue II [Test] (psychiatry)

wb/m²
weber per square meter (chemistry, measurement, and physics)

WBN
wellborn nursery (neonatology)
wide band noise (otorhinolaryngology)

WBPTT
whole blood partial thromboplastin time (hematology and laboratory)

WBR
whole body radiation (radiation therapy)

WBRT
whole blood recalcification time (laboratory)

WBS
whole body scan (radiology)
whole body shower
withdrawal body shakes (chemical dependency)

WBT
wet bulb temperature (measurement)

WC
ward clerk (administration)
water closet [bathroom]
wheelchair
white cell (hematology and laboratory)
white cell cast(s) (hematology and laboratory)
white count (hematology and laboratory)
whooping cough (pediatrics and respiratory)
work capacity (cardiovascular)

W.C.
wheelchair

WC′
whole complement (laboratory)

W/C
wheelchair

W.C.B.
will call back

WCC
white cell count (hematology and laboratory)

WCST
Wisconsin Card Sorting Test (speech and language therapy)

WD
wallerian degeneration (neurology)
warm and dry
well-developed
well-differentiated (laboratory and pathology)
wet dressing (surgery)
Whitney Damon [dextrose agar] (laboratory)
with disease
wrist disarticulation (orthopedics)

W/D
warm and dry
withdrawal

W→D
wet-to-dry [dressing] (surgery)

W—D
wet-to-dry [dressing] (surgery)

W4D
Worth four dot [test] (ophthalmology)

Wd
ward (administration)

wd.
ward (administration)

w/d
well-developed

w-d
well-developed

WDHA
watery diarrhea, hypokalemia, and achlorhydria (gastroenterology)

WDHHA
watery diarrhea, hypochlorhydria, hypokalemia, and alkalosis (gastroenterology)

WDLL
well-differentiated lymphatic lymphoma (oncology)
well-differentiated lymphocytic lymphoma (oncology)

wds
wounds (emergency medicine)

WDWN
well-developed, well-nourished

WD,WN
well-developed, well-nourished

W.D.W.N.
well-developed, well-nourished

WDWNBF
well-developed, well-nourished, black female

WDWNBM
well-developed, well-nourished, black
male

WDWNWF
well-developed, well-nourished, white female

WDWNWM
well-developed, well-nourished, white
male

WE
weekend
Western encephalitis (neurology)
Western encephalomyelitis (neurology)

WEE
Western equine encephalitis (neurology)
Western equine encephalomyelitis (neu-
rology)

WEE virus
Western equine encephalomyelitis virus
(laboratory and neurology)

WEF
war emergency formula (armed forces
and emergency medicine)

WEIL
Weil-Felix [test] (infectious diseases and
laboratory)

WEP
weekend pass (psychiatry and rehabilitation)

WF
Weil-Felix [reaction] (infectious diseases
and laboratory)
wet film (radiology)
white female

W/F
white female

WFE
Williams flexion exercises (orthopedics)

WFI
water for injection (pharmacology)

WFL
within functional limits (orthopedics and
physical therapy)

WFOT
World Federation of Occupational Therapists (occupational therapy)

WFR
Weil-Felix reaction (infectious diseases
and laboratory)
wheal-and-flare reaction (allergy)

WG
water gauge (measurement)
Wegener's granulomatosis (otorhinolaryngology and respiratory)
Wright-Giesma [stain] (laboratory)

WGA
wheat germ agglutinin (laboratory)

wgt
weight (measurement)

WH
well-healed

Wh
white

wh
whispered (otorhinolaryngology and
speech and language therapy)
white

WHAP
Woman's Health and Abortion Project
(gynecology and obstetrics)

WHB
weight-bearing (orthopedics and podiatry)

WhB
whole blood (hematology)

WHCOA
White House Conference on Aging (geriatrics and government)

Whittaker
Whittaker General Medical (pharmacology)

WHML
Wellcome Historical Medical Library (library sciences)

WHMS
well-healed midline scar (surgery)

WHO
World Health Organization (government)
{not an abbreviation} [histological classification system for ovarian tumors] (gynecology, oncology, and pathology)

WHOIRP
World Health Organization International Reference Preparation (government and publications)

Whp
whirlpool (physical therapy and rehabilitation)

whp
whirlpool (physical therapy and rehabilitation)

whr
watt hour (measurement)

WHRC
World Health Research Center (government and research)

WHV
woodchuck hepatic virus (infectious diseases and laboratory)

WHVP
wedged hepatic venous pressure [also called *hepatic wedge pressure*] (cardiovascular and gastroenterology)

WI
walk-in [patient] (administration)
Wisconsin [Postal Service state designation]

WIA
wounded in action (armed forces)

WIC
Women, Infants, and Children [Supplemental Food Program, Centers for Disease Control] (dietary and government)

WID
widow(er)

wid
widow(er)

WIPI
Word Intelligibility by Picture Identification (speech and language therapy)

WISC
Wechsler Intelligence Scale for Children (pediatrics and psychiatry)

WISC-R
Wechsler Intelligence Scale for Children, Revised (pediatrics and psychiatry)

WIST
Whitaker Index of Schizophrenic Thinking (psychiatry)

WJPB
Woodcock-Johnson Psychoeducational Battery (psychiatry)

WK
weak
week
Wernicke-Korsakoff [syndrome] (chemical dependency, geriatrics, and neurology)

wk
weak
week

WKD
Wilson-Kimmelstiel disease (cardiovascular, endocrinology, and nephrology)

WK disease
Wilson-Kimmelstiel disease (cardiovascular, endocrinology, and nephrology)

WKS
Wernicke-Korsakoff syndrome (chemical dependency, geriatrics, and neurology)

wks
weeks

WKY
Wistar-Kyoto [rats] (research)

WL
waiting list (administration)
Wallenstein Laboratory [medium] (laboratory)
wavelength (measurement)
work load (cardiovascular and respiratory)

WLS
wet lung syndrome (respiratory)

WLT
waterload test

WL test
waterload test

WM
ward manager (administration)
white male
whole milk (dietary)
woman

W/M
white male
wound, missile (armed forces and emergency medicine)

wm
whole mount [microscopy] (laboratory)
woman

WMA
wall motion abnormality (cardiovascular)
World Medical Association (government)

WMF
white, middle-aged female

WMM
white, middle-aged male

WMR
Western Medical Review (education)
work metabolic rate (measurement)
World Medical Relief (government and social services)

WMS
Wechsler Memory Scale (psychiatry and speech and language therapy)

WMS-I
Wechsler Memory Scale, Form I (psychiatry and speech and language therapy)

WMSC
Women's Medical Specialists Corps (armed forces)

Wms flex ex
Williams flexion exercises (orthopedics)

WMX
whirlpool, massage, and exercise (physical therapy and rehabilitation)

WN
well-nourished

w/n
well-nourished

WND
wound (emergency medicine)

Wnd
wound (emergency medicine)

wnd
wound (emergency medicine)

WNE
West Nile encephalitis (neurology)

WNF
well-nourished female

WNL
within normal limits

WNM
well-nourished male

WNPW
wide, notched P-wave [on electrocardio-
gram] (cardiovascular)

WNV
West Nile virus (laboratory, neurology)

WO
wash out (radiology)
weeks old [preceded by a number] (neonatology and pediatrics)
without
written order (nursing and pharmacology)

W/O
water in oil [referring to emulsions] (laboratory and pharmacology)
without

w/o
without

WOB
work of breathing (cardiovascular and
respiratory)

WOFL
wound fluid (emergency medicine and
laboratory)

WOP
without pain

WP
weakly positive (laboratory)
wet pack (physical therapy)
wetable powder (pharmacology)
whirlpool (physical therapy)
word processing (business and computer
science)
word processor (business and computer
science)
working point

W.P.
whirlpool (physical therapy)

W/P
water/powder [ratio] (pharmacology)

WPA
World Psychiatric Association (psychiatry)

WPB
whirlpool bath (physical therapy)

WPF
Wright peak flow (respiratory)

WPFM
Wright peak flow meter (respiratory)

WPK
Wright peak flow (respiratory)

WPk
Ward's mechanical tissue pack (dentistry)
wet pack (physical therapy)

W-plasty
{not an abbreviation} [shape of incision]
(plastic surgery)

WPP
Welcher Preschool Primary Scale of Intelligence (pediatrics and psychiatry)

WPPSI
Wechsler Preschool and Primary Scale
of Intelligence (pediatrics and psychiatry)

WPRS
Wittenborn Psychiatric Rating Scale
(psychiatry)

WPSI
Wahler Physical Symptoms Inventory
(psychiatry)

WPT
warbled pure tone (speech and language
therapy)

WPW
Wolff-Parkinson-White [syndrome] (cardiovascular)

WR
washroom

Wassermann reaction [for syphilis] (gynecology, infectious diseases, laboratory, and urology)

water retention

weakly reactive (laboratory)

wiping reaction (neurology)

wiping reflex (neurology)

wrist (orthopedics)

{not an abbreviation} [Walter Reed Army Institute of Research classification system for human T-cell leukemia/lymphoma virus (HTLV-III/LAV); given as WR-0 through WR-6] (immunology, laboratory, oncology, and pathology)

W.R.
Wassermann reaction [for syphilis] (gynecology, infectious diseases, laboratory, and urology)

wr.
wrist (orthopedics)

WRAIR
Walter Reed Army Institute of Research (administration, armed forces, government, and research)

"wrast"
{pronunciation of RAST [radioallergosorbent test]} (allergy) {not an abbreviation}

WRAT
Wide Range Achievement Test (psychiatry)

WRBC
washed red blood cells (hematology)

WRC
washed red cells (hematology)

water-retention coefficient (measurement)

WRE
whole ragweed extract (allergy)

"wrist"
{pronunciation of RIST [radioimmunosorbent test]} (immunology and laboratory) {not an abbreviation}

WRMT
Woodcock Reading Mastery Test (psychiatry and speech and language therapy)

WRVP
wedged renal vein pressure (cardiovascular and nephrology)

WS
ward secretary (administration)

water soluble

water swallow (gastroenterology)

watt seconds (measurement)

Williams syndrome (cardiovascular, genetics, otorhinolaryngology, and neurology)

ws.
watt seconds (measurement)

WSMSA
Washington Standard Metropolitan Statistical Area (statistics)

WSOJ
whole blood serum of a patient with obstructive jaundice (gastroenterology, hematology, and laboratory)

WT
weight (measurement)

whistletip [catheter] (urology)

white

W-T
Warren-Teed [manufacturer] (pharmacology)

Wt
weight (measurement)

wt
weight (measurement)

white

WTAD
Wepman Test of Auditory Discrimination (speech and language therapy)

wt/vol
weight per volume [ratio] (measurement)

wt/wt
weight per weight [ratio] (measurement)

W/U
workup

w/u
workup

WV
West Virginia [Postal Service state designation]
whispered voice (otorhinolaryngology and speech and language therapy)

W/V
weight by volume (measurement)
weight of solute in volume of solvent (measurement)
weight-to-volume [ratio] (measurement)

w/v
weight of solute per volume of solution (measurement)
weight per volume (measurement)

w./v.
weight of solute per volume of solution (measurement)

WV-MBC
walking ventilation to maximum breathing capacity [ratio] (respiratory)

WW
Weight Watchers (dietary)

W/W
weight in weight (measurement)
weight-to-weight [ratio] (measurement)

w/w
weight of solute in weight of solvent (measurement)
weight of solute per weight of total solution (measurement)

WWAC
walk with aid of cane (neurology, orthopedics, podiatry, and rehabilitation)

WWF
World Wrestling Federation (sports medicine)

WxB
wax bite (dentistry)

WxP
wax pattern (dentistry)

WY
Wyoming [Postal Service state designation]

WY/NRT
Weidels Yes/No Reliability Test (speech and language therapy)

WZa
wide zone alpha [hemolysis] (hematology)

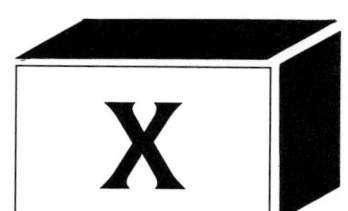

X

break
cross [referring to sections] (laboratory and pathology)
crossed with
crossmatch (blood bank, hematology, and laboratory)
except
exophoria (ophthalmology)
exophoria distance (ophthalmology)
extra
Kienböck's unit [of roentgen ray dosage] (measurement, radiation therapy, and radiology)
magnification sign [for microscopes] (laboratory)
multiplied by (mathematics)
number of times
reactance (measurement and physics)
removal of (surgery)
respirations [on anesthesia chart] (anesthesiology, respiratory, and surgery)
start of anesthesia (anesthesiology and surgery)
ten [Roman numeral]
times [as in "4X" equals "four times"]
transverse [referring to sections] (laboratory and pathology)
Xenopsylla [a genus of fleas] (veterinary medicine)
{not an abbreviation} [homeopathic symbol for decimal scale of potencies]
{not an abbreviation} [symbol for female chromosome] (genetics and laboratory)
{not an abbreviation} [symbol for multiplication] (mathematics)
{not an abbreviation} [symbol for unknown quantity]

X.

Xenopsylla [a genus of fleas] (veterinary medicine)

$\bar{X}$

average of all X's
mean value [indicated by the dash over the symbol] (laboratory and respiratory)
sample mean

$\dot{X}$

time derivative [indicated by the dot above the symbol] (laboratory and respiratory)

$\ddot{X}$

second time derivative [indicated by two dots above the symbol] (laboratory and respiratory)

%X

percentage of the predicted normal value [indicated by the percent sign preceding the symbol] (laboratory and respiratory)

X+#

xiphoid plus number of finger breadths [height of fundus] (obstetrics)

X3

times three [referring to orientation to time, place, and person] (neurology)

x

axis [of a cylindrical lens] (ophthalmology)
except
roentgen [ray(s)] (radiology)
times [as in "4x" equals "four times"]

$\bar{x}$

average of all X's
mean
sample mean

x′

exophoria (ophthalmology)

θx
reaction rate coefficient for red cells (laboratory and respiratory)

XA
xanthurenic acid (laboratory)

Xa
chiasma (anatomy, multiple specialties, and ophthalmology)

Xaa
unknown amino acid (laboratory)

X-A mixture
xylene-alcohol mixture [insecticide] (chemistry)

XAN
xanthine (laboratory, orthopedics, nephrology, pharmacology, and rheumatology)

XANT
xanthochromic (laboratory and neurology)

Xanth
xanthomatosis [excess of lipids in various parts of the body] (cardiovascular, oncology, and ophthalmology) {pronounced "zanth"}

xanth
xanthomatosis [excess of lipids in various parts of the body] (cardiovascular, oncology, and ophthalmology) {pronounced "zanth"}

xantho-
{not an abbreviation} [prefix meaning yellow] {pronounced "zan-tho"}

X-body
{not an abbreviation} [also called *Birbeck granule*] (endocrinology, laboratory, and pathology)

XC
excretory cystogram (radiology and urology)

XCCE
extracapsular cataract extraction (ophthalmology)

X-chrom
female sex chromosome (endocrinology, genetics, and laboratory)

X chromosome
{not an abbreviation} [female sex chromosome] (endocrinology, genetics, and laboratory) {pronounced "X-crow-mah-som"}

"X-crow-mah-som"
{pronunciation of *X chromosome* [female sex chromosome]} (endocrinology, genetics, and laboratory) {not an abbreviation}

X & D
examination and diagnosis

XDH
xanthine dehydrogenase (laboratory, orthopedics, nephrology, pharmacology, and rheumatology)

x disease
{not an abbreviation} [also called *hyperkeratosis* (veterinary medicine) or *aflatoxicosis* (veterinary medicine)]

XDP
xanthine diphosphate (laboratory, orthopedics, nephrology, pharmacology, and rheumatology)
xeroderma pigmentosum (dermatology, genetics, neurology, and ophthalmology)

XDR
transducer (biochemistry, chemistry, electronics, and physics)

Xe
xenon (chemistry)

^{133}Xe
xenon^{133} [also called *radioxenon*] (chemistry)

XEF
excess ejection fraction (cardiovascular)

xeno-
{not an abbreviation} [prefix meaning strange or indicating relationship to foreign material] {pronounced "zen-oh"}

xero
xeromammography (gynecology and radiology) {pronounced "zee-row"}

xero-
{not an abbreviation} [prefix meaning dry or indicating relationship to dryness] {pronounced "zee-row"}

XES
X-ray [roentgen ray] energy spectrometer (radiology)

X-factor
{not an abbreviation} [a coagulation factor; also called *autoprothrombin C, factor X, Prower factor, Stuart factor, Stuart-Prower factor,* and *thrombokinase*] (hematology and laboratory)

XGP
xanthogranulomatous pyelonephritis (nephrology, radiology)

XI
eleven [Roman numeral]

XII
twelve [Roman numeral]

XIII
thirteen [Roman numeral]

XIP
x-ray in plaster (orthopedics and radiology)

xiphi-
{not an abbreviation} [prefix indicating relationship to the xiphoid process] {pronounced "zif-E"}

xipho-
{not an abbreviation} [prefix indicating relationship to the xiphoid process] {pronounced "zif-oh" or "zi-foe"}

XIV
fourteen [Roman numeral]

XIX
nineteen [Roman numeral]

XKO
not knocked out (emergency medicine, neurology, and sports medicine)

XL
extra large (measurement)
xylose-lysine [agar] (laboratory)

XLD
xylose, lysine, desoxycholate [agar] (laboratory)

XLH
X-linked hypophosphatemia (genetics)

X-linked
{not an abbreviation} [gene carried on the X chromosome] (genetics and laboratory)

XLMR
X-linked mental retardation (genetics, neurology, and psychiatry)

XLP
X-linked lymphoproliferative [syndrome] (genetics and laboratory)

XM
crossmatch (blood bank, hematology, and laboratory)

X_m
magnetic susceptibility (physics)

Xmas
Christmas

X-mat.
crossmatch (blood bank, hematology, and laboratory)

X-match
crossmatch (blood bank, hematology, and laboratory)

XMM
xeromammography (gynecology and radiology)

XMP
xanthosine monophosphate [also called *xanthosine-5'-phosphate*] (laboratory)

Xn
Christian (religion)

XO
xanthine oxidase (laboratory)

XO
{not an abbreviation} [symbol indicating the presence of only one sex chromosome, the other *X* or the *Y* being absent] (endocrinology, genetics, and laboratory)

X & O
hug and kiss {slang}

XOP
x-ray out of plaster (orthopedics and radiology)

XOR
exclusive operating room (surgery)

XP
xeroderma pigmentosum (dermatology, genetics, neurology, and ophthalmology)

"X-par-tah-cul"
{pronunciation of *X-particle*} [a hypothetical particle of matter {not an abbreviation}]} (physics) {not an abbreviation}

X-particle
{not an abbreviation} [a hypothetical particle of matter] (physics) {pronounced "X-par-tah-cul"}

X-Prep
{not an abbreviation} [used for bowel evacuation prior to radiographs] (gastroenterology, pharmacology, and radiology)

XR
roentgen ray (radiology)

XRAY
roentgen ray (radiology)

X-ray
roentgen ray (radiology)

x-ray
roentgen ray (radiology)

XRAYS
roentgen rays (radiology)

X-rays
roentgen rays (radiology)

x-rays
roentgen rays (radiology)

XRD
x-ray diffraction (radiology)

XRT
radiotherapy [also called *roentgen ray (X-ray) radiation treatment*] (radiation therapy)
x-ray [roentgen ray] technician (radiology)

XS
cross-section (laboratory and pathology)
excess
xiphisternum [also called the *xiphoid process*] (anatomy)

XS-LIM
exceeds limits of procedure (surgery)

XSLR
crossed straight leg raising [sign] (neurology and orthopedics)

X's & O's
hugs and kisses {slang}

XT
exotropia (distance) [may be written with an *L* or an *R* referring to right or left] (ophthalmology)

X(T)
intermittent exotropia (ophthalmology)

XT'
exotropia (near) (ophthalmology)

Xt
exotropia [may be written with an *L* or an *R* referring to right or left] (ophthalmology)

X₂t.
chi-squared test (statistics)

Xta
chiasma (anatomy, multiple specialties, and ophthalmology)
chiasmata (anatomy, multiple specialties, and ophthalmology)

XU
excretory urogram (radiology and urology)

Xu
x-ray unit (measurement and radiology)

XV
fifteen [Roman numeral]

XVI
sixteen [Roman numeral]

XVII
seventeen [Roman numeral]

XVIII
eighteen [Roman numeral]

X walk
cross walk

x wave
{not an abbreviation} [found on phlebograms] (cardiovascular)

x/week
times/week (rehabilitation)

XX
{not an abbreviation} [normal female sex chromosome type] (endocrinology, genetics, and laboratory)
twenty [Roman numeral]

46XX
{not an abbreviation} [normal female sex chromosome type] (endocrinology, genetics, and laboratory)

XXX
thirty [Roman numeral]

XX/XY
{not an abbreviation} [sex karyotypes] (endocrinology, genetics, and laboratory)

XY
{not an abbreviation} [normal male sex chromosome type] (endocrinology, genetics, and laboratory)

X/Y%
{not an abbreviation} [percent sign following the symbol indicates a ratio function with the ratio expressed as a percentage (Example: $FEV_1/FVC\%$)] (laboratory and respiratory)

46XY
{not an abbreviation} [normal male sex chromosome type] (endocrinology, genetics, and laboratory)

Xyl
xylose (gastroenterology and laboratory)

Xylo
Xylocaine (anesthesiology, pharmacology, and surgery) {pronounced "zi-low"}

xylo-
{not an abbreviation} [prefix indicating relationship to wood] {pronounced "zi-low"}

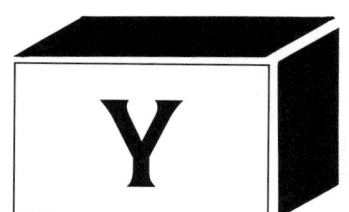

Y
tyrosine (endocrinology and laboratory)
year (measurement)
yellow
Yersinia [a bacterium] (laboratory)
young
yttrium (chemistry and laser surgery)

Y.
Yersinia [a bacterium] (laboratory)

^{90}Y
radioactive yttrium (chemistry)

y
year(s) (measurement)

YACP
young adult chronic patient

YADH
yeast alcohol dehydrogenase (chemistry, gastroenterology, and laboratory)

YAG
yttrium aluminum garnet [crystal laser] (laser surgery and ophthalmology)

Yb
ytterbium (chemistry and laser surgery)

^{169}Yb
ytterbium 169 [a radionuclide] (chemistry and radiology)

Yb-169-DTPA
ytterbium 169 pentetate sodium (chemistry and radiology)

YCB
yeast carbon base (laboratory)

Y chromosome
{not an abbreviation} [male sex chromosome] (endocrinology, genetics, and laboratory)

yd
yard(s) (measurement)

YE
yellow enzyme (laboratory)

YEH$_2$
reduced yellow enzyme (laboratory)

yel
yellow

YELL
yellow

YET
youth effectiveness training (psychiatry)

YF
yellow fever (gastroenterology, hematology, infectious diseases, and neurology)

YJV
yellow jacket venom (allergy, immunology, laboratory, and pharmacology)

Yk
York [antibodies] (laboratory)

-yl
{not an abbreviation} [chemical suffix indicating a radical] (chemistry)

YLC
youngest living child

-ylene
{not an abbreviation} [chemical suffix indicating a bivalent hydrocarbon radical] (chemistry)

YMA
yeast morphology agar (laboratory)

YMCA
Young Men's Christian Association (religion and social services)

YMHA
Young Men's Hebrew Association (religion and social services)

YNB
yeast nitrogen base (laboratory)

YNHH
Yale-New Haven Hospital (administration and education)

YO
years old

Y/O
years old

Y.O.
years old

yo
years old

y/o
years old

y.o.
years old

YOB
year of birth

YORA
younger-onset rheumatoid arthritis (orthopedics and rheumatology)

Y-organ
{not an abbreviation} [moulting gland in crustaceans] (oceanography)

"you-pep"
{pronunciation of *UPEP* [urine protein electrophoresis]} (laboratory) {not an abbreviation}

YP
yield pressure (laboratory)

YPLL
years of potential life lost (measurement and statistics)

YR
year (measurement)

Yr
year (measurement)

yr
year (measurement)

yrs
years (measurement)

YS
yolk sac (embryology, laboratory, and neonatology)

ys
yellow spot [on retina] (ophthalmology)

y.s.
yellow spot [on retina] (ophthalmology)

YSC
yolk sac carcinoma (laboratory, oncology, pathology, and pediatrics)

Y-shaped
{not an abbreviation}

YST
yeast [cells] (laboratory)

Yt
yttrium (chemistry)

yt
yttrium (chemistry)

Y-type
{not an abbreviation}

y wave
{not an abbreviation} [found on phlebograms] (cardiovascular)

YWCA
Young Women's Christian Association
  (religion and social services)

YWHA
Young Women's Hebrew Association
  (religion and social services)

Z

Z
impedance (physics)
ionic charge number (chemistry)
standard score [statistic] (statistics)
zero
zeta [sixth letter of the Greek alphabet]
zone
Zuckung [contraction; Z^I and Z^{II} as well
as Z' and Z'' refer to increasing degrees of contraction] (obstetrics)
{not an abbreviation} [symbol for atomic
number] (chemistry and physics)

Z.
Zuckung [contraction; Z^I and Z^{II} as well
as Z' and Z'' refer to increasing degrees of contraction] (obstetrics)

Z'
[*See Z (Zuckung) above*]

Z''
[*See Z (Zuckung) above*]

z
atomic number (chemistry)
standardized device

"zanth"
{pronunciation of *Xanth* and *xanth*
[xanthomatosis (excess of lipids in
various parts of the body)]} (cardiovascular, oncology, and ophthalmology) {not an abbreviation}

"zan-tho"
{pronunciation of *xantho-* [prefix meaning yellow]} {not an abbreviation}

Z band
{not an abbreviation} [also called *intermediate disk, Z line,* and *Zwischenscheibe disk*] (laboratory)

ZD
zero discharge

Z/D
zero defects
zero discharge

ZDDP
zinc dialkyldithiophosphate (chemistry)

Z-disk
Zwischenscheibe disk [also called *intermediate disk, Z band,* and *Z line*]
(laboratory)

ZDS
Zung Depression Scale (psychiatry)

ZE
Zollinger-Ellison [syndrome] (gastroenterology)

Z-E
Zollinger-Ellison [syndrome] (gastroenterology)

ZEEP
zero end-expiratory pressure (respiratory)

"zee-row"
{pronunciation of *xero* [xeromammogra-
phy (gynecology, radiology, and surgery)] and *xero-* [prefix meaning dry
or indicating relationship to dryness
{not an abbreviation}]} {not an abbre-
viation}

"zen-oh"
{pronunciation of *xeno-* [prefix meaning
strange or indicating relationship to
foreign material {not an abbrevia-
tion}]} {not an abbreviation}

ZES
Zollinger-Ellison syndrome (gastroenterology)

937

Z-ESR
zeta erythrocyte sedimentation rate (hematology and laboratory)

Z-excision
{not an abbreviation} [shape of excision] (surgery)

ZF
zona fasciculata [of adrenal cortex] (anatomy and endocrinology)

Z-flap
{not an abbreviation} [shape of incision] (plastic surgery and surgery)

ZG
zona glomerulosa [of adrenal cortex] (anatomy and endocrinology)

Z/G
zoster serum immune globulin [also called *zoster immunoglobulin*] (immunology, infectious diseases, laboratory, pediatrics, and pharmacology)

ZI
[*Note: See Z (Zuckung) above*]

ZI^a
isotope with atomic number of Z and atomic weight of A (chemistry)

"zif-E"
{pronunciation of *xiphi-* [prefix indicating relationship to the xiphoid process {not an abbreviation}]} {not an abbreviation}

"zi-foe"
{pronunciation of *xipho-* [prefix indicating relationship to the xiphoid process {not an abbreviation}]} {not an abbreviation}

"zif-oh"
{pronunciation of *xipho-* [prefix indicating relationship to the xiphoid process {not an abbreviation}]} {not an abbreviation}

ZIG
zoster serum immune globulin [also called *zoster immunoglobulin*] (im-

munology, infectious diseases, laboratory, pediatrics, and pharmacology)

ZIg
zoster serum immune globulin [also called *zoster immunoglobulin*] (immunology, infectious diseases, laboratory, pediatrics, and pharmacology)

"zi-go"
{pronunciation of *zygo-* [prefix meaning joined or yoked or indicating relationship to a junction {not an abbreviation}]} {not an abbreviation}

ZI^I
[*Note: See Z (Zuckung) above*]

"zi-low"
{pronunciation of *Xylo* [Xylocaine (anesthesiology and pharmacology)], *xylo-* [prefix indicating relationship to wood {not an abbreviation}], and *Zylo* [Zyloprim (pharmacology and rheumatology)]} {not an abbreviation}

"zi-moe"
{pronunciation of *zymo-* [prefix indicating relationship to an enzyme or to fermentation {not an abbreviation}]} {not an abbreviation}

ZIP
Zone Improvement Program [United States Postal Service]
zoster immune plasma (immunology, infectious diseases, laboratory, pediatrics, and pharmacology)

Z line
{not an abbreviation} [also called *Z band, intermediate disk,* and *Zwischenscheibe disk*] (laboratory)

ZMC
zygomatic (otorhinolaryngology and plastic surgery)
zygomaticomaxillary complex (otorhinolaryngology and plastic surgery)

ZN
Ziehl-Neelsen [stain] (laboratory)

Zn
zinc (chemistry, dietary, and laboratory)

Zn. fl.
zinc flocculation [test] (laboratory)

ZnO
zinc oxide [also called *white zinc*] (dermatology and pharmacology)

ZN stain
Ziehl-Neelsen stain (laboratory)

zoo-
{not an abbreviation} [prefix indicating relationship to an animal] {pronounced "zoo"}

"zoo"
{pronunciation of *zoo-* [prefix indicating relationship to an animal {not an abbreviation}]} {not an abbreviation}

Zool
zoological (zoology)
zoology

zool
zoological (zoology)
zoology

ZPG
zero population growth (statistics)

Z-plasty
{not an abbreviation} [shape of incision] (surgery)

ZPLS
Zimmerman Preschool Language Scale (speech and language therapy)

ZPO
zinc peroxide (pharmacology)

ZPP
zinc protoporphyrin (hematology and laboratory)

ZR
zona reticularis [of adrenal cortex] (anatomy and endocrinology)

Zr
zirconium (chemistry)

ZSR
zeta sedimentation ratio [method] (hematology and laboratory)

ZTN
zinc tannate of naloxone (pharmacology)

zygo-
{not an abbreviation} [prefix meaning joined or yoked or indicating relationship to a junction] {pronounced "zigo"}

Zylo
Zyloprim (pharmacology and rheumatology) {pronounced "zi-low"}

zymo-
{not an abbreviation} [prefix indicating relationship to an enzyme or to fermentation] {pronounced "zi-moe"}

zz
zingiber [ginger] (chemistry, dietary, and pharmacology)

Z.Z.'Z."
increasing degrees of contraction [*Zuckung* (contraction); Z^I and Z^{II} as well as Z' and Z'' refer to increasing degrees of contraction] (obstetrics)

APPENDIX A:

CHEMISTRY

A

A	adenine (chemistry and laboratory)
AcAcOH	acetoacetic acid (endocrinology and laboratory)
A, $(C_6H_{10}O_3)_x(C_4H_6O_2)_y(C_{10}H_{14}O_4)_z$	
	ocufilcon [a contact lens material] (ophthalmology)
ACl	aspiryl chloride (laboratory)
AgI	silver iodide (pharmacology)
AgNO$_3$	silver nitrate (pharmacology)
AgNOR	silver-staining nucleolar organizer region (genetics and laboratory)
Ag$_2$O	silver oxide (chemistry)
Ag$_2$SO$_4$	silver sulfate (chemistry)
Al$_2$H$_{14}$Mg$_4$O$_{14}\cdot$2H$_2$O	magaldrate [also called *aluminum magnesium hydroxide*] (pharmacology)
Al$_2$O$_3$	aluminum oxide (chemistry and pharmacology)
Al(OH)$_3$	aluminum hydroxide (chemistry and pharmacology)
3′,5′-AMP	3′,5′-adenosine monophosphate (laboratory)
Arg	arginine (chemistry)
Arg.	arginine (chemistry)
Ars	arsphenamine (chemistry)
Ars.	arsphenamine (chemistry)
As$_2$O$_3$	arsenic trioxide (chemistry)
AT$_7$	hexachlorophene (chemistry)
AT$_{10}$	dihydrotachysterol (chemistry)
^{198}Au	radioactive gold (chemistry)
azo	{not an abbreviation} [indicates the presence of the group −N:N−] (chemistry)

B

B	base [as used in chemical formulas] (chemistry)
	boron (chemistry)
Ba	barium (chemistry and radiology)
BaCl$_2$	barium chloride (chemistry)
BaSO$_4$	barium sulfate (chemistry and radiology)
B, $(C_6H_{10}O_3)_x(C_4H_6O_2)_y(C_{10}H_{14}O_4)_z$	
	ocufilcon [a contact lens material] (ophthalmology)

Be	beryllium (chemistry)
Bi	bismuth (pharmacology)
$(BiO)_2CO_2$	subcarbonate of bismuth (pharmacology)
Bu	butyl (chemistry)

C

C	carbon (chemistry)
	cysteine [an amino acid] (chemistry and laboratory)
	cytidine (genetics and laboratory)
	cytosine (genetics and laboratory)
C-6	hexamethonium (chemistry)
C10	decamethonium (chemistry)
C-10	decamethonium (chemistry)
^{14}C	radioactive carbon (chemistry and laboratory)
CA	carbonic anhydrase (laboratory and nephrology)
	Chemical Abstracts (chemistry)
Ca	calcium (chemistry, laboratory, and pharmacology)
^{45}Ca	radioactive calcium (chemistry and laboratory)
$CaCl_2$	calcium chloride (chemistry)
$CaCl(OCl)$	chlorinated lime (chemistry)
$CaCO_3$	calcium carbonate (chemistry, gastroenterology, and pharmacology)
CaC_2O_4	calcium oxalate (chemistry, laboratory, nephrology, and urology)
CaF_2	calcium fluoride (chemistry)
CaH_2O_2	calcium hydroxide (chemistry)
$Ca(OH)_2$	calcium hydroxide (chemistry)
$Ca_3(PO_4)_2$	tribasic calcium phosphate (chemistry)
$Ca_{10}(PO_4)_6(OH)_2$	hydroxyapatite (laboratory)
$CaSO_4$	calcium sulfate (chemistry)
Cb	columbium [now called *niobium*] (chemistry)
Cbl	cobalamin [a part of vitamin B_{12}] (laboratory and pharmacology)
CBz	carbobenzoxychloride (chemistry)
CC	calcium cyclamate (chemistry)
CCK-179	{not an abbreviation} [methanesulfonate salts of equal parts of dihydroergocornine, dihydroergo-cristine, and dihydroergocryptine] (chemistry)
CCl_4	carbon tetrachloride [a toxin] (chemistry)
C_6Cl_6	hexachlorobenzene (chemistry)
CCl_3CCl_3	hexachloroethane (chemistry)
$CCl_3 \cdot CHO$	chloral (chemistry and pharmacology)
$CCl_3 \cdot CH(OH)_2$	chloral hydrate (chemistry, laboratory, neurology, and pharmacology)
$C_{10}Cl_{10}O$	polychlorinated keton [also called *Keptone*; an insecticide] (chemistry)

CD	carbonate dehydratase (chemistry and laboratory)
Cd	cadmium (chemistry)
^{115}Cd	radioactive cadmium (chemistry)
Ce	cerium (chemistry)
^{58}Ce	radioactive cerium (chemistry)
Cf	californium (chemistry)
CG	phosgene [also called *carbonyl chloride;* a poisonous war gas] (armed forces and chemistry)
CH_2	methylene [the bivalent hydrocarbon radical] (chemistry)
CH_4	methane (chemistry)
C_2H_2	acetylene (chemistry)
C_2H_4	ethylene (chemistry)
C_3H_7	propyl [the univalent chemical radical] (chemistry)
C_5H_8	isoprene (chemistry)
C_5H_{12}	pentane [an aliphatic hydrocarbon] (chemistry, anesthesiology, and pharmacology)
$=C_6H_4$	a divalent radical (chemistry)
C_6H_6	benzene (chemistry)
C_6H_{13}	hexyl (chemistry)
C_6H_{14}	hexane (chemistry)
C_7H_8	toluene (chemistry)
$C_{10}H_7$	naphthyl (chemistry and pharmacology)
$C_{10}H_8$	naphthalene (chemistry and pharmacology)
$C_{10}H_{14}$	myristicene (chemistry)
$C_{10}H_{16}$	myrcene (chemistry and pharmacology)
	phellandrene [a liquid hydrocarbon] (chemistry)
	pinene [also called *firpene;* a terpene] (chemistry)
$C_{10}H_{19}$	menthyl [the monovalent radical] (chemistry)
$C_{14}H_{10}$	anthracene (chemistry)
$C_{21}H_{16}$	methycholanthrene (chemistry)
$C_{21}H_{34}$	pregene [a steroid] (endocrinology and laboratory)
$C_{21}H_{36}$	pregnane [a steroid hydrocarbon] (endocrinology and laboratory)
$C_{26}H_{54}$	hexacosane (chemistry)
$C_{28}H_{58}$	octacosane [an aliphatic hydrocarbon extracted from plant waxes] (chemistry)
$C_{29}H_{60}$	nonacosane (chemistry)
$C_{30}H_{61}$	myricyl (chemistry)
$C_{40}H_{56}$	lycopene [a plant pigment] (chemistry)
cH	hydrogen ion concentration (chemistry)
$C_6H_{16}AlKO_{11}$	potassium glucaldrate [an antacid] (gastroenterology and pharmacology)
CH_3AsCl_2	methyldichlorarsin [a lethal war gas] (armed forces and chemistry)
$C_{13}H_{13}As_2N_2NaO_4S$	neoarsphenamine (pharmacology)
$C_6H_6AsNO_5$	nitarsone (chemistry and veterinary medicine)
$C_6H_6AsNO_2 \cdot HCl$	oxophenarsine hydrochloride [an arsenical] (gyne-

cology, infectious diseases, pharmacology, and urology)

$C_{12}H_{15}AsN_6OS_2$ melarsoprol (pharmacology)

$(CH_3)_2AsOLi$ lithium cacodylate (pharmacology)

C_2H_5Br ethyl bromide (chemistry)

$C_{15}H_{11}BrCl_2N_2$ nolinium bromide (pharmacology)

$C_{20}H_8Br_2HgNa_2O_6$ merbromin (pharmacology)

$C_{12}H_{30}Br_2N_2$ hexamethonium bromide (pharmacology)

$C_{36}H_{12}Br_2N_2$ hexafluorenium bromide (anesthesiology and pharmacology)

$C_5H_8BrNO_4$ nibroxane (pharmacology)

$C_8H_{18}BrNO_2$ methacholine bromide (pharmacology)

$C_{10}H_{16}Br_2N_2O_2$ pipobraman [an antineoplastic agent] (chemotherapy, hematology, oncology, and pharmacology)

$C_{12}H_{19}BrN_2O_2$ neostigmine bromide (pharmacology)

$C_{13}H_9Br_2NO_2$ metabromsalan (pharmacology)

$C_{17}H_{24}BrNO_3$ homatropine methylbromide (pharmacology)

$C_{18}H_{24}BrNO_4$ methscopolamine bromide [also called *scopolamine methylbromide*] (gastroenterology and pharmacology)

$C_{20}H_{30}BrNO_3$ ipratropium bromide (pharmacology)

$C_{21}H_{26}BrNO_3$ mepenzolate bromide (pharmacology)

methantheline bromide (pharmacology)

$C_{21}H_{34}BrNO_3$ oxyphenonium bromide [an anticholinergic] (gastroenterology and pharmacology)

$C_{22}H_{28}BrNO_3$ pipenzolate bromide [an anticholinergic] (gastroenterology and pharmacology)

$C_{23}H_{30}BrNO_3$ propantheline bromide [an anticholinergic] (gastroenterology and pharmacology)

$C_{24}H_{26}BrN_3O_3$ nicergoline (pharmacology)

scopolamine methylbromide [also called *methscopolamine bromide*] (gastroenterology and pharmacology)

$C_{35}H_{60}Br_2N_2O_4$ pancuronium bromide [a skeletal muscle relaxant] (anesthesiology, neurology, pharmacology, and respiratory)

$C_{18}H_{30}BrNO_3S$ penthienate bromide [an anticholinergic] (gastroenterology and pharmacology)

$C_{24}H_{24}CaI_6N_4O_4$ ipodate calcium [radiopaque medium] (chemistry, pharmacology, and radiology)

$C_{14}H_{18}CaN_3Na_3O_{10}$ pentetate calcium trisodium [also called *calcium trisodium penetate;* used as a chelating agent] (chemistry and pharmacology)

$C_{14}H_{24}CaN_4O_8 \cdot 2H_2O$ piperazine edetate calcium [used as an antihelmintic] (pharmacology)

$C_{20}H_{21}CaN_7O_7 \cdot 5H_2O$ leucovorin (chemotherapy, oncology, and pharmacology)

$C_{62}H_{70}CaN_4O_{22} \cdot 2H_2O$ novobiocin calcium (pharmacology)

$C_{44}H_{46}Ca_4O_{18}$ — oxytetracycline calcium [an antibacterial] (pharmacology)

$(CH_3)_2C{:}CH \cdot CH_2 \cdot CH_2 \cdot C(CH_3){:}CH \cdot CH_2OH$
nerol (chemistry)

$(CH_3)_2C{:}C_6H_7 \cdot CHO$ — hyrtenal (chemistry)

$(CH_3)_2C{:}C_6H_7 \cdot CH_2OH$ — myrtenol (chemistry)

$CH_3 \cdot C{:}CH \cdot C(OH){:}C \cdot CHO$
methyl hydroxy-furfurol (chemistry)

$CH_3(C{:}CH \cdot NH{:}CH{:}C)C_2H_5$
methyl ethyl-pyrrole (laboratory)

$(CH_3)_2C{:}C_6H_7(OH){:}CH_2$
pinocarveol [also called *isocarveol*; a terpene alcohol] (chemistry)

$C_2H_5(C \cdot CO \cdot NH \cdot CO)CCH_3$
methyl ethyl-maleicimid (chemistry and laboratory)

$(CH_3)_2CH$ — isopropyl (chemistry)

$C_6H_3(CH_3)_3$ — mesitylene (chemistry)

$(C_6H_4 \cdot CH)_2$ — phenanthrene [a hydrocarbon] (chemistry)

$CH_3CH{=}CH-$ — propenyl [a three-carbon radical with one double bond in between two of the carbons] (chemistry)

$CH_3 \cdot CH{:}CH_2$ — propylene [a gasseous hydrocarbon] (chemistry)

$CH_3 \cdot CH_2 \cdot CH_2$ — propyl [the univalent chemical radical] (chemistry)

$CH_3 \cdot CH_2 \cdot CH_3$ — propane [a gas] (chemistry)

$CH_3(CH_2)_6CH_3$ — octane [an oily hydrocarbon found in petroleum] (chemistry)

$C_3H_5 \cdot C_6H_8 \cdot CH_3$ — limonene (chemistry)

$CH_3[CH(CH_3)(CH_2)_3]_3C(CH_3){:}CH \cdot CH_2OH$
phytol [an alcohol used in preparation of phytonadione and vitamin E] (pharmacology)

$C_3H_5[CH_3(CH_2)_7CH{:}CH(CH_2)_7CO \cdot O]_3$
glycerotrioleate [also called *olein*] (chemistry and pharmacology)

$CH_3 \cdot CH(CH_3)CH_2NCS$ — butyl isothiocyanate (chemistry and pharmacology)

$(CH_3)_2CHCH_2CH_2NH_2$ — isoamylamine (chemistry)

$(CH_3)_2 \cdot CH \cdot CH_2CH(NH_2) \cdot CO_2 \cdot C_2H_5$
leucinethylester (chemistry and laboratory)

$(CH_3CH_2CH_2COO)_2Mn$ — manganese butyrate (pharmacology)

$CH_3 \cdot (CH_2)_3 \cdot CH(NH_2) \cdot COOH$
norleucine [an amino acid] (chemistry and laboratory)

$CH_3(C_2H_5) \cdot CHCH(NH_2) \cdot COOH$
isoleucine (laboratory)

$CH_3CH_2CH_2Cl$ — *n*-propoyl chloride (chemistry)

$CH_3 \cdot CH(C_6H_5)NCS$ — phenyl-ethyl isothiocyanate (chemistry)

$C_6H_5 \cdot CH_2CH(NH_2)COOH$
phenylalanine [an amino acid] (genetics and laboratory)

$CH_3(CH_2)_5CHO$	heptanal [also called *heptoic aldehyde* and *oenanthol*] (chemistry)
$CH_3CHClCH_3$	isopropyl chloride (chemistry)
$CH_3(CH_2)_{14} \cdot CO \cdot (CH_2)_{14} \cdot CH_3$	
	palmitone [a crystalline compound] (chemistry)
$(CH_2-CH_2)_n$	polyethylene [a synthetic plastic material] (chemistry and surgery)
$C_5H_4(CH_3)N$	methylpyridine (chemistry and laboratory)
$CH_2:CHN(CH_3)_3OH$	neurine [a poisonous ptomaine] (chemistry and laboratory)
$CH_3(CH_2)_5NH_2$	*n*-hexylamine (chemistry)
$(CH_3 \cdot CHO)_3$	metaldehyde (pharmacology)
$C_3H_5(C_{14}H_{27}O_2)_3$	myristin (chemistry)
$C_3H_5(C_{16}H_{31}O_2)_3$	palmitin [a fat] (chemistry and laboratory)
$C_{30}H_{61} \cdot C_{16}H_{31}O_2$	myricin (chemistry)
$C_3H_5 \cdot C_6H_3(OCH_3)_2$	methyl eugenol (chemistry)
$CH_3(CHOH)_4CHO$	isorhodeose (chemistry)
$CH_3CHOH \cdot COHN_2$	lactamide (laboratory)
$CH_3 \cdot C_{10}H_4(:O)_2 \cdot OH$	plumbagin [used as an abortifacient] (chemistry, obstetrics, and pharmacology)
$(CH_3C_6H_4 \cdot O)PO$	triorthocresyl phosphate [a poisonous compound] (chemistry)
$CHCl_3$	chloroform (anesthesiology and chemistry)
CH_2Cl_2	methylene chloride [also called *methylene dichloride*] (anesthesiology, chemistry, and pharmacology)
CH_3Cl	methyl chloride (anesthesiology, chemistry, and pharmacology)
$C_2H_4Cl_2$	ethylene chloride (chemistry)
C_2H_5Cl	ethyl chloride (chemistry)
$C_6H_4Cl_2$	orthodichlorobenzene [an insecticide] (chemistry)
$C_6H_6Cl_6$	lindane [an insecticide] (chemistry)
$C_{14}H_{10}Cl_4$	mitotane (chemotherapy, oncology, and pharmacology)
$C_{22}H_{23}ClFN_3O_2$	milenperone (pharmacology)
$C_{28}H_{27}ClF_5NO$	penfluridol [a tranquilizer] (neurology, pharmacology, and psychiatry)
$C_{11}H_{13}ClF_3N_3O_4S_3$	polythiazide [a diuretic and antihypertensive] (cardiovascular and pharmacology)
$C_3H_2ClF_6O$	isoflurane (anesthesiology and pharmacology)
$C_3H_4Cl_2F_2O$	methoxyflurane (anesthesiology and pharmacology)
C_9H_5ClINO	iodochlorhydroxyquin (pharmacology)
$C_9H_{20}ClN$	isometheptene hydrochloride (pharmacology)
$C_{11}H_{10}Cl_2N_4$	metoprine (chemotherapy, oncology, and pharmacology)
$C_{11}H_{17}Cl_2N_2$	proguanil hydrochloride [also called *chloroguanide hydrochloride;* an antimalarial] (infectious diseases, pharmacology, and respiratory)

$C_{12}H_{30}Cl_2N_2$	hexamethonium chloride (pharmacology)
$C_{17}H_{18}ClN_3$	lergotrile (pharmacology)
$C_{17}H_{18}ClN_3 \cdot CH_4O_3S$	lergotrile mesylate (pharmacology)
$C_5H_{11}Cl_2N \cdot HCl$	mechlorethamine hydrochloride (chemotherapy, oncology, and pharmacology)
$C_{12}H_{18}ClN \cdot HCl$	mefenorex hydrochloride (pharmacology)
$C_{16}H_{15}ClN_2 \cdot HCl$	medazepam hydrochloride (pharmacology)
$C_{25}H_{27}ClN_2 \cdot 2HCl \cdot H_2O$	meclizine hydrochloride (pharmacology)
$C_6H_4ClNO_4$	nifurmerone (pharmacology)
$C_7H_9ClN_2O$	pralidoxime chloride (gastroenterology, neurology, and pharmacology)
$C_7H_{10}ClN_3O_3$	ornidazole [an anti-infective] (pharmacology)
$C_8H_{11}Cl_2N_3O_2$	uracil mustard (chemotherapy, oncology, and pharmacology)
$C_8H_{18}ClNO_2$	acetyl-betamethylcholine [also called *methacholine chloride*] (pharmacology)
$C_9H_{16}ClN_3O_2$	lomustine (chemotherapy, oncology, and pharmacology)
$C_{10}H_9ClN_4O$	nimazone (pharmacology)
$C_{11}H_{10}ClNO_3$	meseclazone (pharmacology)
$C_{11}H_{11}Cl_2N_3O$	muzolimine (pharmacology)
$C_{13}H_8Cl_2N_2O_4$	niclosamide (pharmacology)
	nifuroxime (pharmacology)
$C_{13}H_{14}ClNO_2$	pirprofen [an anti-inflammatory] (pharmacology)
$C_{13}H_{18}Cl_2N_2O_2$	melphalan (chemotherapy, oncology, and pharmacology)
$C_{14}H_{16}Cl_2N_4O_3$	obidoxime chloride [a cholinesterase reactivator] (pharmacology)
$C_{15}H_{10}Cl_2N_2O_2$	lorazepam (pharmacology)
$C_{15}H_{11}ClN_2O$	mecloqualone (pharmacology)
$C_{15}H_{11}ClN_2O_2$	oxazepam [a tranquilizer] (chemical dependency, neurology, pharmacology, and psychiatry)
$C_{16}H_{13}ClN_2O$	mazindol (pharmacology)
$C_{17}H_{12}ClN_5O$	intrazole (pharmacology)
$C_{18}H_{14}Cl_4N_2O$	isoconazole (pharmacology)
$C_{18}H_{18}ClN_3O$	loxapine (pharmacology)
$C_{18}H_{26}ClNO_2$	pranolium chloride [a cardiac depressant] (cardiovascular and pharmacology)
$C_{19}H_{16}ClNO_4$	indomethacin (pharmacology)
$C_{19}H_{17}ClN_2O$	prazepam [used as a muscle relaxant and tranquilizer] (neurology, pharmacology, and psychiatry)
$C_{20}H_{17}ClN_2O_3$	ketazolam (pharmacology)
$C_{20}H_{21}Cl_2NO_4$	lifibrate (pharmacology)
$C_{20}H_{24}ClNO_2$	methopholine (pharmacology)
$C_{21}H_{27}ClN_2O_2$	hydroxyzine (pharmacology)
$C_{21}H_{35}ClN_2O_3$	lapyrium chloride (chemistry and pharmacology)
$C_{22}H_{21}ClN_2O_8$	meclocycline (pharmacology)

$C_{27}H_{35}ClN_2O_5$	nisterime acetate (laboratory)
$C_{34}H_{46}ClN_3O_{10}$	maytansine (chemotherapy, oncology, and pharmacology)
$C_{11}H_6ClN_3O_6 \cdot 2C_4H_{11}NO_3$	
	lodoxamide tromethamine (pharmacology)
$C_{18}H_{18}ClN_3O \cdot C_4H_6O_4$	loxapine succinate (pharmacology)
$C_{21}H_{27}ClN_2O_2 \cdot C_{23}H_{16}O_6$	
	hydroxyzine pamoate (pharmacology)
$C_{13}H_{16}ClNO \cdot HCl$	ketamine hydrochloride (anesthesiology and pharmacology)
$C_{13}H_{18}ClNO \cdot HCl$	lometraline hydrochloride (pharmacology)
$C_{13}H_{21}ClN_2O_2 \cdot HCl$	metabutethamine hydrochloride (anesthesiology, dentistry, and pharmacology)
$C_{14}H_{22}ClN_3O_2 \cdot HCl$	metoclopramide hydrochloride (pharmacology)
$C_{17}H_{16}Cl_2N_2O_3 \cdot HCl$	parconazole hydrochloride [an antifungal] (pharmacology)
$C_{18}H_{22}ClNO \cdot HCl$	phenoxybenzamine hydrochloride [an alpha-adrenergic blocking agent used as an antihypertensive] (cardiovascular and pharmacology)
$C_{21}H_{27}ClN_2O_2 \cdot 2HCl$	hydroxyzine hydrochloride (pharmacology)
$C_{22}H_{27}ClN_2O \cdot HCl$	lorcainide hydrochloride (pharmacology)
$C_{22}H_{27}ClN_2O_3 \cdot HCl$	lorajmine hydrochloride (pharmacology)
$C_{29}H_{33}ClN_2O_2 \cdot HCl$	loperamide hydrochloride (pharmacology)
$C_{18}H_{14}Cl_4N_2O \cdot HNO_3$	miconazole nitrate (pharmacology)
$C_{28}H_{44}ClNO_2 \cdot H_2O$	methylbenzethonium chloride [a disinfectant] (chemistry and pharmacology)
$C_{18}H_{26}ClN_3O \cdot H_2SO_4$	hydroxychloroquine sulfate (pharmacology)
$C_7H_{15}Cl_2N_2O_2P$	ifosfamide (chemotherapy, oncology, and pharmacology)
$C_7H_8ClN_3 \cdot O_4S_2$	hydrochlorothiazide (cardiovascular and pharmacology)
$C_9H_{11}Cl_2N_3O_4S_2$	methyclothiazide (pharmacology)
$C_{12}H_{10}Cl_2N_2O_2S$	pazoxide [an antihypertensive] (cardiovascular and pharmacology)
$C_{13}H_{19}ClN_2O_5S_2$	mefruside (pharmacology)
$C_{16}H_{16}ClN_3O_3S$	metolazone (pharmacology)
$C_{21}H_{24}ClN_3OS$	pipamazine [used as an antiemetic] (gastroenterology and pharmacology)
$C_{21}H_{26}ClN_3OS$	perphenazine [used an antipsychotic and antiemetic] (gastroenterology, pharmacology, and psychiatry)
$C_{18}H_{35}ClN_2O_5S \cdot HCl$	mirincamycin hydrochloride (pharmacology)
$C_9H_8ClNS_2$	nimidane (chemistry and veterinary medicine)
$C_{20}H_{24}ClN_3S$	prochlorperazine [also called *prochlorpemazine*; an antiemetic] (gastroenterology and pharmacology)
C_6H_5ClO	parachlorophenol [an antibacterial] (pharmacology)
$C_8H_{12}Cl_3O_6$	paracloralose [a substance in iridescent plates] (chemistry)

$C_{11}H_{15}ClO_2$	phenaglycodol [a tranquilizer] (neurology, pharmacology, and psychiatry)
$C_{13}H_6Cl_6O_2$	hexaclorophene (chemistry and pharmacology)
$C_{13}H_{11}ClO_4$	orpanoxin [an anti-infective] (pharmacology)
$C_{13}H_{16}Cl_{12}O_8$	petrichloral [used as a hypnotic and sedative] (neurology, pharmacology, and psychiatry)
$C_{16}H_{15}Cl_3O_2$	methoxychlor [an insecticide] (chemistry)
$C_{28}H_{33}ClO_{16}$	peonin chloride [a purple dye] (chemistry)
$C_4H_8Cl_3O_4P$	metrifonate [also called *trichlorfon*] (chemistry, pharmacology, and veterinary medicine)
$(CH_3)_3C_4(NH)C_2H_5$	phyllopyrrole [trimethylethylpyrrole from bile pigments] (chemistry and laboratory)
$C_5H_{11} \cdot CO \cdot CH_3$	methyl amylketone (chemistry)
$C_{63}H_{91}CoN_{13}O_{14}P$	mecobalamine (laboratory)
$(C_6H_5 \cdot CO \cdot O)_2Hg + H_2O$	
	mercuric benzoate (pharmacology)
$C_2H_5CO_2NH_2$	ethyl carbamate (chemistry)
$C_{62}H_{89}CoN_{13}O_{15}P$	hydroxocobalamin [also called *vitamin B$_{12b}$*] (pharmacology)
$(CH_3 \cdot CO)_2O$	acetic anhydride (chemistry)
$CH_3 \cdot COOH$	acetic acid (chemistry)
$C_4H_9 \cdot COOH$	valeric acid (chemistry)
$CH_3 \cdot COOK$	potassium acetate (gastroenterology, pharmacology, and urology)
$C_6H_5 \cdot CO \cdot Li$	lithium benzoate (chemistry)
ChE	cholinesterase (laboratory)
$C_2H_2F_4$	norflurane (anesthesiology and pharmacology)
$C_7H_3F_{12}N_3$	midaflur (pharmacology)
$C_{17}H_{16}F_6N_2O$	mefloquine (pharmacology)
$C_{21}H_{30}FN_3O_2$	pipamperone [a tranquilizer] (neurology, pharmacology, and psychiatry)
$C_{22}H_{23}F_2NO_2$	lenperone (pharmacology)
$C_{28}H_{29}F_2N_3O$	pimozide [a tranquilizer] (neurology, pharmacology, and psychiatry)
$C_{28}H_{31}FN_2O$	nivazol (laboratory)
$C_{30}H_{35}F_2N_2O$	lidoflazine (pharmacology)
$C_8H_8F_3N_3O_4S_2$	hydroflumethiazide (pharmacology)
$C_{23}H_{29}FO_6$	isoflupredone acetate (pharmacology)
$C_{24}H_{31}FO_6$	paramethasone acetate [a glucocorticoid] (allergy, orthopedics, pharmacology, and rheumatology)
$C_{27}H_{34}F_2O_7$	procinonide [a steroid] (endocrinology and pharmacology)
$C_6H_{14}FO_3P$	isoflurophate (pharmacology)
C_5HgN_3	histamine (chemistry, laboratory, and pharmacology)
$C_5HgN_3 \cdot 2HCl$	histamine hydrochloride (pharmacology)
$C_6H_5Hg^+$	phenylmercuric ion (chemistry)
$C_{13}H_{16}HgNNaO_6$	mersalyl (pharmacology)

$C_{16}H_{25}HgNNa_2O_6S$	mercaptomerin sodium (pharmacology)
$C_6H_5HgNO_3$	phenylmercuric nitrate [a salt] (chemistry)
$C_7H_5HgNO_3$	nitromersol (dentistry, pharmacology, and surgery)
$C_{16}H_{22}HgN_6O_7$	meralluride (nephrology, and pharmacology)
$C_8H_8HgO_2$	phenylmercuric acetate [a crystalline salt] (chemistry)
$C_{20}H_{26}H_2 \cdot HCl$	mimbane hydrochloride (pharmacology)
CHI_3	iodoform (chemistry and pharmacology)
CH_3I	methyl iodide (pharmacology)
C_2H_5I	ethyl iodide (chemistry)
CH_2INaO_3S	methiodal sodium [a radiopaque medium] (pharmacology and radiology)
$C_{15}H_{10}I_4NNa_4xH_2O$	levothyroxine sodium (chemistry, endocrinology, laboratory, and pharmacology)
$C_8H_3I_2NNaO_5$	iodomethamate sodium [a radiopaque medium] (radiology)
$C_9H_7INNaO_3$	iodohippurate sodium [a radiopaque medium] (radiology)
$(C_{11}H_8I_3N_2NaO_4)$	iothalamate sodium [a radiopaque medium] (radiology)
$C_{12}H_{10}I_3N_2NaO_4$	metrizoate sodium [a radiopaque medium] (pharmacology and radiology)
$C_{12}H_{12}I_3N_2NaO_2$	ipodate sodium [a radiopaque medium] (radiology)
$C_{15}H_{11}I_3NNaO_4$	liothyronine sodium (pharmacology)
$C_{20}H_{12}I_6N_2Na_2O_6$	iodipamide sodium [a radiopaque medium] (radiology)
$C_5H_3I_2NO$	iopydone [a radiopaque medium] (radiology)
$C_7H_9IN_2O$	pralidoxime iodide (pharmacology)
$C_8H_9I_2NO_3$	iopydol [a radiopaque medium] (radiology)
$C_9H_{11}IN_2O_5$	idoxuridine (pharmacology)
$C_9H_{24}I_2N_2O$	propiodal [previously used as a source of iodine] (chemistry)
$C_{10}H_{11}I_2NO_3$	propyliodone [a radiographic medium] (radiology)
$C_{11}H_{16}I_2N_2O_5$	iodopyracet [a radiopaque medium] (radiology)
$C_{12}H_{11}I_3N_2O_4$	iodamide [a radiopaque medium] (radiology)
$C_{12}H_{13}I_3N_2O_2$	ipodate (chemistry)
$C_{15}H_{12}I_3NO_4$	liothyronine (pharmacology)
$C_{15}H_{13}I_2NO_4$	iodoquinol (pharmacology)
$C_{18}H_{22}I_3N_3O_8$	metrizamide [radiopaque medium] (pharmacology and radiology)
$C_{18}H_{26}I_3N_2O_9$	iothalamate meglumine [a radiopaque medium] (radiology)
$C_{18}H_{26}I_3N_3O_9$	iodothalamic acid (cardiovascular, pharmacology, and radiology)
$C_{20}H_{14}I_6N_2O_6$	iodipamide [a radiopaque medium] (radiology)
$C_{23}H_{33}IN_2O$	isopropamide iodide (pharmacology)
$C_{24}H_{20}I_6N_4O_8 \cdot 2C_7H_{17}NO_5$	iocarmate meglumine [a radiopaque medium] (radiology)

$C_{28}H_{28}I_6N_4O_{10}S \cdot C_7H_{17}NO_5$

    iosulamide meglumine [a radiopaque medium] (radiology)

$C_{19}H_{29}IO_2$ iophendylate [a radiopaque medium] (radiology)

$C_4H_4KNaO_6 \cdot 4H_2O$ potassium sodium tartrate [also called *Preston's salt, Rochelle salt,* and *Seignette's salt;* used as a cathartic] (gastroenterology and pharmacology)

$C_4H_6KNO_4 \cdot \frac{1}{2}H_2O$ and $C_8H_{12}MgN_2O_8 \cdot 4H_2O$

    potassium aspartate and magnesium aspartate [used as a nutrient] (dietary, gastroenterology, and pharmacology)

$C_{16}H_{17}KN_2O_4S$ penicillin G potassium [an antibiotic] (pharmacology)

$C_{16}H_{17}KN_2O_5S$ penicillin V potassium [an antibiotic] (pharmacology)

$C_{17}H_{19}KN_2O_5S$ phenethicillin potassium [an antibacterial] (pharmacology)

$C_{18}H_{21}KN_2O_5S$ levopropylcillin potassium [also called *propicillin*] (pharmacology)

$C_{19}H_{22}KN_3O_4S$ hetacillin potassium (pharmacology)

$C_4H_5KO_6$ potassium bitartrate [also called *cream of tartar*] (dietary and veterinary medicine)

$C_6H_{11}KO_7$ potassium gluconate (dietary and pharmacology)

$C_{23}H_{31}KO_4$ prorenoate potassium [an aldosterone antagonist] (endocrinology and pharmacology)

$C_6H_5K_3O_7H_2O$ potassium citrate (cardiovascular, dietary, gastroenterology, pharmacology, respiratory, and veterinary medicine)

$C_{24}H_{33}KO_6 \cdot 2H_2O$ mexrenoate potassium (pharmacology)

$C_3H_7MnO_6P$ manganese glycerophosphate (pharmacology)

$(C_3H_6)_n$ polipropene [a tablet excipient] (pharmacology)

$C_4H_{10}N_2$ piperazine [also called *diethyl diamine, dispermine,* and *piperazine hexahydrate,* the salts of which are used as an antihelmintic] (pharmacology)

$C_4H_{11}N_5$ metformin (pharmacology)

$C_6H_{10}N_4$ pentylenetetrazol [also called *leptazol* and *pentamethylenetetrazol;* a central nervous system stimulant] (neurology, pharmacology, and psychiatry)

$C_6H_{12}N_4$ methenamine (pharmacology)

$C_7H_6N_4$ nifuraldezone (pharmacology)

$C_7H_{17}N$ methyhexamine [also called *methylhexaneamine*] (pharmacology)

$C_8H_{13}N$ hydrocollidine (chemistry)

$C_8H_{19}N$ octodrine [an adrenergic] (anesthesiology, cardiovascular, and pharmacology)

$C_9H_{13}N$	levamfetamine (pharmacology)
	parvoline [a liquid poison] (chemistry)
$C_{10}H_2N$	propylhexedrine [used as a vasocontrictor] (allergy, otorhinolaryngology, and pharmacology)
$C_{10}H_{10}N_2$	β-nicotyrine (chemistry)
$C_{10}H_{14}N_2$	nicotine (chemistry, pharmacology, and veterinary medicine)
$C_{10}H_{15}N$	methamphetamine (pharmacology)
	phentermine [used as an anorexic] (gastroenterology and pharmacology)
$C_{10}H_{21}N$	pempidine tartrate [a ganglion blocking agent used as an antihypertensive] (cardiovascular, neurology, and pharmacology)
$C_{10}H_{21}N_3$	perlapine [a hypnotic] (pharmacology and psychiatry)
$C_{10}H_{24}N_2$	hexamethonium (pharmacology)
$C_{13}H_{11}N_3$	proflavine [also called *diamino-acridine;* a disinfectant] (chemistry and pharmacology)
$C_{19}H_{27}N_3$	morrhuin [a ptomaine] (chemistry and laboratory)
$C_{19}H_{28}N_2$	iprindole (pharmacology)
$C_{20}H_{23}N$	maprotiline (pharmacology)
$C_{21}H_{45}N_3$	hexetidine (pharmacology)
$C_{22}H_{45}N_3$	hexedine (pharmacology)
$C_{27}H_{24}N_4$	mauvein [a violet dye used to determine pH] (chemistry and laboratory)
$C_{36}H_{27}N_3$	nigrosin [a dye] (laboratory)
$C_{14}H_{13}NaO_3$	naproxen sodium (pharmacology)
$C_{25}H_{33}NaO_8$	hydrocortisone sodium succinate (pharmacology)
$C_{25}H_{35}NaO_6$	hydroxydione sodium succinate (anesthesiology and pharmacology)
$C_{26}H_{33}NaO_8$	methylprednisolone sodium succinate (pharmacology)
$CH_4Na_2O_6P_2$	medronate disodium (pharmacology)
$C_6H_6Na_{12}O_{24}P_6$	phytate persodium [a pharmaceutic aid] (pharmacology)
$C_{21}H_{27}Na_2O_8P$	prednisolone sodium phosphate (allergy, chemotherapy, gastroenterology, oncology, ophthalmology, orthopedics, pharmacology, and rheumatology)
$C_{21}H_{29}Na_2O_8P$	hydrocortisone sodium phosphate (pharmacology)
$C_{22}H_{29}Na_2O_8P$	methylprednisolone sodium phosphate (pharmacology)
$C_{11}H_9NaO_5S \cdot 3H_2O$	menadione sodium bisulfite (hematology and pharmacology)
$C_9H_6N \cdot CH_3$	methylquinoline (chemistry)
$CH_3 \cdot N{:}C_6H_8{:}CH \cdot O$	oscine (chemistry and laboratory)
$(CH_3)_2NC_6H_4CHO$	paradimethylaminobenzaldehyde [used in reagents] (laboratory)

$C_5H_4N^+(CH_3)CO_2^-$ homarine (laboratory)

$C_6H_5N(CH_3)NH_2$ methyphenylhydrazine (chemistry and laboratory)

$C_6H_{12}N_4 \cdot C_9H_9NO_3$ methenamine hippurate (pharmacology)

$C_{16}H_{20}N_2 \cdot 2C_{16}H_{18}N_2O_4S \cdot 4H_2O$
penicillin G benzathine [an antibiotic] (pharmacology)

$C_9H_{13}N \cdot C_4H_6O_4$ levamfetamine succinate (pharmacology)

$C_{16}H_{18}N_2 \cdot C_4H_4O_4$ nomifensine maleate (pharmacology)

$C_{16}H_{20}N_2 \cdot C_4H_4O_4$ pheniramine maleate [an antihistaminic] (allergy, otorhinolaryngology, and pharmacology)

$C_{19}H_{19}N \cdot C_4H_6O_6$ phenindamine tartrate [an antihistamine] (allergy, pharmacology, and otorhinolaryngology)

$[(C_{19}H_{18}N_3)_2 \cdot C_{23}H_{14}O_6] \cdot 2H_2O$
pararosaniline pamoate [an antischistosomal] (parasitology and pharmacology)

$(C_4H_{10}N_2)_3 \cdot 2C_6H_8O_7 \cdot xH_2O$
piperazine citrate [used as an antihelmintic] (pharmacology)

$C_5H_{10}N \cdot CO \cdot (CH)_3CH \cdot C_6H_3 \cdot O_2 \cdot CH_2$
piperine [used as an insecticide] (chemistry)

$C_3H_5 \cdot NCS$ allyl isothiocyanate (chemistry)

CH_3NH_2 methylamine (chemistry and laboratory)

$(C_2H_5)_2NH$ diethylamine (chemistry)

$C_6H_4(NH_2)_2$ paraphenylenediamine [a dye] (chemistry)

$C_6H_5NH_2$ aniline (chemistry)

$C_{10}H_{11}NH_2$ hydronaphthylamine (chemistry)

$CH_2 \cdot NH \cdot C(CH_3){:}N \cdot CH_2$
lysidin (laboratory)

$CH_3NHC_3H_7$ methyl propylamine (chemistry)

$C_6H_4 \cdot NH \cdot CH{:}C \cdot C_6H_{11}O_5$
indican (chemistry)

$C_6H_4NH \cdot CH \cdot CO_2 \cdot OK$ potassium indoxyl sulfate (laboratory)

$CH_2NH_2 \cdot CHOH \cdot COOH$
isoserine (chemistry)

$CH_3NHC_6H_4OH \cdot H_2SO_4$ Metol [trademark for a photographic developing solution] (chemistry and dermatology)

$C_8H_8N_4 \cdot HCl$ hydralazine hydrochloride (pharmacology)

$C_{10}H_{15}N \cdot HCl$ methamphetamine hydrochloride (pharmacology)

phentermine hydrochloride [used as an anorexic] (gastroenterology and pharmacology)

phenylpropylmethylamine hydrochloride [also called *phenpromethamine hydrochloride*; an adrenergic used as a vasoconstrictor] (allergy, otorhinolaryngology, and pharmacology)

$C_{10}H_{15}N_5 \cdot HCl$ phenformin hydrochloride [an oral hypoglycemic agent] (endocrinology and pharmacology)

$C_{11}H_{11}N_5 \cdot HCl$ phenazopyridine hydrochloride [an urinary analgesic] (gynecology, pharmacology, and urology)

$C_{11}H_{13}N \cdot HCl$	pargyline hydrochloride [an antihypertensive] (cardiovascular and pharmacology)
$C_{11}H_{13}N_3 \cdot HCl$	imafen hydrochloride (pharmacology)
$C_{11}H_{21}N \cdot HCl$	mecamylamine hydrochloride (pharmacology)
$C_{14}H_{14}N_2 \cdot HCl$	naphazoline hydrochloride (ophthalmology, otorhinolaryngology, and pharmacology)
$C_{15}H_{23}N \cdot HCl$	prolintane hydrochloride [an antidepressant] (neurology, pharmacology, and psychiatry)
$C_{17}H_{25}N \cdot HCl$	phencyclidine hydrochloride [a veterinary analgesic and anesthetic used as an illicit drug (PCP)] (chemical dependency, pharmacology, psychiatry, and veterinary medicine)
$C_{18}H_{20}N_2 \cdot HCl$	mianserin hydrochloride (pharmacology)
$C_{19}H_{21}N \cdot HCl$	indriline hydrochloride (pharmacology)
	nortriptyline hydrochloride (pharmacology and psychiatry)
$C_{19}H_{24}N_2 \cdot HCl$	imipramine hydrochloride (pharmacology)
$C_{21}H_{19}N \cdot HCl$	intriptyline hydrochloride (pharmacology)
$C_{21}H_{25} \cdot NHCl$	melitracen hydrochloride (pharmacology)
$C_6H_5NHCSNH_2$	phenylthiourea [also called *phenylthiocarbamide* or *PTC*; used in genetic research] (genetics, laboratory, and research)
$C_{16}H_{35}N \cdot HF$	hetaflur (dentistry and pharmacology)
$C_6H_5NH \cdot NH_2$	phenylhydrazine [used as a reagent] (endocrinology and laboratory)
$C_{11}H_{16}N_2 \cdot HNO_3$	pilocarpine nitrate [used as a cholinergic] (ophthalmology and pharmacology)
$C_{12}H_8N_2 \cdot H_2O$	orthophenanthrolene (chemistry and laboratory)
$C_5H_9N_3 \cdot 2H_3PO_4$	histamine phosphate (laboratory and pharmacology)
$C_{20}H_{21}N \cdot H_3PO_4$	octriptyline phosphate [an antidepressant] (neurology, pharmacology, and psychiatry)
$C_4H_{10}N_2 \cdot H_3PO_4 \cdot H_2O$	piperazine phosphate [used as an antihelmintic] (gastroenterology and pharmacology)
$C_8H_{12}N_2 \cdot H_2SO_4$	phenelzine sulfate [used as an antidepressant] (neurology, pharmacology, and psychiatry)
$(C_{11}H_{17}N)_2 \cdot H_2SO_4$	mephentermine sulfate (pharmacology)
$C_{25}H_{25}N_2I$	pinacyanole [an aniline dye used as a tissue stain and for red sensitization of photographic plates] (laboratory, pathology, and photography)
$C_{12}H_{11}N_2NaO_3$	phenobarbital sodium [an anticonvulsant, hypnotic, and sedative] (neurology, pharmacology, and psychiatry)
$C_{12}H_{15}N_2NaO_3$	hexobarbital sodium (anesthesiology and pharmacology)
$C_{12}H_{19}N_2NaO_5$	hexethal sodium (pharmacology)
$C_{14}H_{17}N_2NaO_3$	methohexital sodium (anesthesiology and pharmacology)

$C_{15}H_{22}N_2NaO_2$	phenytoin sodium [an anticonvulsant and cardiac depressant] (cardiovascular, neurology, and pharmacology)
$C_{16}H_8N_2Na_2O_8$	indicarmine [also called *indigocarmine, indigotin-disulfonate sodium,* and *soluble indigo blue*] (chemistry and laboratory)
$C_{31}H_{35}N_2NaO_{11}$	novobiocin sodium (pharmacology)
$C_{19}H_{19}N_2NaO_2 \cdot C_3H_8O_3$	
	phenbutazone sodium glycerate [an anti-inflammatory] (pharmacology)
$C_8H_{11}N_2NaO_3 \cdot \frac{1}{2}H_2O$	pentizidone sodium [an antibacterial] (pharmacology)
$C_{11}H_8NNaO_4 \cdot H_2O$	nivimedone sodium (pharmacology)
$C_{12}H_{11}N_2NaO_3H_2O$	nalidixate sodium (pharmacology)
$C_{16}H_{17}N_2NaO_4S$	penicillin G sodium [an antibiotic] (pharmacology)
$C_{17}H_{19}N_2NaO_6S$	methicillin sodium (pharmacology)
$C_{21}H_{21}N_2NaO_5S$	nafcillin (pharmacology)
$C_{23}H_{26}N_5NaO_7S$	piperacillin sodium [an antibacterial] (pharmacology)
$C_{24}H_{25}N_6NaO_5S$	pirbenicillin sodium [an antibacterial] (pharmacology)
$C_{19}H_{18}N_3NaO_5S \cdot H_2O$	oxacillin sodium [a semisynthetic penicillinase-resistant penicillin] (pharmacology)
$C_6H_5 \cdot N{:}N \cdot C_{10}H_4(SO_2 \cdot ONa)_2 \cdot OH$	
	orange G [an acid azo dye] (laboratory)
CH_3NO_2	nitromethane [an explosive] (chemistry)
$CH_4N_2O_2$	hydroxyurea (chemotherapy, oncology, and pharmacology)
C_2H_7NO	colamin [also called *ethanolamine* and *monoethanolamine*] (pharmacology)
	monothioglycerol (pharmacology)
$C_3H_5(NO_3)_3$	glyceryl trinitrate [also called *nitroglycerin*] (chemistry and pharmacology)
$C_3H_5N_3O_9$	nitroglycerin [an explosive as well as a medication] (chemistry, cardiology, and pharmacology)
$C_4H_7N_3O$	isokreatinin (chemistry)
$C_5H_4N_4O$	hypoxanthine (laboratory)
$C_5H_4N_4O_2$	oxypurinol [a xanthine oxidase inhibitor] (pharmacology)
$C_5H_4N_4O_3$	uric acid (chemistry)
$C_5H_5NO_2$	mecrylate [a tissue adhesive] (chemistry and surgery)
$C_5H_8N_4O_{12}$	pentaerythritol tetranitrate [also called *niperty, pentaerythrityl tetranitrate, penthrit, pentrinitrol,* and *PTEN*; an explosive and a vasodilator] (chemistry, cardiovascular, and pharmacology)
$C_5H_9N_3O_{10}$	pentoxifylline [a coronary vasodilator] (cardiovascular and pharmacology)

$C_5H_{11}NO_2$	amyl nitrite (chemistry and pharmacology)
$C_6H_5NO_2$	niacin [also called *nicotinic acid;* a vitamin of the vitamin B complex] (chemistry, dietary, laboratory, and pharmacology)
	nitrobenzene [a poisonous substance also called *nitrobenzol* and *oil of mirbane*] (chemistry)
$C_6H_5(NO_3)_3$	nitroglycerin [also called *glyceryl trinitrate*] (cardiovascular, chemistry, and pharmacology)
$C_6H_5N_5O_3$	leucopterin (chemistry)
$C_6H_6N_2O$	niacinamide [also called *nicotinamide*] (pharmacology)
$C_6H_6N_4O_4$	nitrofurazone (pharmacology)
$C_6H_7N_3O$	isoniazid (pharmacology)
$C_6H_8H_2O_8$	isosorbide dinitrate (pharmacology)
$C_6H_9N_3O_3$	metronidazole (pharmacology)
$C_6H_{11}NO$	nortropinon [a ketone] (chemistry and laboratory)
$C_6H_{11}N_3O_9$	propatyl nitrate [a coronary vasodilator] (cardiovascular and pharmacology)
$C_6H_{13}NO_2$	leucine [an amino acid] (laboratory)
	mydatoxine [a ptomaine] (chemistry and laboratory)
$C_7H_6N_4O_2$	melizame (chemistry)
$C_7H_8N_2O_5$	nifuratrone (pharmacology)
$C_7H_9N_2O^+$	pralidoxime [also called *2-PAM;* a cholinesterase reactivator] (pharmacology)
$C_7H_{11}NO_3$	paramethadione [an anticonvulsant] (neurology and pharmacology)
$C_7H_{11}N_3O_2$	ipronidazole (pharmacology)
$C_7H_{11}N_3O_4$	misonidazole (pharmacology)
$C_7H_{17}NO_5$	meglumine (pharmacology and radiology)
$C_8H_6N_4O_5$	nitrofurantoin (pharmacology)
$C_8H_8N_4O_4$	nifuradene (pharmacology)
C_8H_9NO	acetanilid (chemistry)
$C_8H_{10}N_4O_4$	nifursemizone (chemistry and veterinary medicine)
$C_8H_{11}NO_3$	oxidopamine [an ophthalmic adrenergic] (ophthalmology and pharmacology)
$C_8H_{15}NO_2$	oxanamide [a tranquilizer] (neurology, pharmacology, and psychiatry)
$C_8H_{16}N_2O_6$	piperazine tartrate [used as an antihelmintic] (pharmacology)
$C_8H_{18}NO_2$	methacholine (pharmacology)
$C_9H_8N_2O_2$	pemoline [a central nervous system stimulant] (neurology and pharmacology)
$C_9H_9NO_3$	hippuric acid (chemistry)
$C_9H_{10}N_2O_2$	phenacemide [an anticonvulsant] (neurology and pharmacology)
$C_9H_{11}NO_4$	levodopa (pharmacology)

$C_9H_{13}NO$	norpseudoephedrine [also called *katine*] (chemistry and pharmacology)
$C_9H_{13}NO_3$	homoarterenol hydrochloride [also called *nordefrin hydrochloride*] (pharmacology)
	levonordefrin [an anesthetic] (anesthesiology, dentistry, and pharmacology)
$C_9H_{13}N_3O$	iproniazide (pharmacology)
$C_9H_{14}N_2O_3$	metharbital (pharmacology)
	probarbital [used as a sedative] (neurology, pharmacology, and psychiatry)
$C_9H_{15}N_5O$	minoxidil (pharmacology)
$C_9H_{18}N_2O_4$	meprobamate (pharmacology)
$C_9H_{18}N_4O_4$	nifurimide (pharmacology)
$C_9H_{19}NO_4$	panthenol [also called *pantothenol* and *pantothenyl alcohol*; the alcohol derivative of pantothenic acid] (chemistry, dietary, and pharmacology)
$C_{10}H_7 \cdot NO_2$	nitronaphthalene (chemistry)
$C_{10}H_{10}N_2O_3$	mequidox (pharmacology)
$C_{10}H_{11}N_3O_2$	lobendazole (chemistry, pharmacology, and veterinary medicine)
$C_{10}H_{12}N_4O_4$	nebularine (chemotherapy, oncology, and pharmacology)
$C_{10}H_{12}N_4O_5$	nifurdazil (pharmacology)
$C_{10}H_{13}NO_2$	phenacetin [an analgesic and antipyretic] (pharmacology)
$C_{10}H_{13}NO_3$	metyrosine (pharmacology)
$C_{10}H_{14}N_2O$	nikethamide (pharmacology)
$C_{10}H_{17}NO_2$	methyprylon (pharmacology)
$C_{10}H_{20}N_2O_4$	mebutamate (pharmacology)
$C_{11}H_{11}NO_2$	phensuximide [an anticonvulsant] (neurology and pharmacology)
$C_{11}H_{13}NO_4$	mephenoxalone (pharmacology)
$C_{11}H_{15}NO_2$	isobutamben (anesthesiology and pharmacology)
$C_{11}H_{15}NO_3$	hydroxyphenamate (pharmacology)
$C_{11}H_{15}NO_5$	methocarbamol (pharmacology)
$C_{11}H_{16}N_2O_2$	pilocarpine [an alkaloid used as a cholinergic] (ophthalmology and pharmacology)
$C_{11}H_{17}NO_3$	isoproterenol (pharmacology)
$C_{11}H_{17}N_2O_3$	pentobarbital [a barbiturate used as a hypnotic and sedative] (anesthesiology, neurology, pharmacology, and psychiatry)
$C_{11}H_{28}N_2O_3$	myokinin (laboratory)
$C_{12}H_7N_5O_9$	nifursol (chemistry and veterinary medicine)
$C_{12}H_{10}N_2O_4$	nifurpirinol (pharmacology)
$C_{12}H_{10}N_4O_2$	lumichromic (chemistry and laboratory)
$C_{12}H_{11}NO$	pirfenidone [an anti-inflammatory and antipyretic] (pharmacology)
$C_{12}H_{12}N_2O_3$	phenobarbital [a barbiturate used as an anticonvul-

957

	sant, hypnotic, and sedative] (neurology, pharmacology, and psychiatry)
$C_{12}H_{13}NO_2$	methsuximide (neurology and pharmacology)
$C_{12}H_{13}N_3O_2$	isocarboxazid (pharmacology)
$C_{12}H_{14}N_2O_2$	mephenytoin [an anticonvulsant] (neurology and pharmacology)
	methetoin (pharmacology)
	primidone [also called *desoxyphenobarbital*; an anticonvulsant] (neurology and pharmacology)
$C_{12}H_{15}NO_3$	metaxalone (pharmacology)
$C_{12}H_{15}N_3O_3$	oxibendazole [a veterinary antihelmintic] (pharmacology and veterinary medicine)
$C_{12}H_{16}N_2O_3$	hexobarbital (pharmacology)
$C_{12}H_{19}NO_2$	ocrylate [a tissue adhesive] (pharmacology and surgery)
$C_{12}H_{20}N_2O_2$	isamoxole (pharmacology)
$C_{12}H_{21}N_5O_3$	oxtriphylline [also called *choline theophyllinate* and *theophylline cholinate*; a bronchodilator] (pharmacology and respiratory)
$C_{12}H_{22}N_2O_2$	leucinimide (chemistry and laboratory)
$C_{12}H_{22}N_2O_4$	lorbamate (pharmacology)
$C_{13}H_{11}NO_3$	phenyl aminosalicylate [a tuberculostatic antibacterial] (infectious disease, pharmacology, and respiratory)
$C_{13}H_{12}N_4O_2$	lumiflavin (chemistry and laboratory)
$C_{13}H_{14}N_2O_3$	mephobarbital (pharmacology)
$C_{13}H_{15}NO_2$	octazamide [an analgesic] (pharmacology)
$C_{13}H_{16}N_4O_6$	levofuraltadone (pharmacology)
$C_{13}H_{17}N_3O_2$	parbendazole [a veterinary antihelmintic] (pharmacology and veterinary medicine)
$C_{13}H_{18}N_2O_2$	mingin (laboratory)
$C_{13}H_{18}N_2O_3$	heptabarbital (pharmacology)
$C_{13}H_{18}N_6O_5$	moxnidazole (pharmacology)
$C_{13}H_{20}N_2O_2$	procaine [a local anesthetic] (anesthesiology and pharmacology)
$C_{13}H_{21}NO_3$	isoetharine (pharmacology)
$C_{13}H_{26}N_2O_4$	nisobamate (pharmacology)
$C_{13}H_{36}N_2O_{11}$	novobiocin (pharmacology)
$C_{14}H_{14}N_2O$	mepyrapone [also called *metapyrone, methylpyrapone*, and *metyapone*; a diagnostic aid] (laboratory)
$C_{14}H_{18}N_2O_2$	hypaphorine [a poisonous alkaloid] (chemistry)
$C_{14}H_{18}N_2O_3$	methohexital (pharmacology)
$C_{14}H_{18}N_2O_5$	lidofenin (laboratory)
$C_{14}H_{18}N_4O_2$	ormetoprim [an antibacterial] (pharmacology)
$C_{14}H_{19}NO_2$	piperoxan hydrochloride [an alpha-adrenergic blocking agent] (hematology, pharmacology, and surgery)

$C_{14}H_{20}N_2O_2$	pindolol [a beta-adrenergic blocking agent] (cardiovascular and pharmacology)
$C_{14}H_{20}N_4O_3$	methenamine mandelate (pharmacology)
$C_{14}H_{21}NO_2$	padimate A [an ultraviolet screen] (dermatology and pharmacology)
$C_{14}H_{21}N_3O_3$	oxamniquine [an antischistosomal] (pharmacology)
$C_{14}H_{22}N_2O$	lidocaine [an anesthetic] (anesthesiology and pharmacology)
$C_{14}H_{22}N_2O_2$	naepaine (pharmacology)
$C_{14}H_{22}N_2O_3$	practolol [a beta-adrenergic blocking agent] (cardiovascular and pharmacology)
$C_{15}H_{11}N_3O$	nitrazepam (pharmacology)
$C_{15}H_{12}N_2O_2$	phenytoin [an anticonvulsant and cardiac depressant] (cardiovascular, neurology, and pharmacology)
$C_{15}H_{18}N_4O_5$	mitomycin C (chemotherapy, oncology, and pharmacology)
$C_{15}H_{19}NO$	pronethalol [a beta-adrenergic blocking agent] (cardiovascular and pharmacology)
$C_{15}H_{21}N_3O_2$	physostigmine [also called *eserine;* a cholinergic which functions as an anticholinesterase] (neurology and pharmacology)
$C_{15}H_{22}N_2O_2$	mixidine (pharmacology)
$C_{15}H_{24}N_2O_3$	mefexamide (pharmacology)
$C_{15}H_{25}NO_3$	metoprolol (pharmacology)
$C_{16}H_{10}N_2O_2$	indigo blue [also called *indigotin*] (chemistry and laboratory)
$C_{16}H_{13}N_3O_3$	mebendazole (pharmacology)
$C_{16}H_{14}N_2O$	methaqualone (pharmacology)
$C_{16}H_{15}N_3O_5$	pirolate [an antiasthmatic] (pharmacology and respiratory)
$C_{16}H_{16}N_4O_5$	nifurquinazol (pharmacology)
$C_{16}H_{17}NO_4$	narcissine (chemistry)
$C_{16}H_{18}N_4O_2$	nialamide (pharmacology)
$C_{16}H_{20}N_4O_5$	porfiromycin [an antineoplastic antibiotic] (chemotherapy, oncology, and pharmacology)
$C_{16}H_{21}NO_2$	propranolol [a beta-adrenergic blocking agent] (cardiovascular, neurology, and pharmacology)
$C_{16}H_{21}NO_3$	homatropine (ophthalmology and pharmacology) norhyoscyamine [an alkaloid] (chemistry)
$C_{17}H_{15}NO_3$	indoprofen (pharmacology)
$C_{17}H_{18}N_2O_6$	nifedipine (pharmacology)
$C_{17}H_{19}NO_3$	hydromorphone (pharmacology) morphine (pharmacology)
$C_{17}H_{19}N_3O$	phentolamine [an antiadrenergic] (cardiovascular and pharmacology)
$C_{17}H_{21}NO$	phenyltoloxamine citrate [used as an antihistaminic] (allergy, otorhinolaryngology, and pharmacology)

$C_{17}H_{21}NO_2$	nisoxetine (pharmacology)
$C_{17}H_{23}NO_3$	hyoscyamine (pharmacology)
$C_{17}H_{27}NO_2$	padimate O [an ultraviolet screen] (dermatology and pharmacology)
$C_{18}H_{15}NO_3$	oxaprozin [an anti-inflammatory] (pharmacology)
$C_{18}H_{18}N_2O$	proquazone [an anti-inflammatory] (pharmacology)
$C_{18}H_{23}NO$	mephenamine [also called *orphenadrine*] (neurology and pharmacology)
$C_{18}H_{23}NO_2$	ketazocine [an analgesic] (pharmacology)
$C_{18}H_{24}N_2O_2$	menispermine (chemistry)
$C_{18}H_{25}NO_2$	moxazocine (pharmacology)
$C_{18}H_{26}N_2O_4$	proglumide [an anticholinergic] (pharmacology)
$C_{18}H_{26}N_2O_6$	atropine methonitrate [also called *atropine methylnitrate* and *methylatropine nitrate*] (pharmacology)
$C_{18}H_{27}NO_5$	propanidid [an anesthetic] (anesthesiology and pharmacology)
$C_{19}H_{17}NO_2$	neocinchophen (pharmacology)
$C_{19}H_{20}N_2O_2$	phenylbutazone [also called *diphebuzol;* having analgesic, anti-inflammatory, antipyretic, and uricosuric properties] (orthopedics, pharmacology, and rheumatology)
$C_{19}H_{21}NO_3$	allorphine [also called *antorphine* and *nalorphine*] (pharmacology)
$C_{19}H_{24}N_2O_2$	praziquantel [an antihelmintic] (pharmacology and veterinary medicine)
$C_{19}H_{29}N_3O_4$	pamaquine [an antimalarial] (infectious diseases and pharmacology)
$C_{20}H_{15}NO_3$	oxyphenisatin [a cathartic] (gastroenterology and pharmacology)
$C_{20}H_{20}N_2O_4$	leniquinsin (pharmacology)
$C_{20}H_{22}N_8O_5$	methotrexate (chemotherapy, oncology, and pharmacology)
$C_{20}H_{23}NO_4$	naltrexone (pharmacology)
$C_{20}H_{23}N_3O_2$	oxiperomide [a tranquilizer] (neurology, pharmacology, and psychiatry)
$C_{20}H_{25}N_3O$	prodigiosin [an antibiotic dye] (pharmacology)
$C_{20}H_{26}N_2O$	ibogaine (pharmacology)
$C_{20}H_{27}NO_2$	oxilorphan [a narcotic antagonist] (pharmacology)
$C_{20}H_{44}N_2O_{10}$	hexobendine (pharmacology)
$C_{21}H_{19}NO_4$	oxarbazole [an anti-asthmatic] (pharmacology and respiratory)
$C_{21}H_{21}N_3O_9$	nitrocycline (pharmacology)
$C_{21}H_{27}N_3O_2$	methysergide (pharmacology)
$C_{22}H_{22}N_2O_8$	methacycline (pharmacology)
$C_{22}H_{23}NO_4$	nequinate (chemistry)
$C_{22}H_{23}NO_7$	noscapine (pharmacology)
$C_{22}H_{25}N_3O$	indoramin (pharmacology)

$C_{22}H_{27}NO_2$	alpha-lobeline (pharmacology)
$C_{22}H_{29}NO_2$	propoxyphene [also called *dextropropoxyphene*; an analgesic] (pharmacology)
$C_{22}H_{47}N_3O$	lycetamine (pharmacology)
$C_{23}H_{27}N_3O_7$	minocycline (pharmacology)
$C_{23}H_{29}NO_{12}$	hygromycin [also called *hygromycin A*] (pharmacology)
$C_{23}H_{29}N_3O$	pirolazamide [a cardiac depressant] (cardiovascular and pharmacology)
$C_{23}H_{29}N_3O_2$	oxypertine [an antidepressant] (pharmacology and psychiatry)
$C_{23}H_{31}NO_2$	acetylmethadol [also called *methadyll acetate*] (pharmacology)
	levomethadyl acetate (pharmacology)
$C_{23}H_{31}NO_3$	norgestimate [a progestin] (endocrinology, gynecology, obstetrics, and pharmacology)
$C_{23}H_{42}N_2O_{12}$	pentolinium tartrate [a ganglionic blocking agent used as a antihypertensive] (cardiovascular, neurology, and pharmacology)
$C_{23}H_{45}N_5O_{14}$	paromomycin [an antibiotic] (pharmacology)
$C_{24}H_{19}NO_5$	oxyphenisatin acetate [a cathartic] (gastroenterology and pharmacology)
$C_{24}H_{31}N_3O_3$	milipertine (pharmacology)
$C_{25}H_{29}N_3O$	nufenoxole (pharmacology)
$C_{25}H_{34}N_2O_2$	oxiramide [a cardiac depressant] (cardiovascular and pharmacology)
$C_{25}H_{45}NO_9$	pederin [a toxin isolated from beetles] (chemistry)
$C_{27}H_{27}NO$	pentazocine [a synthetic analgesic] (pharmacology)
$C_{27}H_{30}N_4O$	oxatomide [an antiallergic and antiasthmatic] (allergy, pharmacology, and respiratory)
$C_{27}H_{40}N_2O_2$	pifarnine [an antiulcerative] (gastroenterology and pharmacology)
$C_{27}H_{43}NO_3$	imperialine [an alkaloid] (chemistry)
$C_{28}H_{24}N_2O_7$	orcein [a brown coloring material used as a specific stain for elastic tissue] (laboratory)
$C_{28}H_{41}N_3O_3$	oxethazaine [a topical anesthetic] (anesthesiology, gastroenterology, and pharmacology)
$C_{32}H_{34}N_4O_2$	phylloporphyrin [a compound from chlorophyll] (chemistry)
$C_{32}H_{40}N_4O_7$	hydrobilirubin (laboratory)
$C_{33}H_{47}NO_{13}$	natamycin [also called *pimaricin*] (ophthalmology and pharmacology)
$C_{34}H_{32}N_2O_6$	micranthine (chemistry)
$C_{36}H_{42}N_2O_{10}$	myoctonine [a poisonous alkaloid] (chemistry)
$C_{42}H_{30}N_6O_{12}$	inositol niacinate (pharmacology)
$C_{42}H_{45}N_3O_7$	pamaquine naphthoate [an antimalarial] (infectious diseases and pharmacology)
$C_{42}H_{69}NO_{15}$	josamycin (pharmacology)

$C_{46}H_{77}NO_{19}$ fungicidin [also called *nystatin*] (pharmacology)

$C_{16}H_{18}N_2O_4C_{19}H_{20}ClN_3$ clemizole penicillin [used to produce a form of penicillin G] (pharmacology and research)

$(C_7H_{17}NO_5)_2 \cdot C_{20}H_{14}I_4N_2O_6$
　　iodipamide meglumine [also called *iodipamide methylglucamine*] (radiology)

$C_9H_{13}NO_2 \cdot C_4H_6O_6$ metaraminol (pharmacology)

$C_{12}H_{13}NO \cdot C_4H_6O_5$ nafomine malate (pharmacology)

$(C_{13}H_{16}N_2O)_2 \cdot C_{23}H_{16}O_6$ oxantel pamoate [an antihelmintic] (pharmacology)

$C_{14}H_{14}N_2O \cdot 2C_4H_6O_6$ metyrapone tartrate [a diagnostic aid] (laboratory)

$C_{15}H_{21}N_3O_2C_7H_6O_3$ physostigmine salicylate [a cholinergic] (neurology, pharmacology, and ophthalmology)

$C_{16}H_{25}N_3O \cdot C_4H_4O_4$ propiram fumarate [an analgesic] (pharmacology)

$C_{18}H_{23}NO \cdot C_6H_8O_7$ orphenadrine citrate (neurology and pharmacology)

$C_{19}H_{22}N_2O \cdot C_4H_4O_4$ ketipramine fumarate (pharmacology)

$C_{19}H_{25}NO \cdot C_4H_6O_6$ levallorphan tartrate (pharmacology)

$C_{20}H_{25}N_3O_2 \cdot C_4H_4O_4$ methylergonovine maleate (pharmacology)

$C_{21}H_{21}NO_2 \cdot C_4H_4O_4$ oxetorone fumarate [an analgesic] (neurology and pharmacology)

$C_{21}H_{27}N_3O_2 \cdot C_4H_4O_4$ methysergide maleate (pharmacology)

$C_{24}H_{33}NO_3 \cdot C_2H_2O_4$ nafronyl oxalate (pharmacology)

$C_{27}H_{28}N_2O_4 \cdot C_6H_8O_7$ nitromifene citrate (pharmacology)

$C_6H_{11}NO_3 \cdot C_4H_6O_6 \cdot H_2O$ levarterenol bitartrate [also called *norepinephrine bitartrate*] (pharmacology)

$C_{17}H_{23}NO \cdot C_4H_6O_6 \cdot 2H_2O$
　　levorphanol tartrate (pharmacology)

$C_{18}H_{21}NO_3 \cdot C_4H_6O_6 \cdot 2\frac{1}{2}H_2O$
　　hydrocodone bitartrate (pharmacology)

$C_{18}H_{21}NO_3 \cdot C_4H_6O_6 \cdot 2\frac{1}{2}H_2O$
　　dihydrocodeinone bitartrate (pharmacology)
　　hydrocodone bitartrate (pharmacology)

$C_{16}H_{16}N_4O \cdot 2C_2H_6O_4S$ hydroxystilbamidine isethionate (pharmacology)

$C_{17}H_{19}N_3O \cdot CH_4O_3S$ phentolamine mesylate [an antiadrenergic] (dermatology, hematology, and pharmacology)

$C_{22}H_{27}NO_6 \cdot CH_4O_3S$ nisbuterol mesylate (pharmacology)

$C_{23}H_{30}N_2O_2 \cdot C_2H_6O_3S$ piminodine esylate [a synthetic narcotic analgesic] (pharmacology)

$C_{22}H_{29}NO_2 \cdot C_{10}H_8O_3S \cdot H_2O$
　　levopropoxyphene napsylate (pharmacology)
　　propoxyphene napsylate [used as an analgesic] (pharmacology)

$C_{34}H_{33}N_4O_4FeCl$ hemin (laboratory)

$C_9H_{13}NO \cdot HBr$ hydroxyamphetamine hydrobromide (pharmacology)

$C_{16}H_{21}NO_3 \cdot HBr$ homatropine hydrobromide (pharmacology)

$C_{17}H_{23}NO_3HBr$ hyoscyamine hydrobromide (pharmacology)

$C_{22}H_{27}NO \cdot HBr$ phenazocine hydrobromide [a synthetic narcotic analgesic] (pharmacology)

$C_6H_9N_3O_2 \cdot HCl$	histadine monohydrochloride (pharmacology)
$C_9H_{13}NO \cdot HCl$	phenylpropanolamine hydrochloride [used as a bronchodilator, central nervous system stimulant, and vasoconstrictor] (allergy, neurology, otorhinolaryngology, pharmacology, and respiratory)
$C_9H_{13}NO_2 \cdot HCl$	phenylephrine hydrochloride [an adrenergic] (cardiovascular, otorhinolaryngology, and pharmacology)
$C_{11}H_{15}NO \cdot HCl$	phenmetrazine hydrochloride [a central nervous system stimulant and anorexic] (gastroenterology, neurology, and pharmacology)
$C_{11}N_{16}N_2O_2 \cdot HCl$	pilocarpine hydrocloride [used as a cholinergic] (ophthalmology and pharmacology)
$C_{11}H_{17}NO \cdot HCl$	methoxyphenamine hydrochloride (pharmacology and respiratory)
$C_{11}H_{17}NO_3 \cdot HCl$	isoproterenol hydrochloride (pharmacology)
	methoxamine hydrochloride (pharmacology)
$C_{12}H_{17}NO_4 \cdot HCl$	methyldopate hydrochloride (pharmacology)
$C_{12}H_{19}N_3O \cdot HCl$	procarbazine hydrochloride [an antineoplastic] (chemotherapy, oncology, and pharmacology)
$C_{12}H_{19}NO_4 \cdot HCl$	oxymorphone hydrochloride [used as a narcotic analgesic] (pharmacology)
$C_{12}H_{20}N_2O_3 \cdot 2HCl$	pirbuterol hydrochloride [a bronchodilator] (pharmacology and respiratory)
$C_{13}H_{12}N_4O \cdot HCl$	oxifungin hydrochloride [an antifungal] (pharmacology)
$C_{13}H_{14}N_2O \cdot HCl$	phenyramidol hydrochloride [used as an analgesic and muscle relaxant] (neurology, orthopedics, and pharmacology)
$C_{13}H_{20}N_2O \cdot HCl$	prilocaine hydrochloride [a local anesthetic] (anesthesiology and pharmacology)
$C_{13}H_{20}N_2O_2 \cdot HCl$	procaine hydrochloride [an anesthetic] (anesthesiology and pharmacology)
$C_{13}H_{21}N_3O \cdot HCl$	*procainamide hydrochloride* [also called *procaine amide hydrochloride;* a cardiac depressant] (cardiovascular and pharmacology)
$C_{14}H_{18}N_2O_3 \cdot HCl$	letimide hydrochloride (pharmacology)
$C_{14}H_{19}NO_2 \cdot HCl$	methylphenidate hydrochloride (pharmacology)
$C_{14}H_{21}NO \cdot HCl$	profadol hydrochloride [an analgesic] (pharmacology)
$C_{14}H_{21}NO_2 \cdot HCl$	meprylcaine hydrochloride (anesthesiology and pharmacology)
$C_{15}H_{21}NO_2 \cdot HCl$	isonipecaine [also called *meperidine hydrochloride* and *pethidine hydrochloride*] (pharmacology)
$C_{15}H_{22}N_2O \cdot HCl$	mepivacaine hydrochloride (anesthesiology and pharmacology)
$C_{15}H_{23}NO_2 \cdot HCl$	isobucaine hydrochloride (anesthesiology, dentistry, and pharmacology)

$C_{15}H_{23}NO_3 \cdot HCl$	oxprenolol hydrochloride [a beta-adrenergic blocking agent] (cardiovascular and pharmacology)
$C_{16}H_{14}N_2O \cdot HCl$	methaqualone hydrochloride (pharmacology)
$C_{16}H_{21}NO_2 \cdot HCl$	propranolol hydrochloride [used for treatment of various cardiac conditions and for treatment of migraines] (cardiovascular, neurology, and pharmacology)
$C_{16}H_{23}NO_2 \cdot HCl$	hexylcaine hydrochloride (anesthesiology and pharmacology)
	piperocaine hydrochloride [a local anesthetic] (anesthesiology and pharmacology)
$C_{16}H_{24}N_2O \cdot HCl$	oxymetazoline hydrochloride [an adrenergic] (allergy, otorhinolaryngology, and pharmacology)
$C_{16}H_{24}N_2O_2 \cdot HCl$	molindone hydrochloride (pharmacology)
$C_{16}H_{26}N_2O_3 \cdot HCl$	proparacaine hydrochloride [an anesthetic] (anesthesiology, ophthalmology, and pharmacology)
	propoxycaine hydrochloride [an anesthetic] (anesthesiology and pharmacology)
$C_{17}H_{17}NO_2 \cdot HCl$	memotine hydrochloride (pharmacology)
$C_{17}H_{19}NO \cdot HCl$	nefopam hydrochloride (pharmacology)
$C_{17}H_{19}NO_3 \cdot HCl$	hydromorphone hydrochloride (pharmacology)
$C_{17}H_{19}N_3O \cdot HCl$	phentolamine hydrochloride [used as an antiadrenergic] (cardiovascular and pharmacology)
$C_{17}H_{23}NO \cdot HCl$	pirandamine hydrochloride [an antidepressant] (pharmacology and psychiatry)
$C_{17}H_{27}NO_3 \cdot HCl$	pramoxine hydrochloride [a topical local anesthetic] (anesthesiology and pharmacology)
$C_{17}H_{28}N_2O_3 \cdot HCl$	metabutoxycaine hydrochloride (anesthesiology, dentistry, and pharmacology)
$C_{18}H_{21}NO \cdot HCl$	oxycodone hydrochloride [a morphine derivative] (pharmacology)
	pipradrol hydrochloride [a central nervous stimulant used as an antidpressant] (neurology, pharmacology, and psychiatry)
$C_{18}H_{21}NO_2 \cdot HCl$	naranol hydrochloride (pharmacology)
$C_{18}H_{22}N_2O_2 \cdot HCl$	phenacaine hydrochloride [a topical local anesthetic] (ophthalmology and pharmacology)
$C_{18}H_{23}NO \cdot HCl$	orphenadrine hydrochloride (neurology and pharmacology)
$C_{18}H_{23}NO_3 \cdot HCl$	isoxsuprine hydrochloride (pharmacology)
$C_{18}H_{29}NO_4 \cdot HCl$	iproxamine hydrochloride (pharmacology)
$C_{18}H_{35}NO_2 \cdot HCl$	isomylamine hydrochloride (pharmacology)
$C_{19}H_{20}N_6O \cdot 2HCl$	imidocarb hydrochloride (pharmacology)
$C_{19}H_{21}NO_3 \cdot HCl$	nalorphine hydrochloride (pharmacology)
$C_{19}N_{21}NO_4HCl$	naloxone hydrochloride (pharmacology)
$C_{19}H_{21}N_5O_4 \cdot HCl$	prazosin hydrochloride [used as an antihypertensive] (cardiovascular and pharmacology)
$C_{19}H_{24}N_2O_3 \cdot HCl$	labetalol hydrochloride (pharmacology)

$C_{19}H_{25}NO_2 \cdot HCl$	nylidrin hydrochloride (pharmacology)
$C_{19}H_{26}N_4O_4 \cdot HCl$	piquizel hydrochloride [a bronchodilator] (pharmacology and respiratory)
$C_{19}H_{26}N_4O_5 \cdot HCl$	hoquizil hydrochloride (pharmacology)
$C_{19}H_{29}NO \cdot HCl$	procyclidine hydrochoride [used as a muscle relaxant] (neurology, orthopedics, and pharmacology)
$C_{19}H_{29}NO_2 \cdot HCl$	nexeridine hydrochloride (pharmacology)
$C_{20}H_{21}NO_4 \cdot HCl$	papaverine hydrochloride [used as a smooth muscle relaxant] (cardiovascular, neurology, and pharmacology)
$C_{20}H_{23}NO_2 \cdot HCl$	levoxadrol hydrochloride (anesthesiology and pharmacology)
$C_{20}H_{28}N_2O_3 \cdot HCl$	oxyphencyclimine hydrochloride [an anticholinergic] (gastroenterology and pharmacology)
$C_{21}H_{23}NO_3 \cdot HCl$	proroxan hydrochloride [an antiadrenergic] (pharmacology)
$C_{21}H_{25}NO_2 \cdot HCl$	piperidolate hydrochloride [used as an antispasmodic] (gastroenterology and pharmacology)
$C_{21}H_{25}NO_4 \cdot HCl$	nalmexone hydrochloride (pharmacology)
$C_{21}H_{27}NO \cdot HCl$	methadone hydrochloride (pharmacology)
$C_{21}H_{27}NO_4 \cdot HCl$	nalbuphine hydrochloride (pharmacology)
$C_{22}H_{22}N_2O_8 \cdot HCl$	methacycline hydrochloride (pharmacology)
$C_{22}H_{23}NO_7 \cdot HCl$	noscapine hydrochloride (pharmacology)
$C_{22}H_{24}N_2O_9 \cdot HCl$	oxytetracycline hydrochloride [an antibacterial] (pharmacology)
$C_{22}H_{25}NO_3 \cdot HCl$	pipoxolan hydrochloride [a muscle relaxant] (neurology and pharmacology)
$C_{22}H_{29}NO_2 \cdot HCl$	propoxyphene hydrochloride [an analgesic] (orthopedics and pharmacology)
$C_{22}H_{31}NO_3 \cdot HCl$	oxybutynin chloride [an anticholinergic] (gynecology, neurology, pharmacology, and urology)
$C_{23}H_{27}N_3O_7 \cdot HCl$	minocycline hydrochloride (pharmacology)
$C_{23}H_{29}N_3O \cdot 2HCl$	opipramol hydrochloride (pharmacology and psychiatry)
$C_{24}H_{32}N_2O_5 \cdot HCl$	metoserpate hydrochloride (chemistry and veterinary medicine)
$C_{27}H_{41}NO_6 \cdot HCl$	hydrocortisone (pharmacology)
$C_{29}H_{31}NO_2 \cdot HCl$	nafoxidine hydrochloride (chemotherapy, oncology, and pharmacology)
$C_{14}H_{22}N_2O \cdot HCl \cdot H_2O$	lidocaine hydrochloride (anesthesiology, cardiovascular, and pharmacology)
$C_{17}H_{19}NO_3 \cdot HCl \cdot 3H_2O$	morphine hydrochloride (pharmacology)
$C_{27}H_{58}N_2O_3 \cdot 2HF$	olaflur [a dental caries prophylactic] (dentistry and pharmacology)
$C_{15}H_{32}N_2O \cdot 2HNO_3$	pemerid nitrate [an antitussive] (pharmacology and respiratory)
$C_{10}H_{13}NO_4 1\frac{1}{2}H_2O$	methyldopa (pharmacology)
$C_{27}H_{39}N_5O_5 \cdot 6\frac{1}{2}H_2O$	paucine [an alkaloid] (chemistry)

$C_{19}H_{20}N_2O_3 \cdot H_2O$	oxyphenbutazone [an anti-inflammatory, analgesic, and antipyretic] (pharmacology)
$C_{22}H_{24}N_2O_9 \cdot 2H_2O$	oxytetracycline [an antibiotic] (pharmacology)
$C_{15}H_{21}N_3O \cdot 2H_3PO_4$	primaquine phosphate [an antimalarial] (infectious diseases, pharmacology, and respiratory)
$C_{35}H_{61}NO_{12} \cdot H_3PO_4$	oleandomycin phosphate [an antibacterial] (pharmacology)
$(C_{11}H_{17}NO_3)_2H_2 \cdot SO_4$	metaproterenol sulfate (pharmacology and respiratory)
$(C_{11}H_{17}N_3O_2) \cdot H_2SO_4$	meobentine sulfate (pharmacology)
$(C_{15}H_{21}N_3O_2)_2 \cdot H_2SO_4$	physostigmine sulfate [used as a cholinergic] (ophthalmology and pharmacology)
$(C_{16}H_{26}N_2O_4)_2 \cdot H_2SO_4$	pamatolol sulfate [an antiadrenergic] (pharmacology)
$(C_{18}H_{29}NO_2)_2 \cdot H_2SO_4$	penbutolol sulfate [an antiadrenergic] (cardiovascular and pharmacology)
$C_{18}H_{36}N_4O_{11} \cdot H_2SO_4$	kanamycin sulfate (pharmacology)
$(C_{21}H_{41}N_5O_7)_2 \cdot 5H_2SO_4$	netilmicin sulfate (pharmacology)
$(C_{11}H_{17}NO_3)_2 \cdot H_2SO_4 \cdot 2H_2O$	
	isoproterenol sulfate (pharmacology)
$(C_{17}H_{19}NO_3)_2 \cdot H_2SO_4 \cdot 5H_2O$	
	morphine sulfate (pharmacology)
$(C_{17}H_{23}NO_3)_2 \cdot H_2SO_4 \cdot 2H_2O$	
	hyoscyamine sulfate (pharmacology)
$C_6H_4(NO_2)OH$	nitrophenol (chemistry and laboratory)
$C_{44}H_{80}N_2O_{15} \cdot 2KH_2PO_4$	megalomicin potassium phosphate (pharmacology)
$(C_6H_{11}NO)_n$	policapram [used as a tablet binder] (pharmacology)
$C_6H_2(NO_2)_3OH$	picric acid [also called *trinitrophenal*] (chemistry)
$C_8H_{24}N_4O_3P_2$	octamethyl pyrophosphoramide [also called *schradan;* a systemic insecticide for plants] (chemistry)
$C_{11}H_{22}N_3O_3P$	meturedepa (chemotherapy, oncology, and pharmacology)
$C_{16}H_{16}NO_6P$	naftalofos (veterinary medicine)
$C_{21}H_{27}N_7O_{14}P_2$	nadide (chemistry and laboratory)
$C_{11}H_8N_4O_8P_2 \cdot 6H_2O$	menadiol sodium diphosphate [a synthetic derivative of vitamin K] (hematology and pharmacology)
$C_{10}H_{14}NO_5PS$	parathion [an insecticide] (agriculture and chemistry)
$C_5H_5N_3O_3S$	nithiamide (chemistry and veterinary medicine)
$C_5H_6N_2OS$	methylthiouracil (endocrinology, laboratory, and pharmacology)
$C_5H_6N_4O_3S_2$	methazolamide (ophthalmology and pharmacology)
$C_5H_{11}NO_2S$	methionine [an amino acid] (chemistry, dietary, laboratory)
	penicillamine [a degradation product of penicillin] (orthopedics, pharmacology, and rheumatology)

$C_6H_6N_4O_3S$ niridazole (pharmacology)

$C_7H_{10}N_2OS$ propylthiouracil [a thyroid inhibitor] (endocrinology and pharmacology)

$C_7H_{10}N_2O_2S$ mafenide (pharmacology)

$C_8H_9NO_2S$ oxisuran [an antineoplastic] (chemotherapy, oncology, and pharmacology)

$C_8H_{12}N_2O_4S$ pralidoxime mesylate (pharmacology)

$C_9H_7N_3O_4S_2$ para-nitrosulfathiazole [an antibacterial] (gastroenterology and pharmacology)

$C_{10}H_{10}N_4OS$ methisazone (pharmacology)

$C_{10}H_{11}N_3O_5S$ nifuratel (pharmacology)

$C_{10}H_{14}N_2O_3S$ lydimycin (pharmacology)

$C_{11}H_{16}N_2O_3S$ ozolinone [a diuretic] (cardiovascular, nephrology, pharmacology, and respiratory)

$C_{12}H_{22}N_2O_8S_2$ piposulfan [an antineoplastic] (chemotherapy, oncology, and pharmacology)

$C_{13}H_8N_2O_3S$ nitroscanate (chemistry and veterinary medicine)

$C_{13}H_{19}NO_4S$ probenecid [an uricosuric] (orthopedics, pharmacology, and rheumatology)

$C_{13}H_{22}N_2O_6S$ neostigmine methylsulfate (laboratory and pharmacology)

$C_{14}H_{11}N_3O_3S$ nocodazole (chemotherapy, oncology, and pharmacology)

$C_{14}H_{13}N_3O_5S$ isoxicam (pharmacology)

$C_{14}H_{22}N_2O_3S$ piprozolin [a cholerectic] (gastroenterology and pharmacology)

$C_{15}H_{13}N_3O_3S$ oxfendazole [an antihelmintic] (pharmacology)

$C_{15}H_{13}N_3O_4S$ piroxicam [an anti-inflammatory] (pharmacology)

$C_{16}H_{14}N_2O_6S$ phthalylsulfacetamide [also called *phthalylsulfonazole;* used as an antibacterial] (gastroenterology and pharmacology)

$C_{17}H_{13}N_3O_5S_2$ phthalylsulfathiazole [used as an antibacterial] (gastroenterology and pharmacology)

$C_{17}H_{20}N_2O_5S$ phenethicillin [an antibiotic] (pharmacology)

$C_{18}H_{34}N_2O_6S$ lincomycin (pharmacology)

$C_{19}H_{23}N_3O_4S$ hetacillin (pharmacology)

$C_{19}H_{24}N_2OS$ levomepromazine [also called *methotrimeprazine*] (pharmacology)

$C_{20}H_{33}NO_6S$ pentapiperide methylsulfate [also called *pentapiperium methylsulfate;* an anticholinergic] (gastroenterology and pharmacology)

$C_{21}H_{25}N_5O_8S_2$ mezlocillin (pharmacology)

$C_{21}H_{26}N_2OS_2$ mesoridazide (chemistry)

$C_{21}H_{27}NO_4S$ dimethyl tubocararine iodide [also called *metocurine iodide*] (pharmacology)

$C_{21}H_{36}N_2O_5S$ hexocyclium methylsulfate (pharmacology)

$C_{22}H_{26}N_2O_5S$ methopromazine maleate [also called *methoxypromazine maleate*] (pharmacology)

$C_{22}H_{27}N_3O_3S_2$ metopimazine (pharmacology)

$C_{22}H_{29}NO_7S$ poldine methylsulfate [an anticholinergic] (gastroenterology and pharmacology)

$C_{22}H_{29}N_2O_6S$ pivampicillin hydrochloride [an antibacterial] (pharmacology)

$C_{24}H_{30}N_2O_2S$ piperacetazine [an antipsychotic] (pharmacology and psychiatry)

$C_{40}H_{63}N_3O_4S_3$ pipotiazine palmitate [a tranquilizer] (neurology, pharmacology, and psychiatry)

$C_{46}H_{65}N_{13}O_{12}S$ lypressin (pharmacology)

$C_{51}H_{43}N_{13}O_{12}S_6$ nosiheptide (veterinary medicine)

$(C_{16}H_{18}N_2O_5S)_2C_{16}H_{20}N$ penicillin V benzathine [an antibiotic] (pharmacology)

$(C_{16}H_{18}N_2O_5S)_2 \cdot C_{42}H_{64}N_2$
penicillin V hydrabamine [an antibiotic] (pharmacology)

$C_7H_{10}N_2O_2S \cdot C_2H_4O_2$ mafenide acetate (pharmacology)

$C_{16}H_{18}N_2O_4S \cdot C_{13}H_{20}N_2H_2O$
penicillin G procaine [an antibiotic] (pharmacology)

$C_{43}H_{66}N_{12}O_{12}S_2 \cdot C_6H_8O_7$ oxytocin citrate [used to stimulate labor] (obstetrics and pharmacology)

$C_{21}H_{26}N_2OS_2 \cdot C_6H_6O_3S$ mesoridazole benzenesulfonate [also called *mesoridazole besylate*] (pharmacology)

$C_{20}H_{24}N_2O_2S \cdot CH_3SO_3H$ hycanthone methylate (pharmacology)

$C_7H_{10}N_2O_2S \cdot HCl$ mafenide hydrochloride (pharmacology)

$C_{11}H_{11}N_3O_2S \cdot HCl$ nitramisole hydrochloride (pharmacology)

$C_{12}H_{13}N_5O_2S \cdot HCl$ Prontosil [also called *Prontosil flavum* and *Prontosil rubrum;* no longer used therapeutically] (pharmacology and research)

$C_{19}H_{26}N_2O_5S \cdot HCl$ mesuprine hydrochloride (pharmacology)

$C_{20}H_{24}N_2OS \cdot HCl$ lucanthone hydrochloride (pharmacology)

propiomazine hydrochloride [an antiemetic and sedative] (gastroenterology, neurology, obstetrics, pharmacology, and surgery)

$C_{21}H_{25}N_3O_3S \cdot HCl$ pipazethate hydrochloride [an antitussive] (pharmacology and respiratory)

$C_{25}H_{35}NO_5 \cdot HCl$ mebeverine hydrochloride (pharmacology)

$C_{18}H_{34}N_2O_6S \cdot HCl \cdot H_2O$ lincomycin hydrochloride (pharmacology)

$(C_6H_9NO)_w(C_5H_8O_2)_x(C_7H_{10}O_2)_y(C_{10}H_{14}O_4)_z$
lidofilcon [a hydrophilic contact lens material] (chemistry and ophthalmology)

$C_{23}H_{45}N_5O_{14} \cdot xH_2SO_4$ paromomycin sulfate [an antiamebic] (pharmacology)

$C_{108}H_{360}N_5PO_{35}$ protagon [a crystalline mass] (laboratory and neurosurgery)

$C_4H_6N_2S$ methimazole (endocrinology and pharmacology)

$C_5H_4N_4S$ mercaptopurine (chemotherapy, oncology, and pharmacology)

$C_7H_{14}N_4S_2$ methallibure (chemistry and veterinary medicine)

$C_9H_{16}N_4S_2$ metiamide (pharmacology)

$C_{12}H_9NS$ phenothiazine [also called *dibenzothiazine* and *thiodiphenylamine;* a veterinary antihelmintic] (pharmacology and veterinary medicine)

$C_{14}H_{19}N_3S$ methapyrilene (pharmacology)

$C_{16}H_{19}N_3S$ isothipendyl (pharmacology)

$C_{18}H_{20}N_2S$ methdilazide (pharmacology)

$C_{19}H_{21}NS$ pizotyline [an anabolic, antidepressant, and serotonin inhibitor] (neurology, pharmacology, and psychiatry)

$C_{19}H_{21}N_3S$ metiapine (pharmacology)

$C_{19}H_{22}N_2S$ mepazine acetate (pharmacology)

$C_{12}H_{16}N_2S \cdot C_4H_6O_6$ morantel tartrate (chemistry and veterinary medicine)

$(C_{14}H_{19}N_3S)_2 \cdot 3C_4H_4O_4$ methapyrilene fumarate (pharmacology)

$C_{11}H_{12}N_2S \cdot HCl$ levamisole hydrochloride (pharmacology)

$C_{13}H_{14}N_2S \cdot HCl$ metizoline hydrochloride (pharmacology)

$C_{14}H_{19}N_3S \cdot HCl$ methapyrilene hydrochloride (pharmacology)

$C_{17}H_{20}N_2S \cdot HCl$ promazine hydrochloride [used as an analgesic, antiemetic, antipsychotic, and anesthetic potentiating agent] (anesthesiology, gastroenterology, neurology, pharmacology, and psychiatry)

promethazine hydrochloride [used as an antiemetic, antihistamine, and sedative and to potentiate central depressants] (allergy, gastroenterology, neurology, obstetrics, respiratory, and surgery)

$C_{18}H_{20}N_2S \cdot HCl$ methdilazine hydrochloride (pharmacology)

$C_{20}H_{23}NS \cdot HCl \cdot H_2O$ methixene hydrochloride (gastroenterology and pharmacology)

CH_2O the general formula for monosaccharides [simple sugars] (chemistry)

formaldehyde (chemistry, laboratory, and pharmacology)

CH_2O_2 formic acid (chemistry)

CH_4O methyl alcohol (chemistry)

$C_2H_2O_4$ oxalic acid (chemistry)

$C_2H_4O_2$ acetic acid (chemistry)

diose [a simple sugar] (chemistry)

C_2H_6O ethyl alcohol (chemistry)

$C_3H_4O_2$ propiolactone [also called *beta-propiolactone;* a disinfectant] (chemistry and pharmacology)

C_3H_6O acetone (chemistry)

$C_3H_6O_3$ lactic acid (chemistry)

triose [a simple sugar] (chemistry)

$C_3H_8O_2$ propylene glycol [used in pharmaceutical preparations] (pharmacology)

$C_3H_8O_3$	glycerin (chemistry)
$C_4H_6O_2$	crotonic acid (chemistry)
$C_4H_6O_5$	malic acid (chemistry)
$C_4H_6O_6$	tartaric acid (chemistry)
$C_4H_8O_2$	butyric acid [also called *isobutyric acid*] (chemistry)
$C_4H_8O_4$	tetrose [a simple sugar] (chemistry)
$C_4H_{10}O$	ether [also called *ethyl ether*] (chemistry)
$C_5H_8O_2$	methyl methacrylate (dentistry, orthopedics, and pharmacology)
$C_5H_{10}O_2$	valeric acid (chemistry)
$C_5H_{10}O_5$	pentose [a simple sugar] (chemistry)
$C_5H_{12}O$	amyl alcohol (chemistry)
C_6H_6O	phenol (chemistry)
$C_6H_6O_2$	hydroquinone (pharmacology)
$C_6H_6O_3$	phloroglucin [an aglycone used as a decalcifier in bone specimens] (laboratory and pathology)
$C_6H_7O_2$	potassium sorbate [used as a preservative] (pharmacology)
$C_6H_8O_2$	citric acid (chemistry)
$C_6H_{10}O$	meparfynol [also called *methylparafynol* and *methylpentynal*] (pharmacology)
$C_6H_{10}O_4$	isosorbide (pharmacology)
$C_6H_{10}O_5$	inuloid (laboratory)
	levulin (chemistry)
	meglutol (pharmacology)
$(C_6H_{10}O_5)_4$	inulin (laboratory)
$(C_6H_{10}O_5)_6$	hexamylase (chemistry)
$(C_6H_{10}O_5)_8$	octamylose [a carbohydrate of the starch group] (chemistry)
$C_6H_{12}O$	methyl isobutyl ketone (chemistry and pharmacology)
	paraldehyde [a hypnotic and sedative] (neurology, pharmacology, and psychiatry)
$C_6H_{12}O_4$	kethoxal (pharmacology)
$C_6H_{12}O_6$	dextrose [also called *d-glucose*] (chemistry)
	hexose [a simple sugar] (chemistry)
	inositol (chemistry and laboratory)
	laiose (endocrinology and laboratory)
$(C_6H_{12}O_6)$	mannans (chemistry)
$C_7H_4O_7$	meconic acid (chemistry)
$C_7H_6O_2$	benzoic acid (chemistry)
$C_7H_6O_3$	salicylic acid (chemistry)
$C_7H_6O_4$	patulin [an antibiotic and antimicrobial] (pharmacology)
$C_7H_6O_5$	gallic acid (chemistry)
$C_7H_{14}O_7$	heptose [a simple sugar] (chemistry)
	ketoheptose (chemistry and laboratory)

$C_8H_8O_3$	methyl salicylate (chemistry and pharmacology)
	methylparaben (pharmacology)
$C_8H_{16}O$	methyl heptenone (chemistry)
$C_8H_{16}O_8$	octose [a monosaccharide] (chemistry)
$C_9H_{12}O_2$	methylcreosol (chemistry)
$C_9H_{14}O$	phorone [a ketone] (chemistry, endocrinology, and laboratory)
$C_{10}H_6O_3$	juglone (pharmacology)
	lawsone (pharmacology)
$C_{10}H_8O_3$	hymecromone (pharmacology)
$C_{10}H_8O_4$	lactone (laboratory and pharmacology)
$C_{10}H_{12}O_3$	propylparaben [an antifungal agent also used an a preservative in pharmaceutical preparations] (pharmacology)
$C_{10}H_{12}O_5$	propyl gallate [used in pharmaceutical preparations] (pharmacology)
$C_{10}H_{14}O_2$	nepetalactone [chief component of catnip] (chemistry and veterinary medicine)
$C_{10}H_{14}O_3$	mephenesin (pharmacology)
$C_{10}H_{16}O$	myristicol (chemistry)
$C_{10}H_{20}O$	menthol [an alcohol] (chemistry and pharmacology)
$C_{10}H_{20}O_3$	promoxolane [used as a skeletal muscle relaxant and tranquilizer] (neurology, orthopedics, and pharmacology)
$C_{11}H_8O_2$	menadione [also called *menaphthone* and *vitamin K_3*; a synthetic derivative of vitamin K] (hematology and pharmacology)
$C_{11}H_{20}O_{10}$	primeverose [a disaccharide] (chemistry)
$C_{12}H_8O_4$	methoxsalen (chemistry and pharmacology)
$C_{12}H_{18}O_2$	hexylresorcinol (pharmacology)
$C_{12}H_{22}O_{11}$	cane sugar (chemistry)
	lactose [a disaccharide] (dietary, laboratory, and pharmacology)
	lactulose [a synthetic disaccharide] (pharmacology)
$C_{13}H_{10}O_3$	phenyl salicylate [also called *salol;* used as an analgesic, antipyretic, and antiseptic] (pharmacology and veterinary medicine)
$C_{13}H_{10}O_5$	pimpinellin (chemistry)
$C_{13}H_{12}O_2$	monobenzone (dermatology and pharmacology)
$C_{13}H_{16}O_3$	phenprocoumon [an anticoagulant] (cardiovascular, hematology, and pharmacology)
$C_{13}H_{18}O_2$	ibufenac (pharmacology) {obsolete}
	ibuprofen (pharmacology)
$C_{13}H_{20}O$	ionone (chemistry)
$C_{14}H_{12}O_3$	oxybenzone [a sunscreening agent] (dermatology and pharmacology)
$C_{14}H_{12}O_5$	khellin (pharmacology)
$C_{14}H_{14}O_3$	naproxen (pharmacology)

$C_{14}H_{18}O_8$	peristaltin [a glycoside] (chemistry)
$C_{15}H_{10}O_2$	phenindione [an anticoagulant] (cardiovascular, hematology, and pharmacology)
$C_{15}H_{10}O_4$	chrysophanic acid (chemistry)
$C_{15}H_{14}O$	lactaroviolin [a pigment] (chemistry)
$C_{15}H_{14}O_6$	plumericin (chemistry and research)
$C_{15}H_{18}O_7$	hyenanchin [a poisonous substance] (chemistry)
$C_{15}H_{28}O_{10}$	hygromycin B (pharmacology)
$C_{16}H_{12}O_2$	phenacetolin [used as an indicator] (chemistry and laboratory)
$C_{16}H_{12}O_4$	isoxepac (pharmacology)
$C_{16}H_{12}O_6$	hematein (laboratory)
$C_{16}H_{14}O_3$	ketoprofen (pharmacology)
$C_{16}H_{22}O_3$	homosalate (pharmacology)
$C_{18}H_{20}O_2$	hippulin (chemistry, laboratory, and veterinary medicine)
$C_{18}H_{22}O_2$	hexestrol (pharmacology)
$C_{18}H_{22}O_3$	methallenestril (pharmacology)
$C_{18}H_{26}O_2$	nandrolone [also called *norandrostenolone*] (pharmacology)
$C_{18}H_{32}O_{16}$	manninotriose (chemistry)
	melezitose (chemistry)
$C_{18}H_{34}O_2$	oleic acid (chemistry)
$C_{18}H_{36}O_2$	stearic acid (chemistry)
$C_{19}H_{30}O_3$	oxandrolone [an androgenic steroidal lactone] (pharmacology)
$C_{20}H_{14}O_4$	phenolphthalein [a cathartic] (pharmacology)
$C_{20}H_{18}O_4$	phaseolin [a globulin with antifungal properties] (chemistry and pharmacology)
$C_{20}H_{22}O_3$	nafenopin (pharmacology)
$C_{20}H_{22}O_5$	pleurotin [a toxic antibiotic substance] (pharmacology)
$C_{20}H_{26}O_2$	norethindrone [a progestin] (endocrinology, gynecology, obstetrics, and pharmacology)
	norethynodrel [a progestin] (endocrinology, gynecology, obstetrics, and pharmacology)
$C_{20}H_{28}O$	lynestrenol (pharmacology)
$C_{20}H_{28}O_2$	methandrostenolone (pharmacology)
$C_{20}H_{30}O_2$	methenolone (pharmacology)
	methyltestosterone (endocrinology, laboratory, and pharmacology)
	metogest [a hormone] (endocrinology, laboratory, and pharmacology)
	mibolerone (endocrinology, laboratory, and pharmacology)
	norethandrolone [a synthetic androgen] (endocrinology, laboratory, and pharmacology)
$C_{20}H_{32}O_2$	mesterolone (laboratory and pharmacology)

$C_{20}H_{33}O_7$	melanthin [a poisonous glycoside] (chemistry)
$C_{21}H_{26}O_2$	mestranol (pharmacology)
$C_{21}H_{26}O_3$	octabenzone [an ultraviolet screen] (dermatology and pharmacology)
$C_{21}H_{26}O_5$	prednisone [also called *deltacortisone;* a synthetic glucocorticoid used as an anti-inflammatory] (allergy, chemotherapy, oncology, orthopedics, respiratory, and rheumatology)
$C_{21}H_{28}O_2$	norgestrel [a progestin] (endocrinology, gynecology, obstetrics, and pharmacology)
$C_{21}H_{28}O_5$	prednisolone [a synthetic glucocorticocoid] (allergy, chemotherapy, gastroenterology, hematology, oncology, orthopedics, and rheumatology)
$C_{21}H_{30}O_2$	progesterone [also called *luteohormone* and *progestational hormone;* a hormone] (endocrinology, gynecology, laboratory, obstetrics, and pharmacology)
$C_{21}H_{32}O_3$	oxymetholone [an anabolic-androgenic steroid] (endocrinology and pharmacology)
$C_{22}H_{22}O_8$	picopodophyllin (chemistry and laboratory)
$C_{22}H_{28}O_3$	norethindrone acetate (endocrinology, gynecology, obstetrics, and pharmacology)
$C_{22}H_{28}O_5$	meprednisone (pharmacology)
$C_{22}H_{30}O_5$	methylprednisolone (pharmacology)
$C_{22}H_{32}O_3$	medrysone (ophthalmology and pharmacology)
	methenolone acetate (pharmacology)
$C_{22}H_{36}O_5$	prostalene [a prostaglandin] (endocrinology and laboratory)
	podophyllotoxin [a toxic compound with antineoplastic and cathartic properties] (chemistry, chemotherapy, gastroenterology, oncology, and pharmacology)
$C_{23}H_{16}O_3$	methylaurin (chemistry)
$C_{23}H_{24}O_6$	mangostin [a pigment] (chemistry)
$C_{23}H_{30}O_4$	prednisolone acetate (allergy, chemotherapy, gastroenterology, hematology, oncology, orthopedics, pharmacology, and rheumatology)
$C_{23}H_{32}O_2$	medrogestone (laboratory)
$C_{23}H_{32}O_4$	norgestomet [a progestin] (endocrinology, gynecology, obstetrics, and pharmacology)
$C_{23}H_{32}O_6$	hydrocortisone acetate (pharmacology)
$C_{23}H_{34}O_5$	periplogin [an aglycone sterol derivative] (chemistry)
$C_{23}H_{40}O_5$	nonoxynol 4 [also $C_{15}H_{24}O(C_2H_4O)_4$] (chemistry and pharmacology)
$C_{24}H_{30}O_6$	neoquassin (chemistry)
$C_{24}H_{32}O_5$	marinobufagin [a cardiac poison] (chemistry)
$C_{24}H_{32}O_6$	methylprednisolone acetate (pharmacology)

$C_{24}H_{34}O_4$	medroxyprogesterone acetate (chemotherapy, gynecology, oncology, and pharmacology)
$C_{24}H_{38}O_3$	nabidrox (pharmacology)
$C_{25}H_{28}O_{11}$	nataloin (chemistry)
$C_{25}H_{31}O_3$	nylestriol [an estrogen] (endocrinology, gynecology, laboratory, and pharmacology)
$C_{25}H_{32}O_4$	megestrol acetate (chemotherapy, gynecology, oncology, and pharmacology)
	melengestrol acetate (chemotherapy, gynecology, oncology, and pharmacology)
$C_{25}H_{32}O_8$	prednisolone succinate [used in production of *prednisolone sodium succinate*] (pharmacology)
$C_{25}H_{34}O_4$	methynodiol diacetate (laboratory and pharmacology)
$C_{25}H_{34}O_6$	hydrocortisone hemisuccinate (pharmacology)
$C_{25}H_{36}O_5$	pregnenolone succinate [used in treatment of rheumatoid arthritis] (orthopedics and rheumatology)
$C_{26}H_{34}O_4$	promethestrol dipropionate [also called *methestrol dipropionate;* an estrogenic agent] (chemotherapy, gynecology, obstetrics, oncology, pharmacology, and urology)
$C_{26}H_{34}O_8$	methylprednisolone hemisuccinate (pharmacology)
$C_{26}H_{38}O_6$	hydrocortisone valerate (pharmacology)
$C_{27}H_{34}O_3$	nandrolone phenpropionate (pharmacology)
$C_{27}H_{34}O_{11}$	phillyrin [a crystalline substance with antimalarial properties] (chemistry, infectious diseases, pharmacology, and respiratory)
$C_{27}H_{38}O_6$	prednisolone tebutate [also called *prednisolone butylacetate;* used in production of some injectable prednisolone products] (pharmacology)
$C_{27}H_{40}O_4$	hydroxyprogesterone capraoate (pharmacology)
$C_{27}H_{42}O_3$	methenolone enanthate (pharmacology)
$C_{28}H_{34}O_{15}$	hesperidin (chemistry)
$C_{28}H_{38}O_3$	nandrolone cyclotate (pharmacology)
$C_{28}H_{44}O_3$	nandrolone decanoate (pharmacology)
$C_{29}H_{38}O_3$	oxogestone phenpropionate [a progestin] (endocrinology and pharmacology)
$C_{29}H_{42}O_6$	hydrocortisone cyclopentylpropionate (pharmacology)
	hydrocortisone cypionate (pharmacology)
$C_{30}H_{34}O_{13}$	picrotoxin [also called *cocculin;* a central nervous system stimulant] (chemical dependency, neurology, pharmacology, and psychiatry)
$C_{30}H_{42}O_8$	proscillaridin [used as a cardiotonic] (cardiovascular and pharmacology)
$C_{30}H_{46}O_8$	oleandrin [a cardiac glycoside] (cardiovascular and pharmacology)

	periplocymarin [a cardiac glycoside] (cardiovascular, chemistry, and pharmacology)
$C_{30}H_{50}O$	lanosterol (chemistry and laboratory)
$C_{31}H_{46}O_2$	phytonadione [also called *phylloquinone* and *vitamin K*] (pharmacology)
$C_{32}H_{48}O_9$	oleandrin [an alkaloid] (cardiovascular and pharmacology)
$C_{33}H_{60}O_{10}$	nonoxynol 9 (chemistry and pharmacology)
$C_{34}H_{54}O_8$	lasalocid (chemistry)
$C_{34}H_{62}O_{11}$	octoxynol 9 [also called *octylphenoxy polyethoxyethanol*; a surfactant] (chemistry and pharmacology)
$C_{35}H_{72}O_3$	phthiocerol [an alcohol] (chemistry and laboratory)
$C_{36}H_{56}O_{13}$	periplocin [a glycoside] (cardiovascular, chemistry, and pharmacology)
$C_{36}H_{62}O_{11}$	monensin (pharmacology and veterinary medicine)
$C_{43}H_{72}O_{11}$	narasin (veterinary medicine)
$C_{45}H_{84}O_{16}$	nonoxynol 15 (chemistry and pharmacology)
$C_{48}H_{56}O_2$	lutein (laboratory)
$C_{49}H_{76}O_{20}$	lanatoside C (pharmacology)
$C_{52}H_{72}O_{24}$	mithramycin (pharmacology)
$C_{58}H_{114}O_{26}$	polysorbate 20 [also called *polyoxyethylene 20 sorbitan monolaurate*; a surfactant agent] (chemistry and pharmacology)
$C_{62}H_{122}O_{26}$	polysorbate 40 [also called *polyoxyethylene 20 sorbitan monopalmitate*; a surfactant agent] (chemistry and pharmacology)
$C_{64}H_{124}O_{26}$	polysorbate 80 [also called *polyethylene 20 sorbitan monooleate*; a surfactant agent] (chemistry and pharmacology)
$C_{64}H_{126}O_{26}$	polysorbate 60 [also called *polyethylene 20 sorbitan monostearate*; a surfactant agent] (chemistry and pharmacology)
$C_{75}H_{144}O_{31}$	nonoxynol 30 (chemistry and pharmacology)
$C_{100}H_{94}O_{28}$	polysorbate 65 [also called *polyethylene 20 sorbitan tristearate*; a surfactant agent] (chemistry and pharmacology)
$C_{100}H_{188}O_{28}$	polysorbate 85 [also called *polyethylene 20 sorbitan trioleate*; a surfactant agent] (chemistry and pharmacology)
$CH_2(OCH_3)_2$	methylal (chemistry, laboratory, and pharmacology)
CH_3OCH_3	dimethyl ether (chemistry)
$C_6H_5O \cdot C_2H_5$	phenetole [also called *ethyl phenyl ether*; an oily liquid] (chemistry)
$C_6H_5(OC_2H_5)$	phlorol [an oily liquid] (chemistry)
$(CH_3 \cdot O)_3C_6H_2 \cdot CH_2 \cdot CH_2 \cdot NH_2$	
	mescaline [a psychedelic drug from mescal buttons used as a street drug in the 1960's and 1970's]

(chemical dependency, chemistry, and pharmacology)

$C_6H_4(OC_2H_5) \cdot NH \cdot CO \cdot CH(OH)CH_3$
lactophenin (pharmacology)

$C_{15}H_{24}O(C_2H_4O)_n$
nonoxynol [also called *nonylphenoxypolyethoxyethanol*] (chemistry and pharmacology)

$C_{15}H_{24}O(C_2H_4O)_4$
nonoxynol 4 [also called $C_{23}H_{40}O_5$] (chemistry and pharmacology)

$C_6H_4(OCOCH_3)NH \cdot COOC_2H_5$
neurodin (pharmacology)

CH_3OH methanol (chemistry)

C_2H_5OH ethyl alcohol (chemistry)

$C_6H_5 \cdot OH$ phenol [also called *carbolic acid, hydroxybenzene, oxybenzene, phenic acid, phenylic acid,* and *phenylic alcohol;* an extremely poisonous crystalline compound used as an antimicrobial agent] (chemistry and pharmacology)

$C_{10}H_7 \cdot OH$ naphthol (pharmacology)

$C_{18}H_{35}OH$ oleanol [a solid white alcohol] (chemistry and pharmacology)

$C_{28}H_{57}OH$ octacosanol [a solid white alcohol] (chemistry)

$(CH_2OH)_4C$ pentaerythritol [an alcohol used in synthetic resins and in paints and varnishes] (chemistry)

$CH_2OH \cdot (CHOH)_3 \cdot CHO$
lyxose (laboratory)

$CH_2OH \cdot (CHOH)_4 \cdot CHO$
mannose [an aldohexose sugar] (chemistry)

$CH_2OH(CHOH)_4CH_2OH$
iditol (chemistry)

$CH_2OH(CHOH)_4C[:N \cdot N(CH_3) \cdot C_6H_5] \cdot CHCH \cdot NHN(CH_3) \cdot C_6H_5$
methylphenyl levulosazone (chemistry)

$C_6H_4(OH)CO_2 \cdot C_6H_4NO_2$
nitrosalol (laboratory)

$CH_2OH \cdot CO(CHOH)_4 \cdot CH_2OH$
mannoketoheptose [a natural sugar] (chemistry)
monoketoheptose [a natural sugar] (chemistry)

$C_7H_8O_2 \cdot H_2O$ orcin [also called *orcinol;* used as a reagent] (laboratory)

$C_{12}H_{22}O_{11} + 2H_2O$ mycose [also called *trehalose;* a sugar] (chemistry)

$C_{16}H_{14}O_6 + 3H_2O$ hematoxylin (laboratory)

$C_{18}H_{32}O_{16} + 5H_2O$ melitose (chemistry)

$C_{21}H_{25}O_{10} + 2H_2O$ phlorhizin [a glycoside] (chemistry)

$C_{29}H_{44}O_{12} \cdot 8H_2O$ G-strophanthin [also called *ouabain* and *strophanthin-G*] (cardiovascular and pharmacology)

$C_3H_5(OH)_2 \cdot PO_2(OLi)_2$ lithium glycerophosphate (pharmacology)

$C_6H_5O_7Li_3 + 4H_2O$ lithium citrate (chemistry)

$(C_2H_2O_2)_m(C_3H_4O_2)_n$	polyglactin 910 [a suture material] (surgery)
$(C_4H_6O_2)_m(C_2H_5N)_n$	polyethadene [an antacid] (gastroenterology and pharmacology)
$(C_5H_8O_4)_n$	pentosan [any member of a group of pentose polysaccharides] (chemistry)
$(C_6H_{10}O_3)_n$	polymacon [a contact lens material] (ophthalmology)
$(C_6H_{10}O_5)_n$	irisin (chemistry)
	lichenin (chemistry)
	mannan (chemistry)
	starch, glycogen, or other hexose polymers (chemistry)
$C_8H_5O_2N$	isatin (chemistry)
$C_9H_{20}O_2N$	muscarine (pharmacology)
$(C_{10}H_{16}O_4)_n$	polybutilate [a suture coating] (chemistry and surgery)
$C_{10}H_{17}O_6N$	linamarin (chemistry)
$C_{16}H_{18}ON_2$	paricine [a quinoline alkaloid] (chemistry)
$C_{18}H_{25}O_6N$	jacobine [a poisonous alkaloid] (chemistry)
$C_{18}H_{27}O_5N$	platyphylline [an alkaloid] (chemistry)
$C_{19}H_{12}O_5N_4$	inosine (laboratory)
$C_{19}H_{21}O_3N$	isothebaine (chemistry)
$C_{19}H_{22}ON_2$	homocinchonine (chemistry)
$C_{19}H_{23}O_4N$	porphyroxine [an opium alkaloid] (chemistry and pharmacology)
$C_{19}H_{24}ON_2$	hydrocinchonidine (chemistry)
$C_{22}H_{33}O_3N$	napelline (pharmacology)
$(C_{32}H_{48}O_{16})_n$	porofocon [a contact lens materials designated A or B] (ophthalmology)
$C_{33}H_{42}O_6N_4$	mesobilin (laboratory)
$C_{33}H_{44}O_6N_4$	mesobilirubin (laboratory)
$C_{34}H_{38}O_4N_4$	hemoporphyrin (laboratory)
	mesoporphyrin (laboratory)
$C_{37}H_{38}O_6N_2$	insularine [an alkaloid] (chemistry)
$C_{37}H_{40}O_6N_2$	oxycanthine [an alkaloid causing paralysis] (chemistry and laboratory)
$C_{48}H_{91}O_8N$	nervone (laboratory)
$C_{48}H_{93}O_8N$	kerasin (laboratory)
$C_{48}H_{93}O_9N$	phrenosin [a cerebroside] (laboratory and neurology)
$C_{68}H_{78}O_7N_8$	hematolin (laboratory)
$C_{34}H_{36}O_4N_4FeCl$	mesohemin (laboratory)
$C_{34}H_{33}O_4N_4FeOH$	heme (laboratory)
$C_8H_4O_6N_5 \cdot NH_4 \cdot H_2O$	ammonium purpurate [also called *murexide*] (laboratory)
$C_5H_{11}O_2NS$	penillamine [an amine] (chemistry)
$C_{20}H_{27}O_4P$	octicizer [a plasticizer] (chemistry)

CH $2 \cdot O \cdot PO(OH)_2 \cdot CHOH \cdot CHO$

    3-phosphoglyceraldehyde (laboratory, neurology, and orthopedics)

$C_{19}H_{14}O_5S$ phenolsulfonphthalein [used for tests of renal function] (laboratory, nephrology, and pharmacology)

$C_{31}H_{48}O_2S_2$ probucol [used to reduce serum cholesterol] (cardiovascular and pharmacology)

$C_{20}H_{34}O_3 \cdot HOCl$ oxychlorosene [used as a topical anti-infective] (pharmacology)

$(C_6H_{10}O_3)_v(C_9H_{16}O_2)_w(C_4H_6O_2)_x(C_5H_8O_2)_y(C_{14}H_{12}O_3)_z$

    mafilcon A [a contact lens material] (chemistry and ophthalmology)

$CH_3 \cdot SH$ methylmercaptan (chemistry and laboratory)

$(CH_3)_2Te$ methyl telluride (chemistry)

$(C_6H_{10}O_3)_x(C_8H_{14}O_3)_y$ phemfilcon A [a contact lens materials] (chemistry and ophthalmology)

Cl   chloride (chemistry)

    chlorine (chemistry)

$Cl_3C \cdot CHO$ chloral (chemistry)

$ClCOOCH_3$ methylchloroformate (chemistry)

ClO   chlorine monoxide (chemistry)

Cm   curium (chemistry)

Cn   cyanide (chemistry and pharmacology)

CNCBL   cyanocobalamin (chemistry)

CNCbl   cyanocobalamin (chemistry)

CNOH   cyanic acid (chemistry)

CO   carbon monoxide (chemistry and respiratory)

CO_2 carbon dioxide (chemistry, laboratory, and respiratory)

Co   cobalt (chemistry)

^{60}Co radioactive cobalt (chemistry)

$C_4O_6H_4NaK$ potassium sodium tartrate (chemistry)

$CO(NH_2)_2$ urea (chemistry and laboratory)

COOH   {not an abbreviation} [symbol for the carboxyl group] (chemistry)

CP   chemically pure (chemistry)

    chloropurine (chemistry)

Cr   chromium (chemistry)

^{51}Cr radioactive sodium chromate (chemistry)

    concentrated strength [of solutions] (chemistry and pharmacology)

CS_2 carbon disulfide (chemistry)

Cs   cesium (chemistry)

^{137}Cs radioactive cesium (chemistry)

C-terminal   carboxyl terminal (chemistry)

CTP-^{3}H   cytidine triphosphate tritium-labeled (chemistry)

Cu   *cuprum* [also called *copper*] (chemistry)

^{61}Cu radioactive copper (chemistry)

^{64}Cu	radioactive copper (chemistry)
^{65}Cu	radioactive copper (chemistry)
CuO	cupric oxide (chemistry)
Cu_2O	cuprous oxide (chemistry)
CuSCN	cuprous thiocyanate
Cv	specific heat at constant volume (chemistry)
Cy	cyanogen (chemistry)
	cyclonium (chemistry)
cyclic AMP	cyclic adenosine monophosphate (chemistry)
cyclic GMP	cyclic guanosine monophosphate (chemistry)
CYN	cyanide [a poison] (chemistry)

D

D	cholecalciferol (chemistry)
	deuterium [also called *heavy hydrogen*] (chemistry)
	{not an abbreviation} [a chemical prefix] (chemistry)
	{not an abbreviation} [symbol for vitamin D potency] (chemistry and dietary)
D.	deueron (chemistry)
D-	{not an abbreviation} [a chemical prefix designating: (1) a substance with the configuration of D-glyceraldehyde; (2) the configuration family of the highest numbered asymmetrical carbon atom in carbohydrate nomenclature; and (3) the configuration family of the lowest numbered asymmetrical carbon atom in amino acid nomenclature] (chemistry)
d	deoxyribose (genetics and laboratory)
d-	*dextro-* [chemical symbol meaning to the right or clockwide] (chemistry)
DDT	chlorophenothan [an insecticide] (chemistry)
$DF^{32}P$	di-isopropyl phosphofluoridate (chemistry)
2DG	2-deoxy-D-glucose (chemistry)
D/H	deuterium-to-hydrogen [ratio] (chemistry)
Di	didymium (chemistry)
D_2O	deuterium oxide [also called *heavy water*] (chemistry)

E

E	ester (chemistry)
	ethyl (chemistry)
E_1	estrone (chemistry)
E_2	estradiol (endocrinology, gynecology, laboratory, and obstetrics)

E_3	estriol (endocrinology, gynecology, laboratory, and obstetrics)
E_4	estetrol (endocrinology, gynecology, laboratory, and obstetrics)
EC	electrochemical (chemistry and laboratory)
en	ethylene diamine [in chemical formulas] (chemistry)
Es	einsteinium (chemistry)
Et	ethyl (chemistry)
	ethyl group (chemistry)
eta	{not an abbreviation} [symbol for *viscosity*]
EtO	ethylene oxide (chemistry)
EtOH	ethyl alcohol (chemistry)
Eu	europium (chemistry)

F

F	fluoride (chemistry dentistry, and pharmacology)
	fluorine (chemistry)
	phenylalanine [an amino acid] (laboratory)
f-12	freon (chemistry)
5-FC	5-fluorocytosine [an antifungal] (pharmacology)
Fe	*ferrum* [also called *iron*] (chemistry, laboratory, and pharmacology)
Fe_2	ferrous (chemistry)
Fe^{2+}	ferrous (chemistry)
Fe_3	ferric (chemistry)
Fe^{3+}	ferric (chemistry)
^{59}Fe	radioactive iron (chemistry)
$Fe(C_2H_3O_2)_3$	iron acetate (pharmacology)
$Fe(C_3H_5O_3)_2$	ferrous lactate (hematology and pharmacology)
$FECO_3$	ferrous carbonate (hematology and pharmacology)
$FeCl_2$	an iron chloride (chemistry)
$FeCl_3$	an iron chloride (chemistry)
FeI_2	ferrous iodide [also called *iron iodide*] (chemistry)
Fe(II)	ferrous (chemistry)
Fe(III)	ferric (chemistry)
Fe_2O_3	ferric oxide (chemistry)
Fe_3O_4	ferrosoferric (chemistry)
$Fe(OH)_3$	ferric hydroxide [also called *iron hydroxide*] (chemistry)
$2Fe_2O \cdot 3H_2O$	limonite [also called *hydros ferric oxide*] (chemistry)
Fer	*ferrum* [also called *iron*] (chemistry, laboratory, and pharmacology)
$FePO_4 \cdot 4H_2O$	ferric phosphate [used as a feed and food supplement and as a fertilizer] (agriculture, chemistry, and dietary)

$FeSO_4$	ferrous sulfate (chemistry, laboratory, and pharmacology)
$FeSO_4 \cdot MgSO_4 + 7H_2O$	
	iron magnesium sulfate (pharmacology)
Fm	fermium (chemistry)
FN	fluoride number (chemistry)
FNa	filtered sodium (chemistry)
Fp	filtered phosphate (chemistry)
FPH_2	flavin phosphate, reduced (chemistry)
Fr	francium (chemistry)
F_3T	trifluridine (chemistry)

G

G	glycine (chemistry)
	guanine (chemistry)
	guanosine (chemistry)
G_4	dichlorophen [also called *dihydroxydichlorodiphenyl urethane*] (chemistry)
G-11	hexachlorophene (chemistry)
G_{11}	hexachlorophene (chemistry)
Ga	gallium (chemistry, pharmacology, and radiology)
Gd	gadolinium (chemistry)
Ge	germanium (chemistry)
GIX	{not an abbreviation} [trademark for an insecticidal compound of difluorodiphenyltrichloroethane] (chemistry)
GL54	athomin (chemistry)
GL 54	athomin (chemistry)
Gl	glucinium [also called *beryllium*] (chemistry)
GM	Geiger-Müller [counter] (chemistry)

H

H	hydrogen (chemistry)
	mustard gas (chemistry)
^1H	hydrogen-1 [also called *protium* (ordinary or light hydrogen)] (chemistry)
H1	hydrogen-1 [also called *protium* (ordinary or light hydrogen)] (chemistry)
H^1	hydrogen-1 [also called *protium* (ordinary or light hydrogen)] (chemistry)
^2H	deuterium [also called *hydrogen-2* (heavy hydrogen)] (chemistry)
H2	deuterium [also called *hydrogen-2* (heavy hydrogen)] (chemistry)

H^2	deuterium [also called *hydrogen-2* (heavy hydrogen)] (chemistry)
^{3}H	hydrogen-3 [also called *tritium*] (chemistry)
H3	hydrogen-3 [also called *tritium*] (chemistry)
H^3	hydrogen-3 [also called *tritium*] (chemistry)
H$_3$	procaine hydrochloride (pharmacology)
	tritium [also called *hydrogen-3*] (chemistry)
Ha	hahnium (chemistry)
HAc	acetic acid (chemistry and laboratory)
H$_3$BO$_3$	boric acid (chemistry and pharmacology)
HbO$_2$	oxyhemoglobin (laboratory)
HC	hydrocarbon (chemistry)
H$_2$C:CO	ketene [also called *carbomethane;* a gas] (chemistry and laboratory)
HCl	hydrochloric acid (chemistry, gastroenterology, and laboratory)
	hydrogen chloride (chemistry)
HCN	hydrocyanic acid (chemistry)
	hydrogen cyanide (chemistry)
HCO$_3$	bicarbonate (chemistry, laboratory, and pharmacology)
	bicarbonate ion (chemistry)
	the bicarbonate radical (chemistry)
H$_2$CO$_3$	carbonic acid (chemistry)
HCOOLi + H$_2$O	lithium formate (pharmacology)
Hf	hafnium (chemistry)
Hg	*hydrargyrum* [also called *mercury*] (chemistry)
Hg·C$_6$H$_3$(OH)·COOH	mercury salicylate (pharmacology)
HgCl$_2$	mercuric chloride [also called *mercury bichloride*] (chemistry and pharmacology)
Hg$_2$Cl$_2$	mild mercurous chloride (chemistry)
Hg(CN)$_2$	mercuric cyanide [a poisonous salt] (chemistry and pharmacology)
Hg(CN)$_2$·HgO	mercuric oxycyanide (pharmacology)
HgI	mercurous iodide, yellow (pharmacology)
HgI$_2$	mercuric iodine, red [also called *mercury biniodide*] (pharmacology)
Hg$_2$I$_2$	mercurous iodide (chemistry)
HgNH$_2$Cl	ammoniated mercury (pharmacology)
Hg(NO$_3$)$_2$	mercuric nitrate (chemistry)
HgO	mercuric oxide (ophthalmology and pharmacology)
Hg$_2$O	mercurous oxide (chemistry)
HI	hydriodic acid (chemistry)
	hydroxyindole (chemistry)
Hi	histidine (chemistry)
HIO	hypoiodism
	iodic acid (chemistry)
HIO$_3$	iodic acid (chemistry)

Hippuran-^{131}I	iodohippurate (chemistry)
His	histidine (chemistry and laboratory)
HL	half-life (chemistry and physics)
H/L	hydrophile/lipophile [number] (chemistry)
HN	high nitrogen (chemistry)
HN_2	mechlorethamine hydrochloride (chemistry)
	nitrogen mustard (chemistry)
$H_2N \cdot NH_2$	hydrazine (chemistry)
HNO_2	nitrous acid (chemistry)
HNO_3	nitric acid (chemistry)
H_2O	hydrogen monoxide [also called *water*] (chemistry)
H_2O_2	hydrogen peroxide (chemistry and pharmacology)
H_3O^+	hydronium ion (physics)
	the hydrated proton (chemistry)
Ho	holmium (chemistry)
$H(OCH_2CH_2)_nOH$	polyethylene glycol [also called *macrogal*] [used in pharmaceutical preparations] (chemistry and pharmacology)
$HOCH_2(CHOH)_4CH_2OH$	
	mannitol (laboratory and pharmacology)
$H-O-O-H$	hydrogen peroxide (chemistry and pharmacology)
H_2OsO_4	osmic acid (chemistry)
HPO_3	metaphosphoric acid (chemistry)
H_3PO_2	hypophosphorous acid (chemistry)
H_3PO_3	phosphorous acid (chemistry)
H_3PO_4	orthophosphoric acid (chemistry)
	phosphoric acid (chemistry)
$H_4P_2O_6$	hypophosphoric acid (chemistry)
$H_4P_2O_7$	pyrophosphoric acid (chemistry)
H_2S	hydrogen sulfide [also called *hydrosulfuric acid* and *sulfhydric acid*] (chemistry)
H_2S_2	hydrogen disulfide (chemistry)
$HS \cdot CH_2CH_2 \cdot OH$	mercaptoethanol (chemistry and laboratory)
H_2Se	hydrogen selenide (chemistry)
H_2SiO_3	metasilicic acid (chemistry)
H_4SiO_4	orthosilicic acid (chemistry)
H_2SO_3	sulfurous acid (chemistry)
H_2SO_4	sulfuric acid (chemistry)
hydrarg	*hydrargyrum* [also called *mercury*] (chemistry)

I

I	iodine (chemistry, laboratory, and pharmacology)
I_2	iodine (chemistry, laboratory, and pharmacology)
^{125}I	radioactive iodine (radiology)
^{130}I	radioactive iodine (radiology)
I 131	radioactive iodine (radiology)

I^{131}	radioactive iodine (radiology) {obsolete}
^{131}I	radioactive iodine (radiology)
I 132	radioactive iodine (radiology)
I^{132}	radioactive iodine (radiology) {obsolete}
^{132}I	radioactive iodine (radiology)
IBU	international benzoate unit (chemistry)
IC	inorganic carbon (chemistry)
Il	illinium [previous name for *promethium*] (chemistry)
In	indium (chemistry)
	inulin (chemistry)
Ir	iridium (chemistry)
IUPAC	International Union of Pure and Applied Chemistry

K

k	{not an abbreviation} [one of two immunoglobulin light chains] (laboratory)
K	*kalium* [also called *potassium*] (laboratory and pharmacology)
KBr	potassium bromide [an anticonvulsant and sedative] (chemistry, neurology, pharmacology, and psychiatry)
$KC_2H_3O_2$	potassium acetate (chemistry)
$K_2C_4H_4O_6 + \frac{1}{2}H_2O$	potassium tartrate [used as a cathartic] (gastroenterology and pharmacology)
$K_2C_2H_5(OH)_2PO_4$	potassium glycerophosphate [previously used as a tonic] (chemistry and pharmacology)
KCl	potassium chloride [used as an electrolyte replenisher] (pharmacology)
$KClO_3$	potassium chlorate [an explosive compound used in a solution to treat stomatitis and vaginitis in animals] (chemistry and veterinary medicine)
$KClO_4$	potassium perchlorate [a thyroid inhibitor] (endocrinology and pharmacology)
KCN	potassium cyanide [a poisonous compound] (chemistry)
KCNS	potassium thiocyanate (laboratory)
K_2CO_3	potassium carbonate [used in chemical and pharmaceutical manufacturing] (chemistry and pharmacology)
$K_2C_2O_4 \cdot H_2O$	potassium oxalate [a reagent] (laboratory)
$K_3Fe(CN)_6$	potassium ferricyanide [used in a test for ferrous salts] (chemistry and laboratory)
$KHCO_3$	potassium bicarbonate [used as an antacid, electrolyte replenisher, and urinary alkalizer] (gastroenterology, pharmacology, and urology)

K_2HgI_4 potassium mercuric iodide [used as a germicide and in various reagents] (chemistry, laboratory, and pharmacology)

KH_2PO_2 potassium hypophosphite [previously used in tuberculosis treatment] (infectious diseases, pharmacology, and respiratory)

KH_2PO_4 potassium phosphate, monobasic [also called *potassium dihydrogen phosphate*; used as a buffering agent in pharmaceutical preparations] (chemistry and pharmacology)

K_2HPO_4 potassium phosphate [also called *dipotassium phosphate*; used as a cathartic] (gastroenterology and pharmacology)

KI   potassium iodine [used as an antifungal and used as an iodine source for various thyroid conditions] (endocrinology and pharmacology)

KIO_3 potassium iodate [a source of iodine when added to animal feed] (chemistry and veterinary medicine)

$KMnO_4$ potassium permanganate [used as a topical anti-infective and as a gastric lavage for various poisons] (emergency medicine and pharmacology)

KNO_3 potassium nitrate [previously used as a diuretic] (pharmacology)

KOH   potassium hydroxide [also called *caustic potash, potassa,* and *potassa caustica*; used as an alkalizer in pharmaceutic preparations] (pharmacology)

KPO_3 potassium metaphosphate [used as a buffering agent in pharmaceutical preparations] (chemistry and pharmacology)

K_3PO_4 normal ortho- or tribasic potassium phosphate (chemistry and pharmacology)

Kr   krypton (chemistry)

KSCN   potassium thiocyanate [also called *potassium sulfocyanate*; used as a reagent and previously as an antihypertensive] (cardiovascular, chemistry, laboratory, and pharmacology)

$K_2Si_2O_3$ potassium silicate [used to make rigid dressings] (orthopedics, pharmacology, and surgery)

K_2SO_4 potassium sulfate [used as a cathartic] (gastroenterology and pharmacology)

$K_2SO_3 + 2H_2O$ potassium sulfite [previously used as a cathartic and diuretic] (cardiovascular, gastroenterology, and pharmacology)

K_2TeO potassium tellurate [previously used in tuberculosis treatment] (infectious diseases, pharmacology, and respiratory)

L

l	{not an abbreviation} [chemical symbol for *laevo* (to the left or counterclockwise)] (chemistry)
l-	{not an abbreviation} [chemical prefix] (chemistry and pharmacology)
La	lanthanum (chemistry)
levo-	{not an abbreviation} [chemical prefix and prefix denoting left]
L_g-	{not an abbreviation} [chemical prefix] (chemistry and pharmacology)
Li	lithium (chemistry)
$LiBr \cdot H_2O$	lithium bromide (pharmacology and psychiatry)
Li_2CO_3	lithium carbonate (pharmacology and psychiatry)
$LiIO_3$	lithium iodate (pharmacology and psychiatry)
Li_2O	lithia [also called *lithium oxide*] (pharmacology and psychiatry)
LiOH	lithium hydroxide (pharmacology and psychiatry)
LMW	low molecular weight (chemistry)
LpOH	lysopine dehydrogenase (laboratory)
Lr	lawrencium (chemistry)
L_s-	{not an abbreviation} [chemical prefix] (chemistry and pharmacology)
Lu	lutetium (chemistry)
Lw	lawrencium (physics)

M

M	molecular weight (chemistry)
m-	meta- [prefix in chemical formulas] (chemistry)
Ma	masurium [former name of *technetium*] (chemistry and radiology) {obsolete}
Mag	magnesium (chemistry, laboratory, and pharmacology)
MB	methyl bromide (chemistry)
Md	mendelevium (chemistry)
Me	methyl [also abbreviated as CH_3] (chemistry)
MeOH	methyl alcohol (chemistry)
Met	methionine (chemistry and laboratory)
Mg	magnesium (laboratory and pharmacology)
$Mg_3(C_6H_5O_7)_2 \cdot 14H_2O$	citrate of magnesium [also called *magnesium citrate*] (pharmacology)
$MgCl_2$	magnesium chloride (chemistry)
$MgCl_2 \cdot 6H_2O$	magnesium chloride (pharmacology)
$MgCO_3$	magnesite [also called *native magnesium carbonate*; used in splints and dressings] (orthopedics)

$MgHPO_4 \cdot 3H_2O$	magnesium phosphate, dibasic [used as a laxative] (chemistry, gastroenterology, and pharmacology)
$Mg(NH_4)PO_4 \cdot 6H_2O$	ammoniomagnesium phosphate (chemistry)
MgO	magnesium oxide (pharmacology)
MgO_2	magnesium peroxide (pharmacology)
$Mg(OH)_2$	magnesium hydroxide (pharmacology)
$Mg_3(PO_4)_2 \cdot 5H_2O$	magnesium phosphate, tribasic [also called *trimagnesium phosphate;* used as an antacid] (gastroenterology and pharmacology)
$MgSO_4$	magnesium sulfate (chemistry)
$MgSO_4 \cdot 7H_2O$	magnesium sulfate [also called *Epsom salt*] (pharmacology)
Mn	manganese (chemistry and laboratory)
$Mn(H_2PO_2)_2 \cdot H_2O$	manganese hypophospite (dietary and pharmacology)
$MnSO_4 + 4H_2O$	manganese sulfate (pharmacology and veterinary medicine)
MO	molecular orbit (chemistry)
Mo	molybdenum (chemistry)
mol	molecular (chemistry)
	molecule (chemistry)
molc	molar concentration (chemistry and physics)
Mol. wt.	molecular weight (chemistry)
mol wt	molecular weight (chemistry)
mp	melting point (chemistry)
MSG	monosodium glutamate (chemistry)
MSO_4	morphine sulfate (pharmacology)
Mv	mendelevium (chemistry)
MW	molecular weight (chemistry)

N

N	nitrogen (chemistry)
N_2	molecular nitrogen (chemistry)
^{15}N	radioactive nitrogen (chemistry)
Na	*natrium* [also called *sodium*] (chemistry, laboratory, and pharmacology)
Na^+	*natrium* [also called *sodium*] (chemistry, laboratory, and pharmacology)
^{24}Na	radioactive sodium (chemistry)
$Na_8Al_2(OH)_2(PO_4)_4$	kasal [a food additive] (chemistry)
Na_2ATP	disodium adenosine triphosphate (laboratory)
$Na_2B_4O_7 \cdot 10H_2O$	borax (chemistry)
NaBr	sodium bromide [a sedative] (neurology and pharmacology)
NAC	*N*-acetyl-L-cysteine (laboratory)

NAC-EDTA	N-acetyl-L-cysteine ethylenediaminetetra-acetic acid (laboratory)
NaCl	sodium chloride [also called *salt*] (chemistry, dietary, laboratory, and pharmacology)
NaClO	sodium hypochlorite (pharmacology)
$NaClO_3$	sodium chlorate (pharmacology)
Na_2CO_3	sodium carbonate (pharmacology)
$Na_2C_2O_4$	sodium oxalate [previously used as an anticoagulant in blood collections for laboratory examinations] (hematology and laboratory)
Na_2CTP	disodium cytidine triphosphate (laboratory)
Na_E	exchangeable body sodium (laboratory)
Na_e	exchangeable body sodium (laboratory)
Na_2EDTA	disodium ethylenediaminetetraacetate (laboratory)
NaF	sodium fluoride (chemistry, dentistry, and pharmacology)
$NaHCO_3$	sodium bicarbonate [also called *baking soda* and *bicarbonate of soda*] (dietary, gastroenterology, and pharmacology)
Na_3HEDTA	trisodium ethylenediaminetetraacetic acid (laboratory)
NaH_2PO_4	sodium biphosphate [also called *monosodium acid phosphate*] (pharmacology)
Na_2HPO_2	disodium acid phosphate [also called *sodium phosphate*] (pharmacology)
NaI(Tl)	thallium-activated sodium iodide [crystal] (pharmacology)
NaOH	sodium hydroxide (pharmacology)
NaPG	sodium pregnanediol glucuronide (pharmacology)
Na_2SO_4	sodium sulfate (pharmacology)
$Na_2S_2O_3$	sodium thiosulfate (pharmacology)
$NaVO_3 \cdot 4H_2O$	sodium metavanadate [a poisonous salt] (chemistry)
Nb	niobium [formerly called *columbium*] (chemistry)
^{95}Nb	radioactive niobium (chemistry)
Nd	neodymium (chemistry)
N_d	{not an abbreviation} [symbol for refractive index] (chemistry)
n_D	{not an abbreviation} [symbol for refractive index] (chemistry)
Ne	neon [a gas used in neon lights] (chemistry)
NH_3	ammonia (chemistry, laboratory, and pharmacology)
NH_4	ammonium (chemistry, laboratory, and pharmacology)
NH_4Br	ammonium bromide (chemistry)
$NH_2(CH_2)_3 \cdot CH(NH_2) \cdot CO_2H$	
	ornithine (chemistry, laboratory, and nephrology)

$NH_2(CH_2)_4 \cdot CH(NH_2) \cdot COOH$	
	lysine (laboratory)
$NH_2 \cdot CH_2 \cdot CHOH(CH_2)_2 \cdot CH(NH_2) \cdot COOH$	
	hydroxylysine (laboratory)
$NH_2 \cdot C_6H_4 \cdot CO \cdot CH_3$	paramidoacetophenone [used in Ehrlich's diazo reaction] (gastroenterology, infectious diseases, and laboratory)
$NH_2C_6H_4CO \cdot CH_2CH(NH_4)COOH$	
	kynurenine (laboratory)
$NH_2 \cdot C_6H_4 \cdot CO \cdot O \cdot CH_3$	methyl anthranilate (chemistry)
$NH_2(CH_2)_6NH_2$	hexamethylendiamine (chemistry and laboratory)
$NH_2CH{:}NOH$	isouretin (laboratory)
NH_4Cl	ammonium chloride [also called *ammonium muriate*] (pharmacology)
$NH \cdot C(NH)_2 \cdot CH_3$	methylguanidine [a poisonous ptomaine] (chemistry and laboratory)
NH_4CNO	ammonium cyanate (pharmacology)
$(NH_2)_2CO$	urea (gastroenterology, laboratory, nephrology, and pharmacology)
$(NH_4)_2CO_3$	ammonium carbonate (pharmacology)
$(NH_4)_2C_2O_4$	ammonium oxalate (chemistry and laboratory)
$NH_2 \cdot CO \cdot CO \cdot NH_2$	oxamide [the diamide of oxalic acid] (chemistry, laboratory, nephrology, and urology)
$NH(CO \cdot NH \cdot C_6H_4OH)_2$	
	paradiphenylbiuret (chemistry and laboratory)
$(NH_4)HS$	ammonium hydrosulfide (pharmacology)
NH_4NO_3	ammonium nitrate (pharmacology)
$NH_4O \cdot CO \cdot HN_2$	ammonium carbamate (pharmacology)
$(NH_4)_2 \cdot SO_2$	ammonium sulfate (pharmacology)
NH_4U	ammonium urate crystals (laboratory)
Ni	nickel (chemistry)
$Ni(CO)_4$	nickel carbonyl (chemistry)
$N{:}N$	{not an abbreviated} [indicates the presence of the azo group] (chemistry)
NO	nitric oxide (chemistry)
NO_2	nitrogen dioxide (chemistry)
N_2O	nitrous oxide [also called *dinitrogen monoxide*] (anesthesiology, chemistry, dentistry, and pharmacology)
N_2O_4	nitrogen peroxide [also called *nitrogen tetroxide*] (chemistry)
N_2O_5	nitrogen pentoxide (chemistry)
No	nobelium (chemistry)
$NO_2 \cdot C_6H_4 \cdot C{:}C \cdot COOH{:}$	
	nitropropiol [also called *orthonitrophenylpropiolic acid*] (laboratory)
$NO_2 \cdot C_6H_4 \cdot O \cdot CH_3$	nitro-anisol (chemistry)

$N_2O:O_2$	nitrous oxide-to-oxygen ratio (laboratory and respiratory)
Np	neptunium (chemistry)

O

O	chemical symbol for oxygen (chemistry, laboratory, and respiratory)
$^1O_2$	singlet oxygen (chemistry)
O_2	molecular oxygen (chemistry, laboratory, and respiratory)
	oxygen [diatomic molecule] (chemistry, laboratory, and respiratory)
$O_2{}^-$	superoxide (chemistry)
O_3	ozone (chemistry)
O_4	oxozone [a hypothetical form of oxygen] (chemistry)
o-	{not an abbreviation} [chemical symbol for *ortho-* (prefix in chemical compounds)] (chemistry)
$OCCH_2CO$	malonyl [the divalent radical] (chemistry)
OH	hydroxyl group (chemistry)
	hydroxyl radical (chemistry)
17 OH	17-hydroxycorticosteroids (laboratory)
OH-Cbl	hydroxycobalamin (pharmacology)
$OH \cdot C_6H_4Br$	monobromophenol (chemistry and pharmacology)
$(OH \cdot C_6H_4 \cdot CO_2)_2Hg$	mercuric salicylate (pharmacology)
$OH \cdot C_6H_4 \cdot COOLi$	lithium salicylate (pharmacology)
$OH \cdot C_6H_5I$	iodophenol (pharmacology)
$(OH)_2 \cdot C_6HI_2 \cdot SO_2OK$	picrol [an antiseptic] (pharmacology and surgery)
OHCS	hydroxycorticosteroid (laboratory and pharmacology)
17-OHCS	17-hydroxycorticosteroid (laboratory)
17-OHP	17-hydroxyprogesterone (pharmacology)
$(OH)_2PO \cdot NH \cdot C(:NH) \cdot N(CH_3) \cdot CH_2 \cdot COOH$	
	phosphocreatine [also called *creatine phosphate*] (laboratory, neurology, and orthopedics)
-ol	{not an abbreviation} [a suffix indicating that a substance is an alcohol or phenol] (chemistry and pharmacology)
O,p'-DDD	o,p'-dichloro-diphenyldichlorethane [also called *mitotane*] (chemotherapy, oncology, and pharmacology)
o,p'-DDD	o,p'-dichloro-diphenyldichlorethane [also called *mitotane*] (chemotherapy, oncology, and pharmacology)
Os	osmium (chemistry)

OsO_4	osmium tetroxide [used as a fixative for preparing histologic specimens] (laboratory and pathology)
O_{2v}	superoxide (chemistry)

P

P	phosphate (chemistry and laboratory)
	phosphorus [chemical symbol for] (chemistry, laboratory, and pharmacology)
P 32	radioactive phosphorus (chemistry, nuclear medicine, and radiology)
P^{32}	radioactive phosphorus (chemistry, nuclear medicine, and radiology)
^{32}P	radioactive phosphate [also called *radiophosphate*] (chemistry, nuclear medicine, radiation therapy, and radiology)
P-50	oxygen half-saturation pressure of hemoglobin (laboratory and respiratory)
P-55	hydroxypregnanedione (laboratory)
P231	radioactive phosphorus (chemistry, nuclear medicine, and radiology)
$\tilde{p}$	high-energy phosphate band (chemistry)
p-	para- [prefix in chemical formulas] (chemistry)
Pb	*plumbum* [also called *lead*] (chemistry and laboratory)
PBB	polybromated biphenyls (chemistry)
PBBs	polybromated biphenyls (chemistry)
$Pb(C_2H_5)_4$	ethyl gas [also called *tetra-ethyl lead*] (chemistry)
$Pb(C_2H_3O_2)_2$	lead acetate (chemistry)
$Pb(C_{18}H_{33}O_2)_2$	lead oleate (chemistry)
$Pb(C_2H_3O_2)_2 \cdot 3H_2O$	lead acetate (chemistry)
$PbCl_2$	lead chloride (chemistry)
$PbCO_3$	lead carbonate (chemistry)
$PbCrO_4$	lead chromate (chemistry)
$PbHAsO_4$	lead arsenate (chemistry)
$Pb(NO_3)_2$	lead nitrate (chemistry)
PbO	lead monoxide [also called *massicot*] (chemistry)
Pb_3O_4	lead tetraoxide (chemistry)
PbI_2	lead iodide (chemistry)
$Pb(NO_3)_2$	lead nitrate (chemistry)
PbO	lead monoxide (chemistry)
PbO_2	lead dioxide (chemistry)
PbS	lead sulfide (chemistry)
PbSe	lead selinide (chemistry)
$PbSO_4$	lead sulfate (chemistry)

PCB	pancuronium bromide (anesthesiology, orthopedics, pharmacology, and surgery)
PCB's	polychlorinated biphenyls (chemistry)
Pd	palladium (chemistry)
6-PG	6-phosphogluconate (laboratory)
Ph	phenyl (chemistry and laboratory)
pH	{not an abbreviation} [symbol for expression of hydrogen ion concentration] (chemistry and laboratory)
P_i	inorganic phosphate (chemistry)
pI	{not an abbreviation} [the pH of a solution at its isoelectric point] (chemistry and laboratory)
pK	{not an abbreviation} [the negative logarithm of an ionization constant of an acid] (chemistry)
pKa	negative log of dissociation constant (chemistry)
P-NP	para-nitrophenol (chemistry and laboratory)
$=P:O$	phosphoryl [the trivalent chemical radical] (chemistry)
PO_4	phosphate (chemistry and laboratory)
(PO_4)	calcium phosphate (chemistry)
Po	polonium [a radioactive element] (chemistry)
POC	purgeable organic carbon (chemistry)
pOH	{not an abbreviation} [symbol referring to hydroxyl (OH) concentration or alkalinity of a solution] (chemistry and laboratory)
P-5'-P	pyridoxal-5'-phosphate (laboratory)
PP_i	inorganic pyrophosphate (laboratory)
Pr	praseodymium (chemistry)
	propyl (chemistry and laboratory)
Pt	platinum (chemistry)
$PtCl_4 \cdot 5H_2O$	platinum chloride [a poisonous substance used as a reagent] (chemistry and laboratory)
Pu	plutonium (chemistry)
PVC	polyvinyl chloride (chemistry)

R

R	organic radical [in chemical formulas] (chemistry, laboratory, and pharmacology)
	{not an abbreviation} [any alkyl group of an alkane] (chemistry and laboratory)
	{not an abbreviation} [indicates characteristic side chain in formulas of amino acids] (chemistry and laboratory)
	{not an abbreviation} [symbol for a gas constant (8.315 joules)] (chemistry and laboratory)

Ra	radium (chemistry, radiation therapy, and radiology)
Rad	radium (chemistry, radiation therapy, and radiology)
Rb	rubidium (chemistry)
RD	reaction of degeneration (chemistry and laboratory)
rd	rutherford [unit of radioactivity] (chemistry, radiation therapy, and radiology)
Re	rhenium (chemistry)
Rf	rutherfordium (chemistry)
Rh	rhodium (chemistry)
^{106}Rh	radioactive rhodium (chemistry)
Rn	radon (chemistry)
Ru	ruthenium (chemistry)

S

S	sugar (chemistry)
	sulfur [also called *sulphur*] (chemistry and laboratory)
s	{not an abbreviation} [symbol for atomic orbital with angular momentum quantum number 0] (chemistry and physics)
$SbCl_3$	antimony trichloride (chemistry)
Sb_2O_3	antimony trioxide (chemistry)
Sb_2O_5	antimony pentoxide (chemistry)
Sb_4O_6	anitmony trioxide (chemistry)
Sc	scandium (chemistry)
Se	selenium (chemistry)
^{75}SeM	radioactive selenomethionine (chemistry)
SH	sulfhydryl [also called *sulphydryl*; the univalent radical] (chemistry)
Si	silicon (chemistry)
SiO_2	silica [also called *silicon dioxide*] (chemistry)
Sm	samarium (chemistry)
Sn	*stannum* [also called *tin*] (chemistry)
^{113}Sn	radioactive isotope of stannum (chemistry)
^{121}Sn	radioactive isotope of stannum (chemistry)
SnF_2	stannous fluoride (chemistry, dentistry, and pharmacology)
SO_4	sulfate (chemistry, laboratory, and pharmacology)
Sr	strontium (chemistry)
^{85}Sr	radioactive strontium (chemistry)
Sr^{90}	radioactive strontium (chemistry)
SO_2	sulfur dioxide (chemistry)

T

T	thymine (laboratory)
	tritium (chemistry)
$T\frac{1}{2}$	{not an abbreviation} [symbol for one-half lifetime of radioactive isotope] (chemistry and physics)
$T\frac{1}{2}$	{not an abbreviation} [symbol for one-half lifetime of pharmaceuticals and radioactive isotopes] (chemistry, pharmacology, physics, and radiology)
$t\frac{1}{2}$	{not an abbreviation} [symbol for one-half lifetime of pharmaceuticals and radioactive isotopes] (chemistry, pharmacology, physics, and radiology)
$t\frac{1}{2}$	{not an abbreviation} [symbol for one-half lifetime of pharmaceuticals and radioactive isotopes] (chemistry, pharmacology, physics, and radiology)
Ta	tantalum [used in prostheses and wire sutures] (chemistry, orthopedics, and surgery)
Tb	terbium (chemistry)
Tc	technetium (chemistry and radiology)
^{99m}Tc	technetium 99m [a radioactive technetium] (chemistry and radiology)
Te	tellurium (chemistry)
Th	thorium (chemistry, gastroenterology, and radiology)
$Th(NO_3)_4 \cdot 4H_2O$	thorium nitrate (chemistry, gastroenterology, and radiology)
THO	tritium-labeled water (chemistry and laboratory)
TH_2O	titrated water (chemistry and laboratory)
ThO_2	thorium dioxide (chemistry, gastroenterology, and radiology)
Ti	titanium (chemistry)
TiO_2	titanium dioxide (chemistry, dentistry, dermatology, and pharmacology)
Tl	thallium (cardiovascular, chemistry, and radiology)
Tl-201	thallium-201 [a radioactive isotope] (cardiovascular, chemistry, and radiology)
$^{201}TlCl$	thallium chloride [a radioactive isotope] (cardiovascular, chemistry, and radiology)
Tm	thulium (chemistry)

U

U	uranium (chemistry)
^{235}U	radioactive uranium (chemistry)
$UO_2(C_2H_3O_2)_2 \cdot 2H_2O$	uranyl acetate (otorhinolaryngology, pharmacology, and respiratory)
UO_2SO_4	uranyl sulfate (chemistry and pharmacology)

V

V	vanadium (chemistry and pharmacology)
Vi	virginium (chemistry)

W

W	wolframium [also called *tungsten*] (chemistry)
^{185}W	radioactive wolframium [also called *radioactive tungsten*] (chemistry)

X

Xe	xenon (chemistry)
^{133}Xe	xenon^{133} [also called *radioxenon*] (chemistry)

Y

Y	yttrium (chemistry and laser surgery)
^{90}Y	radioactive yttrium (chemistry)
Yb	ytterbium (chemistry and laser surgery)
^{169}Yb	ytterbium-169 [a radionuclide] (chemistry and radiology)
Yb-169-DTPA	ytterbium-169 pentetate sodium (chemistry and radiology)
-yl	{not an abbreviation} [chemical suffix indicating a radical] (chemistry)
-ylene	{not an abbreviation} [chemical suffix indicating a bivalent hydrocarbon radical] (chemistry)
Yt	yttrium (chemistry)
yt	yttrium (chemistry)

Z

Z	{not an abbreviation} [symbol for atomic number] (chemistry and physics)
z	atomic number (chemistry)
Zn	zinc (chemistry, dietary, and laboratory)
^{65}Zn	radioactive zinc (chemistry)
$Zn(C_2H_3O_2)_2 \cdot 2H_2O$	zinc acetate (pharmacology)
$ZnCl_2$	zinc chloride (dermatology and pharmacology)
$2ZnCO_3 \cdot 3Zn(OH)_2$	zinc carbonate [used in dusting powder] (pharmacology)
ZnI_2	zinc iodide (pharmacology)

$Zn(MnO_4)_2 \cdot 6H_2O$	zinc manganate (pharmacology and urology)
ZnO	zinc oxide [also called *white zinc*] (dermatology and pharmacology)
ZnO_2	zinc peroxide (pharmacology)
$ZnOE$	zinc oxide and eugenol (pharmacology)
$Zn(OH)_2$	zinc hydroxide (pharmacology)
$ZnSO_4$	zinc sulfate (dermatology, gastroenterology, ophthalmology, and pharmacology)
$ZnSO_4 7H_2O$	zinc sulfate [also called *white vitriol* and *zinc zitriol*] (dermatology, gastroenterology, ophthalmology, and pharmacology)
Zr	zirconium (chemistry)
^{95}Zr	radioactive zirconium (chemistry)
ZrO_2	zirconium dioxide [also called *zirconium oxide*] (chemistry)

APPENDIX B:

HEMATOLOGY

BLOOD GROUP SYSTEMS

A-B-O
Auberger
Cartwright
Diego
Dombrock
Duffy
high frequency
I
Kell
Kidd
Lewis
low frequency
Lutheran
M-N-S (also called *MN* and *MNSs*)
P
Rh (also called *Rhesus*)

BLOOD GROUP PHENOTYPES AND GENOTYPES BY BLOOD GROUP SYSTEMS

Blood Group System	Blood Group (Phenotypes)	Blood Group (Genotypes)
A-B-O	A	*AA*
		AO

A Subgroups

A_1
A_2
A_3
A_4
A_{el}
A_{end}
A_i
A_m
A_o
A_x

Blood Group System	Blood Group (Phenotypes)	Blood Group (Genotypes)
	A_1	A^1A^1
		A^1A^2
		A^1O
	A_2	A^2A^2
		A^2O
	AB	AB
	A_1B	A^1B
	A_2B	A^2B
	$A_1{}^b + A_2{}^b$	
	B	BB
		BO
	B Subgroups	
	B_1	
	B_2	
	B_3	
	B_m	
	B_v	
	B_w	
	B_x	
	O	OO
Bombay	O_h	
C-D-E		cde/cde
		Cde/cde
		Cde/Cde
		C^wde/cde
		C^wde/Cde
		C^wde/C^wde
		cdE/cde
		cdE/cdE
		Cde/cdE
		CdE/cde
		CdE/Cde
		CdE/cde
		CdE/CdE
		C^wde/cdE
		C^wde/CdE
		cDe/cde
		cDe/cDe
		CDe/cde
		CDe/cDe

Blood Group System	Blood Group (Phenotypes)	Blood Group (Genotypes)
		cDe/Cde
		CDe/CDe
		CDe/Cde
		C^{w}De/cde
		C^{w}De/cDe
		cDe/C^{w}de
		C^{w}De/CDe
		CDe/c^{w}de
		C^{w}De/Cde
		C^{w}De/C^{w}De
		C^{w}De/C^{w}de
		cDE/cde
		cDE/cDe
		cDe/cdE
		cDE/cDE
		cDE/cdE
		CDe/cDE
		CDe/cdE
		cDE/Cde
		CDE/cde
		CDE/cDe
		cDe/Cde
		CDE/CDe
		CDE/Cde
		CDe/CdE
		CDE/cDE
		CDE/cdE
		Cde/CdE
		CDE/CDE
		CDE/CdE
		C^{w}De/cDE
		C^{w}De/cdE
		cDE/C^{w}de
		C^{w}De/CDE
		C^{w}De/CdE
		CDE/C^{2}de
cis-AB	cis-A$_1$B	
	cis-A$_2$B	
Diego	Di(a+b−)	
	Di(A+b+)	
Duffy	Fy(a+b−)	Fy^2Fy^a
		Fy^2Fy

Blood Group System	Blood Group (Phenotypes)	Blood Group (Genotypes)
	Fy(a+b+)	Fy^aFy^b
	Fy(a−b+)	Fy^bFy^b
		Fy^bfy
	Fy(a−b−)	$fyfy$
I-i	I_1	
	I_2	
	I_3	
Kell	Kell+	KK
		Kk
	Kell−	kk
Kidd	jk(a+b−)	jk^ajk^a
		jk^ajk
	jk(a+b+)	jk^ajk^b
	jk(a−b+)	jk^bjk^b
		jk^bjk
	jk(a−b−)	$jkjk$
Lewis	Le(a−)	
	Le(a+)	
	Le(a−b−)	
	Le(a+b+)	
	Le(a−b+)	
Lutheran	Lu(a+b−)	Lu^aLu^a
	Lu(a+b+)	Lu^aLu^b
	Lu(a−b+)	Lu^bLu^b
	Lu(a−b−)	
M-N-S	M	

<u>M Subgroups</u>

	MS	
	Ms	
	MN	

MN Subgroups

	MNS	
	MNs	
	N	

Blood Group System	Blood Group (Phenotypes)	Blood Group (Genotypes)
N Subgroups		
	NS	
	Ns	
P	P	
	p	pp
	p′	
	P_1	p^1p^1
		p^1p^2
		p^1p^k
		p^1p
	P_2	p^2p^2
		p^2p^k
		p^2p
	p^k	p^kp^k
		p^kp
Rh (Rhesus)	rh	rr
	rh′	$r'r$
		$r'r'$
	Rh_0	R^0r
		R^0R^0
	Rh_1	R^1r
		R^1R^0
		R^0r'
		R^1R^1
	Rh negative	
	rh	
	rh′	
	rh″	
	rh′rh″	
	^{Rh}null	
	Rh_0	R^0r
		R^0R^0
	Rh positive	
	Rh_0	
	Rh_1	
	Rh_2	
	Rh_1Rh_2	
	Rh_1Rh_1	R^1R^1
		R^1r'
	Rh_1Rh_2	R^1R^z
		R^1r''
		R^2r'

Blood Group System	Blood Group (Phenotypes)	Blood Group (Genotypes)
	Rh_2Rh_2	R^2R^2
		R^2r''
	Rh,rh	R^1r
		R^1R^0
		R^0r'
	Rh_2rh	R^2r
		R^2R^0
		R^0r''
	rh'rh	$r'r$
	rh'rh'	$r'r'$
	rh'rh''	$r'r''$
	rh''rh	$r''r$
	rh''rh''	$r''r''$
	$Rh_1^wRh_1$	$R^{1w}R^1$
		$R^1r'^w$
		$R^{1w}r'$
		$R^{1w}R^{1w}$
		$R^{1w}r'w$
	$Rh_1^wRh_2$	$R^{1w}R^2$
		$R^{1w}r''$
		$R^2r'^w$
	rh'^wrh	r'^wr
	rh'^wrh'	r'^wr'
		$r'^wr'^w$
	rh'^wrh''	r'^wr''
	rh_yrh	r^yr
	rh_yrh'	r^yr'
	rh_yrh''	r^yr''
	rh_yrh_y	r^yr^y
	Rh_y^wrh	$R^{1w}r$
		$R^{1w}R^0$
		$R^0r'^w$
	rh_y^wrh'	$r^{1w}r^y$
	Rh_zrh	R^zr
		R^zR^0
		R^0r^y
	Rh_zRh_1	R^zR^1
		R^zr'
		R^1r^y
	Rh_zRh_2	R^zR^2
		R^zr''
		R^2r^y
	Rh_zRh_z	R^zR^z
		R^zr^y

Blood Group System	Blood Group (Phenotypes)	Blood Group (Genotypes)
	$Rh_z{}^wRh_1$	$R^{lw}R^z$
		$R^{lw}r^y$
		$R^z r^{lw}$
Xg		

BLOOD GROUP SYSTEMS WITH ANTIGENIC DETERMINANTS

Blood Group System	Antigenic Determinants
A-B-O	A
	A_1
	B
Auberger	Au^a
Bg	Bg^a
	Bg^b
	Bg^c
	DBG
	Ho
	Ho-like
	Ot
	Sto
Cartwright	Yt^a
	Yt^b
Coltan	Co^a
	Co^b
Cost-Sterling	Cs^a
	Yk^b
Diego	Di^a
	Di^b
Dombrock	Do^a
	Do^b
Duffy	Fy^a (also called *Fy1*)
	Fy^{ab} (also called *Fy3*)

Blood Group System	Antigenic Determinants
	Fy^b (also called *Fy2*) Fy4
Gerbich	Ge1 Ge2 Ge3 [Note: Anti-Ge1 = M.Y.; anti-Ge1,2 = Ge; anti-Ge1,2,3 — Yus.)
H	H
I	I i I^D I^F I^T
Kell	K1 (also called *K*) K2 (also called *k*) K3 (also called *Kp^a*) K4 (also called *Kp^b*) K5 (also called *Ku*) K6 (also called *Js^a*) K7 (also called *Js^b*) K8 (also called *kw*) K9 (also called *KL*) K10 (also called *Ul^a*) K11 K12 K13 K14 K15 K16
Kidd	Jk^a (also called *Jk1*) Jk^{ab} (also called *Jk3*) Jk^b (also called *Jk2*)
Lewis	Le^a (also called *Le1*) Le^b (also called *Le2*) Le^c (also called *Le5*) Le^d Le^x (also called *Le^{ab}* and *Le3*) Mag (also called *Le4*)

Blood Group System	Antigenic Determinants
Lutheran	Lu^a (also called *Lu1*)
	Lu^{ab} (also called *Lu3*)
	Lu^b (also called *Lu2*)
	Lu4
	Lu5
	Lu6
	Lu7
	Lu8
	Lu9
	Lu10
	Lu11
	Lu12
	Lu13
	Lu14 (also called Sw^a)
M-N-S	Cl^a
	Far
	He
	Hill
	Hu
	M
	M_1
	M^A
	M^c
	M^e
	M^g
	Mi^a
	Mt^a
	Mur
	M^v
	N
	N^A
	Ny^a
	Ri^a
	S
	s
	S^B
	Sj
	St^a
	Sul
	Tm
	U
	U^B
	Vr

Blood Group System	Antigenic Determinants
	Vw
	Z
P	P1
	P2 (also called *Tj^a*)
	P3 (also called P^K)
Rh	Rh1 (also called *D* and *Rh~0~*)
	Rh2 (also called *C* and *rh'*)
	Rh3 (also called *E* and *rh''*)
	Rh4 (also called *c* and *hr'*)
	Rh5 (also called *e* and *hr''*)
	Rh6 (also called *ce*, *f*, and *hr*)
	Rh7 (also called *Ce* and *rh~i~*)
	Rh8 (also called *C^w* and *rh^{w1}*)
	Rh9 (also called *C^x* and *rh^x*)
	Rh10 (also called *ce^s*, *hr^v*, and *V*)
	Rh11 (also called *E^w* and *rh^{w2}*)
	Rh12 (also called *G* and *rh^G*)
	Rh13 (also called *Rh^A*)
	Rh14 (also called *Rh^B*)
	Rh15 (also called *Rh^C*)
	Rh16 (also called *Rh^D*)
	Rh17 (also called *Hr~0~*)
	Rh18 (also called *Hr*)
	Rh19 (also called *hr^s*)
	Rh20 (also called *e^s* and *VS*)
	Rh21 (also called *C^G*)
	Rh22 (also called *CE*)
	Rh23 (also called *D^w*)
	Rh24 (also called *E^T*)
	Rh26
	Rh27 (also called *cE*)
	Rh28 (also called *hr^H*)
	Rh29 (also called *RH*)
	Rh30 (also called *Go^a*)
	Rh31 (also called *hr^B*)
	Rh32
	Rh33
Sciana	Bu^a
	Sm
Stoltzfus	Sf^a

Blood Group System	Antigenic Determinants
Vel	Vel 1
	Vel 2
Wright	Wr^a
	Wr^b
Xg	Xg^a

MISCELLANEOUS ANTIGENIC DETERMINANTS

A$_1$Le^b
An^a
At^a

Be^a
Bec
Bi
Big Charles
Bou
Bp^a
Bra
Bx^a
By

Cad
Car
Chido (also called Gursha)
Chr^a
Cip
Coates
Craig

Dahl
Donavieisky
Dp
Driver
Duch

El
En^a
Evans
Evelyn

Fin
Fuerhart

Fuj
Fy5

Gf^a
Gilbraith
Gn^a
Go^b
Good
Green
Gy^a

Hands
Heibel
Hen
Hil
Ht^a
Hy

IA
IB
IH
iH
ILe^{bh}
IP1
iP1
IP2 (also called *ITj^a*)
I^{T}P1

Je^a
Jn^a
Jo^a
Job
Jr

Kam

Kelly
Ken
Knops

Lan
Leu
Luke
Lw^a

Man
Mar
McCall
Mo^a
MZ443

Nij

Ola
Orr

Pea
Pt^a

Rd^a
Reid
Rh25 (also called *LW*)
Rm

Savior
Sch
Sd^a
Simon
Skjelbred

Ters
Th^a
To^a
Todd
Tr^a

Ven
Vennera

Wb
Weeks
Wil
Wilbourne
Ww

Yh^a

Za

754

FACTORS

A
A^1
Auberger (also called *Au*)

Batty (also called *By^a*)
Becker
Berrens (also called *Be^a*)
Bu^a

C
Cartwright (also called *Yt^a*)
Cavaliere (also called *Ca*)

Di^a
Di^b
Dombroch (also called *Do^a*)
Donna

F
f

Gerbich (also called *Ge*)
Gonzales (also called *Go^a*)

Good
Graydon (also called *Gr*)

He
hr
hr′
hr″
hr^v
Hu

I
i
i$_1$
i$_2$
i$_3$
i$_{cord}$
I-i

Jobbins
Js^a
Js^b

K
k

Levay

M^e
M^g
Mi^a

Nyberg (also called *Ny^a*)

P
P^k

$\underline{\underline{Rh}}_0$
$\overline{Rh}_0$
$\mathcal{R}h_0$
rh
rh'
rh''
Rh^A
Rh^B
Rh^C

$\underline{Rh}^D$
$\overline{\overline{Rh}}^w$
rh^w
Ridley
Romunda (also called *Rm*)

Schmidt (also called *Sm*)
Stones (also called *St^a*)
Sutter
Swan (also called *Sw^a*)

Tj
Tj^a

V
Vel (also called *Ve^a*)
Ven
Vr
Vw

Wright (also called *Wr^a*)

MISCELLANEOUS AGGLUTINOGENS

A$_1$	rh''
A$_2$	Rh$_0$
A$_1$;B	Rh$_1$
A$_2$;B	Rh$_2$
B	Rh$_1$^{w}
M	rh'^{w}
N	rh^y
O	S
rh	s
rh'	

MISCELLANEOUS AGGLUTININS

anti-A
anti-A$_1$
(anti-A$_1$)
anti-A$_2$
anti-A$_{hel}$

anti-B

anti-C
anti-c
anti-C^w

anti-D

anti-Di^a
anti-Di^b

anti-E
anti-e

anti-f
anti-Fy^a
anti-Fy^b

anti-H
(anti-H)

anti-He
anti-hr″
anti-Hu

anti-I
anti-i

anti-Jk^a
anti-Jk^b
anti-Js^a

anti-K
anti-k
anti-Kidd

anti-Le
anti-Le$_1$
anti-Le^a
anti-Le^b
anti-Le^H
anti-Le^x
anti-Lu^a
anti-Lu^b

anti-M
anti-M$_1$
anti-M^e
anti-Mi^a

anti-N

anti-P
anti-p′

anti-Rh (also called *antirhesus*)
anti-Rh$_0$
anti-rh′
anti-rh″

anti-S

anti-T
anti-Tj

anti-U

anti-Vw

APPENDIX C:

SYMBOLS

ELEMENTS

Ac	actinium		Ge	germanium
Ag	silver		H	hydrogen
Al	aluminum		Ha	hahnium
Am	americium		He	helium
Ar	argon		Hf	hafnium
As	arsenic		Hg	mercury
At	astatine		Ho	holmium
Au	gold			
			I	iodine
B	boron		In	indium
Ba	barium		Ir	iridium
Bc	beryllium			
Bi	bismuth		K	potassium
Bk	berkelium		Kr	krypton
Br	bromine			
			La	lanthanum
C	carbon		Li	lithium
Ca	calcium		Lu	lutetium
Cd	cadmium		Lw	lawrencium
Ce	cerium			
Cf	californium		Md	mendelevium
Cl	chlorine		Mg	magnesium
Cm	curium		Mn	manganese
Co	cobalt		Mo	molybdenum
Cr	chromium			
Cs	cesium		N	nitrogen
Cu	copper		Na	sodium
			Nb	niobium
Dy	dysprosium		Nd	neodymium
			Ne	neon
Er	erbium		Ni	nickel
Es	einsteinium		No	nobelium
Eu	europium		Np	neptunium
F	fluorine		O	oxygen
Fe	iron		Os	osmium
Fm	fermium			
Fr	francium		P	phosphorus
			Pa	protactinium
Ga	gallium		Pb	lead
Gd	gadolinium			

Symbols

Pd	palladium	Ta	tantalum
Pm	promethium	Tb	terbium
Po	polonium	Tc	technetium
Pr	praseodymium	Te	tellurium
Pt	platinum	Th	thorium
Pu	plutonium	Ti	titanium
		Tl	thallium
Ra	radium	Tm	thulium
Rb	rubidium		
Re	rhenium	U	uranium
Rf	rutherfordium		
Rh	rhodium	V	vanadium
Rn	radon		
Ru	ruthenium	W	tungsten
		Xe	xenon
S	sulfur		
Sb	antimony	Y	yttrium
Sc	scandium	Yb	ytterbium
Se	selenium		
Si	silicon	Zn	zinc
Sm	samarium	Zr	zirconium
Sn	tin		
Sr	strotium		

PULSE GRADING

0	completely absent
+	plus (markedly impaired)
+1	plus one (markedly impaired)
1+	one plus (markedly impaired)
++	two plus (moderately impaired)
+2	plus two (moderately impaired)
2+	two plus (moderately impaired)
+++	three plus (slightly impaired)
+3	plus three (slightly impaired)
3+	three plus (slightly impaired)
++++	four plus (normal)
+4	plus four (normal)
4+	four plus (normal)

REFLEX GRADING

++++	hyperactive or very brisk
4+	hyperactive or very brisk
+++	brisker than average
3+	brisker than average
++	average or normal
2+	average or normal
+	low normal or somewhat diminished
1+	low normal or somewhat diminished
0	no response

HEART MURMUR GRADING

1/6	very faint
I/VI	very faint
2/6	quiet
II/VI	quiet
3/6	moderately loud
III/VI	moderately loud
4/6	loud
IV/VI	loud
5/6	very loud
V/VI	very loud
6/6	extremely loud
VI/VI	extremely loud

LABORATORY QUANTITATIVE TESTING

−	negative
±	very slight reaction or trace
+	slight reaction or trace
1+	slight reaction or trace
++	trace or noticeable reaction
2+	trace or noticeable reaction
+++	moderate amount of reaction
3+	moderate amount of reaction
++++	large amount or pronounced reaction
4+	large amount of pronounced reaction

GREEK ALPHABET AND SYMBOLS

A	alpha
α	alpha
	alpha particle
	is proportional to
B	beta
β	beta
X	chi [also spelled *khi*]
χ	chi [also spelled *khi*]
χ^2	chi square [test]
Δ	anion gap
	centrad prism
	change
	delta
	delta gap
	head
	increment
	occipital triangle
	prism diopter
	sulfur
	temperature

	trine
$\underline{\Delta}$	equiangular
$\overline{\Delta A}$	change in absorbance
ΔdB	difference in decibels (otorhinolaryngology)
H Δ	Hesselbach's triangle (anatomy)
H's Δ	Hesselbach's triangle (anatomy)
ΔP	change in pressure (ophthalmology)
ΔpH	change in pH
Δ scan	delta scan (radiology)
Δt	time interval
$\Delta +$	time interval
δ	delta
E	epsilon
ϵ	epsilon
H	eta
η	eta
Γ	gamma
γ	gamma
	immunoglobulin (immunology and laboratory)
	microgram (measurement)
$m\gamma$	milligamma [also called *nanogram*] (measurement)
I	iota
ι	iota
K	kappa
κ	kappa
Λ	lambda
λ	lambda
	wavelength
M	mu
μ	micro- [prefix for 10^{-6}] (measurement)
	micro- [small when used as prefix]
	micrometer
	micron (measurement)
	mu
μc	microcurie (measurement and radiation therapy)
μEq	microequivalent (measurement)
μf	microfarad (measurement)
μg	microgram (measurement)
μl	microliter (measurement)
μM	micromolar (measurement)
$m\mu$	millimicron (measurement)
$m\mu c$	millimicrocurie [also called *nanocurie*] (measurement and radiation therapy)
$m\mu g$	millimicrogram [also called *nanogram*] (measurement)
μr	microroentgen (measurement)
μsec	microsecond (measurement)
μu	microunit (measurement)
μV	milligamma (also called *micromicrogram* and *picogram*] (measurement)

μv	microvolt (measurement)
μw	microwatt (measurement)
μμ	micromicron [also called *picometer*] (measurement)
μμc	micromicrocurie [also called *picocurie*] (measurement and radiation therapy)
μμg	micromicrogram [also called *picogram*] (measurement)
μγ	microgramma [also called *micromicrogram* and *picogram*] (measurement)
μΩ	microhm (measurement)
N	nu
ν	nu
Ω	ohm
	omega
ω	omega
O	omicron
o	omicron
Φ	phenyl
	phi
φ	phenyl
	phi
Π	pi
π	pi
	3.1416 (ratio of circumference of a circle to its diameter)
Ψ	psi
	psychiatric
ψ	psi
	psychiatric
P	rho
ρ	rho
Σ	sigma
	sum of
σ	difference
	one-thousandth of a second
	sigma
	standard deviation
ς	sigma
T	tau
τ	tau
	{not an abbreviation} [symbol for lifetime of pharmaceuticals and radioactive isotopes] (chemistry, pharmacology, physics, and radiology)
τ½	{not an abbreviation} [symbol for half-life time of pharmaceuticals and radioactive isotopes] (chemistry, pharmacology, physics, and radiology)
Θ	theta
θ	theta
Υ	upsilon
υ	upsilon
Ξ	xi

ξ	xi
Z	zeta
ʃ	zeta

PUNCTUATION AND TYPEWRITER SYMBOLS

#	following a number
	fracture (orthopedics and radiology)
	gauge (measurement and surgery)
	has been done
	has been given
	number (measurement)
	pound (measurement)
	weight (measurement)
+	acid reaction
	added to
	an additional whole (genetics and laboratory)
	convex lens
	decreased [reflexes] (neurology and orthopedics)
	diminished [reflexes] (neurology and orthopedics)
	excess
	less than 50% inhibition of hemolysis (hematology and laboratory)
	mild
	mildly positive
	mildly severe
	plus
	positive
	present
	slight reaction
	sluggish
	trace reaction
+ reaction	acid reaction
(+)	significant
	uncertain mode of inheritance (genetics)
	uncommon mode of inheritance (genetics)
(+)ive	positive
+ +	50% of inhibition of hemolysis (hematology and laboratory)
	moderate
	moderate pain
	moderately positive
	moderately severe
	normally active [reflexes] (neurology and orthopedics)
	notable reaction
	noticeable reaction
	positive moderately
	trace
$\frac{+}{+}$	moderate
	moderately severe

	normally active [reflexes] (neurology and orthopedics)
+++	increased [reflexes] (neurology and orthopedics)
	75% inhibition of hemolysis (hematology and laboratory)
	moderate amount
	moderate reaction
	moderately hyperactive [reflexes] (neurology and orthopedics)
	moderately severe
	moderately severe pain
	positive
++++	complete inhibition of hemolysis (hematology and laboratory)
	large amount
	markedly hyperactive [reflexes] (neurology and orthopedics)
	markedly severe pain with spastic muscles (neurology and orthopedics)
	positive
	pronounced reaction
	severe
	severe pain
±	doubtful
	either positive or negative
	equivocal
	flicker [reflexes] (neurology and orthopedics)
	indefinite
	more or less
	not definite
	plus or minus [also *plus/minus*]
	possibly significant
	questionable
	suggestive
	variable
	very slight
	very slight reaction
	very slight trace
	very slightly severe
	with or without
(±)	possibly significant
± to +	minimal pain
+ to ± ±	slight pain
⊕	plus
	positive
	present
−	absent
	alkaline
	alkaline reaction
	concave lens
	deficiency
	deficient
	minus

	missing a whole of a chromosome [if placed before] (genetics and laboratory)
	missing a part of a chromosome [if placed after] (genetics and laboratory)
	negative
$(-)$	insignificant
$\ominus$	absent
	minus
	negative
$-$ reaction	alkaline reaction
$\underline{\quad}$	mass energy conversion faction
$\mp$	minus or plus
$=$	equal
	equal to
	equals
%	percent (measurement)
?	doubtful
	equivocal
	flicker [reflexes] (neurology and orthopedics)
	question of
	questionable
	suggested
	suggestive
	unknown
[ ]	brackets
	concentration
!	factorial product
✳	birth
	not verified
	presumed
	used as a multiplication sign in genetics (genetics and laboratory)
′	foot (measurement)
	minute (measurement)
	primary accent
	prime
	univalent
″	bivalent
	ditto
	inch (measurement)
	second (measurement)
	secondary accent
/	divided by
	either meaning
	extension
	extensor
	fraction
	of
	organic

	per
	shilling
	slash
	solidus
	to
	virgule
:	is to
	ratio (measurement)
&	and
(	concave

MISCELLANEOUS SYMBOLS

Symbol	Meaning
O	annual
	circle
	daughter
	female
	full moon
	moon
	mother
	octarius [pint] (measurement)
	respirations (anesthesiology)
	sex undetermined
	silver
	sister
Φ	normal
∅	no
	none
⊙	annual
	annual plant
	gold
	start of operation
	sun
OO	male
⊙⊙	biennial
♀	standing
O—	recumbent position
♀	sitting position
□	brother
	father
	male
	quadrature
	son
(□)	adopted
◇	sex unknown
♂	iron
	male
	male sex
	Mars
♀	copper

	female
	female sex
	Venus
♂	earth
	male
	terra
♂ ♀	having male and female flowers separate
♂ - ♀	having male and female flowers on the same plant
♂ : ♀	having male and female flowers on different plants
†	death
	deceased
∞	indefinitely more
	infinity
	is to
↑	above
	alive
	elevated
	elevation
	enlarged
	gas
	greater than
	high
	improved
	increase(d)
	increases
	rising
	superior
	upper
⚛	up
↑↑	Babinski sign extensor response (neurology and orthopedics)
Λ	above
	and
	diastolic blood pressure (anesthesiology, cardiovascular, and surgery)
	elevated
	enlarged
	greater than
	improved
	increased
	more than
	superior
	upper
↑↓	reversible reaction
	up and down
↗	deviated
	displaced
	increase(s)
	increasing
↖	direction

↓	below
	dead
	decrease(d)
	deficiency
	deficit
	depressed
	depression
	deteriorated
	deteriorating
	diminished
	diminution
	down
	falling
	inferior
	less than
	low
	lower
	normal plantar reflex (neurology and orthopedics)
	precipitate(s)
	restricted
V	below
	decreased
	deficiency
	deficit
	depressed
	deteriorated
	deteriorating
	diminished
	diminution
	down
	inferior
	less than
	low
	lower
	or
	systolic blood pressure (anesthesiology, cardiovascular, and surgery)
↘	decrease(s)
	decreasing
↙	decreased
⇕	down
↓↓	down bilaterally
	Babinski sign plantar response
	testes descended (neonatology, pediatrics, and urology)
→	approaches limit of
	causes
	demonstrates
	direction of flow
	direction of reaction

	distal
	followed by
	implies
	indicates
	indicating "from _____ to _____"
	is due to
	leads to
	no change
	produces
	radiates to
	radiating to
	results in
	reveals
	shows
	to
	to the right
	toward
	transfer to
	yields
⇋	electric current
	reversible chemical reaction
	reversible reaction
←	caused by
	derived from
	direction of reaction
	is due to
	produced by
	proximal
	resulting from
	secondary to
	to the left
↔	widened
	width
⌐	not
⇌	reversible reaction
↗	widened
	width
>	from which is derived
	greater than
⊁	not greater than
≧	greater than or equal to
⩾	greater than or equal to
≧	equal to or greater than
	equal to or more than
	greater than or equal to
⇒	implication
	implies
)	causes
	demonstrates

	distal
	followed by
	from which is derived
	greater than
	implies
	indicates
	larger than
	leads to
	more severe than
	produces
	radiates to
	radiating to
	results in
	reveals
	shows
	to
	toward
	worse than
	yields
$<$	less than
	derived from
$\not<$	not less than
$\leqq$	less than or equal to
	equal to or less than
$\leqslant$	less than or equal to
	equal to or less than
$\leqq$	less than or equal to
	equal to or less than
	less than or equal to
$\langle$	caused by
	derived from
	less severe than
	less than
	produced by
	proximal
	smaller than
$\sim$	about
	approximate(ly)
	cycle
	difference
	proportionate to
	similar cycle
$\approx$	approximately
	nearly equal to
$\dot{\sim}$	approximate
$\simeq$	approximately
	approximately equal to
	approximately equals
	congruent to
$\circ$	combined with
$\div$	equivalent

Symbol	Meaning
≆	not equivalent to
°	degree
	hour
	measurement of strabismus angle (ophthalmology)
≑	nearly equal to
≐	approximately equal
≑	approaches
≠	does not equal
	not equal
	not equal to
	unequal
≡	identical
	identical with
≢	not identical
	not identical with
⊥	equilateral
÷	divided by
	division
√	radical
	root
	square root
²√	square root
³√	cube root
⁴√	fourth root
::	as
	describes breakage and reunion (genetics and laboratory)
	equality between ratios
	proportion
	proportionate to
∴	therefore
∵	because
	since
√	check
	observe for
	urine
	voided
√̇	urine and defecation
↱	right turn
⌐	right upper quadrant
∟	factorial product
	right angle
	right lower quadrant
↰	left turn
⌐	left upper quadrant
⌐	left lower quadrant
⊥	perpendicular
‖	parallel
	parallel bars
//	for

	parallel
	parallel bars
|	given
||	absolute value
∠	angle
	flexion
	flexor
∪	logical sum
	union
∩	intersection
	logical product
⊂	is contained in
ᵻ	one
ᵼ	two
‴	line [one-twelfth inch]
	trivalent
. . .	no data
∝	variant
	varies
∂	differential
℥ ᵻ	drachm
	dram
	five milliliters [5 ml]
	teaspoon
℥	drachm
	dram
	five milliliters [5 ml]
	teaspoon
℥	ounce
	thirty milliliters [30 ml]
	ten milliliters [10 ml]
℥ ᵼ	two drams
	two teaspoonfuls
℈	scruple

SYMBOLS WITH LETTERS

Ⓐ	axilla
a̅	before
a	at
@	at
ⒶⓍ	axilla
↑C	increase during assay caused by chemical interference (laboratory)
↓C	decrease during assay caused by chemical interference (laboratory)
c̅	with
✓c̅	check with
✓'d	checked
	examined

	observed
2d	second
3 = D	delayed double diffusion [test]
∠E	angle of entry
f℥	fluid ounce
f℈	fluildrachm
	fluidram
✓g	checking
↓g	decreasing
	diminishing
	falling
	lowering
Ⓗ	hypodermic(ally)
ⓗ	hypodermic(ally)
Ⓜ	intramuscular(ly)
✓ing	checking
Ⓘⓥ	intravenous(ly)
Ⓛ	left
Ⓜ	murmur
ⓜ	by mouth
	mouth
	murmur
✓Ⓜ	factitial murmur
m	minim
m	minim
ⓞ	by mouth
	oral(ly)
p̄	after
✓qs	voided sufficient quantity
©	copyright
®	rectal
	right
®	trademark
Ⓡ	rectally
	rectum
Ⓡ	rectally
℞	prescription
	recipe
	take
/s	angles
	flexors
s̄	without
℥ss	fifteen milliliters [15 ml]
	half-ounce
	tablespoonful
™	trademark
↑V	increase caused by *in vivo* effect (laboratory)
↓V	decrease caused by *in vivo* effect (laboratory)

$\overline{X}$	average of all X's
$\angle X$	angle of exit
$\times$	magnification
	multiplied by
$\textcircled{x}$	biennial plant
	end of anesthesia
	end of operation
$1\times$	once
$\times 2$	twice
$2\times$	twice

NUMBERS

1°	first degree
	one hour
	primary
2°	because of
	due to
	second degree
	secondary
	secondary to
	two hours
3°	tertiary
	third degree
24°	twenty-four hours
606	arsphenamine [formerly used as an antisyphilitic] (pharmacology)
914	neoarsphenamine [formerly used as an antisyphilitic] (pharmacology)

NUMERALS

Arabic	Roman	
0		zero
1	I	one
	i	one
2	II	two
	ii	two
3	III	three
	iii	three
4	IV	four
	iv	four
5	V	five
	v	five
6	VI	six
	vi	six
7	VII	seven
	vii	seven
8	VIII	eight
	viii	eight

Symbols

Arabic	Roman	
9	IX	nine
	ix	nine
10	X	ten
	x	ten
11	XI	eleven
12	XII	twelve
13	XIII	thirteen
14	XIV	fourteen
15	XV	fifteen
16	XVI	sixteen
17	XVII	seventeen
18	XVIII	eighteen
19	XIX	nineteen
20	XX	twenty
30	XXX	thirty
40	XL	forty
50	L	fifty
60	LX	sixty
70	LXX	seventy
80	LXXX	eighty
90	XC	ninety
100	C	one hundred
1,000	M	one thousand
5,000	$\overline{V}$	five thousand
10,000	$\overline{X}$	ten thousand
100,000	$\overline{C}$	one hundred thousand
1,000,000	$\overline{M}$	one million